Family Nurse Practitioner Certification
Prep Plus

Proven Strategies + Content Review + Online Practice

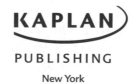

PUBLISHING

New York

ACKNOWLEDGMENTS

Special thanks to the team that made this book possible: Faith Adole, Susan Benesh, Erika Blumenthal, Kim Bowers, Dorothy Cummings, Lola Dart, Patricia DeBruin, Robin Faulk, Selena Gilles, Joanne Greene, Allison Harm, Laura Hollister-Meadows, Judy Hyland, Jody Jones, Ashley Kapturkiewicz, Norma Krantz, Theresa Kyle, Karen Lilyquist, Heather Maigur, Allyson Neal, Monica Ostolaza, Melissa Rendeiro, Catherine Richmond, Christine Ricketts, Susan Sanders, Jenifer Schmitz, Kendra Spaulding, Pedro Villanueva, Michael Wolff, Deanna Womble, Jessica Yee, and many others.

The Mini Prep Tests that accompany this text are based upon the published test plans of the American Association of Nurse Practitioners (AANP™) and the American Nurses Credentialing Center (ANCC©), neither of which sponsors nor endorses this product.

This publication is designed to provide accurate information in regard to the subject matter covered as of its publication date, with the understanding that knowledge and best practice constantly evolve. The publisher is not engaged in rendering medical, legal, accounting, or other professional service. If medical or legal advice or other expert assistance is required, the services of a competent professional should be sought. This publication is not intended for use in clinical practice or the delivery of medical care. To the fullest extent of the law, neither the Publisher nor the Editors assume any liability for any injury and/or damage to persons or property arising out of or related to any use of the material contained in this book.

Kaplan Publishing print books are available at special quantity discounts to use for sales promotions, employee premiums, or educational purposes. For more information or to purchase books, please call the Simon & Schuster special sales department at 866-506-1949.

TABLE OF CONTENTS

Part Two. Body Systems

Part Three. Pediatrics to Geriatrics

Part Four. Professional Practice and Advanced Practice Considerations

Welcome to Your Kaplan Studies!

Thank you for choosing Kaplan to help you study for the Family Nurse Pracitioner certification exam. We are honored to be part of your preparation for this critical next step in your career. You will soon join thousands of other family nurse practitioners who are making a significant positive impact on the lives of families around the world.

YOUR KAPLAN RESOURCES

Your Kaplan book contains:

- A comprehensive overview of the AANP and ANCC Family Nurse Practitioner certification exams
- Lessons that cover the concepts you will see on your test
- Key takeaway summaries
- 500+ practice questions with detailed explanations

Your Student Homepage offers the following:

- Bonus content that covers assessment and developmental considerations across the life span
- A 75-question Mini Prep Test based on the AANP exam with an explanation of every question
- A 100-question Mini Prep Test based on the ANCC exam with an explanation of every question

Register Your Book

To access your Student Homepage, visit **kaptest.com/booksonline**. Choose "Family Nurse Practitioner" from the list of tests at the top and answer the questions that appear.

Once you have created your username and password, you'll be able to log in to your resources at **kaptest.com**. When you're ready to use your Mini Prep Tests, click **Sign In** at the upper right of the page and enter your username and password. Then click on your Family Nurse Practitioner product to open it.

> **Getting Started**
> - Go to **kaptest.com/booksonline** to register your book.
> - Use this book to learn, practice, and review.
> - Log in to your Student Homepage at **kaptest.com** to access your two Mini Prep Tests for additional practice and review.

How to Use This Book

Congratulations! You have taken an important step in preparing yourself for the Family Nurse Practitioner certification exam. This book contains the information you want and need to earn your certification.

To get you started, Part 1 of this book offers a complete overview of the different versions of the Family Nurse Practitioner certification exam, as well as valuable test-taking strategies to drive your success. Additionally, you will find an introduction to the foundational healthcare and pharmacology topics that you will need to master for Test Day.

Part 2 offers a comprehensive overview of every major body system. Each chapter includes key definitions, assessment protocols, guidelines for diagnoses, and treatment plans that will reinforce your family nurse practitioner studies.

Part 3 focuses on the health of infants, children, and adolescents as well as the specialized needs of elderly patients. From growth and development to age specific ailments and disorders, this section reviews the critical information needed to care for patients across the life span.

Finally, Part 4 discusses the professional considerations that are pertinent to the family nurse practitioner and also the advanced topics that will appear on your test. These chapters will not only prepare you to earn your certification but will also enrich your professional practice and enhance the care you give to all your patients.

Nearly every chapter in this book concludes with a set of practice questions that allows you to review the concepts covered in that chapter. After completing all of the lessons in a particular chapter, take your time working through its accompanying practice question set. This approach will allow you to apply the test-taking strategies you have learned and to identify both the areas in which you have improved and the areas that require further study. Each question has a detailed explanation to help check and guide your reasoning, so be sure to study the explanation for each question as a regular part of your test prep.

HOW TO USE YOUR ONLINE RESOURCES

Your Student Homepage offers valuable bonus lessons on assessment and developmental considerations across the life span, as well as test-like practice quizzes to help you review. Use these anytime in partnership with this book to expand your studies. After thoroughly reviewing the comprehensive lessons and completing the practice sets in this book and online, you are ready to take your online Mini Prep Tests.

These tests have been designed as half-sized versions of the AANP and ANCC Family Nurse Practitioner certification exams to allow for more efficient practice.

We recommend that you take each test timed so that your practice will mimic your official Test Day experience as closely as possible. Once you have completed the first test, be sure to thoroughly review its answers and explanations before taking the second test. As you review your results, focus on the content areas in which you have room to grow and use your book as a reference and review guide.

ONWARD TO YOUR PREP!

By using Kaplan's *Family Nurse Practitioner Certification Prep Plus* book and online resources, you are taking a critical step toward your rewarding new career. We wish you the best of luck on Test Day and beyond!

kaptest.com/publishing

The material in this book is up-to-date at the time of publication. However, changes may have been instituted in the tests after this book was published.

If there are any important late-breaking developments—or changes or corrections to the Kaplan test preparation materials in this book—we will post that information online at **kaptest.com/publishing**. Check this link during your studies for possible updates or changes to this publication.

PART ONE

Test & Content Overview

CHAPTER 1

Test Overview

If you are reading this book, it is very likely that you (a) are thinking of becoming a Family Nurse Practitioner, (b) have recently enrolled in an FNP program, or (c) are nearing the end of your FNP curriculum. Graduating from your program is something to be proud of, but you now need to take one more step—sit for and pass a certification exam.

Certification and licensure are two different things. Licensure requirements vary state by state, but can include proof of education, clinical hours, an agreement with an overseeing physician, and proof of national certification before you are allowed to practice. Certification is part of APRN licensure in most U.S. states.

The Family Nurse Practitioner certification examination is an entry-level, competency-based examination reflective of clinical knowledge in family/individual health across the life span. It focuses on requirements for safe clinical practice and is limited to content that can be tested in an objective format.

Certification Options

You have the option to certify through either the American Nurses Credentialing Center (ANCC) or the American Association of Nurse Practitioners (AANP). Either test will certify you as an FNP. The exams are overall very similar, but small differences may help you make a decision about which to take.

Eligibility Requirements

You must meet eligibility requirements to sit for the exam. These include:

- RN licensure
- Master's, postgraduate, or doctoral degree from a family nurse practitioner program accredited by the Commission on Collegiate Nursing Education (CCNE) or the Accreditation Commission for Education in Nursing (ACEN)
- Completion of at least 500 hours of faculty-supervised clinical practice
- Completion of separate, graduate level courses in advanced physiology/pathophysiology, advanced health assessment, and advanced pharmacology, including pharmacodynamics, pharmacokinetics, and pharmacotherapeutics of all broad categories of agents

Prior to degree conferral and graduation, authorization to sit for the exam may be granted; this is dependent on completion of all coursework, clinical hours, and other eligibility requirements. Exam results will be held until the final degree is conferred and all other requirements are met. Be sure to read the candidate handbook carefully for this option.

Application

The ANCC requires an online application. The AANP allows for paper applications, but an additional fee is assessed.

Digital Resource

You may complete an application online through either certification program's website:

- ANCC: **www.nursingworld.org/our-certifications/family-nurse-practitioner/**
- AANP: **www.aanpcert.org/signin**

It may take up to six weeks after a completed application is submitted to receive an eligibility notice, the authorization to test (ATT), and instructions for signing up for a testing location, date, and time. With ANCC, you have up to 90 days to take the test once you receive the authorization to test (you can make a one-time request to extend this 90-day testing window). AANP allows 120 days to take the test before another application (and payment) is needed. A one-time 60-day extension may be granted with sufficient justification.

Special testing accommodations are available for candidates with documented disabilities as defined by the Americans with Disabilities Act. If eligible, you must notify either certifying body before scheduling a test appointment.

Each organization offers a discount for membership in specific nursing organizations. Consider joining a national organization—not just for the discount on the certification test, but also for savings on continuing education and the opportunity to network with colleagues. Also, consider recertification costs, as every five years FNPs must recertify.

Digital Resource

Both exams are computer-based tests and administered at independent testing centers (Prometric) throughout the country (**www.prometric.com/en-us/Pages/home.aspx**). Not all testing centers have the same exams, so you will need to see if your preferred location offers the test you want.

Test Content

American Nurses Credentialing Center (ANCC)

This exam has 200 questions. You have four hours to complete the test, which includes time for reading instructions and working through a practice session at the computer (the actual test time is 3.5 hours). On the exam are 25 pilot questions that are unscored, experimental questions. Your final results are based on the 175 scored questions. You have, on average, 50 seconds to answer each question. There is no penalty for guessing, so manage your time in order to answer every question.

Composition (from Test Content Outline effective date: 2/9/16)

Compared to the AANP exam, the ANCC exam typically has more questions focused on professional practice, including issues such as healthcare policy and ethics. The three main content areas are laid out in the following table.

Content area	# items	% items
Foundations for Advanced Practice	64	37%
Professional Practice	30	17%
Independent Practice	81	46%
TOTAL	175	100%

Table 1.1.1 Content of AANC Certification Exam

Specific topics found within each content area are as follows:

1. Foundations for Advanced Practice (37%)
   - Advanced Physiology/Pathophysiology Across the Life Span
   - Advanced Pharmacology for Treating Patients Across the Life Span
   - Advanced Health/Physical Assessment Across the Life Span
   - Clinical Prevention and Population Health for Improvement of Outcomes
   - Research Methodology
   - Informatics

2. Professional Practice (17%)
   - Leadership, Advocacy, and Inter-Professional Collaboration
   - Quality Improvement and Safety
   - Healthcare Economics, Policy, and Organizational Practices
   - Scope and Standards of Practice

3. Independent Practice (46%)
   - Health Promotion and Maintenance Across the Life Span
   - Illness and Disease Management
   - Care of Diverse Populations
   - Translational Science/Evidence-Based Practice
   - Advanced Diagnostic Reasoning/Critical Thinking

> **Digital Resource**
>
> Specific details here regarding test content can be found here: **www.nursingworld. org/~4acd24/globalassets/certification/certification-specialty-pages/resources/ test-content-outlines/familynp-tco.pdf**.

American Association of Nurse Practitioners (AANP)

This test has 150 questions; 15 of these are unscored pilot questions. Your final results are based on the 135 scored questions. You have three hours to take the exam. Prior to the exam, you can spend up to 15 minutes on a tutorial that shows how to use the computer and keyboard; this time is not part of the three-hour test time.

Composition (2015 Family Nurse Practitioner Practice Analysis)
Test specifications are based on two domains: Domain I (Practice—Assessment, Diagnose, Plan, Evaluate) and Domain II (Patient Age—Developmental Parameters). Test items are distributed across Domain I and further divided across Domain II.

Domain I	# items	% items
Assess	48	36%
Diagnose	33	24%
Plan	31	23%
Evaluate	23	17%
TOTAL	135	100%

Table 1.1.2 AANP Domain I

Domain II	# items	% items
Prenatal	4	3%
Pediatric (includes newborn & infant)	19	14%
Adolescent (early/late)	24	18%
Adult	50	37%
Geriatric	29	21%
Elderly	9	7%
TOTAL	135	100%

Table 1.1.3 AANP Domain II

Specific topics found within each domain are as follows:

1. Assess
   - Obtain subjective patient information including, but not limited to, relevant medical history (including bio-psychosocial, economic, environmental, family, military, travel, occupational, and preventive components), chief complaint, history of present illness, and review of systems to determine health needs and problems
   - Obtain objective information based on patient age/developmental level, health history, and comorbidities to further define and evaluate health needs and problems
2. Diagnose
   - Formulate differential diagnoses
   - Establish definitive diagnoses

3. Plan
   - Establish a safe plan of patient-centered treatment and care that is individualized, cost-effective, consistent with best evidence, age appropriate, and culturally sensitive in order to address the diagnoses

4. Evaluate
   - Determine the effectiveness of the plan of treatment and care based on outcomes
   - Modify the plan of treatment and care as appropriate based on outcomes

The AANP materials include a list of FNP procedures: **minor lesion removal, incision and drainage, microscopy, pap tests, joint aspirations and injections, skin biopsy, therapeutic injections, wound closure, splinting, casting, wound management, diagnostic interpretation of ECG and x-ray, cerumen removal, pulmonary function testing and office spirometry, fluorescein staining, long-term contraceptive management, long-term hormonal implantation, foreign body removal, and nail removal.**

Digital Resource

Specific details regarding test content can be found here: **www.aanpcert.org/resource/ documents/AGNP%20FNP%20Candidate%20Handbook.pdf**.

Scoring Information

Test results for both exams are given in a pass/fail format immediately upon completion of the test. Candidates who do not pass their exam will receive a score report that indicates strength and weakness on each of the major content areas of the test.

For the ANCC exam, a candidate's raw score (e.g., 125/175) is converted into a scaled score. Test results are reported on a scale with a maximum scaled score of 500. A minimum, scaled score of 350 or higher must be achieved in order to pass the exam.

As previously mentioned, you should not leave any question blank, as blank answers will count against you. There is no penalty for guessing. If you are uncertain of your answer, the test will allow you to "mark" these questions. You may go back and review/change the answers, provided you have not exceeded the allotted testing time.

Candidates who do not pass the ANCC certification exam may apply to retake the test after 60 days from the last testing date. The exam cannot be taken more than 3 times in any 12-month period.

As with the ANCC certification exam, the AANP exam is a criterion-referenced test. The exam's scoring system is complex; its goal is to define what a minimally competent entry-level FNP will know and answer correctly. Total raw scores are converted to a scaled score ranging from 200–800 points; a minimum score of 500 is sufficient to pass the examination.

Candidates who do not pass the exam may apply to retake the test after completing 15 hours of continuing education in the area(s) of weakness identified on the score report. The AANP certification exam may not be taken more than two times in any calendar year.

Test Day Rules

- If you arrive late for or miss your scheduled examination time or arrive without the required identification, you will not be able to take the examination as scheduled. You will forfeit your fee and be required to submit a new registration. You will be required to pay any applicable fees related to registration and testing. You are able to cancel and reschedule at least 24 hours in advance of the scheduled examination time without any additional fee (if that retest date and time is within the initial authorization time frame)

- No personal items may be brought into the testing area. The testing center provides lockers for such items

- No food or drink may be brought into the testing area. You may take a break at any time, but you will need to sign out (and back in), and total testing time will not be adjusted to accommodate a break

- The center provides paper and pencil (or similar), which may be used during the exam

- You may not ask questions about content during the exam. You cannot give or get help from others during the exam

- Candidates are required to sign a confidentiality agreement, stating they will not release any details about test questions

---

Digital Resource

Additional testing center regulations are published on Prometric's website: **www. prometric.com/en-us/for-test-takers/prepare-for-test-day/documents/ TestCenter Regulations.pdf**.

The FNP certification exam is an important test. You have dedicated the last few years to obtaining your education and clinical experience and now have to clear this last hurdle. Take the time to understand the logistics of the test, and approach the application process with care. Take the time to read instructions closely and complete applications judiciously to minimize the risk of having to do things a second time.

Digital Resource

Additional information for the examinations can be found in the candidate handbook:

- AANC: **www.nursingworld.org/~4ac3ba/globalassets/certification/renewals/ GeneralTestingandRenewalHandbook**
- AANP: **www.aanpcert.org/resource/documents/AGNP%20FNP%20Candidate%20 Handbook.pdf**

CHAPTER 2

Test-Taking Strategies

Both the AANP and ANCC certification exams are standardized tests, meaning that each will be predictable in terms of format and content. As with any standardized exam, you can increase your odds of being successful by not only reviewing the tested content, but also by knowing about the construction of the test and the types of questions you will face.

Know the Test

Purpose

The AANP national certification examinations are competency-based examinations for nurse practitioners to reflect knowledge and expertise in the role and population area of education (**www.aanpcert.org/certs/program**). The ANCC Family Nurse Practitioner board certification examination is a competency-based examination that provides a valid and reliable assessment of the entry-level clinical knowledge and skills of nurse practitioners (**nursecredentialing.org/FamilyNP**). The test has an evidence-based, scientific foundation.

Neither the AANP nor the ANCC exam is a specialty or acute care-based examination. The examination will determine if you have and can apply the knowledge and skills needed to be a safe and effective entry-level NP in primary care. Having that mindset is important when preparing for your exam.

About Standardized Examinations

Teacher-generated tests are designed to evaluate students' learning of the material presented in class. These tests are designed for a single class (and often certain topics or weeks of school). Questions have limited focus and emphasize specific details. These questions require lower-level thinking, including recalling and recognizing facts and specific details and understanding specific concepts. Many study by memorizing notes and study guides, making flashcards, and taking multiple-choice tests by selecting familiar answers. This strategy will not work for the certification exam.

Standardized tests are designed to measure knowledge across different courses and disciplines, covering a much broader domain of information. Questions have a global focus and emphasize application, integration, and association. These questions require higher-level thinking including problem solving, application to new situations, and critical reasoning. The questions are written by a team of experts to eliminate the candidate's use of cues and clues to determine the correct answers. Standardized tests will ask you to apply your knowledge in a context different from the one in which you studied to test your clinical judgment and application skills.

Test questions require higher-level thinking, so memorizing data (knowing what to do) will not be sufficient for this exam. Few questions will focus on facts, details, and particular sets of knowledge. The NP certification examination expects you to understand concepts and apply your clinical expertise (know what to do and why) just as you would in the patient exam room. The questions will present brief scenarios. You cannot ask clarifying questions; you need to think like an expert. As you review, focus on the following concepts:

- Risk factors for a condition and how the condition may have developed
- Common signs and symptoms of a condition

- Typical interventions and the rationale behind a given option
- Expected outcome

Test Plan

The previous chapter discussed the test plans for both the AANP and ANCC Family Nurse Practitioner exams. A cursory review will suffice for the content areas of strength; for the content areas of weakness, you will need a concentrated review. Prepare a study plan. This book provides a review of the essential areas of study. It will focus your studies, but not provide all the details that you may need. Use the table of contents from this review book or your primary care textbook as an outline or guide for your study plan. Identify the areas on which you want to focus and set a date and time to review that material. A comprehensive review will include more than this review book.

Question Structure and Design

Both the AANP and AANC have multiple-choice questions. The AANC includes alternate type questions, including (1) multiple response, (2) drag and drop, and (3) hot spot, but most of the test questions are multiple choice. Regardless of question type, identifying the structure of the question can assist you in determining the best approach to the question and answer choices.

Multiple Choice

Multiple-choice questions are made up of a stem (scenario and question) and answer choices. Typical answer choices include one correct answer, one incorrect answer, and two partially correct answers or plausible incorrect answers. You will learn to distinguish partially correct responses (sometimes correct or with an exception) from the best answer choice, given the context. There may be more than one question related to a given scenario. Negatively phrased questions ("all of the following except") questions are rare.

While some test items evaluate factual knowledge (e.g., selecting a common sign or symptom of a given condition), the majority of questions measure higher-level thinking and reasoning and will ask you to apply your clinical expertise with assessment or intervention to a clinical situation. The information you need to answer a multiple-choice question is included in the question and answer choices, but you need to know the content to understand the question and the nuances of each of the answer choices. The test is not testing content per se, but rather your ability to use it in a new situation to make a safe and effective decision.

With every multiple-choice question, the answer is provided. You simply have to identify the correct answer by eliminating the incorrect ones. Your job is to determine the correct answer (the safest, most effective answer).

Key words can help you determine the type of question. For example, priority questions include words like *first, next, best, most important*, etc. You are asked for the best answer; think: "if I can do one thing." The best answer may not be exactly what you are looking for, may not be perfect, but will be better than the rest. Evaluation questions include words such as "indicate an understanding" or "further teaching is needed." You are asked to find the correct (true) or incorrect (false) answer in relation to the topic.

- Be mindful of the nursing process as you answer each question. Make sure your assessment is complete before you diagnose, plan, or intervene. Determine the purpose of the question. Is it to test your ability to gather subjective and objective information, develop a diagnosis, implement a plan of care, or evaluate care given? Read each answer choice only after you understand the context of the question
- Consider the underlying pathophysiology and how it affects presentation and selection of intervention
- Read every answer choice carefully. Look for clue words and numbers. These modifiers can assist in selecting or eliminating answer choices
- Never select an answer without reading all the choices

- Make a decision about each possible answer choice as you read it. Evaluate what the answer choices mean (some gather information; some implement based on that information—determine what you need). Determine what the answer choice means within the context of the question. Does this answer choice lead to the desired or best possible outcome for the patient or scenario? If it is incorrect, unsafe, or does not address the topic, eliminate it from consideration. Or, choose the answer option that is inclusive (of other choices)

- The response with the most common presentation is likely correct. For example, a person with alcohol withdrawal can present with fine motor tremors and motor seizures. Because fine motor tremors are seen in most adults with alcohol withdrawal and motor seizures are far less common, fine motor tremors is a better choice

- Avoid selecting an answer because it contains familiar words from a lecture or reading. Avoid selecting an answer because it is a true statement. Just because an answer choice is true does not mean it is the correct answer to a given question. The correct answer relates back to the topic/context

- Select the answer representing the safest action in relation to the topic of the question

- Don't agonize over any one question; it can upset your pacing and confidence. If you read a question and don't know the answer, just take a deep breath and start eliminating options

- Nursing is seldom black and white. As such, a correct answer will usually contain relative qualifiers that allow for exception (e.g., *may be, may, few, rarely*). The correct answer rarely includes absolute qualifiers (e.g., *always, never, must*), as they do not allow for exceptions

- Be careful of negatively phrased questions—those that ask which is NOT true, require an intervention, or ask for all of the following "except." These ask you to pick an incorrect, false, or unsafe statement. You will be given three true/good statements and one incorrect statement. Put an "F" (for false) on your white board so that you do not forget that you are looking for an incorrect/false statement

- Answer every question. Questions left blank are marked with a zero. You can and should guess—with a random guess, you have a 25% chance of getting the question correct; with educated guessing, that jumps to 50–75%

Here is an example of a priority question:

1. A family nurse practitioner examines a 24-year-old female patient, 12 weeks pregnant, who is experiencing dysuria and urinary urgency and frequency. The patient reports that her roommate gave her some doxycycline 100 mg tablets, and she has taken three pills over the last three days, with little relief of her symptoms. What is the nurse practitioner's best response?

   A. Inform the patient to avoid taking prescription drugs prescribed for another person

   B. Prescribe trimethoprim-sulfamethoxazole 800–160 mg orally every 12 hours for 10 days

   C. Continue with doxycycline 100 mg orally for 7 days

   D. Request a urine sample from the patient for a culture and sensitivity

This is an action-oriented question. You are asked to consider the patient's symptoms and care and determine the best answer. From this scenario, you can make some assumptions.

You are told the patient is pregnant, but no other chronic illnesses are mentioned. You can assume that this pregnant young woman is in otherwise good health. Dysuria and urinary frequency are common symptoms of a urinary tract infection (UTI), and UTIs are common in pregnancy. Usual bacteria include *Escherichia coli, Klebsiella, Proteus mirabilis, and Staphylococcus saprophyticus.* UTIs are commonly diagnosed and treated after a culture and sensitivity. Common antibiotics include trimethoprim-sulfamethoxazole, fosfomycin, nitrofurantoin, ciprofloxacin, levofloxacin, cephalexin, azithromycin, and doxycycline.

Which answer choice is the best course of action for this patient?

Let's look at choice A—Inform the patient to avoid taking prescription drugs prescribed for another person. While this is a true statement, the outcome does nothing for the patient's current symptoms. This meets a psychosocial need of the patient (teaching information). The underlying cause of a UTI is physical; you want a physical answer.

Now let's look at choice B—Prescribe trimethoprim-sulfamethoxazole 800–160 mg orally every 12 hours for 10 days. Trimethoprim-sulfamethoxazole is frequently used to treat UTIs, yet this is not the best answer. First, the patient is pregnant, and trimethoprim must be used cautiously during the first trimester of pregnancy. Second, this selection represents treatment, and evidence-based practice dictates a culture and sensitivity to diagnose and appropriately treat. It is not known if the bacteria are susceptible to trimethoprim-sulfamethoxazole.

Choice C is next—Continue with doxycycline 100 mg orally for 7 days. Doxycycline is commonly used to treat UTIs, but this is not the best answer. First, it is prescribed every 12 hours, not daily. Second, as stated above, evidence-based practice dictates a culture and sensitivity to diagnose and appropriately treat. It is not known if the bacteria are susceptible to doxycycline.

Finally, choice D—Request a urine sample from the patient for a culture and sensitivity. This is an assessment answer. Diagnosis and treatment of a UTI are based on culture and sensitivity. This is the safest answer for this patient.

Now, consider this question:

2. A 25-year-old patient presents to the clinic with what his friends suspect to be alcohol withdrawal. Which of the following would be the most likely finding?

    A. Visual hallucinations

    B. Fine motor tremors

    C. Nausea and vomiting

    D. Motor seizures

This is an evaluation question. You are asked to consider the patient's symptoms and determine which represents the most likely finding. It is a true/false (correct/incorrect) question. Consider the answers.

Answer choices (A), (B), and (D) may be seen in alcohol withdrawal. However, fine motor tremors (B) are by far the most common. Choice (C), nausea and vomiting, is more commonly found in alcohol intoxication.

Multiple Response

Multiple-response (select all that apply) questions have more than four possible answer choices. For the question to be scored as correct, you must select *all* of the answer choices that apply, not just the *best* response. No partial credit is given. When more than one correct answer is required, the number of correct answers to be selected is stated in the question. Read the stem thoroughly to determine what the question is asking. Look at each item one at a time, independent of the other answer choices. Don't group answer choices; read each as if it is the only piece of information being evaluated. It does not work to compare and contrast the answer choices, as you would when answering a multiple-choice question. Change each answer choice into a statement, and then determine if the statement is correct or incorrect in relation to the topic. A statement may be a correct (true) statement, but it needs to be viewed within the context of the question asked.

Ordered Response

Drag and drop, or ordered-response questions, ask you to place answers in a specific order. The strategy to use when answering this kind of question is to picture yourself performing the procedure. Or, find the first step, then the last, and then fill in the center steps last. All the steps of the task may not be included in the answer options. In these cases, you need to correctly order the steps that are listed. No partial credit is given for this type of question.

Hot Spot

Hot-spot questions ask you to identify a location on a graphic (image) or table. This is not a test of your fine motor skills; this question type is designed to evaluate your knowledge of nursing content, anatomy and physiology, and pathophysiology. Select the area on the image that best describes the answer to the question asked.

Study Plan

Don't worry about how or what others are doing. You should tailor your study plan to your specific needs.

Review of Content

Review areas of weakness first—these are areas that may not make sense, areas that do not click in your brain, and areas in which you struggle. It might be tempting to put these aside and review a familiar topic, or one that comes easily to you. Don't do it. To be successful on the certification exam, you need an understanding of all the test areas. First, complete the rigorous task of reviewing the more troublesome areas, and then reward yourself by studying your areas of strength.

Kaplan's review approach starts out with a didactic overview of tested areas; each chapter is then followed by a set of practice questions. If, after reviewing a chapter, the information sounds familiar and you answer the practice questions readily, the topic is likely an area of strength and you can get by with a cursory review. If, after reviewing a particular section, the content is not clear or you struggle with the questions, you likely need further study. Pull out your textbooks and review that specific content area.

Practice Questions: Quality over Quantity

Don't time yourself on the practice questions at the end of each of these chapters. It is more important to understand how the questions work—the structure, the content, and the thinking process.

Identify what the question is asking. What is the NP's focus? What is the patient's problem, issue, or "chief complaint"? If you struggle with finding the topic, read the last sentence first and then read the stem or scenario again. This "backwards approach" ensures you know what the question is asking before you read the whole question. When you read it again "normally," you will recognize important clues that may make answering the question easier. Differentiate between the actual topic and the distracting information. Review each answer choice carefully and determine whether or not it answers the question asked.

The certification exam is timed; you have ~60 seconds per question. However, you should take your time answering the questions at the end of each chapter. Slow down. Pay attention. This initial practice allows you to focus on question structure and the logic behind answering the question.

Take the online Mini Prep Tests once you have learned, practiced, and reviewed all of the content material presented in this book. Taking a comprehensive set of test questions helps you in four ways:

1. It reinforces the skills and strategies you've learned
2. It helps you work on timing
3. It gives you a sense of how you're doing on the various topics and what you need to work harder on
4. It helps you learn to cope with test fatigue

Take each Mini Prep Test in one sitting, in a test-like environment—that means you are not allowed snacks, beverages, phones, or any documents with you when you take the test.

When you take the Mini Prep Tests, pay close attention to the time. You may take the tests in a timed or untimed mode. Two hours is allotted for the ANCC Mini Prep Test (100 questions) and 1.5 hours for the AANP (75 questions). Poor pacing causes candidates to spend too much time on certain questions and possibly run out of time before being able to answer every one. If you pace yourself, you will be able to answer each question in the allotted time.

Review of Questions

After every set of questions, stop and review. Review how you are feeling, review the test in general, and review each question.

Self-Reflection

After completing each set of questions, whether it be a practice set at the end of a chapter or a Mini Prep Test, stop and reflect before you move on. What is going well? (Keep doing it.) What is not working well? (Stop. Implement a plan of change.) Then, continue to evaluate whether the process is effective after the next set of questions. Learn from what you do so that you can improve what you do next. This is the nursing process—you have used it throughout your career, and now you need to apply it to your own approach to test taking. This purposeful reflection will help you make needed changes as you move through your studies.

Reflect on the Test-Taking Experience

Pay attention to the setting—each step of your preparation should be focused on Test Day. For example, complete practice questions sitting at a desk, in a quiet environment, without distractions including your phone, music, snacks, and drinks. Do not check other websites when you are taking practice tests.

Note your answer patterns—sets of incorrect answer choices can indicate places where you lost focus. Consider: were you distracted? Did your anxiety rise to a level that impacted your performance? What time during the test did the run of incorrect answers take place? Is this consistent with the previous test(s)? Identify the pattern of the runs (if there is one) and take a break before this occurs. For example, if a set of incorrect answers happens around question 40, take a break at question 35. You do not need to get up and walk around; sit quietly in your chair, take a deep breath, and let your brain and body rest. Do not push through questions if you need a break. Mental fatigue can have a seriously negative impact on your test performance, so breaks are essential.

What is your timing like? Did you take longer than 90 seconds per question, on average? Did you take less than 30 seconds per question, on average? Are there questions on which you vacillated between two answer choices? Did you consider information that was not in the question? Did you read the full stem and answer choices before selecting an answer? Did you select only familiar answers? Take the time to read each question and answer choice, and select the best answer related to the topic of the question.

Pay attention to your pattern of changing answers. Change your answer only if you have a good reason to do so—when you know you misread the question, or a detail about the topic pops into your mind that leads you to read the answer choices differently. Look back at the test to see if you changed answers from correct to incorrect, or incorrect to correct. If the former is true, try a set of questions without changing your answer. See if your score increases. If so, don't change your answers. If the latter is true, the technique works for you.

Reflect on the Questions

Reflect on the questions—consider content, topic, and thinking process. If you are not familiar with the content, the question and answers may not make sense (i.e., you may not understand the intent of the words).

- When you complete these sets of practice questions, don't just tally up how many you got correct and incorrect. Rather, review the feedback for every practice question

- Understand why the correct answer is correct and the incorrect answers are incorrect. If you answered the question incorrectly, consider where your thinking went astray. Then, use this information as you move forward in your studies

- Active reflection is the key to success. Ask yourself questions. Is this material relevant? Does it relate to what I know? How do I incorporate this information into what I know already? Do not skip over words, thinking you can review the information later—look them up and make sure you understand the word in context

- After reviewing content, ask yourself if every question/answer now makes sense. Once you understand a certain question type, you will improve your chances of answering it correctly in the future

- After reviewing the rationale, ask if you now understand the specific topic of each question. If you have not identified the correct topic, it is difficult to eliminate incorrect answer choices and select the best answer

- After reviewing the rationale, ask if you used the correct thinking process when working through each question. Did you recognize patterns in the answer choices? Did you differentiate between gathering more data (assessment) and doing something based on that data (implementation)? Consider if the information provided in a question stem is incomplete or vague; if so, ask yourself if the assessment answers would provide the needed information. A good assessment is one that confirms what is going on with the patient or one that determines your next step of action. Did you differentiate between a psychosocial and a physical answer choice? A physical problem (topic) likely requires a physical answer choice. Did you prioritize answer choices with the ABCs? Within the context of the topic of the question, you can prioritize respiratory answers over circulatory answers over everything else. Last, did you evaluate the answer choices and ask the outcome of each? Did the intended outcome match the topic of each question?

This purposeful review of your thinking process will assist you in developing habits that will help you be successful on Test Day and change those habits that won't. The best learning takes place with self-reflection.

Managing Your Anxiety

The certification exam can be stressful, but you can practice now to keep your emotions in check. You know about the levels of anxiety. If anxiety is high, then thinking is not clear and you will not be as effective when problem solving. Uncontrolled anxiety can disrupt your ability to focus and stay calm. While you may not be able to completely eliminate feelings of anxiety, you can reduce their intensity as well as their impact on your test performance.

Self-Regulation

There are two parts to self-regulation: behavior and emotion. From the behavioral perspective, choose actions that support your goal, such as developing an individualized study plan and following it. From the emotional side, manage your emotions and anxiety when you are facing this exam. You want to manage your emotional response to the test so you can focus, concentrate, and use your critical thinking at its highest level. When you are too anxious, your ability to stay calm, on task, and focused is limited, and it is harder to achieve your goal.

Identify your "tells" when you your anxiety is building. For some, this translates as tachycardia, heart palpitations, difficulty focusing, and nausea. Next, define what you can do to manage those symptoms. You may lean back in the chair and take a deep breath, use relaxed breathing techniques, or visualize success. It is important to practice these actions before you take the certification examination to find out which implementations work best for you.

Be Confident

Having the right mindset plays a large part in how well people do on a test. Those who are nervous about the exam and hesitant to make guesses often fare much worse than students with an aggressive, confident attitude. Students who start with question 1 and plod on from there don't score as well as students who pick and choose the easy questions first before tackling the harder ones. People who take a test cold have more problems than those who take the time to learn about the test beforehand. In the end, factors like these determine if people are good test takers or if they struggle even when they know the material.

Test Day

Pacing: plan to use the entire test time. The ANCC allows four hours for 200 questions. The AANP allows three hours for 150 questions. If you finish early, great; but don't fall short in preparing mentally and physically for this marathon exam.

Two-pass system: using the two-pass system is one way to help your pacing on a test. The key idea is that you don't simply start with question 1 and trudge onward from there. Instead, start at the beginning but take a first pass through the test, first answering all the questions that are easy for you. If you encounter a tough problem, spend only a small amount of time on it and then move on in search of easier questions. This way, you don't get bogged down on a tough problem when you could be earning points answering later problems that you do know. On your second pass, go back through the section and attempt all the tougher problems that you passed over the first time. You should be able to spend a little more time on them, and this extra time might help you answer the problem. Even if you don't reach an answer, you might be able to employ techniques like process of elimination to cross out some answer choices or just take a guess, since incorrect answers are not penalized.

- Go through the exam and answer those items about which you are confident. This saves time and builds your confidence. Next, go back and focus on the marked or skipped questions. Use the same strategies: identify the topic of the question, eliminate likely incorrect answers (those that are not safe and not effective), and make an educated guess

- Budget your time. If you are taking more than two minutes on a question, answer it and move on. Make an educated guess. Go back later to questions you do not know; don't waste time. Guess if you have to; do not leave any question blank

Process of elimination: select the correct answer by eliminating the choices that are not safe, not effective, and do not match the topic of the question.

Take a break: the countdown clock in the computer continues to count down, even if you stop for a break. Nonetheless, consider a break if you are mentally or physically fatigued. Go to the bathroom. Get a drink or a quick snack. Walk up and down the halls a few times. Return to the test refreshed and start back in on the questions.

Conclusion

Memorizing content will not work for this exam. Questions emphasize application, problem solving, and critical reasoning—rather than knowing facts. Study content in such a way that you understand the physiology behind the common signs, symptoms, and interventions so that you can reason your way through a test question.

It may be likely that you cannot select the correct answer on each question, but you should be able to eliminate the incorrect answer choices (those that are not safe, not effective, not related to the topic). You cannot cram for this test; you must use a logical approach that includes both reviewing content and taking practice tests. Answering questions is not enough. You must take the time to review each question, review each answer, and understand the rationale behind each option. Understand the correct answer and you can answer the same question if asked again. Understand how to apply your knowledge correctly, and you can answer questions that are similar in structure and approach on your official test.

Trust the process. Be confident. Take the time to complete a comprehensive review. You can do this—you will be an FNP!

CHAPTER 3

Clinical Prevention and Population Health for Improvement of Outcomes

LESSON 1: HEALTHY PEOPLE 2020

Learning Objectives

■ Identify the history and development of Healthy People 2020
■ Understand the Healthy People 2020 framework, topic areas, and objectives
■ Integrate concepts related to Healthy People 2020 into practice

Healthy People 2020 is a national agenda that communicates a vision for improving the health of the U.S. population and achieving health equity for all. It provides a set of specific, measurable objectives with targets to be achieved over the decade. These objectives are organized within distinct topic areas.

Initiatives are organized by general health and wellness topics (e.g., respiratory health or mental health) and also by age group (such as teen health or older adult health). There are sections directed to special populations such as mothers (maternal health) or disadvantaged populations. Finally, there are sections directed at social/community concerns, infrastructure, health advances/technology, and global issues.

Digital Resource

For up-to-date information, visit the U.S. Department of Health and Human Services website at **www.healthypeople.gov**.

Besides initiatives, the Healthy People 2020 website also offers webinars/e-learning resources for clinicians and the general public, links to state-related resources, and health data for researchers.

History and Development

Healthy People 2020 is based on the accomplishments of four previous Healthy People initiatives:

- 1979 Surgeon General's Report: *Healthy People: The Surgeon General's Report on Health Promotion and Disease Prevention*
- *Healthy People 1990: Promoting Health/Preventing Disease: Objectives for the Nation*
- *Healthy People 2000: National Health Promotion and Disease Prevention Objectives*
- *Healthy People 2010: Objectives for Improving Health*

Healthy People 2020 is the result of a multi-year process that was developed with input from a diverse group of individuals and organizations.

The Federal Interagency Workgroup (FIW) initiated the Healthy People 2020 development effort, basing the guidelines on data from public comments, past Healthy People efforts, and the work of 12 nationally known experts in public health that serve on the U.S. Department of Health and Human Services Secretary's Advisory Committee on National Health Promotion and Disease Prevention Objectives for 2020.

Framework, Topic Areas, and Objectives

There are more than 1,200 objectives in Healthy People 2020. Each objective has reliable data, baseline measurements, and targets for specific health goals that can be achieved by 2020.

Experts from multiple lead federal agencies helped prepare each objective, which were then made available for public feedback. A final set of objectives was selected by the FIW.

Many objectives include interventions that are designed to reduce or eliminate illness, disability, and premature death on both the individual and community level. Others focus on broader issues such as:

- Reducing health disparities
- Focusing on social determinants of health
- Improving access to quality healthcare
- Reinforcing public health services
- Advancing the availability and dissemination of health-related information

Initiatives

Healthy People is led by the Department of Health and Human Services (HHS), with an Advisory Committee providing input to the Secretary of HHS. It has been used as a strategic management tool by the federal government, states, communities, and many other stakeholders. These stakeholders have a direct influence on and provide ongoing input to the Healthy People development and implementation process.

Healthy People 2020 Initiatives

General Healthy People Initiatives include arthritis, osteoporosis, and chronic back conditions; blood disorders and blood safety; cancer; etc.

Disorders	Initiatives
Arthritis, osteoporosis, and chronic back conditions	These are three common conditions that can adversely affect the quality of life and reduce productivity and patients' sense of well-being; they can affect people throughout the life span.
Blood disorders and blood safety	Focuses on bleeding and clotting disorders, as well as blood handling safety. Some blood-related disorders discussed include DVT, hemophilia, and sickle-cell disease.
Cancer	Cancer continues to be a leading cause of morbidity and mortality; Healthy People 2020 objectives include reducing the number of cases, disability, and mortality.
Chronic kidney disease	Chronic kidney disease is recognized as a significant contributor to disability, mortality, and economic burden; Healthy People 2020 offers screening and dietary recommendations among other resources.
Diabetes	Diabetes affects almost 30 million Americans; Healthy People 2020 addresses DM1, DM2, and gestational diabetes. Diabetes can lead to multi-organ damage and produces a tremendous health burden, with sequelae including blindness, kidney damage, and cardiac involvement. Combating the U.S. obesity epidemic, providing education, managing already existing cases, and uncovering many undiagnosed cases are among Healthy People 2020 goals.

Table 3.1.1 Summary of Healthy People 2020 Initiatives

Disorders	Initiatives
Dementias, including Alzheimer disease	Dementias (including Alzheimer's) represent a significant emotional and medical burden for sufferers and their caretakers, as well as costly treatment and care. Key goals for Healthy People 2020 include providing adequate medical management for this group of conditions and giving adequate support to dementia sufferers and their caretakers.
Healthcare-associated infections	Healthcare-associated infections (HAIs) are an emerging source of concern in the U.S.; the World Health Organization and other entities warn that antibiotic resistance is becoming so prevalent that there are concerns some infections may become untreatable. Interventions include healthcare worker training (reinforcing basic measures such as handwashing) and avoidance of preventable HAIs such as catheter-related urinary tract infections.
Hearing and other sensory or communication disorders	About 16% of Americans will experience communication or sensory disorders in their lifetime. For hearing disorders, screening (such as for children), prevention (including the use of earplugs), and management (such as providing hearing aids for those with hearing loss) are some Healthy People 2020 goals.
Heart disease and stroke	About 33% of Americans have cardiovascular disease. One focus of Healthy People 2020 is to educate the public on modifiable cardiac risks such as undiagnosed hypertension, smoking, and obesity.
HIV	HIV represents an ongoing crisis in the U.S., with one million Americans diagnosed and many thousands more unaware of their HIV status. The main Healthy People 2020 goals are reducing new HIV infections, increasing access to care, improving health outcomes, and reducing health inequity.
Immunization and infectious diseases	Healthy People 2020 highlights vaccine-preventable diseases, noting that influenza, viral hepatitis, and tuberculosis (TB) continue to cause significant mortality and health burdens in the U.S.
Mental health and mental disorders	About 18% of American adults report mental health conditions. Unfortunate sequelae of mental health disease can include suicidality and loss of role function (such as inability to maintain employment). Special populations adversely affected by mental illness can include adolescents, older adults (for comorbid dementia and behavioral disturbance), and veterans.
Respiratory disease	Chronic obstructive pulmonary disease and asthma are two widespread conditions that account for a significant respiratory health burden in the U.S. Healthy People 2020 goals for these include prevention, diagnosis, management, and education.
Sexually transmitted diseases	STDs constitute a continuing public health problem in the U.S., with sequelae including fetal abnormalities, reproductive difficulties, and increased cancer risk. Issues such as disparities in health access and education are two priorities of Healthy People 2020.
Sleep health	Up to one-fourth of Americans report sleep disturbances. Inadequate sleep has implications for driving safety, work productivity, health outcomes, and quality of life.
Substance abuse	It is estimated that >20 million Americans suffer from a substance abuse issue. Ramifications of substance abuse include loss of work productivity, unsafe sex, motor vehicle accidents, and crime. The prevalence of opioids is also of special concern. Improving prevention, education, and drug treatment are three Healthy People 2020 objectives.
Tobacco use	Though the dangers of tobacco have been extensively publicized, Americans continue to use tobacco products. Healthy People 2020 objectives include continued education (including on the dangers of secondhand smoke) and smoking cessation initiatives.
Vision	Healthy People 2020 vision objectives focus on evidence-based interventions protecting eye health and preventing vision loss. Common conditions implicated in vision loss include diabetes and glaucoma.

Table 3.1.1 Summary of Healthy People 2020 Initiatives (Continued)

Early and middle childhood	The early and middle childhood years are recognized as setting the stage for healthy physical and mental development. To that end, Healthy People 2020 concerns for this age group include improving school success and identifying and treating children with developmental challenges.
Adolescent health	This section is actually devoted to both teen and young adult concerns. One reason for this focus on adolescents (10–19) and young adults (20–24) who make up about one-fifth of the U.S. population is that, at these ages, young people are developing the health beliefs and habits that will serve them for the rest of their lives. Illicit drug use, unprotected sex, and unsafe driving habits are just some of the issues that can add or detract from the future well-being of this age group.
Older adults	The aging of the American population—with about 15% of the population aged 65 years or older—poses a significant challenge. Older adults tend to be affected by multiple chronic diseases, are more prone to cancer, experience mobility issues, and suffer cognitive losses (such as dementia). Healthy People 2020 goals for this population include improving healthcare availability such as Medicare access, addressing concerns such as elder abuse, and providing resources for older adults with mental or physical limitations.

Table 3.1.2 Age-Related Healthy People 2020 Initiatives

Healthy People 2020 covers multiple safety-related initiatives:

- Environmental Health concerns include indoor and outdoor air quality, hazardous and toxic contaminants, and ground water quality
- Food Safety includes the reduction of foodborne illnesses and recommendations for the handling and storage of food
- Healthy People 2020's section on Injury and Violence Prevention notes that injury is the leading cause of death for Americans up to age 44 and a top contributor to disability. Causes of injury include falls, drowning, and violence
- Medical Product Safety covers topics such as reducing medical errors, reducing opioid deaths/overdoses, and reducing preventable medication-related deaths from medications such as anti-coagulants and narrow therapeutic index medications
- Occupational Safety and Health covers issues such as reducing work-related diseases, injuries, and mortality
- Preparedness addresses disaster readiness/major health incidents

Access to health services (disadvantaged populations)	Healthy People 2020 notes that many Americans suffer reduced access to healthcare. Reasons for health access disparity include poverty, living in poorly served rural areas, and a lack of culturally competent services. These problems can lead to Americans putting off or never receiving needed healthcare, which can lead to poorer health outcomes.
Disability and health	People with disabilities represent nearly 20% of the U.S., but disability can strike up to one-third of Americans at some point. Disability-related health issues can include reducing physical barriers to care/health access and providing adequate social and emotional support.
Lesbian, gay, bisexual, and transgender health	The LGBT community can experience social barriers to healthcare caused by discrimination. LGBT youth can be at special risk, with increased suicide rates (2–3 times higher than the general population), among other disparities.
Maternal, infant, and child health	Pregnant women and their infants/children comprise a population deserving special attention. Pregnant women can suffer issues such as preeclampsia/eclampsia, and infants/children are at risk for health concerns like sudden infant death syndrome (SIDS) and developmental issues.

Table 3.1.3 Healthy People 2020 Special Populations

Social/Community Concerns, Infrastructure, Health Advances/Technology, and Global Concerns	
Educational and community-based programs	Education and community-based interventions can improve the health awareness and health outcomes—not just of individual patients but also of the community at large.
Family planning	Family planning ranks as an important health concern. Issues such as contraception, unintended pregnancy, and infertility greatly impact individuals and the family unit.
Genomics	Healthy People 2020's focus on genomics derives in part from the fact that 90% of the leading causes of death—including diseases such as heart disease and diabetes—have a genetic component. Objectives include genetic testing for gene-related ovarian, breast, and colon cancers.
Global health	Global health is an increasingly important component of the national health strategy, as outbreaks of diseases elsewhere in the world (such as Ebola or Zika) can lead to outbreaks in the U.S. Partnering internationally to help detect and treat illnesses makes all populations safer.
Health communication and health information technology	Topics in this section include improved communication between healthcare providers and between healthcare facilities, appropriate safe use of personal health information, more efficient management of healthcare information, and using technology to aid in healthcare detection, management, and treatment.
Health-related quality of life & well-being	Health-related quality of life and well-being is Healthy People 2020's section addressing quality of life issues including life expectancy, physical/mental/social health, and health behaviors across the life span.
Public health infrastructure	Infrastructure is needed in order to plan, deliver, evaluate, and improve public health. Three key components include: competent workforce, state-of-the-art data & information systems, and agencies that evaluate/respond to public health needs.
Social determinants of health	Healthy People 2020 recognizes that good health is not only to be promoted in healthcare centers, but also promoted in schools, workplaces, and communities. But Healthy People 2020 notes that not all Americans have equal access to healthcare resources. Various social determinants—such as where one is born, where one lives/works/plays, and the resources available in one's neighborhood (such as access to healthy food, emergency services, safe affordable housing, social support)—all factor into the effectiveness of one's health services.

Table 3.1.4

Looking to the Future

The next decade's framework (Healthy People 2030) is already being developed. General concepts include creating social and physical environments that provide health and well-being and supporting healthy development, behaviors, and well-being across the life span.

Takeaway

Healthy People 2020 initiatives address specific diseases, age-related concerns, safety-related concerns, social/community concerns, infrastructure, health advances/technology, and global concerns that the nurse practitioner can expect will be the foci of that decade.

LESSON 2: PREVENTIVE SERVICES

Learning Objectives
- Review the economic impact of preventable chronic diseases on the U.S. healthcare system
- Understand the importance of using evidence-based preventive health guidelines
- Analyze the potential improved health outcomes through use of effective preventive health services
- Review validated tools for development of preventive health protocols

In the U.S., chronic diseases and conditions such as heart disease, stroke, cancer, type 2 diabetes, obesity, chronic lung conditions, and arthritis are the leading health issues and causes of death. One in two adults have one or more chronic health conditions, and one in four adults have two or more chronic health conditions. Preventable chronic diseases and the health risk behaviors that cause them account for most healthcare costs.

Most chronic diseases are attributed to the following risk factors, and according to the CDC, most adults in the U.S. have more than one of these risk factors:

- Tobacco use and exposure to secondhand smoke
- Excessive alcohol use
- Obesity (high body mass index)
- Lack of exercise and physical inactivity
- Diets low in fruits and vegetables
- Diets high in sodium and saturated fats

Prevention science: a multidisciplinary field devoted to the scientific study of the theory, research, and practice related to the prevention of social, physical, and mental health problems, including etiology, epidemiology, and intervention.

Prevention Science Term	Definition
Incidence	The number of new events (for example, new cases of a disease) in a defined population, occurring within a specified period of time
Prevalence	The proportion of people in a population who have some attribute or condition at a given point in time or during a specified time period
Morbidity	The illness or lack of health caused by disease, disability, or injury
Mortality	The measure of the incidence of deaths in a population
Reportable Disease	Health conditions that are required through statute, ordinance, or administrative rule to be reported to a public health agency when it is diagnosed in an individual
Epidemic	A group of cases of a specific disease or illness clearly in excess of what one would normally expect in a particular geographic area
Endemic	Prevalence in or peculiarity to a particular locale or people
Screening	The use of technology and procedures to differentiate individuals with signs or symptoms of disease from those less likely to have the disease
Surge Capacity	The ability to expand care or service capabilities in response to unanticipated or prolonged demand
Surveillance	The ongoing, systematic collection, analysis, and interpretation of health data. This activity also involves timely dissemination of the data and use for public health programs.

Table 3.2.1 Preventive Science Terminology

Levels of Prevention

Health prevention interventions are activities aimed at eradicating, eliminating, minimizing the impact, or slowing the progress of disease and disability. The concept of prevention is best defined in the context of levels. Traditionally, the levels of prevention are referred to as primary, secondary, and tertiary.

Primary prevention: prevent the disease or injury before it occurs. Strategies include minimizing exposure to hazards that cause disease or injury, altering unhealthy or unsafe behaviors that can lead to disease or injury, and increasing resistance to disease or injury should exposure occur. Examples include:

- Legislation and enforcement to ban or control the use of hazardous products (e.g., asbestos, air pollution, food contaminants) or to mandate safe and healthy practices (e.g., use of seat belts, car seats, motorcycle helmets)
- Health education (e.g., lifestyle modifications such as proper diet and exercise, smoking cessation)
- Immunization against infectious diseases

Secondary prevention: reduce the impact of a disease or injury that has already occurred. Strategies include early detection with prompt intervention to slow or stop disease progression. Examples include:

- Regular mammograms for early detection of breast cancer
- Daily, low-dose aspirin and/or diet and exercise programs to prevent subsequent heart attack or stroke
- Workplace assignment adjustments so injured or ill workers can return safely to their jobs

Tertiary prevention: stop the progression of an ongoing illness or injury that has lasting effects. Strategies include managing chronic health problems and long-term injuries through patient education and rehabilitation for those with impairments to improve function, quality of life, and life expectancy. Examples include:

- Cardiac or stroke rehabilitation programs, chronic disease management programs (e.g., for diabetes, arthritis, depression)
- Monitoring of prescribed medication to make sure the patient is taking them
- Crisis intervention and therapy (e.g., following a suicide attempt)

Successful prevention depends upon:

- Understanding of causation
- Dynamics of transmission
- Identification of risk factors and risk groups
- Early detection testing
- Effective treatment measures
- Systematic application of these elements to appropriate persons or groups
- Continuous evaluation of epidemiology, efficacy of treatment measures, and development of new procedures for detection and treatment

National Involvement in Prevention

The costs of chronic and preventable diseases are a huge burden on our economy and on our healthcare system. Public and private organizations in the U.S. have worked to develop an infrastructure designed to prevent these diseases and/or mitigate the toll they take on the population.

National Prevention Strategy

The Office of the Surgeon General released a National Prevention Strategy in 2011 that encompasses the visions and goals of many public and private healthcare initiatives. Research from this office has determined that effective healthcare prevention programs lower healthcare costs and increase productivity.

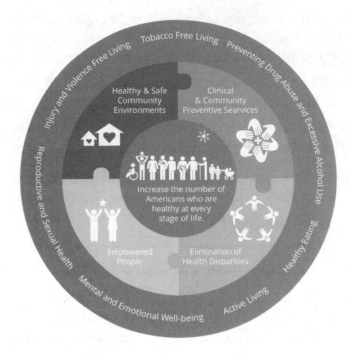

Figure 3.2.1 National Prevention Strategy

Office of Disease Prevention and Health Promotion

Congress created the Office of Disease Prevention and Health Promotion (ODPHP) in 1976 to lead disease prevention and health promotion efforts in the U.S. It is part of the U.S. Department of Health and Human Services under the Office of the Assistant Secretary for Health. The ODPHP plays a vital role in keeping the nation healthy, and accomplishes this by setting national health goals and objectives and supporting programs, services, and education activities that improve the health of all Americans.

The ODPHP collects and analyzes data and also manages three independent websites:

- **health.gov**—the home of ODPHP and an essential resource for health information
- **healthypeople.gov**—tools and resources for professionals about Healthy People 2020 health objectives
- **healthfinder.gov**—evidence-based, actionable health guidance for consumers

This information is retained and reported back to relevant agencies. One of the most important functions of the ODPHP is to maintain a repository of training modules for healthcare professionals and the public.

> **Pro Tip**
>
> The ODPHP provides free health and wellness information, which can be found at Health Topics A to Z (**healthfinder.gov/HealthTopics/**). This offers the most current health and prevention information available on more than 120 topics. There is a web badge link so healthcare providers can add the myhealthfinder.gov tool to their websites in order to help disseminate preventive health screening and education to consumers.

The recommendations found on **healthfinder.gov** come from the U.S. Preventive Services Task Force (USPSTF), the CDC Advisory Committee on Immunization Practices (ACIP), and the Health Resources and Services Administration (HRSA) as advised by organizations including the American Academy of Pediatrics (through the Bright Futures cooperative agreement) and the National Academies of Sciences, Engineering, and Medicine (formerly the Institute of Medicine). The Affordable Care Act (ACA) requires most insurance plans to cover preventive services at no cost to the healthcare consumer.

U.S. Preventive Services Task Force

Created in 1984, the U.S. Preventive Services Task Force (USPSTF) is an independent, volunteer panel of national experts in prevention and evidence-based medicine. It makes evidence-based recommendations about clinical preventive services such as screenings, counseling services, and preventive medications. There are currently 98 recommendations that cover diseases and healthy aging from a wide range of specialties (internal medicine, family medicine, pediatrics, behavioral health, obstetrics and gynecology, and nursing).

These recommendations are based on a rigorous review of existing peer-reviewed, evidence-based population studies and data. They are intended to help primary care clinicians and patients decide together whether a preventive service is right for a patient's needs.

Each year, the task force publishes a report that identifies critical gaps in research related to clinical preventive services and recommends research priorities for further examination. The task force assigns recommendations, via a letter grade (A, B, C, or D grade, or "I statement"), which aim to balance the risks and benefits of a preventive service. The recommendations address services offered in primary care and apply to people with no signs or symptoms of the disease or condition. Cost is not a consideration when determining a recommendation grade.

The work of the USPSTF is recognized by the Affordable Care Act, and under the law, preventive services with a task force grade of A or B must be covered without cost sharing (e.g., copayment or deductible) by new health insurance plans or policies.

> **Digital Resource: USPSTF Final Recommendations**
>
> Recommendations can be found at **www.uspreventiveservicestaskforce.org/BrowseRec/Index/browse-recommendations** and/or in peer-reviewed journals.

Grade level	Definition	Suggestions for practice
A	• Good research-based evidence to support the recommendation • USPSTF recommends the service • High certainty that the net benefit is substantial	Offer or provide this service
B	• Fair research-based evidence to support the recommendation • USPSTF recommends the service • High certainty that the net benefit is moderate or there is moderate certainty that the net benefit is moderate to substantial	Offer or provide this service
C	• Expert opinion and panel consensus to support recommendations • USPSTF recommends selectively offering or providing this service to individual patients based on professional judgment and patient preferences • Moderate certainty that the net benefit is small	Offer or provide this service for selected patients depending on individual circumstances
D	• Evidence of harm from this intervention • USPSTF recommends against the service • Moderate or high certainty that the service has no net benefit or that the potential harm outweighs the benefits	Discourage the use of this service
I Statement	• Evidence is lacking, of poor quality, or conflicting • Evidence is insufficient to assess the balance of benefits and harms of the service • Balance of benefits and harms cannot be determined	If the service is offered, patients should understand the uncertainty about the balance of benefits and harms. Clinicians are advised to review the clinical considerations section of USPSTF recommendations statement for any service

Table 3.2.2 USPSTF Recommendation Grading System

Healthy People Initiative

The Healthy People Initiative, in tandem with the CDC, has developed a model that addresses prevention at the individual and population level. It has identified four domains of prevention health efforts:

1. Epidemiology and surveillance—to monitor trends and track progress
2. Environmental approaches—to promote health and support healthy behaviors
3. Healthcare system interventions—to improve the effective delivery and use of clinical and other high-value preventive services
4. Community programs linked to clinical services—to improve and sustain management of chronic conditions

Takeaways

- Chronic, preventable illnesses account for the majority of healthcare expenditures and deaths of adults in the U.S.
- There are well-developed definitions and prevention strategies with national, state, and local initiatives that address prevention on both individual and population levels.

LESSON 3: SCREENING TESTS

Learning Objectives

■ Understand sensitivity and specificity

■ Identify valid sources of recommended screening tests and schedules for men, women, and special populations

■ Identify generally accepted recommendations for screening tests

Screening tests are either primary, secondary, or tertiary measures (*see Chapter 3, Lesson 2*). Screening tests must be sensitive and specific, which speaks to the validity and reliability of the test. The USPSTF makes recommendations for primary screening based on these principles and methodology.

- **Specificity:** the ability of a test to identify those who do not have a given disease—the probability that if a person does not have a disease, the test will be negative. In other words, if the result for a highly specific test is positive, one can be nearly certain the disease is present. Specificity rules in (SPIN) disease with a high degree of confidence.

- **Sensitivity:** the ability of a test to correctly identify patients who have a given disease—the probability that if a person has a disease, the test will be positive. In other words, if the result for a highly sensitive test is negative, you can be nearly certain the disease is absent. Sensitivity rules out (SNOUT) disease with a high degree of confidence.

Test	Age
Abdominal aortic aneurysm	One-time screening by ultrasonography for men ages 65–75 years who have ever smoked
Alcohol misuse	• 18 years or older for alcohol misuse; provide counseling for persons engaged in risky or hazardous drinking • CAGE Questionnaire is a valid tool
Asymptomatic bacteriuria screening with urine culture	Pregnant women at 12–16 weeks gestation or at the first prenatal visit, if it occurs later
Blood pressure screening	Start at age 18 and older

Colonoscopy (preferred)	Initial testing:
	
	• Age 45 for African American women, then every 10 years
	  Age 50 for Non-African American women, then every 10 years
	• Alternatives to colonoscopy:
	  – Flexible sigmoidoscopy: every 5 years
	  – Double contrast barium enema test: every 5 years
	  – Commuted tomography: every 5 years
	  – Guaiac-based fecal occult blood test (gFOBT): yearly

Diabetes	Age 40–70 years who are overweight or obese
Fall risk assessment	• Start at age 65 or older • Implement exercise interventions if high risk
Hepatitis C	Done once for women born between 1945–1965 with an unknown infection status

Table 3.3.1 USPSTF A and B Primary Screening Recommendations

Test	Age
HIV	• Yearly for any age of patients participating in unsafe sex practices or sharing injection drug equipment • Once for age 13–64, and reassess risk yearly
Latent tuberculosis infection	All children and adults in a high-risk population
Low-dose aspirin use for the primary prevention of cardiovascular disease and colorectal cancer	Start at age 50–59 years for those who have a 10% or greater 10-year cardiovascular risk, are not at increased risk for bleeding, have a life expectancy of at least 10 years, and are willing to take low-dose aspirin daily for at least 10 years
Lung cancer	• Age 55–80 years who have a 30 pack-year smoking history and currently smoke or have quit within the past 15 years • Discontinue once a person has not smoked for 15 years or has limited life expectancy
Major depressive disorder (MDD) screen	• Start at age 18 and older including pregnant and postpartum women • Use a validated screening tool specific for adolescent, adult, geriatric, postpartum, and general adult populations
Obesity	• Start at age 6 years and older and continue to assess throughout the life of a patient • Refer patients with a body mass index of 30 kg/m^2 for behavioral interventions
Osteoporosis	• Initial bone density screening at age 65 or for any postmenopausal woman with clinical risk factors for a fracture • Repeat every two years; consider more often only if other illness develops
Prostate cancer	• Begin screening at age 50; African American males or men with a FH of prostate cancer in a first-degree relative under age 65, initial test at age 45 • PSA of less than 2.5 ng/mL, retest every two years • Screening should be done yearly for men whose PSA level is 2.5 ng/mL or higher
Skin cancer	• Counsel patients and parents of those age 10–24 and fair-skinned

Statin therapy to reduce CV risk	• Start low to moderate dose statin in ages 40–75 years if the following criteria are met:
	  – No history of cardiovascular disease (CVD)
	  – One or more CVD risk factors (e.g., dyslipidemia, diabetes, hypertension, or smoking)
	  – Calculated 10-year CVD event risk of 10% or greater

Tobacco use screen, counseling, and interventions	All adolescents and adults
TSH	Initial test at age 50 then every five years
Type 2 diabetes	40–70 years as part of cardiovascular risk assessment for those who are overweight or obese
Vision screening	At least once from age 3–5, then annually in age 65 and older
Excludes recommendations for STI screening, PAP smears, pelvic/breast exams, mammograms, and pregnancy-related screening (*see Chapter 9, Lessons 3, 4, and 5*); immunizations (*see Chapter 3, Lesson 4*); and primary screening recommendations for children and newborns (*see Chapter 17*)	

Table 3.3.1 USPSTF A and B Primary Screening Recommendations (Continued)

Additional Recommendations

The USPSTF also utilizes input from healthcare specialty organizations when making recommendations. In an effort to compile these additional recommendations, the Choosing Wisely campaign was created. More than 70 specialty societies have identified commonly used tests or procedures within their specialties that are possibly overused. The campaign aims to promote conversations between clinicians and patients by helping patients choose care that is:

- Supported by evidence
- Not duplicative of other tests or procedures already received
- Free from harm
- Truly necessary

Digital Resource

Recommendations from the USPSTF and the Choosing Wisely campaign are updated at least annually, so they are handy reference tools for healthcare providers who want to remain current. These are available here: **www.choosingwisely.org**.

Special Considerations in Screening Tests

Many specialty medical organizations and professional associations have screening recommendations that are different than the USPSTF. For example, the American Cancer Society (ACS) recommends that men have a chance to make an informed decision with their healthcare provider about whether to be screened for prostate cancer. The decision should be made after getting information about the uncertainties, risks, and potential benefits of prostate cancer screening, after which men can decide to proceed with a prostate-specific antigen (PSA) blood test and/or digital rectal examination (DRE). Men should not be screened unless they have received this information.

Takeaways

- Screening protocols and tests are recommended for patients based on age, gender, and past medical and family history, and are based on a review of research which meets stringent criteria.
- Screening test recommendations are graded. Grades are based on elements of population studies and relevant net health benefits, which minimizes risk and promotes early detection of a disease process.
- The USPSTF recommendations A and B are to be covered services by all insurers.
- Many professional healthcare organizations have recommendations that may differ from the USPSTF guidelines and may offer the clinician additional guidance in provision of screening services.

LESSON 4: VACCINATIONS/IMMUNIZATIONS

Learning Objectives

■ Discuss general considerations related to immunizations
■ Identify age-appropriate recommendations for immunizations
■ Define side effects of and contraindications to immunizations

Immunization allows for a focus on disease prevention. Though a key health promotion activity during childhood health supervision visits, immunizations are also recommended for adults. Active immunity occurs in response to immunization.

Definitions

- **Acellular:** contains only those fragments of bacterial cells best suited to stimulating an immune response
- **Active immunity:** immunity acquired when a person's immune system generates an adaptive immune response to antigen exposure, generating immunologic memory
- **Conjugate vaccine:** vaccines in which the bacterial cell wall polysaccharide is linked with proteins, dramatically increasing the immune response
- **Killed vaccine:** contains whole dead organisms incapable of reproducing, yet produces an immune response
- **Live attenuated vaccine:** vaccine containing weakened modified living organisms capable of producing an immune response without the complications of the illness
- **Polysaccharide vaccine:** inactivated subunit vaccine containing long chains of sugar molecules composing certain bacteria's surface capsule
- **Recombinant vaccine:** DNA encoding an antigen is inserted into bacterial or mammalian cells; antigen is expressed in the cells and then purified from them
- **Toxoid vaccine:** vaccine with a toxin that is heat-treated to weaken its effect, yet still allows production of an immune response

General Considerations

Immunization Handling and Administration

Immunization efficacy is affected by vaccine storage and handling. Vaccines must be stored as recommended and reconstituted as directed to maintain their effectiveness. The correct route of administrations is also critically important. Live vaccines may be administered on the same day as one another, but if they are not given on the same day, they must be separated by at least 28 days in order to ensure efficacy.

Side Effects of Immunizations

Any immunization may produce side effects, and most of them are mild. Localized reactions may occur such as redness, tenderness, and swelling at the site. A cool compress at the site may be helpful. Systemic effects such as low-grade fever or fussiness may also occur and be eased with oral acetaminophen. These effects usually resolve within a few days.

Vaccine Information Statements

Vaccine information statements (VIS) must be provided to parents before an immunization is administered to a child (as required by the National Childhood Vaccine Injury Act). Each VIS provides information about the benefits, risks, and side effects specific to the particular vaccine.

> **Pro Tip**
> A recent study determined there is no link between immunization and the development of autism spectrum disorder, as was previously thought.

Precautions and Contraindications

Precautions are conditions that increase the risk of an adverse reaction or may impair the person's ability to acquire immunity from the vaccine. Temporary precautions include moderate to severe illness, immunosuppression, pregnancy, and recently received blood products or other antibody-containing products. Postponing immunization is recommended in these instances. The vaccines may be given later when the immunocompromise is resolved or the woman is no longer pregnant.

Contraindications are conditions that justify withholding an immunization. Anaphylactic or systemic allergic reaction to a vaccine component is a permanent contraindication to that vaccine. Encephalopathy without an identified cause within seven days of pertussis immunization permanently contraindicates further immunization with pertussis-containing vaccine. Live vaccines should not be given to significantly immunocompromised individuals nor to pregnant women (due to risk to the fetus).

Minor respiratory illness or a low-grade fever does not usually warrant vaccine postponement. Always ask about previous vaccine reactions and screen for precautions and contraindications prior to administration of each vaccine immunization.

Vaccine Adverse Event Reporting

In the event of a clinically significant adverse occurrence following an immunization, report the occurrence to the Vaccine Adverse Event Reporting System (VAERS) by utilizing the required form. VAERS may be reached by phone (800) 822–7967 or online: **www.vaers.hhs.gov**.

Immunization Schedules

A branch of the Centers for Disease Control (CDC), the Advisory Committee on Immunization Practices (ACIP) annually reviews the recommended immunization schedules and updates the schedules to reflect current best practices. The schedules are approved by the CDC, American Academy of Family Physicians, American Academy of Pediatrics, American College of Nurse-Midwives, American College of Obstetricians and Gynecologists, and the American College of Physicians.

The Recommended Immunization Schedule for Children and Adolescents Aged 18 Years or Younger, United States, 2018 is available at **www.cdc.gov/vaccines/schedules/downloads/child/0-18yrs-child-combined-schedule.pdf**. The schedule provides standard recommendations for all children, as well as recommendations for catching up on missed vaccines and additional information on medical indications for particular vaccines.

The Recommended Immunization Schedule for Adults Aged 19 Years or Older, United States, 2018 is available at **www.cdc.gov/vaccines/schedules/downloads/adult/adult-combined-schedule.pdf**. Similar to the child and adolescent schedule, standard recommendations for all adults, as well as additional information on medical indications for particular vaccines, are included.

App Alert

Download the free CDC Vaccine Schedule app for iOS and Android to stay up-to-date with immunization schedules and footnotes. You can find more immunization schedules and a link for the app here: **www.cdc.gov/vaccines/schedules/hcp/child-adolescent.html#schedule**.

Immunization Descriptions

Hepatitis B (Hep B)

Hep B is a recombinant vaccine used to prevent hepatitis B virus infection, which can affect the liver. Spread through contact with blood and body fluids, hep B can be transmitted from an infected mother to a newborn at birth, as well as via contaminated needles. The recommended childhood schedule is one dose at birth (preferably within the first 12 hours), then at age 1–2 months and 6–18 months. Verify immunity status of adolescents and adults, and in the non-immune, provide a 3-dose series: first dose, 1 month later, and 6 months following the first dose.

Rotavirus

The vaccine prevents infection with rotavirus, which is the most common cause of severe gastroenteritis among infants and young children, leading quickly to dehydration and significant morbidity. Rotavirus vaccine may not be given until the infant is at least 6 weeks of age and is contraindicated in infants with a history of intussusception or who have severe combined immunodeficiency syndrome and is precautionary in other immunocompromised states. It is not given past 8 months of age. The recommended childhood schedule depends upon the brand of vaccine:

- Rotarix, 2 doses: ages 2 months and 4 months
- RotaTeq 3 doses: ages 2 months, 4 months, and 6 months

Diphtheria, Tetanus, Acellular Pertussis (DTaP)

DTaP contains pertussis cell wall proteins and diphtheria and tetanus toxoids in a combination vaccine, providing protection against diphtheria, tetanus, and pertussis disease in children younger than 7 years of age. The recommended schedule is 5 doses, at age 2 months, 4 months, 6 months, 15–18 months, and 4–6 years. Children who have a contraindication to the pertussis component receive the diphtheria-tetanus (DT) vaccine at the same ages instead.

> **Pro Tip**
> The older vaccine, diphtheria, pertussis, tetanus (DPT), contained killed whole cells of pertussis bacteria and caused more frequent and severe adverse reactions than DTaP.

Tetanus, Diphtheria, Acellular Pertussis (Tdap)

TdaP contains tetanus toxoid, reduced diphtheria toxoid, and acellular pertussis. The recommended schedule is as a tetanus booster at age 11–12 years, also providing a boost to diphtheria and pertussis immunization. Tdap is also administered any time a tetanus shot is recommended in children 7 to 18 years of age. Provide one dose of Tdap for each pregnancy. Use Tdap once as a tetanus booster in adulthood.

Tetanus and Diphtheria (Td)

Td contains tetanus toxoid and reduced diphtheria toxoid. Td is recommended as a tetanus booster every 10 years, after Tdap is given once in adulthood.

Haemophilus Influenzae Type B (Hib)

Haemophilus influenzae type B causes life-threatening illnesses (meningitis, epiglottitis, septic arthritis) in children younger than 5 years of age. HiB vaccination has been very effective at reducing rates of these diseases in children. It is not given past the age of 5 years and is contraindicated in infants younger than 6 weeks of age. The number of doses recommended is based upon the conjugate vaccine brand utilized:

- PedvaxHIB at ages 2 months, 4 months, and 12–15 months OR
- ActHIB, MenHibrix, Hiberix, or Pentacel at ages 2 months, 4 months, 6 months, and 12–15 months

Pneumococcal Vaccines

The pneumococcal vaccine is used for prevention of *Streptococcus pneumoniae* (pneumococcus) infection. Pneumococcus is the most common cause of pneumonia, sepsis, meningitis, and otitis media in young children, as well as community-acquired pneumonia and sepsis in adults. The pneumococcal conjugate vaccine, PCV13, contains 13 strains of pneumococcus and stimulates an immune response in infants (minimum age is 6 weeks). The pneumococcal polysaccharide vaccine (PPSV) contains 23 strains of *S. pneumoniae* and does not provoke an immune response in children younger than 2 years of age. The recommended schedule for pneumococcal vaccine is as follows:

- Children <2 years of age—PCV13 (4 doses) at ages 2 months, 4 months, 6 months, and 12–15 months
- Children >2 years of age who are at high risk for pneumococcal sepsis, which includes asplenia, cerebrospinal fluid leak, chronic heart disease (2–5 years only), chronic lung disease (2–5 years only), chronic renal failure or nephrotic syndrome, cochlear implant, congenital immunodeficiency, diabetes mellitus, HIV infection, sickle cell disease, treatment with immunosuppressive drugs or radiation therapy, or solid organ transplantation—PPSV23
- Immunocompetent adults aged 65 years and older—PCV13 (1 dose), then at least 1 year later PPSV
- Adults aged 19–64 years with chronic heart, lung, or liver disease, diabetes mellitus, or who smoke cigarettes—PPSV23
- Adults 19 years of age or older with asplenia, cerebrospinal fluid leak, cochlear implant, or immunocompromising conditions—PCV13 followed by PPSV23 at least 8 weeks later

Inactivated Poliovirus (IPV)

IPV is a killed virus vaccine protecting against the paralyzing polio virus, which poses no risk for vaccine-acquired disease. The recommended childhood schedule is at ages 2 months, 4 months, 6–18 months, and 4–6 years.

Influenza

The inactivated influenza vaccine (IIV) and the recombinant influenza vaccine (RIV) protect against four strains of influenza. Annual influenza vaccination is recommended for all persons 6 months of age or older. Children 6 months to 8 years of age receiving influenza vaccine for the first time need two doses, four weeks apart. RIV is approved for use in adults over 19 years of age only.

Persons whose egg allergy is only demonstrated by hives may receive age-appropriate IIV or RIV. Persons with a history of significant egg allergy or anaphylaxis may receive the influenza vaccine in a healthcare facility where severe reaction may be identified and immediately managed. Pregnant women or women intending to become pregnant before the next flu season should only receive IIV.

Measles, Mumps, Rubella (MMR)

MMR is the combination vaccine of the live attenuated viruses for measles, mumps, and rubella. MMR is contraindicated during pregnancy and immunocompromised states. The recommended dosing schedule is as follows:

- Children—2 doses, at ages 12–15 months and again at 4–6 years
- Women who are determined to be rubella non-immune while pregnant—1 dose of MMR after delivery or termination of pregnancy
- Adults born after 1957 without documented evidence of immunity—1 dose of MMR

> **Pro Tip**
> MMR is not prepared from the allergenic albumin portion of the egg, so an egg allergy is no longer a contraindication for measles vaccination. Anaphylactic reactions may be associated with the neomycin or gelatin components of the vaccine.

Varicella Zoster

Varicella zoster vaccine is a live attenuated vaccine providing protection against chickenpox. The recommended childhood schedule is 2 doses, at age 12–15 months and 4–6 years. Additionally, in the non-immune person who is exposed to varicella, the vaccine provides effective post-exposure prophylaxis when given with 3–5 days of the exposure. Adults without evidence of immunity to varicella need 2 doses, at least 4–8 weeks apart. If 1 dose has been received in the past and the adult remains non-immune, only 1 additional dose is needed.

Hepatitis A (Hep A)

Hep A is an inactivated whole virus vaccine and prevents infection with hepatitis A, which is primarily transmitted via the fecal-oral route. It can also be spread by eating or drinking contaminated food or water or through close physical contact with an infected individual.

The recommended childhood schedule is 2 doses, at age 12 months followed by a second dose 6–18 months later. Adults with chronic liver disease who receive clotting factor concentrates, use injection or non-injection drugs, work with Hep A-infected primates or in a Hep A research lab setting, have contact with individuals from a Hep A-endemic area, or are men who have sex with men should also receive the Hep A series.

Meningococcal

The meningococcal vaccine protects against infection with *Neisseria meningitidis,* which causes meningitis, meningococcemia, and pneumonia. The recommended childhood schedule is 2 doses, one at age 11–12 years and one at age 16 years. The meningococcal conjugate vaccine is needed by children and adults with asplenia, HIV, persistent complement component deficiency, or sickle cell disease, as well as military recruits and previously unimmunized first-year college students aged 21 years or younger.

Human Papillomavirus (HPV)

The HPV vaccine prevents human papillomavirus infection transmitted through direct skin-to-skin contact, most often during vaginal or anal penetrative sexual acts. The recommended childhood schedule is 2 doses beginning at 11–12 years of age, with the second dose following 6–12 months later. HPV vaccine may be given as early as 9 years of age. Previously unimmunized adult females up to 26 years of age and males up to 21 years of age should receive a 3-dose series (UPDATE: as of 10/2018, the FDA approved the HPV vaccine for adult patients between the ages of 27 and 45). It is not recommended for administration during pregnancy.

Herpes Zoster Virus (HZV)

A new shingles vaccine called Shingrix (recombinant zoster vaccine) was licensed by the USFDA in 2017. Shingrix provides strong protection against shingles and post herpetic neuralgia. Both the CDC and the ACIP recommended immunocompetent adults aged ≥50 years get two doses of Shingrix, 2 to 6 months apart. There is not available human data to establish associated risk in pregnant women.

Takeaways

- Live vaccines are contraindicated in immunocompromised individuals and during pregnancy.
- Minor side effects such as low-grade fever or localized redness, tenderness, or edema may occur following immunization.
- Federal law requires vaccine information statements be provided to parents of children receiving immunizations.
- Refer to the ACIP immunization schedule updated annually for the most current immunization recommendations.

PRACTICE QUESTIONS

Select the ONE best answer.

Lesson 1: Healthy People 2020

1. All of the following are true of Healthy People 2020 except:

   A. It is funded by the pharmaceutical industry

   B. It is a national agenda that communicates a vision for improving health and achieving health equity of the U.S. population

   C. It provides a set of more than 1,200 specific, measurable objectives with targets to be achieved over the decade

   D. Initiatives are organized by general health and wellness topics, age, and special needs populations such as maternal health or vulnerable population groups

2. The Lesbian, Gay, Bisexual, and Transgender (LGBT) population is included as a special population in the Healthy People 2020 initiative due to which of the following health concerns?

   A. LGBT population experiences few social barriers to healthcare caused by discrimination

   B. LGBT youth can be at special risk, with increased suicide rates 2–3 times higher than the general population

   C. LGBT individuals have less access to healthcare due to living in poorly served rural areas

   D. LGBT individuals experience a lower risk of violence and victimization, which has long-lasting effects on the individual and the community

3. Many objectives of Healthy People 2020 focus on broader population issues including which of the following?

   A. Increasing health disparities

   B. Reducing equal access to quality healthcare

   C. Increasing services to identified minority populations

   D. Decreasing the availability and dissemination of health-related information

4. Improvement in sleep health is an objective of Healthy People 2020 for what reason?

   A. Inadequate sleep has implications for driving safety, work productivity, and quality of life

   B. 75% of adult population in the U.S. reports some sort of sleep disturbance

   C. Sleep apnea can be successfully treated with zolpidem

   D. Sleep apnea significantly increases the risk of diabetes and glaucoma

Lesson 2: Preventative Services

5. Which organization, created by Congress in 1984, is an independent, volunteer panel of national experts that develops screening recommendations based on evidence-based medicine?

    A. The World Health Organization

    B. American Association of Family Physicians

    C. National Screening Program

    D. The U.S. Preventive Services Task Force (USPSTF)

6. Daily exercise and staying current with routine-recommended immunizations are examples of what level of prevention?

    A. Primary prevention

    B. Secondary prevention

    C. Tertiary prevention

    D. Primordial prevention

7. A patient with type 2 diabetes who sees a podiatrist for monthly foot examinations is practicing what type of prevention?

    A. Tertiary prevention

    B. Primary prevention

    C. Secondary prevention

    D. Diabetic surveillance

8. A patient who has experienced a stroke with hemiparesis and is now participating in occupational therapy is practicing what type of prevention?

    A. Tertiary prevention

    B. Secondary prevention

    C. Primary prevention

    D. Disease mitigation

9. The CDC reports that the costliest healthcare expenditures in the U.S. are attributed to:

    A. Ebola and dengue fever

    B. Chronic, preventable diseases

    C. Tick-borne diseases, such as Lyme disease

    D. Motor vehicle accidents

10. The term *prevalence* refers to:

    A. Health conditions required through statute, ordinance, or administrative rule to be reported to a public health agency when diagnosed in an individual

    B. A group of cases of a specific disease or illness clearly in excess of what one would normally expect in a particular geographic area

    C. Illness or lack of health caused by disease, disability, or injury

    D. The proportions of people in a population who have some attribute or condition at a given point in time, or during a specified time period

Lesson 3: Screening Tests

11. Which of the following tests carries a grade A recommendation for a 67-year-old male who has smoked a pack of cigarettes every day for the last 25 years?

    A. Abdominal ultrasound

    B. Chest CT

    C. PSA

    D. Pulmonary function test

12. The ability of a test to correctly identify those with the disease (true positive rate) is known as:

    A. False positivity

    B. Incidence rate

    C. Sensitivity

    D. Specificity

13. The ability of a test to correctly identify those without the disease (true negative rate) is known as:

    A. Mortality rate

    B. Prevalence rate

    C. Sensitivity

    D. Specificity

14. According to the USPSTF, which population has the highest risk of contracting HIV and should be screened?

    A. A 25-year-old patient with a negative HIV test last year

    B. A 35-year-old patient recently diagnosed with hepatitis B contracted from IV drug use

    C. A 42-year-old patient with a 10-year history of smoking marijuana

    D. A 72-year-old patient in a monogamous sexual relationship

Lesson 4: Vaccinations/Immunizations

15. Which of the following is not a permanent contraindication to vaccination?

    A. Systemic allergic reaction to a vaccine component

    B. Encephalopathy following pertussis immunization

    C. Pregnancy in a younger female

    D. Anaphylaxis to a vaccine component

16. Which type of vaccine involves manipulation of the bacterial cell wall to make the immune response more effective in infancy?

    A. Conjugate

    B. Live

    C. Polysaccharide

    D. Toxoid

17. In which of the following scenarios might it be acceptable to postpone immunization?

    A. Low-grade fever or mild illness

    B. Moderate to severe illness

    C. Prior localized reaction

    D. All of the above

18. Which type of vaccine is always contraindicated in pregnancy?

    A. Polysaccharide

    B. Toxoid

    C. Killed

    D. Live

ANSWERS AND EXPLANATIONS

Lesson 1: Healthy People 2020

1. A

Healthy People 2020 is *not* funded by the pharmaceutical industry **(A)**. It does, however, communicate a vision for improving health and achieving health equity for the U.S. population (B), provide measurable objectives for the decade (C), and have both general and specific population initiatives (D).

2. B

LGBT health concerns include youth being at special risk, with suicide rates 2–3 times higher than the general population **(B)**. LGBT populations does experience social barriers caused by discrimination that would not be characterized as "few" (A). LGBT individuals do not primarily live in poorly serviced rural areas (C); this statement is true of all disadvantaged populations having less access to healthcare services. Finally, LGBT individuals experience higher, not lower (D), risk of violence and victimization, which has lasting effects on both the individual and community.

3. C

One objective of Healthy People 2020 is to increase services to identified minority populations **(C)**, including, but not limited to, disadvantaged populations; those with disabilities; the LGBT population; and mothers, infants, and children. The objectives include reducing health disparities, not increasing them (A); improving equal access to quality healthcare, not reducing it (B); and advancing the availability and dissemination of health-related information, not decreasing it (D).

4. A

It is true that inadequate sleep has implications for driving safely, work productivity, and quality of life **(A)**. Twenty-five percent, not 75% (B), of the adult population in the U.S. reports some sort of sleep disturbance. Sleep apnea is treated with weight loss and CPAP at night; zolpidem (C) is a short-term sleep aid for insomnia. Sleep apnea significantly increases the risk of heart attacks and stroke, not diabetes and glaucoma (D).

Lesson 2: Preventative Services

5. D

The U.S. Preventive Services Task Force (USPSTF) **(D)** is the agency that develops screening recommendations based on evidence-based medicine. The World Health Organization (A), established in 1948 in Switzerland, is an agency of the United Nations that is concerned with international public health. The American Association of Family Physicians (B), founded in 1947, is the largest medical organization in the U.S. Its goal is to promote the science and art of family medicine. The National Screening Program (C) has developed the infrastructure and clinical guidelines for comprehensive national screening programs to enable early detection of priority chronic diseases.

6. A

Daily exercise and staying current with routine immunizations is primary prevention **(A)**. Primary prevention is aimed at preventing disease before it occurs. Secondary prevention (B) is aimed at decreasing the impact of disease that has already occurred. Tertiary prevention (C) is aimed at stopping the progression of ongoing disease. Primordial prevention (D) is aimed at preventing risk factors.

7. C

A diabetic patient who sees a podiatrist for monthly foot exams is practicing secondary prevention **(C)**. Tertiary prevention (A) is aimed at stopping the progression of ongoing disease. Primary prevention (B) is aimed at preventing disease before it occurs. Diabetic surveillance (D) involves gathering data on diabetes and diabetic complications.

8. A

Occupational therapy after a stroke with hemiparesis would be considered tertiary prevention **(A)**. Tertiary prevention is aimed at stopping the progression of disease or injury. This activity is not secondary prevention (B) or primary prevention (C). Disease mitigation (D) is aimed at stopping disease-specific risk through early diagnosis and treatment.

9. B

Chronic, preventable diseases **(B)** contribute to the costliest healthcare expenditures in the U.S. Ebola and dengue fever (A), tick-borne diseases (C), and motor vehicle accidents (D) are not among the most costly healthcare expenditures.

10. D

Prevalence refers to the proportions of people in a population who have some attribute or condition at a given point in time or during a specified time period **(D)**. Health conditions required through statute, ordinance, or administrative rule to be reported to a public health agency when diagnosed in an individual (B) are called reportable communicable diseases and conditions. A group of cases of a specific disease or illness clearly in excess of what one would normally expect in a particular geographic area (C) is an epidemic. The illness or lack of health caused by disease, disability, or injury in a period of time (C) is incidence.

Lesson 3: Screening Tests

11. A

The USPSTF recommends one-time screening for abdominal aortic aneurysms with abdominal ultrasonography **(A)** in men ages 65–75 years who have ever smoked. The USPSTF recommends annual screening for lung cancer with low-dose chest CT (B) in adults aged 55–80 years who have a 30 pack-a-year smoking history and currently smoke or have quit within the past 15 years. The USPSTF recommends against PSA (C) screening. The USPSTF recommends against screening, including pulmonary function tests (D), for chronic obstructive pulmonary disease in asymptomatic adults.

12. C

The ability of a test to correctly identify those with the disease (true positive rate) is known as sensitivity **(C)**. A false positive (A) is a test result that incorrectly indicates a condition is present when it is not. Incidence rate (B) is the number of new cases per population at risk in a given time period. Specificity (D) is the extent to which a diagnostic test is specific for a particular condition, trait, etc.

13. D

The ability of the test to correctly identify those without the disease (true negative rate) is specificity **(D)**. Specificity is the extent to which a diagnostic test is specific for a particular condition, trait, etc. Mortality rate (A) is the relative frequency of deaths in a specific population (death rate). Prevalence rate (B) is the proportion of people in a population who have some attribute or condition at a given point in time or during a specified time period. Sensitivity (C) is the ability of a test to correctly identify those with the disease (true positive rate).

14. B

A 35-year-old patient recently diagnosed with hepatitis B contracted from IV drug use **(B)** should be screened for HIV. The IV drug use puts them at high risk of contracting HIV. A 25-year-old patient with a negative HIV test last year (A) only needs to be rescreened if they start participating in high-risk behaviors. A 42-year-old patient with a 10-year history of smoking marijuana (C) is at no greater risk than the general population. They should have a one-time test and risk reassessment yearly. A 72-year-old patient in a monogamous relationship (D) is not at high risk and falls out of the age range (13–64) recommendations for HIV screening.

Lesson 4: Vaccinations/Immunizations

15. C

Pregnancy **(C)** is a temporary condition, so it may be considered a *temporary* precaution or contraindication for particular vaccinations. Permanent contraindications to vaccination are systemic allergic reaction to a vaccine component (A), encephalopathy following pertussis immunization (B) (contraindicates further pertussis vaccination), and anaphylaxis to a vaccine component (D).

16. A

Conjugate **(A)** vaccines are better at producing an immune response in infancy due to manipulation of the bacterial cell wall. Live (B) vaccines are available for certain viruses, not bacteria. Polysaccharide (C) vaccines are less efficient at producing immune responses in infants. Toxoid (D) vaccines contain a bacterial toxin.

17. B

Vaccines may be postponed when the patient has a moderate to severe illness **(B)**. Immunizations may be given in the presence of low-grade fever or mild illness (A) or in the instance of prior localized reaction (C).

18. D

Live **(D)** vaccines are contraindicated in pregnancy (as well as in immunocompromised individuals). Polysaccharide (A), toxoid (B), and killed (C) vaccines are generally safe for use in pregnancy.

CHAPTER 4

Pharmacology Overview

LESSON 1: PHARMACOLOGY BASICS

Learning Objectives
- Understand pharmacology basics
- Apply knowledge regarding pharmacokinetics and pharmacodynamics to improve medication management and health outcomes

Pharmacokinetics

Pharmacokinetics is the study of how medication passes through the body (i.e., what the body does to the drug), including absorption, distribution, metabolism, bioavailability, and excretion.

Absorption

Absorption is the mechanism by which medication moves from its site of entry into the bloodstream. Drugs cross biological membranes to be absorbed, which can be accomplished by diffusion or active transport.

- **Passive diffusion:** when medication simply moves across a gradient from an area of higher concentration to an area of lesser concentration
- **Active transport:** when the drug moves against the concentration gradient, energy expenditure is required (i.e., protein transport of the molecule to cross the cell membrane)

Other issues that may affect absorption include the size of the drug molecule (larger molecules have a harder time crossing membranes), food in the gut (which may slow absorption), the presence of other medications (as medications may compete for absorption sites), and the surface area available to absorb the medication (less surface area leads to less absorption).

Distribution

Distribution occurs when medication is delivered into body tissues and extracellular spaces. A number of issues can affect distribution, including, but not limited to, molecule size, pH, lipophilicity (the ability of a molecule to dissolve in fat), and vascularity/perfusion.

Protein vs. Tissue Binding

Distribution is also affected by how easily medications are bound by plasma binding proteins. Medication that is "bound" is essentially held in "reservoir," as it is not readily available. The more of a drug that is bound, the longer the duration of action of the drug, as it will be slowly released; this increases the drug's half-life (the time it takes for a given amount of medication to be reduced by half). Fluoxetine (Prozac) is a medication with a long half-life. As such, in instances when a patient stops this medication suddenly, the patient will not suffer a discontinuation effect.

Volume of distribution entails distribution of a drug within body tissues. For a drug that is highly tissue-bound, very little drug remains in the circulation; thus, plasma concentration is low and volume of distribution is high.

Blood-Brain Barrier

The blood-brain barrier—a semi-permeable diffusion barrier—prevents uptake of most pharmaceuticals within the brain. Lipid mediated diffusion assists some small molecule drugs to cross the blood-brain barrier.

Metabolism

Metabolism is the biotransformation of a drug into a form that can be excreted by the body. The most active organ in metabolism is the liver. Metabolism rates are influenced by coexisting morbidities (i.e., liver disease), drug-drug interactions, and genetic factors.

Cytochrome P450 is the most important enzyme involved in drug metabolism. The gut is secondarily involved, and there are small levels of CYP450 activity in the lungs, placenta, and kidneys. There are over 50 CYP enzymes, but 3A4 and 2D6 are generally the most important.

Drug-drug interactions can occur in which the CYP450 enzyme can be *induced*, causing a given drug substrate to be metabolized more rapidly (causing reduced action of that medication). Alternatively, the P450 enzymes can be *inhibited*, causing increased serum levels of the drug substrate.

Some people are genetically prone to be rapid metabolizers; regular dosages may actually be sub-therapeutic for these people, since medications are so swiftly excreted from their systems. Other people are poor metabolizers; medications linger in their systems, potentially causing increased adverse effects or even toxicity. For example, about 20% of Asians poorly metabolize drugs dependent on the 2C19 enzymes. These enzymes are involved in metabolizing many common medications, such as clopidogrel (Plavix) and omeprazole (Prilosec).

Ingested foods/drinks can also affect the CYP450 enzyme system. One well-known culprit, grapefruit juice, reduces cytochrome P450 3A4 (CYP3A4) enzyme activity and causes difficulty with eliminating certain medications. These medications can remain in circulation (bioavailable), making it more likely for the patient to experience adverse effects. Grapefruit juice has been implicated in slowing metabolism of estrogens (thus causing more estrogen absorption) and increasing the absorption of buspirone (Buspar) and carbamazepine (Tegretol).

Bioavailability

Bioavailability is the degree and rate at which a drug enters systemic circulation, ultimately accessing the site of action. Most drugs go through "first pass metabolism," in which they are acted upon by the liver (and gut) enzymes before they reach systemic circulation. Whatever medication remains becomes "bioavailable."

> **Pro Tip**
> Some medications, such as insulin, would be completely inactivated during first-pass metabolism and are thus administered parenterally.
>
> Some medications are not metabolized at all, such as metformin, which is excreted unchanged by the kidneys.

Excretion

Excretion is removal of a drug from the body and primarily occurs via the kidneys. Other mechanisms of excretion include sweat, exhaled air, feces, saliva, and breast milk.

Renal dosing is an important prescribing consideration that must be considered in patients whose kidney function is not optimal. Such patients may include elderly patients, patients with kidney disease, patients dependent on one kidney or some form of dialysis, and patients taking an existing nephrotoxic medication.

Digital Resource

The American Geriatric Society's Beers Criteria® provides lists of potentially problematic medications for older adults that can be accessed online here: **https://geriatricscareonline. org/ProductAbstract/american-geriatrics-society-updated-beers-criteria-for-potentially-inappropriate-medication-use-in-older-adults/CL001.**

This information is available for free; the site requires the user to create a username and password.

Prescribing Considerations

Besides efficacy and concerns about pharmacokinetics, other considerations for medication prescription include:

- Generic vs. brand/trade medication
- Route of medication
- Therapeutic window
  - Antiarrhythmics, antineoplastics, digoxin, lithium, theophylline, and warfarin have narrow therapeutic windows
- Current medication regimen of the patient, including over-the-counter medications and alternative and complementary medications/supplements
- Patient demographics: age, gender, ethnicity
- Likelihood of patient compliance
- Patient allergies
- Drug-drug interactions

Digital Resource

Online resources provided by Drug.com and RxList.com are helpful tools in checking drug-drug interactions:

- **www.drugs.com/drug_interactions.html**
- **www.rxlist.com/drug-interaction-checker.htm**

Pro Tip

The nomogram method using body surface area (BSA) is used to determine the correct pediatric medication dosage based on body surface area:

- child's BSA m^2 × adult dose/1.73 m^2

Pharmacodynamics

Pharmacodynamics is the study of the mechanism of action of medications and their effects on the body (i.e., what a drug does to the body), including receptor binding, postreceptor effects, and chemical reactions.

Drugs show affinity for certain receptors. The drug/receptor binding reaction leads to receptor activation and cellular response, resulting in the drug's action. The magnitude of this receptor activation is related to the concentration of the activating drug (the agonist).

The dose-response curve plots the concentration of a drug against its effect. This relationship can be influenced by the patient (age, disease) and the presence of other competing drugs. Drug molecules acting on the same receptor differ in the biological response (the efficacy) and in the amount of drug required to achieve the desired effect (the potency).

- **Agonist:** a chemical that binds to a receptor and elicits an appropriate response
- **Antagonist:** chemical that binds to a receptor but elicits no response and blocks access to the receptor by an agonist

When a beta receptor in the heart is stimulated by an agonist, such as epinephrine, there is an increase in the rate/force of cardiac contractions. A beta-blocker antagonist prevents this from occurring.

Full agonists have maximum efficacy activating their matching receptors. Hydrocodone, heroin, and methadone are full opioid agonists. The antagonist naloxone (Narcan) binds to opioid receptors without activating them and may be used to reverse opioid overdose.

Chirality

Chirality refers to the shape of a drug molecule. Medications that display chirality essentially have mirror-image versions of a given molecule (called enantiomers). Though they are mirror images, the two versions of the medication can have drastically different effects.

Mismatch of drug molecules with receptor sites may result in undesirable effects such as increased toxicity and increased dose requirement.

Pro Tip

A racemic mixture (racemate) is one with equal amounts of left-handed and right-handed enantiomers. Most medications are dispensed in this manner.

Some pharmaceutical companies have sought to create single enantiomer versions of medications, citing the fact that sometimes one version has increased efficacy and binds more effectively to the desired receptors, thus allowing for less medication to be prescribed. In turn, this allows for reduced side effects. One well-known example of this is citalopram (Celexa), a racemic mix, and its "sister" medication escitalopram (Lexapro), which is single-enantiomer.

Takeaways

- Pharmacokinetics is what the body does to the drug (absorption, distribution, metabolism, bioavailability, and excretion).
- Pharmacodynamics is what the drug does to the body (receptor binding, postreceptor effects, and chemical reactions).
- It is important to know cytochrome P450's enzymatic effect on certain medications, as this factors into prescribing considerations.

LESSON 2: ANTI-INFECTIVES

Learning Objectives
- Identify the three types of anti-infectives and their target pathogens
- Identify the major types of antibiotics, anti-infectives, and antivirals by drug class
- Understand the implications of antibiotic overuse

Note: the tables below offer truncated drug profiles and do not cover all medications in each category. For complete drug information, consult a medication manual.

Anti-infective is the general term used to describe any medicine that can inhibit the spread of an infectious organism or kill the infectious organism. Anti-infective medications encompass antibiotics, antifungals, and antivirals.

The effectiveness of anti-infective medications depends on many factors, some of which are pharmacokinetics, pharmacodynamics (*see Chapter 4, Lesson 1*), drug interactions, and host defense mechanisms (immune system and underlying health of the host).

Definitions

- **Anti-mycobacterial:** targets mycobacterium, including tuberculosis and leprosy
- **Bactericidal:** kills bacteria; some bactericidal medications may not completely eradicate virulent or resistant pathogens; bactericidal antibiotics may be preferred for patients who have infections that impair host defenses locally (e.g., meningitis, endocarditis) or who are immunocompromised (e.g., neutropenic)
- **Bacteriostatic:** stops bacterial growth; some bacteriostatic medications may kill susceptible bacterial species
- **Broad spectrum:** targets many types of bacterial pathogens
- **Narrow spectrum:** targets few types of bacterial pathogens
- **Narrow therapeutic index (NTI):** defined as those drugs where small differences in a dose or blood concentration may lead to concentration-dependent and serious therapeutic failures or adverse side effects; drugs with this classification often require close monitoring and peak and trough blood levels
- **Peak and trough blood levels:** blood serum samples collected to determine the level of an antibiotic (or sometimes other medications) as it moves through the body; medications that require peak and trough testing are generally those which have a short half-life, with an NTI and high-risk adverse side-effect profiles; peak specimens represent the highest concentration in the body and are drawn 30 minutes to two hours after administration of the medication (depending on the medication and the route of administration); trough specimens represent the lowest concentration and are generally drawn 30 minutes prior to administration of the next dose of the medication
- **Synergism:** a more rapid and complete bactericidal action from a combination of antibiotics than occurs with either antibiotic alone; a common example is a cell wall–active antibiotic (e.g., a β-lactam, vancomycin) plus an aminoglycoside; this type of antibiotic combination is used for treatment of infections such as *H. pylori*

Antibiotics

Antibiotics work by blocking vital processes in the bacteria cells, killing the bacteria or stopping them from multiplying.

Selection and Use of Antibiotics

Antibiotics should be used only if clinical or laboratory evidence suggests bacterial infection due to the risk of promoting antibiotic resistant pathogens. Antibiotics kill sensitive bacteria, but may leave resistant bacteria to multiply. Antibiotic resistance is of greatest concern in children and older adults, given their high rates of antibiotic use.

At least 30% of antibiotics prescribed in the outpatient setting (for acute respiratory conditions such as colds, bronchitis, sore throats caused by viruses, and even some sinus and ear infections) are unnecessary. Unnecessary and inappropriate use (wrong selection, dose, and duration) of antibiotic use may approach 50% of all outpatient antibiotic use.

Note: certain bacterial infections (e.g., abscesses, infections with foreign bodies) require surgical intervention and do not respond to antibiotics alone.

Spectrum of Antibiotic Activity

While cultures and antibiotic sensitivity testing are essential for selecting a drug for serious infections, initial treatment must often begin before culture results are available. Empiric antibiotic selection involves selecting antibiotics based on the most likely pathogen.

For empiric treatment of serious infections that may involve any one of several pathogens (e.g., fever in neutropenic patients) or that may be due to multiple pathogens (e.g., polymicrobial anaerobic infection), a broad spectrum of activity is desirable. The most likely pathogens and their susceptibility to antibiotics vary according to geographic location (within cities or even within a hospital) and can change from month to month.

Digital Resource

The CDC has developed an Antibiotic Resistance Map program to see the latest antibiotic resistance threats in an area: **www.cdc.gov/drugresistance/index.html**.

While empiric therapy (treatment of the most likely organisms for a specific infection) has its place, it may be prudent to opt for definitive therapy: selecting an antibiotic after the organism is identified (with or without information on susceptibility and resistance). Antibiotics are generally selected based on their type (gram-positive/negative), location in the body (e.g., urinary, respiratory, spinal and brain, skin, soft tissue, and GI tract), and resistance or sensitivity (definitive treatment) based on the results of the culture and sensitivity testing.

Drugs with the narrowest spectrum of activity that can control the infection should be used. For serious infections, combinations of antibiotics are often necessary because multiple species of bacteria may be present or because combinations act synergistically against a single species of bacteria.

Like all medicines, antibiotics have the potential to cause side effects. When antibiotics are necessary, the benefits far outweigh the risks; when they are not needed, you are taking an unnecessary risk.

Antibiotic Classes

Medication	Mechanism of action and indications	Side effects/adverse reactions and prescribing considerations
Aminoglycoside Remember GNATS: G: gentamicin N: neomycin A: amikacin T: tobramycin S: streptomycin	• Bactericidal • Gram (−) bacteria • Especially useful in treating infections such as meningitis, endocarditis, tuberculosis, and plague	• GI upset, anorexia • **Black box warning:** irreversible ototoxicity due to concentration at 8th cranial nerve (observe for early signs) • Nephrotoxic (monitor kidney function) • amikacin and gentamicin commonly have peak and trough levels drawn
Penicillin 1st generation: penicillin G • Target: narrow spectrum and indicated mostly for gram (+) infections and certain gram (−) bacilli 2nd generation: ampicillin, amoxicillin • Target: wider spectrum that includes most common gram (+/−) bacterial infections 3rd generation: carbenicillin and ticarcillin and 4th generation: piperacillin • Target: broad spectrum; are effective against most gram (−) bacteria (e.g., meningococci)	• Bactericidal • 1st generation: certain gram (−) bacilli such as non-β-lactamase–producing *H. influenzae, E. coli,* and *P. mirabilis*; salmonella; and shigella • ampicillin is indicated primarily for infections typically caused by susceptible gram (−) bacteria such as meningococcal meningitis, UTIs, biliary sepsis, respiratory infections, listeria meningitis, enterococcal infection, some typhoid fever, and typhoid carriers • The addition of a β-lactamase inhibitor allows use against methicillin-sensitive staphylococci, *H. influenzae, M. catarrhalis,* bacteroides sp, *E. coli,* and *K. pneumoniae*	• Rash, anaphylaxis, CNS toxicity at high doses (especially with renal insufficiency), nephritis, *C. difficile* induced diarrhea, leukopenia, thrombocytopenia, Coombs positive hemolytic anemia • Pregnancy category B • amoxicillin has generally replaced ampicillin for PO use because it is absorbed better, has fewer GI effects, and can be given less frequently

Table 4.2.1 Antibiotics by Class

Medication	Mechanism of action and indications	Side effects/adverse reactions and prescribing considerations
Cephalosporin 1st generation: cefazolin (Kefzol), cephalexin (Keflex) • Target: gram (+) cocci bacteria with susceptibility to methicillin, including *Staphylococcus aureus* and a few gram (−) bacteria like *Proteus mirabilis* and *Klebsiella pneumoniae* 2nd generation: cefaclor (Keflor), cefonicid (Monocid) • Target: less effective against gram (+) than first generation; more effective against gram (−) like Enterobacter and Haemophilus 3rd generation: cefotaxime (Claforan), ceftriaxone (Rocephin) • Target: less effective against gram (+) than second generation; broad-spectrum against gram (−), especially GI tract infections 4th generation: cefpirome (Cefrom), cefepime (Maxipeme) • Target: most beta-lactamase producing gram (+) bacteria; broad-spectrum against gram (−) species similar to 3rd generation 5th generation: ceftobiprole • Target: methicillin resistant staphylococcus (MRSA)	• Bactericidal • Effective against gram (+/−) bacteria depending on the generation • 3rd generation antibiotics are used to treat non-enterobacter infections that tend to be resistant to many other antibiotics	• Nausea, diarrhea, rash, electrolyte imbalances (monitor BMP), pain at the injection site if the drug is administered through a vein or into a muscle • 10% of people who are allergic to penicillin are also allergic to first-generation cephalosporin (the later generations are safer for those with a penicillin allergy)
Fluoroquinolone ciprofloxacin (Cipro), levofloxacin (Levaquin) • Target: gram (−) bacteria	• Bactericidal • Prostatitis, UTIs, pneumonia, salmonella, bone and joint infections	• CNS alterations, GI upset, increased AST, photosensitivity, rash, allergic rhinitis, prolonged QT interval • Avoid using in pregnancy, lactation, and children <18 years (affects cartilage development) • **Black box warning:** Achilles tendon rupture, tendonitis, seizures, increased intracranial pressure, toxic psychosis
Tetracycline doxycycline (Vibramycin), minocycline (Minocin), and tetracycline (Achromycin) • Target: broad-spectrum antibiotics used to treat gram (+/−) pathogens • Aerobic bacteria are more susceptible to tetracyclines than anaerobic bacteria	• Bacteriostatic • Used to treat moderate to severe acne and rosacea (minocycline), UTI, URI, GI infections, and STDs (chlamydia-doxycycline); prophylaxis for *Bacillus anthracis* (anthrax) and malaria, *Yersinia pestis* (plague), typhus fever, and diseases caused by rickettsiae, such as Rocky Mountain spotted fever	• GI upset, sun sensitivity, neutropenia, esophagitis, headache, reversible tooth discoloration in adults • Pregnancy category D due to evidence of embryotoxicity and teratogenicity, including toxic effects on skeletal formation • Contraindicated in breastfeeding and children <8 years of age (stains actively growing tooth enamel) • Do not take with milk or dairy products

Table 4.2.1 Antibiotics by Class (Continued)

Medication	Mechanism of action and indications	Side effects/adverse reactions and prescribing considerations
Sulfonamide co-trimoxazole (Septrin), sulfadiazine, sulfamethoxazole (Gantanol), trimethoprim-sulfamethoxazole (Bactrim, Bactrim DS, Septra, Septra DS), trimethoprim (Trimpex, Proloprim, Primsol), sulfasalazine (Azulfidine EN-tabs, Azulfidine, Sulfazine), sulfisoxazole (Gantrisin) • Target: broad-spectrum antibiotics used to treat gram (+/−) pathogens	• Bacteriostatic • sulfonamides are mainly indicated for treatment of urinary tract and skin infections • trimethoprim/sulfamethoxazole has a broad antibacterial spectrum and many indications	• Asthma exacerbation, GI upset, hypersensitivity, hyperkalemia in the elderly population, peripheral, neuropathy, photosensitivity, proteinuria, rash • sulfisoxazole, a folate inhibitor, can cause hemolysis in patients with glucose-6-phosphate dehydrogenase activity; other drugs that produce similar effects include other sulfonamides, nitrofurantoin, furazolidone, chloramphenicol, pyrimethamine, and sulfones • nitrofurantoin also has sulfa and should be avoided in the last month of pregnancy (hyperbilirubinemia)
Macrolide azithromycin (Zithromax), clarithromycin (Biaxin), erythromycin • Target: gram (+) coverage and limited gram (−) coverage (*H. influenzae*, *B. pertussis*)	• Bactericidal or bacteriostatic depending on concentration and susceptibility • Community acquired pneumonia, chlamydia, treatment of streptococcal tonsillitis in penicillin allergic patients, COPD exacerbation, pertussis	• Diarrhea, nausea, vomiting, pruritis, headache, increased risk of arrhythmias, QT prolongation, torsades de pointes, pancreatitis • warfarin (increased risk of bleeding), HMG-CoA reductase inhibitors (increased risk of rhabdomyolysis), quinidine (risk of arrhythmia)

Table 4.2.1 Antibiotics by Class (Continued)

Miscellaneous Antibiotics

Medication	Mechanism of action and indications	Side effects/adverse reactions and prescribing considerations
Other antibacterials metronidazole (Flagyl)	• Bactericidal • Effective against anaerobic bacteria, gram (+) clostridium (*C. difficile*), and protozoa such as *Giardia*, amebiasis, trichomoniasis • Used topically for rosacea; also used for bacterial vaginosis, GI infection	• Abdominal cramps, nausea, vomiting, metallic taste, dark red-brown urine, leukopenia, hepatotoxicity, carcinogenic (in animals) • **Black box warning:** avoid unnecessary use because carcinogenic in mice • Do not take with alcohol or drink alcohol for 3 days after last dose due to potential for decreased hepatic metabolism and risk of increased acetaldehyde in the bloodstream causing SOB, arrhythmias, hypotension, nausea, and vomiting

Table 4.2.2 Other Antibiotics

Medication	Mechanism of action and indications	Side effects/adverse reactions and prescribing considerations
Other antibacterials nitrofurantoin (Macrobid) • Active against some gram (+) pathogens such as *S. aureus*, *S. epidermidis*, *S. saprophyticus*, *enterococcus faecalis*, *S. agalactiae*, group D *Streptococci*, *viridans streptococci*, and corynebacterium • Active against some gram (−) pathogens: *E. coli*, enterobacter, neisseria, salmonella, and shigella	• Bactericidal • nitrofurantoin may be used as an alternative to trimethoprim/ sulfamethoxazole for treating urinary tract infections in females and as a prophylaxis against recurrent cystitis related to coitus	• Dizziness, headache, confusion, yellow/brown urine, myalgia, anemia, peripheral neuropathy, pseudotumor cerebri • Use cautiously if renal impairment and in patients with limited renal function • Can cause hemolytic anemia of a newborn if administered close to delivery
Anti-tuberculosis isoniazid, rifampin, pyrazinamide, ethambutol	• rifampin: bactericidal • isoniazid, pyrazinamide: bactericidal or bacteriostatic • ethambutol: inhibits metabolite synthesis • Combination of these medications is first-line drug regimen • After 2–4 months of treatment, ethambutol and pyrazinamide are usually eliminated • isoniazid and rifampin therapy is continued for 6–12 months	• rifampin causes orange-colored urine, nausea, vomiting, oral contraceptive failure • isoniazid causes burning sensation in feet; pyrazinamide causes joint pain • Use alternative birth control method when using rifampin for the duration of the cycle • Adverse side effects are not serious but are the main cause of noncompliance • Drug resistance is common
Other antibacterials mupirocin (Bactroban) • Target: primarily effective against gram (+) bacteria	• Bacteriostatic at low concentrations and bactericidal at high concentrations; inhibits bacterial protein/RNA synthesis • Treats skin conditions like impetigo	• Burning, itching, hives, anaphylaxis, hypersensitivity, superinfection • Do not use on large wounds because it contains polyethylene glycol, and excessive absorption can cause kidney dysfunction • Few issues with antibiotic cross-resistance • Pregnancy category B

Table 4.2.2 Other Antibiotics (Continued)

Antibiotic Use in Pregnancy

In general, antibiotics cannot be classified as teratogens or nonteratogens without consideration of the gestational timing, dose, route, and duration of the treatment. Talking about a "safe" list is somewhat misleading, as it implies the agents on the list are indeed safe, yet very few agents have been evaluated to the extent required to provide that statement. Anecdotal information is available as is general information. Often it is a question of risk vs. benefit.

Thus, in general:

- Penicillins, cephalosporins, and erythromycin have not been found to be associated with an increased risk of birth defects
- Avoid tetracyclines (stains develop on bones and teeth and when administered IM, and have occasionally produced maternal liver failure), quinolones, aminoglycosides, macrolides (excluding erythromycin), and high-dose metronidazole (2 g stat) unless the benefits outweigh the risks

- The evidence regarding an association between the nitrofuran and sulfonamide classes of antibiotics and birth defects is mixed; however, prescribing sulfonamides or nitrofurantoin in the first trimester is still considered appropriate when no other suitable alternative antibiotics are available; trimethoprim is a folate antagonist and its use is questioned in the first trimester; however, it is also unlikely to cause problems unless poor dietary folate intake or the patient is taking another folate antagonist

Antifungal

There are two main types of antifungal medications:

1. **Fungicidal:** capable of killing fungi; bind to fungal membranes and increase permeability; nutrients leak out, and fungi die; major drugs in this class are amphotericin B, ketoconazole, miconazole, and nystatin

2. **Fungistatic:** limits the growth of active fungi but does not eradicate the microorganisms; binds to keratin in the skin and hair so fungi cannot enter the tissue and undergo further growth; griseofulvin is the major drug in this category

Medication	Indications	Side effects/adverse effects and prescribing considerations
amphotericin B, ketoconazole, miconazole, nystatin, terbinafine (Lamisil), tolnaftate (Tinactin), griseofulvin, clotrimazole, ketoconazole shampoo (Nizoral)	• Systemic fungal infections of blood, brain, lungs; amphotericin B: aspergillosis; ketoconazole: histoplasmosis; miconazole: candidiasis; nystatin: cryptococcus • Dermatophytic, local fungal infections of hair, skin, nails; terbinafine: tinea pedis, onychomycosis, tinea corporis, tinea cruris; tolnaftate: tinea corporis/pedis/cruris • Fungal infection of mucous membranes: miconazole, ketoconazole, clotrimazole, and nystatin: oropharyngeal candidiasis; vaginal candidiasis; nasal and sinus fungal infections • griseofulvin (PO) is used for dermatophytosis with nail, scalp, or large body surface involvement	• amphotericin B: hypokalemia, cardiac arrest, renal impairment or failure, hallucinations, pulmonary edema, anemia, insomnia, elevated LFTs, constipation, hematuria • ketoconazole (**Black box warning:** hepatotoxicity and QT prolongation, thrombocytopenia, hemolytic anemia, leukopenia, gynecomastia, pruritus, abdominal pain) • miconazole, terbinafine, clotrimazole and nystatin topical, vaginal and oropharyngeal preparations: burning, itching, erythema • nystatin: abdominal pain, nausea, vomiting, diarrhea • griseofulvin is contraindicated in patients with hepatic failure and should not be used during pregnancy (category X); may cause oral contraceptive failure; taken with a fatty meal yields increased absorption; do not take with alcohol (disulfiram type reaction)

Table 4.2.3 Antifungal Medications

Antiviral

Viruses are opportunistic and rely on the inability of the host cell to prevent infection (passive or active immunity) or destroy the virus. Immunocompromised patients have frequent infections. A well-functioning immune system will eliminate or effectively destroy the replication of most viruses. The currently available antiviral drugs target three main groups of viruses: influenza, herpes, and hepatitis viruses.

Mechanism of Action

Antiviral medications either interfere with DNA or RNA viral replication, or they interfere with the ability of the virus to bind to host cells.

Medication	Mechanism of action and indication	Side effects/adverse side effects and prescribing considerations
amantadine (Symmetrel), rimantadine (Flumadine)	• Non-antiretroviral • Narrow antiviral spectrum—active only against influenza A • Used prophylactically when vaccine is not available or cannot be given; therapeutic use can reduce recovery time	• Anorexia, nausea, vomiting • CNS effects: insomnia, nervousness, lightheadedness (rimantadine has fewer CNS effects)
Synthetic nucleoside analog: acyclovir (Zovirax), valacyclovir (Valtrex), famciclovir (Famvir)	• Non-antiretroviral • Used to suppress replication of HSV-1 (oral herpes), HSV-2 (genital herpes), VZV (varicella: chickenpox or shingles) • acyclovir and valacyclovir are drugs of choice for treatment of initial and recurrent episodes of these infections • Start therapy at the earliest sign of recurrent episodes of genital herpes or herpes zoster	• Jaundice, bruising, kidney injury, nausea, vomiting, diarrhea, headache, joint aches • Renal and hepatic dosing important
Synthetic nucleoside analog: ganciclovir (Cytovene)	• Non-antiretroviral • Used to treat infection with cytomegalovirus (CMV)	• Bone marrow toxicity (dose-dependent)
Neuraminidase inhibitor: oseltamivir (Tamiflu), zanamivir (Relenza)	• Non-antiretroviral • Active against influenza types A and B • Reduces duration of illness	• oseltamivir: nausea, vomiting • zanamivir: diarrhea, nausea, sinusitis • Treatment must begin within 48 hours (preferably 24 hours) of onset of symptoms
Synthetic nucleoside analog: ribavirin (Virazole—inhalation; Rebetol—oral)	• Non-antiretroviral • Inhalation form (Virazole) used for hospitalized infants with respiratory syncytial virus infections • Oral form (Rebetol) dosed on patient weight and used together with an interferon alfa product (such as Peg-Intron or Intron A) to treat chronic hepatitis C	Nausea, vomiting, diarrhea, abdominal pain, headache, dizziness, fatigue; mood changes such as irritability, anxiety, suicidal thoughts

Table 4.2.4 Antiviral Medications

Medication	Mechanism of action and indication	Side effects/adverse side effects and prescribing considerations
Hepatitis medications: Hepatitis C virus (HCV)—most common, current treatments are combination medications • ombitasvir/paritaprevir/ ritonavir (Technivie) • ombitasvir/paritaprevir/ ritonavir and dasabuvir (Viekira Pak) • daclatasvir (Daklinza)—an NS5A inhibitor, for use with sofosbuvir (Sovaldi) for chronic HCV genotype 3 infections • ledipasvir/sofosbuvir (Harvoni)	• Non-antiretroviral; HCV protease and polymerase inhibitors with or without PED IFN alfa and ribavirin have become the new standard of care for the treatment of chronic HCV infection • Protease inhibitors interfere with HCV replication by inhibiting a key viral enzyme, NS3/4A serine protease; simeprevir (Olysio) • HCV polymerase inhibitors: HCV NS5B polymerase plays an essential role in HCV replication; sofosbuvir (Sovaldi) • HCV NS5A inhibitors: NS5A is integral for HCV RNA viral replication; daclatasvir (Daklinza)	• Asthenia, fatigue, headache, cough, increased bilirubin and lipase, myalgia, irritability • **Black box warning:** test all patients for evidence of current or prior HBV before treating with HCV direct acting antivirals (DDAs); without treatment HBV in HCV/HBV, coinfected patients may be reactivated; initiate HBV treatment as indicated
Reverse transcriptase inhibitors: abacavir (Ziagen), delavirdine (Rescriptor), didanosine (Videx), lamivudine (Epivir), stavudine (Zerit), tenofovir (Viread)	• Antiretroviral; HIV is the indication for this class as HIV is a retrovirus • Block activity of the enzyme reverse transcriptase, preventing production of new viral DNA	• Numerous adverse side effects, which vary with each drug • Drug therapy may need to be modified because of adverse effects • Goal of HIV antiretroviral therapy is to find the regimen that will best control the infection (based on viral load, immune studies) with a tolerable adverse effect profile • Medication regimens change during the course of the illness based on viral load and immune studies
Protease inhibitors: amprenavir (Agenerase), indinavir (Crixivan), nelfinavir (Viracept), ritonavir (Norvir), saquinavir (Invirase)	• Antiretroviral; indicated for HIV as HIV is a retrovirus • Inhibits the protease retroviral enzyme, preventing viral replication	• Numerous adverse side effects, which vary with each drug • Drug therapy may need to be modified because of adverse effects • Goal of HIV antiretroviral therapy is to find the regimen that will best control the infection (based on viral load, immune studies) with a tolerable adverse effect profile • Medication regimens change during the course of the illness based on viral load and immune studies
Fusion inhibitor: enfuvirtide (Fuzeon)	• Antiretroviral; indicated for HIV treatment • Inhibits viral fusion, preventing viral replication • Newer class of HIV medications	• Flu-like symptoms, elevated liver enzymes, weight loss, cough, pneumonia, glomerulonephritis, hypotension, HSV infection • Medication regimens change during the course of the illness based on viral load and immune studies

Table 4.2.4 Antiviral Medications (Continued)

Education

- Do not stop medications prior to finishing full course unless serious adverse events occur
- Report disabling side effects as an alternative medication can often be used
- Many of the medications in the antibiotic classes can interfere with the effectiveness of oral contraceptives; counsel to use alternative birth control through the remainder of the cycle during which the antibiotic is given

Takeaways

- If penicillin-allergic, can use macrolides, cephalosporins, and newer quinolones (age 18 or older).
- Macrolides have more drug-drug interactions compared with the other classes of antibiotics.
- Penicillins, cephalosporins, and erythromycin have not been found to be associated with an increased risk of birth defects.
- Avoid sulfas in pregnant women in the first trimester (folate antagonist) and third trimester (hyperbilirubinemia).
- Fluoroquinolones have a lot of drug interactions and cause prolongation of QT interval.
- Use the antibiotic with the narrowest spectrum that will be effective in eradicating an organism.
- Antifungal medications come in tablet, cream, liquid, injection, spray, and shampoo; the type chosen depends on the infection.
- Most viral diseases, with the exception of those caused by HIV, are self-limited illnesses that do not require specific antiviral therapy.

LESSON 3: ANTINEOPLASTICS

Learning Objectives
- Discuss the major classes of chemotherapeutic agents
- Review common and major side effects of chemotherapeutic agents
- Identify clinical considerations for care of patients undergoing chemotherapy

Note: the table below offers truncated drug profiles and does not cover all medications in each category. For complete drug information, consult a medication manual.

Cancer treatment is a dynamic process that often involves numerous members of the healthcare team (medical oncology, surgical oncology, radiation oncology, dietary, physical/occupation therapy, etc.). The patient's treatment plan may involve PO, IM, and/or IV medications as part of systemic therapy, commonly referred to as chemotherapy. Systemic therapy recommendations vary and are influenced by factors such as cancer type/stage, tumor biology, tumor genomics, and patient dynamics (age, presence of comorbidities, etc., as well as patient preference/goals of treatment).

Antineoplastics either interfere with the process of DNA replication or directly damage DNA to the degree that the cell must go through apoptosis. Antineoplastics damage any cells that are actively going through cell division, not just cancer cells. Intestinal, skin, hair, and blood cells also replicate rapidly and can be damaged by chemotherapy, which produces many of the bothersome or even dangerous side effects patients may experience. Despite these side effects, the benefits of treatment often outweigh the risks and ultimately improve patient outcomes.

Cancer treatment is constantly evolving, with new agents moving from clinical trials to standard protocols. The following table is not a comprehensive list of all antineoplastics; rather, it is an overview of select agents.

CHAPTER 4 | **PHARMACOLOGY OVERVIEW**

Medication indication	Precautions and considerations
Alkylating agents altretamine, busulfan, carboplatin, carmustine, chlorambucil, cisplatin, cyclophosphamide, dacarbazine, lomustine, melphalan, oxaliplatin, temozolomide, thiotepa Treat many different cancers, including cancers of the lung, breast, and ovary, as well as leukemia, lymphoma, Hodgkin disease, multiple myeloma, and sarcoma	• Potential for bone marrow suppression • There is a dose-dependent increase in risk of leukemia with alkylating agents; risk of leukemia is highest 5–10 years after treatment
Antimetabolites 5-fluorouracil (5-FU), 6-mercaptopurine (6-MP), capecitabine (Xeloda), cytarabine (Ara-C), floxuridine, fludarabine, gemcitabine (Gemzar), hydroxyurea, methotrexate, pemetrexed (Alimta) Commonly used to treat leukemia and cancers (breast, ovarian, and intestinal tract)	• Antimetabolites can seriously weaken the immune system • Bone marrow suppression, causing hemorrhage, liver damage, kidney damage, neutropenia/leukopenia, and acute pancreatitis
Antitumor antibiotics • Anthracyclines: daunorubicin, doxorubicin, epirubicin, idarubicin • Antitumor antibiotics that are not anthracyclines: actinomycin-D, bleomycin, mitomycin-C, mitoxantrone (also acts as a topoisomerase II inhibitor) Widely used for a variety of cancers: breast, endometrial, ovarian, testicular, thyroid, stomach, bladder, liver, lung, soft tissues, and several childhood cancers	Anthracyclines are potentially cardiotoxic
Topoisomerase inhibitors • Topoisomerase I inhibitors: topotecan, irinotecan (CPT-11) • Topoisomerase II inhibitors: etoposide (VP-16), teniposide, mitoxantrone (also acts as an antitumor antibiotic) Used to treat certain leukemia and cancers: lung, ovarian, and gastrointestinal	Topoisomerase II inhibitors can increase the risk of acute myelogenous leukemia (AML) 2–3 years after the drug is given
Mitotic inhibitors docetaxel, estramustine, paclitaxel, vinblastine, vincristine, vinorelbine Indicated for non-small cell lung cancer (NSCLC), myelomas, lymphomas, leukemia, and cancer of the breast	Dose-dependent neuropathy can occur, limiting the amount and/or number of doses that can be administered
Differentiating agents • retinoids: skin cancer • bexarotene (Targretin): cutaneous T-cell lymphoma • arsenic trioxide (Trisenox) and tretinoin (ATRA or Atralin): acute promyelocytic leukemia	Retinoids and tretinoin have additional medical uses (acne, treating fine lines/wrinkles, skin damage related to sun exposure)

Table 4.3.1 Antineoplastic Medications

Medication indication	Precautions and considerations

Hormone (or endocrine) therapy
 	
• Antiestrogens:
  – Selective estrogen receptor downregulators: fulvestrant (Faslodex)—breast cancer
  – Aromatase inhibitors: letrozole, anastrozole, exemestane—breast cancer
  – Selective estrogen receptor modulators (SERM): tamoxifen, raloxifene (Evista), toremifene (Fareston)—breast cancer
• LNRH agonists (or analogs): leuprolide, goserelin—breast and prostate cancer
• LHRH antagonists: degarelix—prostate cancer
• Antiandrogens: flutamide, bicalutamide, nilutamide, and enzalutamide—prostate cancer
• Androgen synthesis inhibitors: ketoconazole, aminoglutethimide, and abiraterone acetate—prostate cancer
	• Vasomotor symptoms and arthralgias are common side effects
	• Risk for osteoporosis with aromatase inhibitors
	• Risk of thrombus formation with SERMs
	• Risk of endometrial cancer with tamoxifen

Immunotherapy: monoclonal antibodies There are several types of immunotherapy: monoclonal antibodies, non-specific immunotherapies, oncolytic virus therapy, T-cell therapy, and cancer vaccines • nivolumab (Opdivo): unresectable or metastatic melanoma, squamous non-small cell lung cancer (NSCLC) • pembrolizumab (Keytruda): metastatic melanoma, lung cancer • atezolizumab (Tecentriq): advanced NSCLC after chemotherapy • durvalumab (Imfinzi): bladder cancer • rituximab (Rituxan): CLL and non-Hodgkin lymphoma • ofatumumab (Arzerra): refractory CLL • trastuzumab, pertuzumab: HER2 positive breast cancer	Many immunotherapies can cause decreased immune response overall and increase the risk of infection; caution patients to avoid crowds, obviously sick individuals, and others that are immune compromised
CDK-4 Inhibitors palbociclib (Ibrance): metastatic breast cancer	• Potential for neutropenia • Given in combination with letrozole

Table 4.3.1 Antineoplastic Medications (Continued)

Treatment and Survivorship

For the nurse practitioner in the primary care setting, you can anticipate working with patients somewhere along the cancer treatment spectrum. Being knowledgeable of side effects, adverse effects, and long-term effects of systemic therapy will assist you in caring for these patients in a comprehensive manner.

- Commonly associated chemotherapy induced side effects may include nausea/vomiting, stomatitis, diarrhea, arthralgias, bone pain, peripheral neuropathy, skin/nail changes, alopecia, and/or secondary infections (i.e., fungal). There are exceptions—for example, alopecia is not common with capecitabine (Xeloda), hormone blocking therapy, or immunotherapy

- Due to these side effects, watch for dehydration, altered electrolyte balance, malnutrition, and fatigue

- Steroids are commonly used to help prevent chemo-induced nausea and vomiting and also utilized to prevent allergic reactions. Patients may experience increased appetite, fluid retention, mood changes, elevated serum glucose, immune suppression, and difficulty sleeping

- Benzodiazepines are considered first-line therapy to address nausea/vomiting. Treat the night before chemotherapy and on the day of chemotherapy; use in conjunction with other antiemetics as needed. If a patient were in recovery at the time of diagnosis, using benzodiazepines could contribute to relapse

- Hair loss can be a side effect of many chemo agents. New prevention strategies such as scalp cooling (which utilizes specialist caps worn during chemo infusions) can help mitigate this issue

- If immunocompromised: depending on the severity of leukopenia, patient may need to avoid crowds as much as possible (if in a crowd, wear a mask); encourage good handwashing, immunization of close contacts, proper nutrition and hydration, and proper oral hygiene. Clean toothbrush daily in hot water or the dishwasher; do not drink water, other fluids, or foods that have been left out more than one hour; do not eat fresh fruit, uncooked herbs, undercooked meat, and raw fish or vegetables

- If possible, encourage the patient to have a dental cleaning and inspection prior to initiating chemotherapy

- Bone metastasis is common with breast and prostate cancer. These patients may be treated with meds such as denosumab or zoledronic acid; patients taking zoledronic acid can develop osteonecrosis of the jaw (a rare but serious adverse effect)

- Other common patient complaints include weight gain, which can be significant (often related to steroid therapy), and "chemo brain" (memory and cognition problems experienced after initiation of treatment, sometimes long-lasting)

Takeaways

- Chemotherapy targets rapidly replicating cells of the cancer. Additionally, these agents have some effects on other rapidly replicating cells throughout the body, such as the GI tract, hair, and bone.

- Chemotherapy has numerous side effects: immune suppression, alopecia, stomatitis, GI complaints, fatigue, undernutrition, and weight loss.

- Chemotherapy agents are often given with other chemotherapeutic agents or other drugs to target the cancer or minimize adverse side effects.

- Patients undergoing treatment for cancer need close observation including physical assessment and lab and other diagnostic studies to monitor for disease progression and adverse side effects.

LESSON 4: CARDIOVASCULAR

Learning Objectives
- Define drug classes of the cardiovascular system and the conditions for which they are indicated
- Demonstrate understanding of the mechanism of action of cardiovascular drugs and safe prescribing habits
- Identify the cardiovascular agents requiring close surveillance

Note: the tables below offer truncated drug profiles and do not cover all medications in each category. For complete drug information, consult a medication manual.

This lesson outlines the essentials of cardiovascular pharmacology and reviews those agents typically used in the treatment of hypertension, hyperlipidemia, cardiac arrhythmias, congestive heart failure, and hypercoagulable state. Each of these therapies should be rendered as recommended by the various guidelines including JNC 8, ASCVD Risk Algorithm, and CHADS$_2$ Stroke Risk Assessment.

Diuretics

Mechanism of Action

The four major subclasses of diuretics decrease sodium reabsorption, and hence promote water excretion at different sites along the nephron.

Subclass and site of action within the nephron	Indications	Prescribing considerations	Adverse effects/side effects

Thiazide/thiazide-like act on distal convoluted tubule:
 	
• hydrochlorothiazide (HydroDIURIL)
• chlorothiazide (Diuril)
 	
Loop diuretics act on the loop of Henle:
 	
• furosemide (Lasix)
• bumetanide (Bumex)
• torsemide (Demadex)
 	
Carbonic anhydrase inhibitors act on the proximal tubule:
 	
• acetazolamide (Dazamide, Diamox)
 	
Potassium sparing act on the collecting tubule:
 	
1. Sodium channel blockers
  – triamterene (Dyrenium)
2. Aldosterone antagonists
  – spironolactone (Aldactone)
  – eplerenone (Inspra)
	• Hypertension
	• Refractory edema in CHF, cirrhosis, and renal failure
	• Reduction of stone formation in idiopathic hypercalciuria
	• Decreased urine volume in nephrogenic diabetes insipidus
	• Meniere's disease
		Contraindications:
		
		• Hypersensitivity to sulfonamides
		• eGFR <30 mL/minute;
		• Volume depleted patients
		• Electrolyte imbalances: hyponatremia, hypokalemia, hyperkalemia
		
		Precautions:
		
		• Monitoring of serum electrolytes recommended
		• May trigger episodes of gout
		• May induce hypercalcemia (especially in hyperparathyroidism)
		• May increase LDL levels
		• May induce hyperglycemia
		• May worsen SLE
			Orthostatic hypotension, dizziness, drowsiness, syncope, weakness, nausea, GI irritation, ototoxicity
			
			spironolactone may cause gynecomastia, breast pain, decreased libido, hirsutism, menstrual irregularities

Table 4.4.1 Diuretic Subclasses

Education

- Emphasize the importance of dietary sodium restriction to maximize diuretic effectiveness
- Review signs and symptoms of hypovolemia including weakness, dizziness, and orthostatic hypotension, which would warrant a dose adjustment
- Review signs and symptoms of hypokalemia (loop diuretics or thiazides) and hyperkalemia (potassium-sparing diuretics) including weakness, muscle cramping, cardiac palpitations, and dizziness, which should be reported promptly
- Warn patient urinary volume is expected to increase. Counsel patient to avoid taking their diuretics late in the day or at bedtime to minimize sleep disturbances
- May need to monitor daily weight; rapid water weight loss (>1–2 lb/day) could be harmful

Calcium Channel Blockers

Mechanism of Action

Calcium channel blocker (CCB) activity is aimed at modifying the electrophysiologic properties of cardiac and smooth muscle cells by blocking inward movement of calcium through the cell membrane. The drugs differ in the type of tissue cells upon which they act.

Subclass	Cardiac contraction	Cardiac conduction (SA and AV nodes)	Vascular smooth muscle
Dihydropyridines	Small decrease	Little or no effect	Strong effect
Phenylalkylamines	Large decrease	Large effect	Moderate effect
Benzothiazepines	Moderate decrease	Large effect	Moderate effect

Table 4.4.2 Effects of Calcium Channel Blockers

Subclass	Indications	Prescribing considerations	Side effects/adverse effects
Dihydropyridines • nifedipine (Procardia) • nifedipine ER (Procardia XL) • amlodipine (Norvasc) • felodipine (Plendil) • nicardipine (Cardene) • nicardipine (Cardene SR) **Phenylalkylamines** • verapamil hydrochloride (Calan) • verapamil SR (Isoptin SR) **Benzothiazepines** • diltiazem SR (Cardizem) • diltiazem ER (Tiazac) • diltiazem CD (Cartia XT)	• Hypertension • Vasospastic angina • Arrhythmias	Contraindications: • Hypotension (SBP <90) • Sick sinus syndrome • Second-degree AV block • Third-degree AV block • Wolff-Parkinson-White syndrome Precautions: • May worsen or precipitate CHF due to negative inotropic effect • Hypotension may occur with initial dosing or when combined with a beta-blocker • May cause first-degree AV block or bradycardia • May cause liver enzyme elevation	Rash-including erythema multiforme and Stevens-Johnson syndrome, dyspnea, hypotension, bradycardia, pedal edema, headache, nausea, diarrhea, constipation, impotence

Table 4.4.3 Calcium Channel Blocker Subclasses

Education

- Counsel patients that they may experience hypotensive effects during dose titration
- Emphasize the importance of reporting side effects, including signs of CHF (e.g., swelling of feet, shortness of breath), irregular heartbeat, nausea, constipation, dizziness, and hypotension
- Advise to avoid grapefruit juice, which can cause an increase in the amount of CCB in the body

Beta-Blockers

Mechanism of Action

Beta receptors exist in the heart, lung, and peripheral vascular tissue. Beta-1 receptors are found mainly in the heart, whereas beta-2 receptors are found both in the lungs and peripheral vascular smooth muscle. Alpha receptors exist within vascular smooth muscle tissue. All beta and alpha blockers work similarly: they act as a competitive blockade of the beta- (and alpha-) adrenergic receptors. Inhibition causes a decrease in heart rate, myocardial contractility, blood pressure, and myocardial oxygen demand. Beta-blockers also impede the vasodilating and bronchodilating actions of catecholamines and suppress renin release.

Subclass	Indications	Prescribing considerations	Side effects/adverse effects
Nonselective • propranolol (Inderal) • nadolol (Corgard) • penbutolol (Levatol) • timolol (Betimol) **Beta 1-selective** • atenolol (Tenormin) • metoprolol (Lopressor) • bisoprolol (Zebeta) • nebivolol (Bystolic) **Alpha-beta-blocker** • labetalol (Trandate) • carvedilol (Coreg)	• Hypertension • Angina, long-term management: atenolol, metoprolol, nadolol, propranolol • CHF: metoprolol, carvedilol, bisoprolol • Prophylaxis of migraine: propranolol, timolol • MI prophylaxis, acute MI: atenolol, metoprolol, carvedilol	Contraindications: • Uncompensated heart failure • Bradycardia • Heart block (second- or third-degree) • Pulmonary edema • Severe asthma or COPD Precautions: • May suppress signs and symptoms of hypoglycemia • May mask clinical signs of hyperthyroidism • May increase triglycerides and total cholesterol and LDL levels while decreasing HDL levels • May exacerbate variant angina • May worsen muscle weakness	Bradycardia, depression, impotence, diarrhea, dizziness, drowsiness, fatigue, muscle weakness, nausea, vomiting, insomnia

Table 4.4.4 Beta-Blocker Subclasses

Receptor	Location	Stimulation effects
Beta-1	Cardiac	Increased heart rate and force of cardiac contractility
	Kidney	Increased renin secretion
Beta-2	Bronchial, vascular, coronary arteriole, uterine smooth muscle, skeletal muscle	Vasodilation
	Pancreas	Decreased insulin secretion
	Liver	Increased gluconeogenesis
Alpha-1	Vascular smooth muscle	Vasoconstriction
	Stomach, intestine	Decreased motility and tone
	Kidney	Increased renin secretion
	Liver	Increased gluconeogenesis
Alpha-2	Vascular smooth muscle	Vasodilation

Table 4.4.5 Alpha- and Beta-Adrenergic Receptor Sites

Education

- Counsel patients to report symptoms of shortness of breath, nocturnal cough, and lower extremity edema
- Medication should not be discontinued abruptly
- Be sure to advise patients to inform all healthcare providers of beta-blocker use, including ophthalmologists and dentists
- Teach patients how to check their pulse and to call the office if their heart rate falls below 50 beats per minute or if dizziness, near syncope, or orthostatic hypotensive symptoms emerge
- Counsel diabetic patients about the dangers of beta-blockers masking symptoms of hypoglycemia
- Caution patient that exercise-induced fatigue may develop
- Alpha-blockers need to be taken at bedtime

Ace Inhibitors and Angiotensin Receptor Blockers

Mechanism of Action

ACEIs block the production of the angiotensin converting enzyme. This enzyme triggers the conversion of angiotensin I to angiotensin II. Angiotensin II induces vasoconstriction and stimulates aldosterone production by the adrenal glands. By reducing aldosterone secretion, water absorption lessens, and its effects in the distal renal tubule cause a slight increase in serum potassium levels.

ARBs also diminish the effects of angiotensin II, but achieve this by blocking angiotensin II receptors. Since they act as receptor blockers, ARBs have no effect on bradykinin breakdown and levels, eliminating exposure to the cough trigger.

Subclass	Indications	Prescribing considerations	Side effects/adverse effects
ACEIs • lisinopril (Prinivil, Zestril) • benazepril (Lotensin) • enalapril (Vasotec) • quinapril (Accupril) • ramipril (Altace) **ARBs** • losartan (Cozaar) • candesartan (Atacand) • irbesartan (Avapro) • olmesartan (Benicar) • telmisartan (Micardis) • valsartan (Diovan) *recalled in 2018 due to safety concerns	• Hypertension • Heart failure • Acute myocardial infarction • Diabetic nephropathy • Left ventricular dysfunction	Contraindications: • Hereditary or idiopathic angioedema • Bilateral renal artery stenosis • Pregnancy Precautions: • May induce neutropenia and agranulocytosis; monitor WBCs • Anaphylactic reaction includes angioedema, which is a swelling of the face, extremities, lips, mucous membranes, tongue, glottis, or larynx • May induce proteinuria or nephrotic syndrome; monitor urinary microalbumin levels • May induce hyperkalemia or increased serum creatinine, especially in patients with chronic kidney disease; monitor electrolyte and creatinine levels	Dry cough, orthostatic hypotension, leukopenia, headache, myalgia, renal insufficiency, hyperkalemia, impotence

Table 4.4.6 ACEI and ARB Subclasses

Education

- Counsel patient to seek emergency care if any of the following should occur: swelling of the face, mouth, hands, tongue; difficulty breathing or swallowing; sudden onset of abdominal pain, diarrhea, and/or vomiting
- Counsel patient on signs and symptoms of excess potassium including irregular heartbeat, leg weakness, numbness/tingling of hands or feet, and/or unexplained nervousness
- Report a dry, hacking cough on an ACEI, so the ACEI can be discontinued and another class of meds started

Antiarrhythmic Agents

Mechanism of Action

Class I antiarrhythmic drugs (quinidine, procainamide) slow cardiac conduction by extending the refractory period of atrial and ventricular myocardium cells.

Class II antiarrhythmic drugs (beta-blockers) block sympathetic activity on the heart, which reduces the sinus node rate and increases the refractory period of the AV node.

Class III antiarrhythmic drugs (amiodarone) block sodium channels, which slows conduction and increases the refractory period of the AV node. It also possesses vasodilatory action to decrease myocardial oxygen needs.

Class IV antiarrhythmic drugs (nondihydropyridine CCBs) act by inhibiting calcium ion influx, which results in slowing AV conduction and prolonging the refractory period of the AV node.

Digoxin works by slowing AV node conduction and extending the AV node refractory, and achieves this via vagal stimulation. Furthermore, its enhanced excitation-contraction coupling trait heightens an inotropic effect on the cardiac cell, resulting in an increased force of myocardial contraction.

Subclass	Indications	Prescribing considerations	Side effects/adverse effects
Class IA • quinidine (Quinidex) • procainamide (Procan) **Class IB** • lidocaine (Xylocaine) • tocainide (Tonocard) **Class IC** • flecainide (Tambocor) • propafenone (Rythmol) **Class II** (beta-blockers) • propranolol (Inderal) • metoprolol (Lopressor, Toprol XL) **Class III** • amiodarone (Cordarone) **Class IV** (CCBs) • verapamil (Calan) • diltiazem (Cardizem) **Other** • digoxin (Lanoxin) • adenosine (Adenocard)	• Atrial fibrillation • Paroxysmal supraventricular tachycardia • Premature ventricular contractions • Heart failure	Contraindications: • Severe sinus node dysfunction • Marked sinus bradycarda • Second- and third-degree AV block Precautions: • quinidine, amiodarone, and digoxin all require regular monitoring to ensure plasma levels are therapeutic and minimize risk for toxicities development • amiodarone can alter thyroid, lung, and optic functions, as well as raise liver enzymes • digoxin toxicity increases risk for ventricular tachycardia and ventricular fibrillation arrhythmias	Bronchospasms, respiratory distress, bradycardia, fatigue, dizziness, headache, blood dyscrasias, ventricular arrhythmias, rash, photosensitivity

Table 4.4.7 Antiarrhythmic Subclasses

Education

- Recommend patients carry medical alert card, bracelet, etc., to identify themselves as taking an antiarrhythmic drug
- Encourage patients to report any uncomfortable or new symptoms to their healthcare provider such as cough (amiodarone toxicity) or decreased appetite, nausea, vomiting, diarrhea, and visual changes such as yellow halos around lights (digoxin toxicity)
- Avoid grapefruit juice with amiodarone and CCBs
- Remind and emphasize to patients the need for regular visits and blood testing to monitor for toxic effects

Antihyperlipidemic Agents

Mechanism of Action

HMG-CoA reductase inhibitors (statins) inhibit the HMG-CoA reductase enzyme, which is the catalyst for cholesterol production in the liver, specifically LDL synthesis.

Bile acid sequestrants bind to bile acids and transform into an insoluble complex. These complexes result in increased fecal excretion of bile acids. Reduction in bile acid levels result in two compensatory changes: increased removal of LDL from plasma and decreased intracellular stores of cholesterol.

Niacin acts on lipase, which inhibits the release of fatty acids from adipose tissue. Decreased fatty acid activity results in decreased synthesis of VLDL and LDL by the liver. It is believed niacin's ability to promote HDL levels is due to its reduction of lipid transfer from HDL to VLDL and delayed HDL clearance within the liver.

Ezetimibe acts on intestinal epithelial cells to inhibit cholesterol from both dietary and biliary sources.

Subclass	Indications	Prescribing considerations	Side effects/adverse effects
HMG-CoA reductase inhibitors • atorvastatin (Lipitor) • fluvastatin (Lescol) • pravastatin (Pravachol) • rosuvastatin (Crestor) • simvastatin (Zocor) **Fibric acid derivatives** • gemfibrozil (Lopid) • fenofibrate (Tricor) **Bile acid sequestrants** • cholestyramine (Questran) • colestipol (Colestid) • colesevelam (Welchol) **Other agents** • nicotinic acid, niacin (Niaspan) • ezetimibe (Zetia)	• Hyperlipidemia • Hypertriglyceridemia	Contraindications: • Acute liver disease • Pregnancy and lactation • Severe renal dysfunction Precautions: • Incidence of rhabdomyolysis is rare, but symptoms of muscle pain, tenderness, or weakness should be reported by patient immediately • Patients may be at increased risk of rhabdomyolysis when gemfibrozil is administered concomitantly with HMG-CoA reductase inhibitor	Fatigue, rash, nausea, vomiting, diarrhea, dyspepsia, myalgia, arthralgia, headache, increased LFTs

Table 4.4.8 Antihyperlipidemic Subclasses

Education

- HMG-CoA reductase inhibitors: patients should promptly report muscle pain, tenderness, and weakness to prescriber; may also cause photosensitivity. Avoid grapefruit juice, which can cause increased drug levels
- Bile acid sequestrants: can interfere with absorption of other drugs, so other medications should be taken 1 hour prior or 3–4 hours after bile acid sequestrant administration
- Nicotinic acid (Niacin): often causes facial and upper extremity flushing; taking med with hot fluids may worsen flushing; taking aspirin (81–325 mg) 30 minutes prior to niacin may help reduce flushing episodes

Agents That Act on Blood

Mechanism of Action

Heparin prevents and slows the formation of new thrombi. It achieves this by binding with antithrombin III (AT-III) at two specific sites. The first AT-III binding site alters factor X ability to affect the clotting cascade. The second AT-III binding site inhibits conversion of prothrombin to thrombin, which results in reduced fibrin availability and reduced fibrinogen production.

Low molecular weight heparin (LMWH) differentiates itself from unfractionated heparin (UFH) by inhibiting thrombin generation higher in the clotting cascade. LMWH has a more predictable anticoagulant effect and has a great affinity for anti-factor Xa rather than anti-factor IIa.

Warfarin inhibits the synthesis of coagulation factors VII, IX, X, and II (prothrombin) by the liver. It achieves this through antagonistic activity on vitamin-K binding sites within the liver. Warfarin also reduces the synthesis of anticoagulant proteins C and S. It is important to remember oral anticoagulants do not affect existing clotting factors; rather, they prevent extension of an existing thrombus and new thrombi formation. For this reason, its efficacy can take several days to achieve and should be monitored closely.

Direct thrombin inhibitors (DTIs), like Pradaxa, are oral anticoagulants that block thrombin activity to prevent clot formation. Their greatest attribute is that, unlike warfarin, DTIs do not require regular INR monitoring.

Aspirin, a platelet aggregation inhibitor, prevents the synthesis of thromboxane A_2 and prostacyclin, which are key components of platelet aggregation and vasoconstriction. Dipyridamole, another type of platelet aggregation inhibitor, induces vasodilation and reduces levels of cAMP that are associated with platelet adhesiveness.

ADP induced platelet-fibrinogen binding inhibitors such as clopidogrel (Plavix) block the binding of ADP to its platelet receptor, which in turn prevents activation of the GPIIb/IIIa complex necessary for clot formation.

Platelet glycoprotein IIb/IIIa inhibitors (GPIIb/IIIa) like abciximab (ReoPro) block the GPIIb/IIIa binding site to inhibit platelet aggregation. Whereas anagrelide (Agrylin), a phosphodiesterase 3 (PDE3) inhibitor, induces both thrombocytopenic effects as well as prevention of platelet aggregation.

Thrombolytic agents are aimed at the conversion of plasminogen to plasmin. The plasmin enzyme breaks down fibrin as well as fibrinogen, resulting in dissolution of the blood clot.

Subclass	Indications	Prescribing considerations	Side effects/adverse effects

Heparin
• heparin sodium
 	
Low molecular weight heparin (LMWH)
• enoxaparin (Lovenox)
 	
Oral anticoagulants
• Classic—warfarin (Coumadin)
• Direct thrombin inhibitor (DTI)
  – dabigatran (Pradaxa)
  – rivaroxaban (Xarelto)
 	
Platelet aggregation inhibitors
• Traditional
  – acetylsalicylic acid (aspirin)
  – dipyridamole (Persantine), aspirin/ dipyridamole ER (Aggrenox)
• ADP induced platelet-fibrinogen binding inhibitors
  – clopidogrel (Plavix)
  – ticlopidine (Ticlid)
• Platelet glycoprotein IIb/IIIa inhibitors (GPIIb/IIIa)
  – abciximab (ReoPro)
  – tirofiban (Aggrastat)
• Platelet aggregation inhibitors— phosphodiesterase 3 (PDE3) inhibitors
  – anagrelide (Agrylin)
  – cilostazol (Pletal)
 	
Thrombolytic agents
• alteplase-tPA (Activase)
• reteplase (Retavase)
• streptokinase (Streptase)
	• Prevention or treatment of venous thromboembolism (VTE) including deep vein thrombosis and pulmonary emboli
	• Prevention of arterial ischemic events including cerebrovascular attack (CVA), acute myocardial infarction (MI), and intermittent atrial fibrillation
	• Prevention and treatment of peripheral arterial thrombosis
		Contraindications:
		• Uncontrolled active bleeding
		• Pregnancy (heparin, enoxaparin can be used in pregnancy)
		• Hemorrhagic blood dyscrasias
		
		Precautions:
		• All patients should be monitored closely for uncontrolled bleeding
		• There are an extensive number of drug-to-drug, drug-to-food, and drug-to-disease interactions that may occur; close INR monitoring may be required
		• May cause increase in liver enzymes and impair hepatic function
			Localized injection site irritation, hemorrhage, easy bruising, headache, dyspepsia, epistaxis, abdominal pain, diarrhea

Table 4.4.9 Agents That Act on Blood Subclasses

Education

- Counsel patients on the gravity of any signs or symptoms of bleeding—when to call 911 vs. contacting primary care provider
- Assess patient's fall risk; review with safety measures and fall prevention strategies
- Highlight the vast number of drugs, foods, and supplements that can interact with efficacy of anticoagulant therapy. Emphasize the importance of lab monitoring as appropriate

Takeaways

- Know important teaching points for each class.
- Orthostatic hypotension is a concern with diuretics and antihypertensive medications, especially if a patient is being treated with meds from both classes.
- Beta-blockers lower the heart rate and blood pressure, can mask signs of hypoglycemia, and induce bronchospasm.
- Angioedema can occur with ARBs and ACEIs.
- Dry cough can occur with ACEIs; the patient needs to be treated with a different class of antihypertensive.
- Grapefruit juice is problematic with statins, amiodarone, and CCBs.
- Warfarin is contraindicated in pregnancy.

LESSON 5: RESPIRATORY

Learning Objectives

- Understand medications commonly used to treat disorders of the respiratory system
- Develop a patient education plan specific to respiratory medications

Note: the tables below offer truncated drug profiles and do not cover all medications in each category. For complete drug information, consult a medication manual.

Medications used to treat the respiratory system are aimed at treating and minimizing symptoms, preventing complications, and decreasing the progression or rate of progression of diseases of the respiratory tract (e.g., asthma, COPD). This lesson covers medications used to treat conditions of the lower respiratory tract. Often lower respiratory tract symptoms are exacerbated by upper respiratory disorders (i.e., allergic rhinitis). The upper respiratory disorder must be treated appropriately to get optimal treatment of the lower respiratory tract disorder. *See Chapter 4, Lesson 12, regarding antihistamines and nasal corticosteroids.*

Definitions

- **Metered dose inhaler (MDI):** distributes medication in a liquid form with each inhalation
- **Hydrofluoroalkane (HFA):** propellant used in MDI to propel the medication out of the canister
- **Dry powder inhaler (DPI):** distributes medication in a powder form; medication is either kept in a reservoir or a capsule/tablet is loaded into the inhaler for each dose

Bronchodilators (Beta 2-Agonists) and Antimuscarinics

Mechanism of Action

Beta-2 agonists cause relaxation of smooth muscle via stimulation of the $beta_2$-adrenergic receptors, which antagonize bronchoconstriction activity. There are two types: short-acting (SABA) and long-acting (LABA).

Antimuscarinic (anticholinergic) agents block the bronchoconstrictor effects of acetylcholine on M3 muscarinic receptor of airway smooth muscle. There are two types of antimuscarinic agents: short-acting (SAMA) and long-acting (LAMA).

Examples	Indications	Prescribing considerations	Side effects/adverse effects

Beta-2 agonist
 	
• SABA
  – albuterol (Proair, Proventil, Ventolin)
  – levalbuterol (Xopenex)
• LABA
  – salmeterol (Serevent Diskus)
  – indacaterol (Arcapta)
  – olodaterol (Striverdi)
  – arformoterol (Brovana)
	Asthma, COPD, relief of airway constriction, and shortness of breath caused by airway constriction	• Caution if HTN, arrhythmias, hypokalemia, ischemic heart disease, diabetes
		• The SABA can be given in an inhaler and/or a nebulized form
		• LABA **Black box warning:** increase risk of asthma-related deaths in patients not on long-term asthma control
		• Pediatric patients should use a spacer with all inhalers to ensure adequate inhalation of medication
			• Side effects: nervousness, palpitations, headache, cough, dizziness, bad taste, tremor
			• Adverse effects: tachycardia, paradoxical bronchospasm, cardiac arrhythmia, hypokalemia

Antimuscarinic (anticholinergic)
 	
• SAMA
  – ipratropium bromide (Atrovent)
• LAMA
  – tiotropium (Spiriva)
  – aclidinium bromide (Tudorza Pressair)
  – glycopyrrolate (Seebri Neohaler)
  – umeclidinium (Incruse Ellipta)
	Asthma, COPD, relief of airway constriction, and shortness of breath caused by airway constriction	• Caution if angle closure glaucoma, enlarged prostate, or obstruction of the bladder neck
		• SAMA can be prescribed in inhaler or nebulized form
			• Side effects: dry eyes, dry mouth, urinary retention, constipation, worsening glaucoma, nervousness, dyspepsia, cough
			• Adverse effects: angle closure glaucoma, paradoxical bronchospasm

Table 4.5.1 Bronchodilators

Education

- Teach the importance of keeping a short-acting beta agonist available at all times for relief of acute symptoms
- Patients should report frequent or scheduled use of SABA or SAMA, as this is not recommended; frequent or scheduled use indicates the underlying disorder is not adequately controlled

Anti-Inflammatory Agents

Inhaled Corticosteroids (ICS)

Most studies have found regular use of ICS alone does not alter the long-term decline of FEV_1, nor mortality among patients with COPD. COPD patients with moderate to very severe symptoms and/or frequent exacerbations benefit more from combination ICS and LABA therapy than from either component alone.

Mechanism of Action

Reduce inflammation in the airways by inhibiting inflammatory cytokines. They have glucocorticoid and mineralocorticoid effects. The potency of the inhaled corticosteroid is directly related to the dosage given.

Phosphodiesterase-4 (PDE4) Inhibitor

Mechanism of Action

Reduce inflammation by increasing intracellular cyclic AMP levels through inhibition of PDE4.

Oral Glucocorticoids

- *See Chapter 4, Lesson 10,* for mechanism of action, prescribing considerations, side effects/adverse effects for corticosteriods
- Appropriate for the treatment of acute exacerbations, but have no role in chronic daily management of COPD or asthma

Mast Cell Stabilizers

Mechanism of Action

Decreases inflammation by inhibiting the degranulation of mast cells, preventing the release of histamine. Not frequently used because of limited efficacy.

Examples	Indications	Prescribing considerations	Side effects/adverse effects
ICS • beclomethasone dipropionate (Qvar) • budesonide (Pulmicort) • ciclesonide (Alvesco) • fluticasone propionate (Flovent, ArmonAir) • mometasone (Asmanex)	Asthma, COPD	• Caution if acute asthma or bronchospasm, TB infection, glaucoma, osteoporosis, measles, or varicella exposure • Caution if hypersensitivity to milk protein (DPI form) • fluticasone propionate and budesonide only inhaled steroid indicated for <5 years old; all others are indicated for ≥5 • budesonide is the only ICS that comes in nebulizer form	• Side effects: hoarse voice, skin bruising, headache, pharyngitis, sinusitis, rhinitis, cough • Adverse effects: oral candidiasis, pneumonia, adrenal suppression, growth suppression, osteoporosis
PDE4 inhibitor roflumilast (Daliresp)	COPD (severe to very severe) with history of frequent exacerbations; especially for chronic bronchitis	• Oral medication • Caution if history of depression, suicidal ideation, or acute bronchospasm	• Side effects: diarrhea, nausea, reduced appetite, weight loss, abdominal pain, sleep disturbances, headache • Adverse effects: pancreatitis, suicidal ideation, renal failure
Mast cell stabilizers cromolyn sodium (Intal)	Asthma	Not to be used for acute attacks	• Side effects: bad taste, cough, post nasal drip, headache • Adverse effects: bronchospasm

Table 4.5.2 Inhaled Corticosteroids

Education

• ICS should be used daily as prescribed and should not be used to relieve acute symptoms
• Should be used with spacers to prevent deposition of medication in oropharynx
• Patients should rinse out their mouth after using ICS to prevent oral candidiasis
• Cromolyn sodium is not for acute symptoms, and maximum efficacy can take 2–4 weeks

Combination Inhalers

Various combination inhalers are used to treat COPD and asthma. The combination can include an ICS + LABA or SABA + SAMA. Prescribing considerations, side effects/adverse effects, and patient education coincides with the ingredients in each inhaler. See the above tables for this information.

ICS + LABA	SABA + SAMA
• fluticasone + salmeterol (Advair Diskus, Advair HFA) • mometasone + formoterol (Dulera HFA) • budesonide + formoterol (Symbicort HFA)	albuterol + ipratropium (Combivent Respimat, Duoneb)

Table 4.5.3 Combination Inhalers

Methylxanthines

Mechanism of Action

Increases cyclic AMP and antagonizes adenosine receptors. Causes bronchodilator and anti-inflammatory effect although exact mechanism unknown.

Examples	Indications	Prescribing considerations	Side effects/adverse effects
theophylline (SlowBid, Theo-Dur)	Asthma	• Narrow therapeutic window (monitor drug levels) • Metabolized by cytochrome P450, so high drug interaction profile as well as decreased drug clearance with age • Multiple food interactions • Not frequently prescribed because of risk of toxicity	• Side effects: insomnia, heartburn, nausea, headache, irritability, tremor • Adverse effects: cardiac arrhythmia, grand mal seizures, hypotension

Table 4.5.4 Methylxanthines

Education

- Educate regarding signs of toxicity and need to avoid foods and medications that may cause interactions
- Keep regular follow-up appointments to check drug levels

Leukotriene Receptor Antagonist (LTRA)

Mechanism of Action

Decrease inflammation and mucus production and cause bronchodilation by selectively binding leukotriene receptors.

Examples	Indications	Prescribing considerations	Side effects/adverse effects
• montelukast (Singulair) • zafirlukast (Accolate) • zileuton (Zyflo CR)	Asthma, allergic rhinitis (montelukast only)	• Caution with zileuton if elevated liver enzymes, hepatic disease, or alcohol abuse • montelukast and zafirlukast have an indication for children	• Side effects: headache, cough, nausea, sleep disorders, restlessness • Adverse effects: thrombocytopenia, depression, suicidal ideation, hallucinations

Table 4.5.5 LTRAs

Education

- Zafirlukast should be taken on an empty stomach

Anti-IgE Therapy

Mechanism of Action

Inhibits binding of IgE to receptors on mast cells and basophils, causing decreased release of mediators in allergic response.

Examples	Indications	Prescribing considerations	Side effects/adverse effects
omalizumab (Xolair)	Asthma (uncontrolled with other therapies)	• Anaphylaxis can occur at any time with this medication • Caution if anaphylaxis history, acute symptoms	• Side effects: injection site pain, headache, nausea, fatigue, dizziness, pruritus, myalgia, arthralgia • Adverse effects: anaphylaxis, malignancy, vascular event

Table 4.5.6 Anti-IgE Therapy

Education

- Educate regarding signs and symptoms of anaphylaxis and when to seek emergency care

Takeaways

- Although similar drug therapy is used for both asthma and COPD, the introduction of medications varies: in asthma, the lowest dose of ICS to maintain control should be prescribed and treatment stepped down once control has been achieved; in COPD, ICS should be an "add-on" therapy for people with COPD who have two exacerbations of COPD in one year, and high-dose usage is recommended.

- Patients should leave the clinic with a good understanding of what side effects may occur, the seriousness of those side effects, and what to do if a given side effect occurs.

- Non-pharmacological interventions remain essential components of a COPD treatment strategy.

LESSON 6: ENDOCRINE

Learning Objectives

■ Demonstrate knowledge of medications associated with treatment of Addison disease, diabetes mellitus, and thyroid supplementation and suppression

■ Identify the drug subclasses of diabetes mellitus medication and their associated mechanisms of action

■ Identify safe prescribing practices associated with endocrine medications

Note: the tables below offer truncated drug profiles and do not cover all medications in each category. For complete drug information, consult a medication manual.

Medications for Addison's Disease

Mechanism of Action

The drugs required to effectively treat Addison disease depend on the hormones that are no longer being produced by the adrenal glands. Corticosteroids, in physiologic doses, are administered to replace deficient endogenous hormones. Corticosteroids have a role in reducing inflammation, maintaining blood glucose levels, and managing stress (*see Chapter 4, Lesson 10, for more information on corticosteroids*). Mineralocorticoids with high glucocorticoid activity promote reabsorption of sodium and excretion of potassium from renal distal tubules.

Medication	Indication	Prescription considerations	Side effects/adverse effects
Glucocorticoid hormones • hydrocortisone • prednisone • cortisone acetate	Daily cortisol replacement (hydrocortisone is also useful in acute adrenal crisis)	• Avoid concomitant use with immune modulators • Numerous drugs increase or decrease drug levels/effects	• Side effects: depression, euphoria, mood swings, hyperglycemia, acne, headache, abdominal distention, thinning skin; stimulates appetite • Adverse effects: arrhythmia, pulmonary edema, suppression of hypothalamic-pituitary axis, reduction of growth velocity, osteoporosis, psychiatric disturbances, venous thrombosis
Mineralocorticoid hormones • fludrocortisone	Aldosterone replacement	• Provide additional dosing during times of stress • Avoid use in pregnant and nursing women if possible • Numerous drug interactions	• Side effects: hypertension, edema, muscle weakness, impaired wound healing • Adverse effects: hypokalemia, heart enlargement, CHF, peptic ulcer

Table 4.6.1 Hormone Replacement in Addison Disease

Education

- Dosages are adjusted during pregnancy, times of stress, illness, or surgery
- These medications may mask signs of infection or increase risk of developing a serious illness
- Do not abruptly stop taking the medication

Thyroid Medications

Thyroid Supplements

Mechanism of Action

Thyroid supplements replace low levels of endogenous T_3 and T_4. They are also used to suppress levels of thyroid stimulating hormone (TSH) and thyroid-releasing hormone (TRH).

Thyroid Suppressants

Mechanism of Action

Thyroid suppressants inhibit iodine absorption, resulting in reduced thyroid hormone synthesis. These agents do not inhibit stored or circulating levels of T_3 and T_4, nor do they affect oral and parenteral supplements. Propylthiouracil (PTU) also blocks peripheral tissues from converting T_4 into T_3.

Examples	Indications	Prescription considerations	Side effects/ adverse effects
Thyroid supplements • levothyroxine sodium (Synthroid, Levoxyl) • liothyronine (Cytomel) • lotrix (Thyrolar, Euthyroid)	• Hypothyroidism • Pituitary TSH suppression • Treatment or prevention of euthyroid goiters • Management of thyroid cancer	• Start with a low dose, monitor closely, and advance dose slowly in frail elderly and patients with cardiovascular disease • May aggravate or worsen symptoms of diabetes mellitus and diabetes insipidus • Higher doses may be needed in severe hypothyroid states and other conditions such as pregnancy	• Side effects: diaphoresis, tachycardia, abdominal cramps, diarrhea, irregular menses, heat intolerance, weight loss, headache, insomnia, nervousness • Adverse effects: palpitations, chest pain, arrhythmia
Thyroid suppressants • methimazole (Tapazole) • propylthiouracil (PTU)	• Hyperthyroidism • Thyrotoxicosis prior to subtotal thyroidectomy or radioactive iodine therapy	• May cause bone marrow depression • May prolong bleeding	• Side effects: rash, diarrhea, nausea, vomiting, headache, vertigo • Adverse effects: hepatitis, agranulocytosis, hypoprothrombinemia

Table 4.6.2 Thyroid Medications

Education

Thyroid Supplements

- Response to medication is not immediate and must be taken for 6–8 weeks before TSH levels are reassessed
- Discourage alteration and abrupt cessation of medication without consulting provider
- Change in brand of medication should be avoided because bioequivalence among brands can vary
- Encourage patient to take medication at the same time each day—preferably before breakfast on an empty stomach to increase absorption

Thyroid Suppressants

- Avoid consumption of agents that contain iodine
- Immediately report to provider symptoms of fever, sore throat, malaise, unusual bleeding, headache, rash, or lymphadenopathy

Diabetes Mellitus Medications

Mechanism of Action

- **Biguanide:** decreases hepatic production of glucose, minor effects on insulin sensitivity in liver, and peripheral tissue; no direct effect on pancreas
- **Second-generation sulfonylurea:** enhances insulin secretion by binding to pancreatic beta cell receptor sites
- **Thiazolidinedione:** increases glucose sensitivity in muscle and liver, decreases gluconeogenesis
- **Nonsulfonylurea secretagogue (meglitinides):** short-acting stimulant of insulin secretion
- **Alpha-glucosidase inhibitor:** reduces glucose resorption in GI tract
- **Glucagon-like peptide:** stimulates glucose-dependent endogenous insulin secretion, inhibits glucagon secretion, slows gastric emptying
- **Dipeptidyl peptidase-4 inhibitor:** inhibits enzyme, DPP-4, which inactivates GLP-1, resulting in increased insulin secretion
- **Sodium-glucose co-transporter 2 inhibitor:** blocks SGLT2 protein, which promotes glucose resorption in renal tubule, increases insulin sensitivity, and decreases gluconeogenesis
- **Insulin:** mimics endogenous insulin activity by binding to cell wall receptors to allow cellular utilization of glucose

Examples	Indications	Prescription considerations	Side effects/adverse effects
Biguanide • metformin, metformin ER (Glucophage, Glucophage XR)	Type 2 diabetes mellitus, insulin-resistance	• Use cautiously in patient with chronic kidney disease (CKD), hepatic dysfunction, or congestive heart failure (CHF) • Can induce lactic acidosis • Can decrease vitamin B12 absorption	• Side effects: abdominal cramps, diarrhea, flatulence, heartburn, headache • Adverse effects: cholestatic and hepatocellular liver injury
Second-generation sulfonylurea • glipizide (Glucotrol) • glimepiride (Amaryl) • glyburide (DiaBeta)	Type 2 diabetes mellitus	• Use cautiously in patients with hepatic or renal dysfunction • Use cautiously in patients with hypersensitivity to sulfa drugs	• Side effects: hypoglycemia, weight gain, tinnitus, skin rash • Adverse effects: cholestatic jaundice, suppression of all blood cell lines
Thiazolidinedione • pioglitazone (Actos)	Type 2 diabetes mellitus	• **Black box warning:** increased risk of ischemic events and CHF associated with concomitant use of insulin or nitrates	• Side effects: weight gain, edema, headache • Adverse effects: CHF, fracture
Non-sulfonylureas secretagogue (meglitinides) • nateglinide (Starlix) • epaglinide (Prandin)	Type 2 diabetes mellitus	• Drug is safe in mild renal dysfunction but should be avoided in severe CKD • Hepatic dysfunction can increase concentration • May cause hypoglycemia	• Side effects: upper respiratory infection (URI), flu-like symptoms, weight gain, diarrhea, arthropathy, dizziness, increased uric acid • Adverse effects: jaundice, hypersensitivity reactions

Table 4.6.3 Diabetes Mellitus Medications—Oral

Examples	Indications	Prescription considerations	Side effects/adverse effects
Alpha-glucosidase inhibitor • acarbose (Precose)	Type 2 diabetes mellitus	• Renal dysfunction can increase concentration • Increases incidence of renal tumors • May cause hypoglycemia	• Side effects: flatulence, diarrhea, abdominal pain, increased liver function tests (LFT) • Adverse effects: fulminant hepatitis, skin hypersensitivity reaction
Glucagon-like peptide (GLP-1) • liraglutide (Victoza) • exenatide (Byetta)	Type 2 diabetes mellitus	• Must be taken 1 hour before a meal • May cause pancreatitis • May cause hypoglycemia	• Side effects: rash, nausea, vomiting, dyspepsia, dizziness, headache • Adverse effects: antibody formation, increased resting heart rate
Dipeptidyl peptidase-4 (DPP-4) inhibitor • linagliptin (Tradjenta) • saxagliptin (Onglyza) • sitagliptin (Januvia)	Type 2 diabetes mellitus	• May be associated with thyroid cancer • May cause pancreatitis • May cause hypoglycemia	• Side effects: rash, nasopharyngitis, nausea/vomiting, dyspepsia, dizziness, headache • Adverse effects: anaphylaxis, angioedema, acute pancreatitis
Sodium-glucose co-transporter 2 (SGLT2) inhibitor • canagliflozin (Invokana) • dapagliflozin (Farxiga) • empagliflozin (Jardiance)	Type 2 diabetes mellitus	• May increase risk for osteoporosis • May increase potassium levels • May increase risk for bladder cancer • May cause diabetes ketoacidosis	• Side effects: increased urination, constipation, genital yeast infections, urinary tract infections • Adverse effects: increased serum potassium, hypersensitivity reaction, renal impairment

Table 4.6.3 Diabetes Mellitus Medications—Oral (Continued)

Examples	Indications	Prescription considerations	Side effects/adverse effects
Rapid-acting • insulin lispro (Humalog) • insulin aspart (Novolog) • insulin glulisine (Apidra) • insulin inhalation (Afrezza)	Type 1 and type 2 diabetes mellitus	• Use as standing doses or sliding scale based on blood sugar readings • Add to regimen as pre-meal or bolus administered to largest meal • Afreeza: for patients 18 or older; contraindcated in smokers, smokers who recently quit, patients with chronic lung disease	• Side effects: weight gain, rash, injection site irritation, hypoglycemia • Adverse effects: anaphylaxis, profound hypoglycemia, Somogyi effect

Table 4.6.4 Diabetes Mellitus Medications—Insulin

Examples	Indications	Prescription considerations	Side effects/adverse effects
Short-acting • regular insulin (Humulin R, Novolin R)	Type 1 and type 2 diabetes mellitus	• Use as standing doses or sliding scale based on blood sugar readings • Add to regimen as pre-meal or bolus administered to largest meal	• Side effects: weight gain, rash, injection site irritation, hypoglycemia • Adverse effects: allergic reaction, profound hypoglycemia
Intermediate-acting • NPH insulin (Humulin N, Novolin N)	Type 1 and type 2 diabetes mellitus	• Start at 0.2 units per kg as total daily dose • Administer before breakfast and dinner • Two-thirds of dose is given in the morning, one-third is given before dinner	• Side effects: weight gain, rash, injection site irritation, hypoglycemia • Adverse effects: allergic reaction, profound hypoglycemia
Long-acting • insulin glargine (Lantus) • insulin detemir (Levemir)	Type 1 and type 2 diabetes mellitus	• Start with 10 units or 0.2 units per kilogram at bedtime • Increase dose by 2–4 units every 3–5 days to achieve fasting sugar goal	• Side effects: weight gain, rash, injection site irritation, hypoglycemia • Adverse effects: allergic reaction, profound hypoglycemia

Table 4.6.4 Diabetes Mellitus Medications—Insulin (Continued)

See Chapter 13, Lesson 2, Table 13.2.7, for onset, peak, and duration of insulin.

Education

- Teach about signs and symptoms of hypoglycemia including feeling jittery, headache, nausea/vomiting, and dizziness
- Instruct how to take the medication in relation to meals in order to avoid hypoglycemia
- Review how to perform a glucose check and how often to measure glucose levels
- Educate how to adjust medications as needed for sick days

Takeaways

- Patients on thyroid hormone supplementation should not change medication brands in order to avoid changes in hormone levels.
- Iodine-containing foods should be avoided when thyroid-suppressing medications are being taken.
- Oral hypoglycemic agents are used in insulin-resistance and type 2 diabetes, not type 1 diabetes.
- Insulin dosage regimens are individualized based on patient needs.

LESSON 7: EYE AND EAR

Learning Objectives
- Demonstrate knowledge of medications associated with treatment of eye and ear disorders
- Identify safe prescribing practices associated with eye and ear medications

Note: the tables below offer truncated drug profiles and do not cover all medications in each category. For complete drug information, consult a medication manual.

Certain ear infections are treated with systemic antibiotics (*see Chapter 4, Lesson 2*), while other ear disorders require topical otic medication. Eye disorders vary greatly and as such may require treatment from a variety of ophthalmic classifications.

The following classes are frequently encountered in family practice:

- Antibiotics (ophthalmic and otic)
- Miotic, mydriatric, vasoconstricting, and miscellaneous ophthalmic agents
- Analgesic and cerumenolytic otic agents

Opthalmic & Otic Antibiotics

Ophthalmic and otic antibiotic preparations display either a bacteriostatic or bactericidal action (*see Chapter 4, Lesson 2, for additional information*). Similar to systemic antibiotics, avoid use in persons with allergy.

Examples	Indications	Prescription considerations	Side effects/adverse effects
Macrolide • erythromycin	Prophylaxis of neonatal conjunctivitis; treatment of conjunctivitis	Apply a thin ribbon of ointment to lower conjunctiva	• Side effects: vision is briefly blurred • Adverse effects: hypersensitivity
Fluoroquinolone • ciprofloxacin	Conjunctivitis, corneal ulcers; otitis externa	• Ophthalmic ointment approved for use in >2 years of age, eye drops in >1 year of age • Otic: 1 single use container into ear canal BID (a wick may improve action)	• Side effects: vision briefly blurred with ophthalmic ointment; pruritus or pain (otic) • Adverse effects: serious hypersensitivity (ophthal); fungal superinfection, headache (otic)
Aminoglycoside • gentamicin	Ophthalmic infection	Ointment applied to lower conjunctiva 2–3 times daily; drops 1–2 drops every 4 hours	• Side effects: burning, irritation • Adverse effects: allergic reaction, corneal ulceration
Mixed • bacitracin and polymyxin B	Superficial infections of conjunctivae or cornea	• May decrease levels of BCG • Apply 1/4–1/2 inch to lower conjunctiva every 3–4 hours	• Side effects: burning, itching • Adverse effects: edema, conjunctival erythema, anaphylactoid reactions

Table 4.7.1 Ophthalmic and Otic Antibiotic Preparations

Patient Education

Avoid touching the tip of the ointment tube or dropper bottle to anything. Ophthalmic ointment should be applied from inner to outer canthus. For ear drops, instruct parents to straighten the ear canal by pulling the ear down and back in children under 3 years of age; up and back in older children.

Miotic Agents

Prescribed for patients with glaucoma. These agents produce miosis and constriction of the iris, opening the blocked channels, which allows normal outflow of aqueous humor and decreases intraocular pressure.

Example	Prescription considerations	Side effects/adverse effects
pilocarpine	• Use cautiously in patients with hypertension though systemic absorption may be minimal • 1 drop in affected eye up to 4 times daily	• Side effects: headache, temporary reduction in visual acuity • Adverse effects: allergic reaction

Table 4.7.2 Mitotic Ophthalmic Agents

Education

Wash hands before and after use. Make sure vision is clear prior to driving or using machinery.

Mydriatic Agents

These agents dilate the pupil, decrease formation of aqueous humor, and vasoconstrict the superficial scleral blood vessels.

Example	Prescription considerations	Side effects/adverse effects
phenylephrine	• 1 drop before procedure; may repeat every 10–60 minutes PRN • Do not use in patients <1 year of age due to increased systemic absorption	• Side effects: burning, irritation, vision changes, rebound miosis • Adverse effects: rarely hypertension syncope

Table 4.7.3 Mydriatic Ophthalmic Agents

Education

Do not use with an eye injury or infection.

Medications Specific to Glaucoma

In addition to miotic agents (*see Table 4.7.2*), alpha adrenergic agents, beta-adrenergic antagonists (beta-blockers), prostaglandin analogs, and carbonic anhydrase inhibitors (CAIs) are used to treat glaucoma. Combination meds combine two agents into one drop (such as Combigan, an alpha agonist and beta-adrenergic antagonist).

- Alpha-adrenergic agents, beta-adrenergic antagonists, and CAIs reduce aqueous humor production; alpha-adrenergic agents also increase outflow
- Prostaglandin analogs increase aqueous humor outflow

Examples	Prescription considerations	Side effects/adverse effects
Alpha-adrenergic agents brimonidine tartrate	• Contraindicated in patients taking MAO inhibitors • 1 drop in affected eye 3 times daily	• Side effects: stinging or itching/local irritation; headache, dry mouth • Adverse effects: blurred vision, abnormal taste
Beta-adrenergic antagonists timolol	1 drop daily or BID; contraindicated with asthma	• Side effects: possible bradycardia/ hypotension; can mask s/s of hypoglycemia • Adverse effects: contraindicated with asthma; sudden d/c may worsen symptoms of hyperthyroidism
Prostaglandin analogs latanoprost	1 drop daily (in evening)	Side effects: may have change in iris color and growth of eyelashes; stinging or itching/local irritation
CAIs dorzolamide	Avaliable as drops and PO formulation	Side effects: stinging or itching/local irritation

Table 4.7.4 Medications to Treat Glaucoma

Education

- With any eye dropper, be careful not to touch applicator tip to any surface to avoid contamination
- **Alpha-adrenergic agents:** patients should wait 15 minutes after administration prior to inserting contact lenses to avoid absorption of the drug by the lenses
- **Beta-adrenergic antagonists:** patients should occlude the inner canthus during drop administration (diminish systemic absorption); wait 15 minutes before inserting contact lenses

Miscellaneous Agents

Ocular lubricants form an occlusive film on the surface of the eye to prevent drying of its surface. Immunosuppressant ophthalmic preparations (cyclosporin) increase tear production in previously inflamed eyes.

Example	Prescription considerations	Side effects/adverse effects
Ocular lubricants	Apply 1/4 inch of lubricant to lower conjunctiva	Side effects have not been noted; discontinue use if eye pain, visual changes, redness, or eye irritation occur
cyclosporin	1 drop twice daily	• Side effects: burning or eye discomfort • Adverse effects: hypersensitivity

Table 4.7.5 Miscellaneous Ophthalmic Agents

Education

Do not use ocular lubricants with contact lenses. Do not touch applicator tip to any surface to avoid contamination. After administering cyclosporin, close the eyes with head tipped down for 2–3 minutes. Do not blink or squint during this time.

Otic Agents

Analgesic Agents

Provide pain relief and inflammation reduction in serous otitis media, otitis externa, or when cerumen removal is needed.

Example	Prescription considerations	Side Effects/adverse effects
antipyrine and benzocaine	• Fill ear canal or moistened cotton pledget and insert • May repeat every 1–2 hours	• Side effects: none known • Adverse effects: allergy—severe redness, burning, stinging, new pain

Table 4.7.6 Analgesic Otic Agents

Education

Avoid dizziness caused by instillation of cold ear drops by warming the container in the hands a few moments prior to administration. To use for ear wax removal, administer for 2-3 days, then use a bulb syringe with warm water to irrigate the cerumen from the ear canal. Do not touch the dropper to any surface to avoid contamination.

Cerumenolytic Agents

Cerumenolytic agents serve to emulsify and disperse ear wax.

Example	Prescription considerations	Side effects/adverse effects
carbamide peroxide	• Younger children: 3 drops BID up to 4 days • Older children and adults: 5–10 drops BID up to 4 days	• Side effects: rash, redness • Adverse effects: superinfection

Table 4.7.7 Cerumenolytic Agents

Education

Instill drops into affected ear canal. Lie on side or keep head tilted for several minutes (placing cotton in the ear and being upright does not work as well). Gently irrigate ear with warm water via bulb syringe to loosen cerumen.

Takeaways

- When instilling ear drops, straighten the ear canal by pulling the ear down and back in the child <3 years of age and up and back in the older child.
- Patients need to understand the importance of avoiding touching ophthalmic ointment or bottle applicators or ear droppers to any surface in order to maintain cleanliness.
- Patients should use ophthalmic and otic medications only as prescribed; with ophthalmic meds, report any visual changes to the provider.

LESSON 8: GASTROINTESTINAL

Learning Objectives
- Demonstrate knowledge of the medications associated with gastrointestinal (GI) health
- Recognize safe prescribing practices associated with GI medications

Note: the tables below offer truncated drug profiles and do not cover all medications in each category. For complete drug information, consult a medication manual.

Gastrointestinal Medications Overview

GI conditions may alter responses to drug therapy; drugs used in digestive disorders primarily alter GI secretion, absorption, or motility. They may act systemically or locally in the GI tract.

The drug groups included in this lesson are drugs used for acid-peptic disorders, laxatives, antidiarrheals, and antiemetics. Other drug groups used in GI disorders include cholinergics, anticholinergics, corticosteroids, and anti-infectives. While many of these are discussed in this lesson, some of these medications may be discussed in other lessons, as noted.

Many common symptoms relate to GI dysfunction. These symptoms may result from a disorder in the digestive system, disorders in other body systems that are affecting the GI tract (such as the CNS), or drug therapy (such as opioids, which affect Mu receptors and cause constipation).

Many GI symptoms and disorders alter the ingestion, dissolution, absorption, and metabolism of drugs. Drugs may be administered to relieve these symptoms and disorders, but drugs administered for conditions unrelated to the digestive system may also cause such symptoms and disorders.

Antidiarrheal Medications

See Chapter 4, Lesson 12, for information related to over-the-counter (OTC) antidiarrheal medications.

Antidiarrheals can generally fall into several categories:

- **Adsorbents:** coat the walls of the GI tract, and/or bind to the causative bacteria or toxin, which are then eliminated through the stool
  - Examples: bismuth (Kaopectate)
- **Anticholinergics:** decrease intestinal muscle tone and peristalsis of GI tract, thereby slowing the movement of fecal matter through the GI tract
  - Examples: belladonna alkaloids (Donnatal), atropine, hyoscyamine
- **Intestinal flora modifiers:** bacterial cultures of lactobacillus organisms or other beneficial bacteria (probiotics) that work by supplying missing bacteria to the GI tract and/or suppressing the growth of diarrhea-causing bacteria
  - Examples: lactobacillus acidophilus (Lactinex); fecal transplants for intractable *Clostridium difficile*

Mechanism of Action

Opiates block Mu receptors in the GI tract or directly slow muscle spasms or contractions; they decrease bowel motility and relieve rectal spasms, decrease transit time through the bowel, and allow more time for water and electrolytes to be absorbed. Examples are paregoric, opium tincture, codeine, loperamide, and diphenoxylate.

Medication	Indication	Prescription considerations	Side effects/adverse effects
diphenoxylate hydrochloride and atropine sulfate (Lomotil)	Acute or chronic non-bloody diarrhea	Class V controlled medication	• Side effects: diphenoxylate (narcotic-type effects such as drowsiness, dizziness, and additive effect to CNS depressants) and atropine (delirium, pyrexia, hypohydrosis, dry eyes, dry mouth) • Adverse effects: anaphylaxis, angioedema, pancreatitis, respiratory distress, anticholinergic toxidrome
eluxadoline (Viberzi)	Irritable bowel syndrome with diarrhea	Contraindicated with liver problems, previous pancreatitis, or cholecystectomy	• Risk of pancreatitis in first week, especially in those who have had cholecystectomy and/or who drink >3 alcoholic drinks per day • Sphincter of Oddi spasm in those without a gall bladder

Table 4.8.1 Antidiarrheal Medications

Education
Notify provider if diarrhea persists longer than two days or if blood is present in the stool.

Laxative (Anti-Constipation) Medications
See Chapter 4, Lesson 12, for information related to OTC anti-constipation (laxative) medications.

Constipation is defined as the abnormally infrequent and/or difficult passage of feces through the lower GI tract. Constipation is a symptom of another pathology and not a disease in and of itself, and can be caused by a variety of diseases or medications.

Mechanisms of Action
- **Bulk-forming:** absorbs water to increase bulk and distends bowel to initiate reflex bowel activity
- **Surfactant (stool softeners):** uses a surfactant that helps soften the stool and lubricate the intestinal wall
- **Osmotic:** draws fluid from the lining of the GI tract into the lumen, thereby increasing fluid volume and softening the stool
- **Stimulant:** encourages bowel movements by acting on the intestinal wall to increase the muscle contractions that move along the stool mass
- **Guanylate cyclase-C (G-CC) agonist:** promotes intestinal secretions in response to a meal
- **CIC-2 (chloride channel-type 2) activator:** enhances intestinal fluid secretion to improve motility, which helps pass stool

Medication	Indication	Prescription considerations	Side effects/adverse effects
Bulk forming • psyllium (Metamucil), polycarbophil (FiberCon), methylcellulose (Citrucel)	Constipation, postpartum, elderly patients, IBS	• Those with high sugar content should be avoided • Space 2 hours from other medication	• Side effects: dose-dependent flatulence, bloating • Adverse effects: abdominal obstruction or impaction if not taken with adequate fluid
Surfactant • docusate (Colace), mineral oil	Constipation where straining with stool should be avoided	• May decrease absorption of digoxin; mineral oil may decrease absorption of OCPs • May increase anticoagulant effect due to low vitamin K	• Side effects: incontinence • Adverse effects: long-term use can impair absorption of nutrients and fat-soluble vitamins
Osmotic • Fleet phospho soda, milk of magnesia, magnesium citrate • GoLYTELY, GlycoLax, MiraLax • lactulose (Cephulac), sorbitol	• Constipation, bowel cleansing for procedures • lactulose: encephalopathy of portal system	• Avoid in patients with renal or cardiac impairment • lactulose: avoid in persons requiring low galactose diet; use with caution in patients with diabetes	• Side effects: nausea, vomiting, bloating, flatulence, cramping • Adverse effects: fluid and electrolyte disturbances
Stimulant • aloe cascara (Nature's Remedy) • senna compounds (Ex-Lax, Senokot), bisacodyl (Dulcolax)	Constipation	Contraindicated in those with abdominal pain, nausea, and vomiting	• Side effects: abdominal pain, nausea, vomiting • Adverse effects: muscle weakness, electrolyte imbalance
Guanylate cyclase-C (G-CC) agonist • linaclotide (Linzess)	IBS with constipation, chronic constipation	Do not prescribe if bowel obstruction is a possibility	Side effect: diarrhea
Chloride channel-type 2 (ClC-2) activator • lubiprostone (Amitiza)	IBS with constipation, chronic constipation, opioid induced constipation	Do not prescribe if bowel obstruction is a possibility	Side effect: diarrhea

Table 4.8.2 Anti-Constipation Medications

Education

- Ensure adequate hydration while using these medications in order to prevent dehydration and electrolyte imbalance
- Stimulant laxatives are popular OTC treatments but are more likely to cause side effects
- Do not crush or chew tablets

Antiemetic and Antinausea Medications

See Chapter 4, Lesson 12, for information related to OTC antinausea medications.

Antiemetic medications are grouped by their action on one of the five neurotransmitter receptor sites that are of primary importance in the vomiting reflex:

- M1—muscarinic: scopolamine (TransDerm Scop)
- D2—dopamine: chlorpromazine (Thorazine), droperidol (Inapsine), metoclopramide (Reglan), prochlorperazine (Compazine), promethazine (Phenergan)
- H1—histamine: meclizine (Antivert), diphenhydramine
- 5-hydroxytryptamine (HT)-3—serotonin: ondansetron (Zofran), granisetron (Kytril), dolasetron (Anzemet)
- Neurokinin 1 (NK1) receptor—substance P: aprepitant (Emend)

Mechanism of Action

Below are some common antiemetics and their mechanisms of action, indications, and side effects:

- **Chlorpromazine:** depresses reticular activating system to suppress emesis
- **Promethazine:** dopamine receptor blocker, H1 blocker
- **Ondansetron:** serotonin type 3 receptor antagonist
- **Metoclopramide:** potent dopamine receptor blocker, accelerates gastric emptying
- **Lorazepam:** enhances the effect of gamma-aminobutyric acid (GABA)
- **Dexamethasone:** unclear regarding antiemetic effect, decreases inflammation

Medication	Indication	Prescription considerations	Side effects/adverse effects
chlorpromazine (Thorazine)	Treatment of nausea and vomiting	• Avoid in pregnant or lactating women • Not recommended in infants <6 months or in geriatric patients	• Side effects: dizziness, drowsiness, tachycardia, orthostatic hypotension • Adverse effects: akathisia, tremors, dystonia, tardive dyskinesia, neuroleptic malignant syndrome
promethazine (Phenergan)	Treatment of nausea and vomiting	• Contraindicated in children <2 years of age • Risk of extravasation with intravenous use	• Side effects: bradycardia, tachycardia, orthostatic hypotension, dizziness, confusion • Adverse effects: akathisia, tardive dyskinesia, apnea, neuroleptic malignant syndrome
ondansetron (Zofran)	Prevention of nausea and vomiting associated with chemotherapy	Use with caution in patients with risk of prolonged QT interval	• Side effects: anxiety, drowsiness, diarrhea, constipation, fatigue • Adverse effects: anaphylaxis, bradycardia or other arrhythmia, cardiopulmonary arrest

Table 4.8.3 Antiemetic and Antinausea Medications

Medication	Indication	Prescription considerations	Side effects/adverse effects
metoclopramide (Reglan)	Prevention and treatment of nausea and vomiting, treatment of gastroparesis *Note that erythromycin (an antibiotic) is a prokinetic agent that can speed gastric emptying*	Use with caution in geriatric patients, neonates, or patients with renal impairment, HTN, depression	• Side effects: confusion, dizziness, drowsiness, diarrhea • Adverse reactions: tardive dyskinesia (often irreversible), suicidal ideation, extrapyramidal symptoms
lorazepam (Ativan)	Adjunct to antiemetic therapy	• May cause significant respiratory depression, especially when used with other CNS depressants • Not recommended in patients with depression or psychosis	• Side effects: confusion, sedation, weakness, hypotension, additive effects with other depressants • Adverse effects: respiratory depression, coma, tolerance/abuse potential with higher doses or long-term use
dexamethasone (Decadron)	Adjunct to antiemetic therapy	• Avoid concomitant use with immune modulators • Numerous drugs increase or decrease drug levels/ effects	• Side effects: depression, euphoria, mood swings, acne, headache, abdominal distention • Adverse effects: arrhythmia, anaphylaxis, pulmonary edema
scopolamine (M1-muscarinic receptor antagonist and anticholinergic)	Antiemetic	• May raise the chance of seizures in some people • Sensitivity to bright lights • Sudden cessation of use after prolonged daily use can cause scopolamine withdrawal syndrome: consistent with rebound cholinergic activity and includes dizziness, nausea, vomiting, paresthesia of the hands and feet, dysphoria, and hypotension	Side effects: dizziness, drowsiness, orthostatic hypotension

Table 4.8.3 Antiemetic and Antinausea Medications (Continued)

See Chapter 4, Lesson 3, for a more in-depth discussion of chemo-induced nausea and vomiting medications.

Antireflux Medications

See Chapter 4, Lesson 12, for information related to H2 blockers, proton pump inhibitors, and antacids.

Prostaglandin analogs: prostaglandin therapy counteracts the systemic effects of NSAIDs and enhances epithelial cell growth and repair. Misoprostol is the only prostaglandin E2 analog approved by the FDA for the prevention of NSAID-related ulcers and is designed to help overcome the NSAID-induced deficiency of prostaglandins in the gastric mucosa.

Mechanism of Action

Reduces acid secretion by competing with histamine at H2 receptors of gastric parietal cells.

Education

- Inform provider of all prescription and OTC medications being taken
- If a rash develops, notify provider immediately

Ulcerative Colitis/Crohn's Disease Medications

Immunosuppressive, immune-modulating medications, and corticosteroids are used to treat ulcerative colitis and Crohn's disease. *See Chapter 4, Lesson 10, for information related to corticosteroids.*

Mechanism of Action

- **Infliximab:** monoclonal antibody binding to tumor necrosis factor alpha
- **Mesalamine:** modulates local chemical mediators (especially leukotrienes) of the inflammatory response
- **Sulfasalazine:** inhibits prostaglandins, cytokine synthesis, and immunosuppressive activity

Medication	Indication	Prescription considerations	Side effects/adverse effects
infliximab (Remicade)	Crohn's disease, arthritis, psoriasis in adults	• Not recommended for use in lactating women • Use with caution in persons otherwise predisposed to infection or with heart failure • Avoid concomitant use with other immune modulators	• Side effects: headache, fever, pain, hypertension, cough, rash, pruritus • Adverse effects: bronchospasm, arrhythmia, anaphylaxis, Stevens-Johnson syndrome
mesalamine (Asacol, Pentasa, Rowasa)	Treatment and remission maintenance for ulcerative colitis	Use cautiously in persons with renal or hepatic impairment	• Side effects: chills, dizziness, fatigue, fever, headache, rash, pruritus, pain, gastrointestinal upset • Adverse effects: chest pain, abnormal T waves on ECG
sulfasalazine (Azulfidine)	Ulcerative colitis, Crohn's disease	Use cautiously in persons with renal or hepatic impairment	• Side effects: fever, dizziness, gastric distress, anorexia, pruritus, urticaria • Adverse effects: cyanosis, Stevens-Johnson syndrome, jaundice

Table 4.8.4 Ulcerative Colitis/Crohn's Disease Medications

Education

- Medications used for ulcerative colitis and Crohn's disease result in immunosuppression, placing those persons at increased risk for infection
- Avoid exposure to tuberculosis and other infections
- Discontinue sulfasalazine at first sign of rash

Antispasmodics

Mechanism of Action

Antispasmodics block the action of acetylcholine at parasympathetic sites in smooth muscle and secretory glands.

Medications	Indication	Prescription considerations	Side effects/adverse effects
dicyclomine (Bentyl), hyoscyamine (Anaspaz, Levsin, Symax)	Irritable bowel syndrome	Do not use in lactating women nor during pregnancy	• Side effects: tachycardia, palpitations, dizziness, drowsiness, headache, bloating • Adverse effects: allergy, decreased diaphoresis, apnea

Table 4.8.5 Antispasmodic Medications

Education

Use caution during exercise and/or hot weather to avoid heat prostration. Maintain adequate hydration and avoid overheating.

Antiparasitic Medication

Mechanism of Action

- **Metronidazole:** antibiotic with amebicidal effects; inhibits protein wall synthesis, causing cell death in susceptible organisms such as the protozoa *Giardia*
- **Ivermectin:** anthelmintic, binds to glutamate-gated chloride ion channels in invertebrate muscle and nerve cells to kill parasites

Medication	Indication	Prescription considerations	Side effects/adverse effects
metronidazole (Flagyl)	Giardiasis, other protozoal infections	• Teratogenic effects with use during pregnancy • Use cautiously in persons with hepatic impairment	• Side effects: confusion, dizziness, constipation, diarrhea, metallic taste, vaginal itching, sore tongue, dark urine, disulfiram-like reaction if taken with alcohol • Adverse effects: seizure, aseptic meningitis, peripheral and optic neuropathy
ivermectin (Stromectol)	Worm infestation	• Do not use in lactating women • Repeat treatment may be needed if immunocompromised	• Side effects: orthostatic hypotension, edema, dizziness, pruritus, fever, arthralgia • Adverse effects: hives, dyspnea, seizure, Mazzotti reaction (when treating onchocerciasis), Stevens-Johnson syndrome

Table 4.8.6 Antiparasitic Medications

Education

- Administer ivermectin with a high-fat meal to increase bioavailability

Gallstone Dissolution Agents

Medication	Mechanism of action	Adverse reactions
ursodeoxycholic acid (Ursodiol, Actigall)	Decreases absorption of cholesterol by the intestines and secretion of cholesterol by the liver	>10%: headaches, dizziness, diarrhea, constipation, nausea, back pain

Table 4.8.7 Gallstone Dissolution Agent

Helicobacter Pylori-Associated Peptic Ulcer Disease Medications

- Combination of two antimicrobials (such as amoxicillin, clarithromycin, metronidazole, or tetracycline (*see Chapter 4, Lesson 2*) and a protein pump inhibitor (PPI) or a histamine-2 receptor antagonist (H2RA)
- Bismuth compound is added for its antibacterial effects, as well as increasing the $HCO3^-$ and mucous contents of the stomach

Takeaways

- Encourage hydration and monitor for dehydration/electrolyte with anticonstipation medication use.
- Be cautious with antiemetic medications in pregnant women, young children, and older adults, and in patients with risk of prolonged QT interval, renal impairment, altered mood, and psychosis.
- When treating *H. pylori*, more than one antimicrobial is indicated to prevent resistance; adding a PPI or H2RA decreases signs and symptoms and hastens healing.

LESSON 9: GYN/GU

Learning Objectives

- Demonstrate knowledge of the medications associated with men's health, urology, gynecology, and pregnancy
- Recognize safe prescribing practices associated with these medications

Note: the tables below offer truncated drug profiles and do not cover all medications in each category. For complete drug information, consult a medication manual.

Medications that target the GU/GYN system fall into broad treatment categories:

- Hormones and modifiers
- Benign prostatic hyperplasia (BPH)
- Urinary incontinence/frequent urination
- Urinary pain and analgesia

Hormones and Modifiers

The mechanism of action of hormone therapy is to augment normal hormone cycles and levels. They are used to treat the following conditions:

- Females: hormone replacement therapy, contraception, treatment of some tumors, and treatment of infertility
- Males: hormonal replacement therapy, benign prostatic hypertrophy, erectile dysfunction, treatment of tumors of the testicles and prostate

Medication	Mechanism of action	Side effects/adverse events
Intrauterine device (IUD) - Copper IUD (ParaGard): nonhormonal - levonorgestrel IUD (Mirena, Skyla, Liletta, and Kyleena): hormonal	- Copper IUD interferes with both sperm transport and egg fertilization; implantation may be prevented - Hormonal IUD mechanism unknown but may alter endometrium, inhibit sperm survival, or thicken cervical mucus, preventing sperm from passing into the uterus	- Adverse events that cause removal of IUD: pregnancy, expulsion, pain/bleeding - Copper IUD: anemia, backache, dysmenorrhea, dyspareunia, leukorrhea, prolonged menstrual flow, menstrual spotting, cramping, urticarial skin reaction, vaginitis - Hormonal IUD: ovarian cyst, ectopic pregnancy, uterine perforation, thromboembolism, abdominal or pelvic pain, weight gain
Estrogen estradiol (Estrace), ethinyl estradiol	- Used for birth control by preventing luteinizing hormone (LH) surge, which prevents ovulation - Used for hormone replacement therapy (HRT) by replacing estrogen that is rapidly declining in menopause; counteracts the symptoms of menopause	- Blood clots, MI, breast or ovarian cancer, gallbladder disease, migraine, breast pain, HTN, mood changes, glucose intolerance, melasma, musculoskeletal pain, alterations to lipid levels, GYN cancers - **Black box warnings as HRT:** should not be used without progestin in patients with a uterus because of increased risk of endometrial cancer; should not be used to prevent dementia or cardiovascular disease
Human chorionic gonadotropin (HCG)	Used for hypogonadism by stimulating the testes to make testosterone	Minimal reactions reported
misoprostol (synthetic prostaglandin E1 analog)	Used for cervical ripening prior to delivery by inducing uterine contractions	- Abdominal pain, diarrhea, hypotension or HTN, headache, MI - **Black box warning:** not for use in pregnant women (premature birth, abortion, uterine rupture)
Progesterone levonorgestrel, desogestrel, drospirenone, norethindrone, medroxyprogesterone acetate	Thickens cervical mucus, which acts as a barrier to sperm and thins the uterine lining, preventing implantation; there is evidence to suggest that progesterone may also incapacitate sperm	Abdominal/pelvic pain/cramping, acne/skin changes, headaches, irregular menstrual bleeding, ovarian cyst(s), vulvovaginitis

Table 4.9.1 Hormones and Modifiers

Medication	Mechanism of action	Side effects/adverse events
Testosterone • Injectable: testosterone enanthate (Delatestryl), testosterone cypionate-injectable, testosterone undecanoate (Aveed)-injectable • Transdermal: AndroGel, Fortesta, Axiron	Used for hypogonadism by replacing testosterone in men with deficiency	• Increased prostate-specific antigen, benign prostatic hypertrophy, MI, priapism, hepatitis, venous thromboembolism, acne, hirsutism, male pattern baldness, gynecomastia • **Black box warnings:** risk of virilization in children who accidentally come in contact with transdermal application; pulmonary oil microembolism (testosterone undecanoate only) **Considerations** • Caution if cardiovascular disease, diabetes, polycythemia, hyperlipidemia, CHF • Monitor Hgb/Hct to test for erythropoiesis; prostate-specific antigen (PSA) needed at baseline and routine testing for length of therapy • Schedule III medication • Aveed under restricted distribution in U.S.

Table 4.9.1 Hormones and Modifiers (Continued)

Education

• Baseline pregnancy test is necessary prior to contraceptive therapy; notify immediately if pregnancy occurs on hormone therapy

• Keep follow-up appointments to monitor for side effects and for required lab/diagnostic testing (Pap smear, mammogram, hormone levels, Hgb/Hct, liver function test, PSA, and lipids)

• Take medications as prescribed, or hormone levels may be altered resulting in return of symptoms, pregnancy

• Go to the ER if on hormonal therapy and symptoms of adverse event occur

> **Pro Tip**
>
> The ACHES acronym indicates possible symptoms of a thromboembolism:
>
> • **A**bdominal pain: mesenteric or pelvic embolism
> • **C**hest pain: myocardial infarction (MI) or pulmonary embolism (PE)
> • **H**eadache: cerebrovascular accident (CVA)
> • **E**ye problems: retinal thrombosis
> • **S**evere leg pain: deep vein thrombosis (DVT) or thrombophlebitis

Combined Oral Contraceptives

Combination oral contraceptives (COCs) are a highly reliable form of contraception. The perfect-use failure rate is 0.1%, but the typical-use failure rate is approximately 8%, due primarily to missed pills or failure to resume therapy after the seven-day pill-free interval. COCs have some cardiovascular adverse side effects. However, as the estrogen and progestin content has decreased over the last decade, there has been a reduction in both side effects and cardiovascular complications. COCs can be safely used in nonsmoking women until menopause.

Mechanism of Action

COCs suppress hypothalamic gonadotropin-releasing hormone (GnRH) and pituitary gonadotropin secretion. The most important mechanism for providing contraception is inhibition of the mid-cycle luteinizing hormone (LH) surge, so that ovulation does not occur. Another mechanism of contraceptive action is suppression of ovarian folliculogenesis (via suppression of pituitary follicle-stimulating hormone [FSH] secretion). However, a substantial number of women can develop follicles while taking a COC that contains lower doses of ethinyl estradiol (20–35 mcg). Progestin-related mechanisms that contribute to the contraceptive include:

- Rendering the endometrium less suitable for implantation
- Alterations in cervical mucus to make it less permeable to penetration by sperm
- Impairment of normal fallopian tube motility and peristalsis

In addition to using COCs for contraception, they can also be useful for the treatment of women with hyperandrogenism (polycystic ovarian syndrome).

Initiation of Treatment with COCs

There are several options for starting COCs.

- **Quick start:** begin taking COCs on the day the prescription is filled, as long as pregnancy has been reasonably excluded
- **Sunday start:** start taking the pills on the first Sunday after the period begins; most pill packs are arranged for a Sunday start to avoid withdrawal bleeding on a weekend
- **First day start:** begin the pill on the first day of menses; this approach provides the maximum contraceptive effect in the first cycle, and backup contraception for the first seven days of use is not needed

With the quick start and Sunday start, the pill is often started more than than five days after the onset of menses. For this reason, backup contraception is suggested for the first seven days. Follicular development and breakthrough ovulation is more common in women who delay starting the pill after menses when compared with women who start on day one.

Contraindications

Absolute Contraindications to Estrogen-Containing Contraceptives

- Migraine with aura
- Ischemic heart disease, past or current (or multiple risk factors: smoking, diabetes, hypertension, hyperlipidemia, older age)
- Smoking: in women >35 years of age who smoke >15 cigarettes/day
- Hypertension: poorly controlled (systolic >160 mmHg or diastolic >100 mmHg)
- Stroke
- Deep venous thrombosis, past or current

- Major surgery with prolonged immobilization (estrogen-containing contraceptives should be stopped 4–6 weeks before such surgery)
- Breast cancer (diagnosis ≤5 years ago)
- Endometrial cancer
- Known or suspected pregnancy
- Postpartum: first 3 weeks (if not breastfeeding), first month (if breastfeeding)
- Active liver disease: viral hepatitis, cirrhosis, or tumor

Relative Contraindications to Estrogen-Containing Contraceptives
- Migraine without aura
- Smoking: in women >35 years of age who smoke <15 cigarettes/day
- Hypertension: well-controlled or moderately well-controlled (systolic 140–159 mmHg or diastolic 90–99 mmHg)
- Diabetes (with end organ damage)
- Superficial thrombophlebitis
- Breast cancer, more than 5 years in the past
- Postpartum: 3–6 weeks
- Liver disease (viral hepatitis, severe cirrhosis, hepatocellular adenoma, malignant tumors)
- Concurrent treatment with certain anticonvulsants (including phenytoin, carbamazepine, barbiturates, primidone, topiramate, oxcarbazepine, lamotrigine)
- Hormone-related cholestasis in the past
- Symptoms of gallstones

Absolute Contraindications to Progestin-Only Contraceptives
- Breast cancer
- Known or suspected pregnancy
- Unexplained vaginal bleeding

Relative Contraindications to Progestin-Only Contraceptives
- Concurrent medication that cause progestins to be metabolized more rapidly: (1) anti-seizure medications: phenytoin, carbamazepine, primidone, phenylbutazone, felbamate, oxcarbazepine, and lamotrigine (lamotrigine levels decreased by progestins); (2) antibiotics: rifampin/rifampicin; (3) ritonavir-boosted protease inhibitors
- Women who have undergone bariatric surgery (may have difficulty with absorption)

For most women, the benefits of hormonal contraceptives exceed their potential risks.

Education

- Patient should be aware of method of COC initiation and need for backup contraception. Many antibiotics interfere with the efficacy of COCs and backup contraception is needed

- Encourage smoking cessation in women who smoke and abstinence in those who do not

- Patient should consider a dual protection strategy (condom plus a second method), as hormonal contraceptives offer no protection from sexually transmitted infections

Urinary Tract, Erectile Dysfunction, and Prostate Agents

Medications in this class treat patients who initially present with lower urinary tract symptoms (LUTS). LUTS refers to symptoms associated with overactive bladder (frequency, urgency, and nocturia). It includes symptoms relating to storage and/or voiding disturbances and the pain associated with their etiology. These symptoms are common among aging men. The aging male may also have a loss of erectile function from hypogonadism, T2DM, cardiovascular disease, and neurological disorders.

Medication	Mechanism of action	Side effects/adverse reactions
5-alpha-reductase inhibitors finasteride, dutasteride (Avodart)	• Indicated for BPH • Suppresses dihydrotestosterone (DHT) levels by preventing the conversion of testosterone into DHT, which shrinks the size of the prostate	Orthostatic hypotension, dizziness, decreased sexual desire, inability to maintain an erection or ejaculate, and generalized weakness
Alpha-1-receptor antagonists alfuzosin (Uroxatral), doxazosin (Cardura), tamsulosin (Flomax), terazosin (Hytrin), silodosin (Rapaflo)	• Indicated for BPH • Decreases bladder outlet obstruction by relaxing the smooth muscle tissue of the bladder neck (is available in long action form)	Dizziness and abnormal muscle weakness
Anticholinergic agents darifenacin (Enablex), fesoterodine (Toviaz), oxybutynin (Ditropan), tolterodine (Detrol), trospium, solifenacin (Vesicare), hyoscyamine (Anaspaz)	• Used as urinary antispasmodic • Muscarinic receptor antagonist, which relaxes the smooth muscle of bladder	Constipation, dry mouth, blurry vision, dizziness, dyspepsia, headache, urinary retention, UTI, and weakness **Considerations:** oxybutynin and tolterodine available in immediate and long acting forms
Analgesics Azo Dye (OTC), phenazopyridine	Anesthetizes the urinary tract	Dizziness, headache, and GI upset, orange urine **Considerations** • If taken prior to urinalysis (U/A), will alter results of U/A • Available OTC phenazopyridine (Azo) in 95 mg tablets; available as prescription in 100–200 mg tablets
Phosphodiesterase-5 inhibitors avanafil (Stendra), sildenafil (Viagra), tadalafil (Cialis), vardenafil (Staxyn)	• Indicated for erectile dysfunction • Causes relaxation of smooth muscles and increases blood flow to the corpus cavernosum	Flushing, headaches, GI upset, muscle aches, back pain, respiratory infection, nasopharyngitis **Considerations:** contraindicated in men who are taking nitrates; concurrent use may lead to hypotension

Table 4.9.2 Urinary Tract and Prostate Agents

Takeaways

- Selecting an appropriate contraceptive method requires a thorough medical history, with a focus on ruling out the most common contraindications.

- Depo-Provera has a black box warning related to risk of possible bone mineral density loss. It should only be used for longer than two years if no other method of contraception is possible.

- With combined hormonal contraception, cardiovascular side effects increase with number of cigarettes smoked. This risk increases proportionately with age.

- When prescribing COCs, use the lowest effective estrogen dose to decrease cardiovascular risk.

- ED and LUTS develop from common pathophysiological mechanisms; patients seeking consultation for one condition should always be screened for the other condition.

LESSON 10: MS/ANALGESIC

Learning Objectives

- Demonstrate knowledge of medications associated with treatment of musculoskeletal disorders and use of analgesic medications

- Identify safe prescribing practices associated with analgesics and medications used to treat musculoskeletal disorders

Note: the tables below offer truncated drug profiles and do not cover all medications in each category. For complete drug information, consult a medication manual.

Pain is a complex, multidimensional, subjective phenomenon that can be associated with disease or injury encompassing physiologic, sensory, emotional, behavioral, cognitive, and cultural dimensions. Whether pain is visceral, somatic, neuropathic, acute, or chronic, different approaches can be taken to manage pain.

Anti-Inflammatory Agents

Inflammation occurs in response to tissue injury and infection. Fluid, leukocytes, and chemical mediators accumulate at the area of injury. As one of the five characteristics of inflammation, pain can be treated with anti-inflammatory agents. Anti-inflammatory agents not only have analgesic abilities, but also have antipyretic and anticoagulant properties.

Non-Steroidal Anti-Inflammatory Drugs (NSAIDs)

Mechanism of Action

The first-generation NSAIDs inhibit prostaglandin synthesis. In addition, salicylates and propionic acid derivatives inhibit the hypothalamic heat-regulator center. Second-generation NSAIDs are COX-2 inhibitors, which decrease the inflammatory response.

Medication (examples)	Indication	Prescription considerations	Side effects/adverse effects
First-Generation NSAIDs			
Salicylates aspirin (ASA, Bayer, Ecotrin)	For mild to moderate pain, fever, TIA/thromboembolic conditions, and arthritis	• Contraindicated in flu or virus symptoms in children (risk of Reye syndrome), anticoagulant therapy, GI bleeding, bone marrow suppression, third trimester of pregnancy • Caution with renal or hepatic disorders, gout (may exacerbate), alcoholism • Increased risk of hypoglycemia with oral hypoglycemic drugs; increased ulcerogenic effect with glucocorticoids • Decrease cholesterol and potassium, T3, T4 levels; increase PT, bleeding time, uric acid • Prescribe with caution in patients with asthma	• Side effects: hypotension, tachycardia, agitation, dizziness • Adverse effects: ulcer, bleeding, anaphylaxis, hemolytic anemia, bronchospasm, thrombocytopenia, Reye syndrome, hepatotoxicity
Para-chlorobenzoic acid derivatives, or indoles indomethacin (Indocin), sulindac (Clinoril)	For mild to moderate pain; acute and chronic arthritis	Highly protein bound (90%) and displaces other protein-bound drugs, resulting in potential toxicity	• Side effects: hypertension, edema, abdominal distress, dizziness • Adverse effects: anaphylaxis, acute respiratory distress
Phenylacetic acids diclofenac sodium (Voltaren), etodolac (Lodine), ketorolac tromethamine (Toradol)	For mild to moderate pain; acute and chronic arthritis; post-surgical pain (ketorolac)	• diclofenac is available in PO, extended-release, and topical 1% gel preparations • ketorolac is available in PO, IV, IM, ophthalmic, and intranasal preparations and should only be used short-term	• Side effects: dizziness, edema, hypertension, pruritus, abdominal distress, tinnitus • Adverse effects: anaphylaxis, nephrotoxicity
Propionic acid derivatives ibuprofen (Motrin, Advil), ketoprofen (Nexcede), naproxen (Naprosyn, Aleve), oxaprozin (Daypro)	For mild to moderate pain; acute and chronic arthritis	• Highly protein bound • It may take several days for the anti-inflammatory effect to be evident • Can increase the effects of warfarin (Coumadin), sulfonamides, many of the cephalosporins, and phenytoin • High risk of toxicity when ibuprofen is taken concurrently with calcium channel blockers	• Side effects: dizziness, edema, hypertension, pruritus, abdominal distress, tinnitus • Adverse effects: anaphylaxis, Stevens-Johnson syndrome, acute renal failure, hemolytic anemia

Table 4.10.1 NSAIDs

Medication (examples)	Indication	Prescription considerations	Side effects/adverse effects
Fenamates meclofenamate sodium monohydrate (Meclomen), mefenamic acid (Ponstel)	For mild to moderate pain; acute and chronic arthritis	• Avoid in patients with history of peptic ulcer disease • Contraindicated with CABG	• Side effects: edema, hypertension, bleeding • Adverse effects: cardiovascular thrombotic event, Stevens-Johnson syndrome, anaphylaxis
Oxicams piroxicam (Feldene), meloxicam (Mobic)	For mild to moderate pain; acute and chronic arthritis	• Full clinical response to piroxicam may take 1–2 weeks • piroxicam is highly protein bound and should not be taken with aspirin or other NSAIDs	• Side effects: edema, hypertension, bleeding • Adverse effects: cardiovascular thrombotic event, GI perforation
Second-Generation NSAIDs			
COX-2 inhibitors celecoxib (Celebrex)	For acute and chronic arthritis; dysmenorrhea	• Contraindicated in advanced renal disease, severe hepatic failure, anemia, concurrent use of diuretics and ACE inhibitors • Caution in renal or hepatic dysfunction, hypertension, fluid retention, heart failure, infection, history of GI bleeding or ulceration, concurrent anticoagulant therapy, steroids, or alcohol use • Decrease effect of ACE inhibitors; increased INR and GI bleeding with warfarin; may increase toxicity with lithium; fluconazole increases celecoxib levels	• Side effects: cough, fever, rash, sneezing, edema • Adverse effects: cardiovascular thrombotic event, GI perforation

Table 4.10.1 NSAIDs (Continued)

Combination drugs of an NSAID and an opioid analgesic may be used to treat moderate to severe pain. An example includes hydrocodone/ibuprofen (Isoprene). Combination drugs of an NSAID and medications used to treat gastric irritation (PPI, H2 antagonist) may be used to prevent gastrointestinal upset while treating pain. Examples include ibuprofen/famotidine (Duexis) and naproxen/esomeprazole (Vimovo). NSAIDs are also common in several OTC medications (e.g., Excedrin, Alka-Seltzer Plus Cold).

> **DANGER SIGN** NSAIDs are contraindicated in severe renal or liver disease, or the presence of ulcers or bleeding disorders (elderly patients are at greater risk for serious GI events). NSAIDs may increase risk of serious cardiovascular thrombotic events; therefore, prescribe with caution in patients with cardiovascular risk factors (i.e., history of MI, cerebrovascular, or peripheral vascular disease).

Education

- Notify provider if stools are black and tarry
- Take with food to decrease the risk of GI upset
- Avoid taking aspirin with NSAIDs (could cause GI upset and possible GI bleeding)
- Avoid alcoholic beverages (increases gastric irritation and can lead to GI bleeding)
- Inform the dentist or surgeon before a procedure when taking ibuprofen or other NSAIDs
- Avoid use during pregnancy
- It may take several weeks to experience desired drug effect of some NSAIDs
- Herbal remedies such as dong quai, feverfew, garlic, ginger, and ginkgo may cause bleeding when taken with NSAIDs

Corticosteroids

Mechanism of Action

Suppresses migration of polymorphonuclear leukocytes and reverses increased capillary permeability, thereby decreasing inflammation.

Medications	Indication	Prescription considerations	Side effects/adverse effects
prednisone, prednisolone (Orapred, Pediapred), methylprednisolone (A-Methapred, Medrol)	• Systemic lupus erythematosus (SLE); adjunct for rheumatoid arthritis, reactive arthritis, acute gout glares; adjuvant for cerebral or spinal cord edema pain or peripheral nerve pain • Strong anti-inflammatory action, appetite stimulant, mood elevation • High dose for severe exacerbations of SLE	• Avoid concomitant use with immune modulators; numerous drugs increase or decrease drug levels/effects • Baseline and ongoing labs: hemoglobin, occult blood, electrolytes, blood glucose; test for occult blood • Use lowest effective dose for shortest duration possible due to potential for adverse effects, particularly with elderly patents • Prescribe with caution with glaucoma (obtain IOP with therapy >6 weeks)	• Side effects: depression, euphoria, mood swings, hyperglycemia, acne, headache, abdominal distention, thinning skin, stimulates appetite, hypokalemia • Adverse effects: immunosuppression, arrhythmia, pulmonary edema, suppression of hypothalamic-pituitary axis, Cushing syndrome, reduction of growth velocity (monitor growth with long-term use in pediatric patients), osteoporosis, psychiatric disturbances, venous thrombosis (rare)

Table 4.10.2 Corticosteroids

Education

- Instruct patient to avoid exposure to tuberculosis and other infections
- Teach your patient about signs of infection, hyperglycemia, and adrenal gland dysfunction and to report these immediately
- Ensure patient understands to not stop drug abruptly; rather, follow weaning schedule as prescribed

Disease-Modifying Antirheumatic Drugs (DMARDs)

DMARDs treat pain and protect joint function by preventing inflammation; they are prescribed for patients with rheumatoid arthritis, ankylosing spondylitis, psoriatic arthritis, juvenile idiopathic arthritis, and lupus. DMARDs are also called immune modulators or biologics. Immune modulators, such as azathioprine (Imuran), are prescribed to treat ulcerative colitis/Crohn's disease.

Mechanism of Action

- **Hydroxychloroquine:** action resulting in anti-inflammatory and immune modulating effects is unknown
- **Leflunomide:** inhibits pyrimidine synthesis
- **Methotrexate:** exhibits adenosine-mediated anti-inflammatory effects
- **Sulfasalazine:** exact action not understood, but has immunosuppressive, antibacterial, and anti-inflammatory effects; inhibits prostaglandin synthesis in the colon
- **Tumor necrosis factor inhibitors:** suppress natural response to tumor necrosis factor (TNF) involved in early inflammatory response
- **Non-TNF agents:** monoclonal antibodies directed against certain portions of T-cells (abatacept), B-cells (rituximab), or antagonists of interleukins (tocilizumab, anakinra)

Medication	Indication	Prescription considerations	Side effects/adverse effects
hydroxychloroquine	Rheumatoid arthritis, systemic lupus erythematosus	• Baseline ocular exam • Many drug interactions	• Side effects: headache, tinnitus, vertigo, anorexia, weight loss, mood changes, rash • Adverse effects: severe hypoglycemia, irreversible retinal damage, QT prolongation, cardiomyopathy
leflunomide	Rheumatoid arthritis	• Obtain a baseline PPD prior to initiating therapy • Contraindicated in pregnancy or those wishing to become pregnant	• Side effects: stomach pain, diarrhea, weight loss, headache • Adverse effects: hepatotoxicity, severe immune suppression, Stevens-Johnson syndrome
methotrexate	Rheumatoid arthritis, Crohn's disease	• Baseline and ongoing labs: CBC, liver, and kidney function tests • Concurrent administration with NSAIDs not recommended • Contraindicated in pregnancy or those wishing to become pregnant	• Side effects: appetite loss, nausea/vomiting, rash, diarrhea, blood in urine or stools, difficulty urinating • Adverse effects: anaphylaxis, cirrhosis, shortness of breath, seizures, infection

Table 4.10.3 DMARDs

Medication	Indication	Prescription considerations	Side effects/adverse effects
sulfasalazine	Rheumatoid arthritis, ulcerative colitis, Crohn's disease	Monitor CBC, reticulocyte count, liver function tests	• Side effects: dizziness, fever, headache, rash, GI symptoms • Adverse effects: anaphylaxis, aplastic anemia, hepatotoxicity
Biologic response modifiers tumor necrosis factor (TNF) inhibitors (etanercept, adalimumab, infliximab, certolizumab golimumab) and non-TNF agents (abatacept, rituximab, tocilizumab, anakinra)	• TNF inhibitors: rheumatoid and juvenile arthritis, psoriasis, Crohn's disease, ulcerative colitis • Non-TNF agents: rheumatoid arthritis (also JIA and psoriatic arthritis for abatacept)	• Baseline and ongoing labs: CBC, liver, and kidney function tests • Update immunizations prior to initiation • Chest x-ray prior to initiation • Screen for TB, HBV, HCV • Multiple drug and natural supplement interactions	• Side effects: headache, dizziness, rash, nausea, cough, fatigue • Adverse effects: serious infection, infusion-related fever, malignancy (lymphoma)

Table 4.10.3 DMARDs (Continued)

Education

- Avoid exposure to know infectious persons
- Teach your patient about signs of infection (including fungal) and to report these immediately (important prior to, during, and after therapy)

Anti-Gout Drugs

Mechanism of Action

- **Allopurinol, febuxostat:** limit uric acid production
- **Colchicine:** blocks neutrophil-mediated inflammatory responses induced by the presence of uric acid
- **Pegloticase:** converts uric acid to allantoin
- **Probenecid:** inhibits tubular reabsorption of uric acid

Medication	Indication	Prescription considerations	Side effects/adverse effects
allopurinol, febuxostat	Chronic gout management	• Prescribe maintenance doses of colchicine when started • Use with caution in renal disease • Do not use with azathioprine or mercaptopurine	• Side effects: rash, nausea/vomiting (febuxostat) • Adverse effects: Stevens-Johnson syndrome, hepatotoxicity, bone marrow depression (allopurinol)
colchicine	Decreases gout flares when initiating chronic gout treatment	• Most effective when started within 12–24 hours of gout attack • Stop when symptom-free 2–3 days • Use caution with renal or liver disease	• Side effects: nausea, vomiting, diarrhea • Adverse effects: fatal overdose, bone marrow suppression

Table 4.10.4 Anti-Gout Drugs

Medication	Indication	Prescription considerations	Side effects/adverse effects
pegloticase	Refractory gout	• Give as an intravenous infusion every 2 weeks • Use with caution in CHF • Do not use with allopurinol, febuxostat, or probenecid	• Side effects: urticaria, gout flares, nausea, bruising • Adverse effects: anaphylaxis, infusion reaction, exacerbation of CHF
probenecid	Chronic gout	• Begin after acute gout attack ends • Do not use with salicylates (antagonizes action) • Increases methotrexate levels	• Side effects: rash, headache, nausea/vomiting • Adverse effects: anaphylaxis, kidney stones

Table 4.10.4 Anti-Gout Drugs (Continued)

Education
- Discontinue allopurinol at the first sign of a rash
- Optimum benefit for allopurinol takes 2–6 weeks
- Maintain adequate hydration

Non-Opioid Analgesics: Acetaminophen

Acetaminophen is a para-aminophenol derivative that does not have anti-inflammatory properties. Combination drugs of acetaminophen and an opioid analgesics may be used to treat moderate to severe pain (e.g., oxycodone/APAP [Percocet], hydrocodone/APAP [Vicodin]). Acetaminophen is common in many OTC medications (e.g., Excedrin, Midol, Vicks Cold & Flu, NyQuil).

Mechanism of Action
- Weakly inhibits prostaglandin synthesis and inhibits the hypothalamic heat-regulating center

Medication	Indication	Prescription considerations	Side effects/adverse effects
acetaminophen (APAP, Tylenol, Tylenol ES, Ofirmev IV)	Mild to moderate pain, fever, osteoarthritis	• Maximum dose of 4 g/day • Contraindicated in severe hepatic or renal disease, alcoholism • Decreased effect with oral contraceptives, antacids, anticholinergics, cholestyramine, charcoal • Assess liver enzymes and bilirubin in patients taking high doses	• Side effects: anorexia, nausea, vomiting, rash, insomnia, oliguria, urticaria • Adverse effects: hepatotoxicity, anemia, blood dyscrasias, Stevens-Johnson syndrome

Table 4.10.5 Acetaminophen

> **Pro Tip**
> Acetylcysteine (Mucomyst) is the antidote for acetaminophen toxicity (>50 mcg/mL).

Education

- Avoid excessive alcohol intake (may lead to liver injury)
- Check acetaminophen dosage on package label of combination OTC drugs
- Do not exceed the recommended dosage of no more than 4 g/day to avoid liver damage (adults)
- Be careful to distinguish between pediatric elixir and infant drops, as they are different dosing concentrations

Opioid Analgesics

Opioids are prescribed for moderate to severe pain. The Controlled Substances Act of 1970 classified opioids in five schedule categories according to their potential for drug abuse. Schedule II drugs have a high potential for abuse, which may lead to significant drug dependence. Schedule III drugs have a somewhat lesser potential for abuse, which may lead to moderate drug dependence. Schedule IV drugs have a low potential for abuse, which may lead to moderate drug dependence.

Medications	Controlled substance schedule
codeine codeine in combination with APAP (Tylenol with Codeine [#3, #4])	Class II Class III
fentanyl (Astral, Actiq, Duragesic, Sublimaze)	Class II
hydrocodone (Hysingla ER, Zohydro ER); in combination with APAP (Lortab, Norco, Vicodin), ibuprofen (Reprexain, Vicoprofen)	Class II
hydromorphone (Dilaudid)	Class II
meperidine (Demerol)	Class II
methadone (Dolophine)	Class II
morphine (Duramorph, MS Contin)	Class II
oxycodone (Oxycontin, Roxicodone); in combination with APAP (Percocet), ASA (Percodan)	Class II
tramadol (Ultram)	Class IV

Table 4.10.6 Controlled Substance Schedules for Opioids

Mechanism of Action

Opioid analgesics act on the CNS primarily by activating the μ receptors, while weakly activating the kappa (κ) receptors. Analgesia, respiratory depression, euphoria, and sedation are effects of μ activation, while activation of κ receptors leads to only to analgesia and sedation. Opioids suppress respiration and coughing by acting on the respiratory and cough centers in the medulla of the brainstem. Most opioids, with the exception of meperidine (Demerol), have an antitussive effect.

Prescription Considerations

Use with caution in persons with renal or hepatic involvement, respiratory disease, increased intracranial pressure, altered level of consciousness, or history of substance abuse/addiction. Individualize the dosing regimen based on the patient's needs. Do not use codeine (pain or cough) or tramadol (pain) in children under 12 years of age. Meperidine is also not recommended for use in children due to increased risk for neurotoxicity. Note: the FDA prohibits prescription of codeine- and hydrocodone-containing cough and cold medicines in children younger than 18 years of age, as their safety risks outweigh the potential benefits in this age group.

Side Effects/Adverse Effects

In addition to sedation, euphoria, and analgesia, use of opioid analgesics may also result in itching, constipation, urinary retention, tremor, and weakness. Usage may lead to respiratory/cardiac arrest, coma, or physical dependence. Withdrawal symptoms may occur if medication is stopped abruptly following long-term use. Transdermal fentanyl may cause a local reaction of erythema, irritation, and pain.

Education

- Opioids taken with kava kava, valerian root, and St. John's wort may increase sedation
- Do not operate machinery or make important decisions when initially starting an opioid medication, in order to determine the extent of its effect first
- Maintain a high-fiber diet with adequate hydration in order to combat the constipating effects

Adjuvant Medications

The purpose of adjuvant medications is to enhance analgesic efficiency of opioid and non-opioid medications, potentially allowing for a decrease in the amount of pain medication required with an increase in pain control. Acting as synergists to analgesics, they are also used to treat symptoms that might exacerbate pain, reduce side effects common to analgesics, as well as provide analgesia for specific types of pain.

Mechanism of Action

- **Tricyclic antidepressants:** direct analgesic effect, enhances opioids, elevates mood by increasing concentrations of serotonin/norepinephrine at synapses and inhibiting their reuptake
- **Anticonvulsants:** suppress spontaneous nerve stimuli

Medication	Indication	Prescription considerations	Side effects/adverse effects
Tricyclic antidepressants amitriptyline, doxepin, imipramine, nortriptyline	Neuropathic pain	• Start with a low dose and increase slowly to avoid adverse effects • Taper the dosage to discontinue • Do not use with recent/concurrent MAO inhibitors	• Side effects: blurred vision, constipation, nausea/vomiting, dry mouth, urinary retention, sedation, increased appetite leading to weight gain, confusion, sexual dysfunction, diaphoresis, and tremor • Adverse effects: cardiac arrhythmia, delirium, decreased seizure threshold
Anticonvulsants carbamazepine, gabapentin, lorazepam, phenytoin, topiramate	• Neuropathic pain • topiramate also used for migraine prophylaxis	• Use caution with patients on high doses of opioids and in patients with liver or kidney disease • lorazepam may cause profound sedation and respiratory depression when used with opioids, and is contraindicated in acute narrow angle glaucoma	• Side effects: sedation, dizziness, confusion, nausea/vomiting, constipation, urinary retention, vision issues (topiramate) • Adverse effects: Stevens-Johnson syndrome, suicidal thoughts

Table 4.10.7 Adjuvant Medications

See Chapter 4, Lesson 11, for additional information regarding anticonvulsants and Chapter 12, Lesson 3, for tricyclic antidepressants.

Education

- Avoid alcohol intake with tricyclic antidepressants and anticonvulsants
- Take regularly and do not stop abruptly
- It may take several weeks to reach maximum effectiveness

Takeaways

- Avoid the use of aspirin in children due to the risk of Reye syndrome.
- NSAIDs often negatively affect the GI tract and can also prolong bleeding.
- DMARDs place the patient at risk for serious infection.
- Acetaminophen has an analgesic, but not an anti-inflammatory, effect.
- Opioid use should be prescribed with caution/reserved for moderate to severe pain.

LESSON 11: NEUROLOGIC

Learning Objectives

■ Demonstrate knowledge of medications associated with treatment of neurological disorders

■ Identify safe prescribing practices associated with neurological medications

Note: the tables below offer truncated drug profiles and do not cover all medications in each category. For complete drug information, consult a medication manual.

Medications affecting the central nervous system (CNS) modify a portion of the neurotransmission process. They may exert an effect on a neurotransmitter's release, production, or storage, or they may act to block or activate postsynaptic receptors. CNS medications include antiepileptic medications, sedatives/hypnotics, psychotropic medications, and medications used for the treatment of headaches, neurogenerative disorders, and substance abuse. Opioids are discussed in *Chapter 4, Lesson 10. See Chapter 12, Lessons 2 and 3*, for information related to selective serotonin reuptake inhibitors (SSRIs) and serotonin-norepinephrine reuptake inhibitors (SNRIs). For atypical antidepressants, tricyclic antidepressants, and serotonin modulators, *see Chapter 12, Lesson 3*. Mood stabilizers and first/second generation antipsychotics are discussed in *Chapter 12, Lesson 5. See Chapter 12, Lesson 7*, for information on medications used to treat attention deficit hyperactivity disorder (stimulants, non-stimulants, and alpha 2 agonists).

Antiepileptic Medications

Choice of antiepileptic medication is dependent upon seizure classification, characteristics of the drug, and variables such as patient age, lifestyle, preference, and comorbid conditions. Major considerations are patient characteristics and drug toxicity. Faster drug absorption times, higher peak medication concentrations, and more rapid clearing of antiepileptic drugs in pediatric patients leads to an increase in adverse effects and less effective seizure control in this population. Monotherapy is preferred in both children and adults when it is successful at reducing seizure episodes.

Mechanism of Action

Antiepileptic medications achieve seizure reduction through:

- Blocking sodium or calcium voltage-gated channels
- Inhibiting excitatory glutamate transmission
- Improving inhibitory γ-aminobutyric acid (GABA) impulses

Medication	Indication	Prescribing considerations	Side effects/adverse effects
carbamazepine (Tegretol)	Focal or generalized seizures, bipolar disorder, chronic pain syndromes, mood management	• Measure serum level at 3, 6, and 9 weeks • Use with caution in the elderly, Asian, and those with a history of blood dyscrasia • Contraindicated with TCAs or MAOI use past 14 days • Therapeutic level: 4–12 mcg/mL • Many drugs affect serum concentration	• Side effects: hyponatremia, fluid retention, nausea, vomiting, diarrhea, rash, pruritus • Adverse effects: blurred/double vision, lethargy, headache, drowsiness, dizziness, blood dyscrasia, Stevens-Johnson syndrome (SJS), toxic epidermal necrolysis (TEN)
gabapentin (Neurontin, Gralise)	Refractory focal seizures, peripheral neuropathy	Cautious use with opioids, benzodiazepines, and in persons with renal disease	• Side effects: sedation, dizziness, ataxia, weight gain • Adverse effects: abnormal thinking, emotional lability
lamotrigine (Lamictal)	Focal, generalized, or mixed seizure disorders, severe seizures	• Extended release formulation provides more stable serum concentrations • Drug levels increased with concomitant valproic acid, decreased with numerous drugs • Excreted in breast milk • Titrate dose up slowly to avoid rash	• Side effects: rash, nausea • Adverse effects: dizziness, somnolence, angioedema, increased risk in children of SJS and TEN
levetiracetam (Keppra)	Variety of seizures	Metabolism independent of CYP system (fewer drug interactions)	• Side effects: nausea, fatigue, dizziness, headache, respiratory infection • Adverse effects: diplopia, somnolence, SJS, non-psychotic behavioral disturbance, anaphylaxis, angioedema
phenobarbital (Luminal)	Focal and generalized seizures, status epilepticus	• Use with caution if acute/chronic pain or current alcohol use • Reduces effects of hormonal conception • Check serum concentration 3–4 weeks after initiation • Therapeutic serum concentration: 10–40 mcg/mL • Avoid use in pregnancy • Schedule IV drug	• Side effects: sedation, marked excitement, depression, confusion, nausea, vomiting • Adverse effects: CNS and respiratory depression, apnea, circulatory collapse

Table 4.11.1 Antiepileptic Medications

Medication	Indication	Prescribing considerations	Side effects/adverse effects
phenytoin (Dilantin)	Focal and generalized seizures, status epilepticus	• Broad spectrum CYP inducer (numerous drug interactions) • Therapeutic serum concentration: 10–20 mcg/mL • Bioavailability differs between brands • Supplement with folic acid to decrease gingival hypertrophy	• Side effects: gingival hypertrophy, hirsutism, rash, decreased bone density • Adverse effects: confusion, slurred speech, diplopia, ataxia
topiramate (Topamax)	Focal and other seizures, migraine prevention	• Reduces effects of hormonal conception • Measure serum bicarb at initiation and every 2–4 months • Avoid use in pregnancy (birth defects)	• Side effects: weight loss, decreased sweating, metabolic acidosis • Adverse effects: impaired cognition and expressive language, acute myopia, secondary angle glaucoma
valproic Acid (Depakote)	Generalized and focal seizures, status epilepticus, manic depression, migraine prevention	• Inhibits CYP system (numerous drug interactions) • Avoid use in pregnancy (multiple fetal ill effects) • Monitor liver function tests • Recommended serum concentration for epilepsy: 50–100 mcg/mL	• Side effects: nausea, vomiting, easy bruising, hair loss, tremor, weight gain • Adverse effects: insulin resistance, metabolic syndrome, thrombocytopenia, pancreatitis

Table 4.11.1 Antiepileptic Medications (Continued)

> **Pro Tip**
>
> Individuals developing a rash with carbamazepine are more likely to develop one with lamotrigine, phenytoin, phenobarbital, or oxcarbazepine (Trileptal), and vice versa.

Education

- Avoid abrupt withdrawal of antiepileptic medication (keep track of supply/refills to avoid running out of drug)
- Continue medication even when seizures subside
- Notify provider prior to starting other medications

Sedatives/Hypnotics

Mechanism of Action

The barbiturates and benzodiazepines selectively enhance GABAergic transmission. Benzodiazepines have an effect on the brain's limbic system, reducing anxiety at lower doses and causing sedation/hypnosis at higher doses. Barbiturates have extensive neuronal effects, resulting in a calming effect and reduced excitement at lower doses and hypnosis at higher doses. The non-benzodiazepine sedatives selectively bind to benzodiazepine receptors, yielding sedation.

Medication	Indication	Prescribing considerations	Side effects/adverse effects
Barbiturates Short-acting: amobarbital (Amytal), butalbital (Fioricet, Fiorinal), pentobarbital (Nembutal), secobarbital (Seconal) Ultra-short-acting: thiopental (Pentothal)	Anxiety, sedation, hypnosis, insomnia, headache (butalbital)	• Multiple drug interactions • Contraindicated in hepatic impairment, dyspnea, airway obstruction, and porphyria	• Side effects: headache, confusion, bradycardia, hypotension, respiratory depression, impaired concentration • Adverse effects: angioedema, tolerance, physical dependence, severe withdrawal symptoms
Benzodiazepines alprazolam (Xanax), clonazepam (Klonopin), diazepam (Valium), flurazepam (Dalmane), lorazepam (Ativan)	Anxiety, sleep disorders, skeletal muscle spasms (diazepam)	Use cautiously in hepatic impairment, and concomitantly with alcohol and other CNS depressants	• Side effects: drowsiness, confusion, ataxia • Adverse effects: dependence withdrawal seizures
Non-benzodiazepine sedatives eszopiclone (Lunesta), zolpidem (Ambien, Zolpimist), zaleplon (Sonata)	Insomnia	Side effects may be more pronounced in the elderly	Side effects: headache, GI upset, dizziness, daytime drowsiness, amnesia, complex sleep related behavior, lethargy, palpitations

Table 4.11.2 Sedatives/Hypnotics

Education

- Avoid using alcohol while taking a sedative/hypnotic medication
- Do not abruptly stop long-term use of barbiturates or benzodiazepines
- There is a risk of impaired driving the morning after taking these medicines

Medications for Headaches

Headaches are generally managed with acetaminophen or nonsteroidal anti-inflammatory drugs (*see Chapter 4, Lesson 10*). However, cluster and migraine headaches often need further management. Migraines may be prevented via the use of beta-blockers, tricyclic antidepressants, anticonvulsants, or calcium-channel blockers. The addition of caffeine to NSAIDs, opioids, or ergotamine may increase the medications' efficacy in treating headaches.

Mechanism of Action

The triptans act as serotonin agonists on small peripheral nerves innervating the intracranial vasculature. This results in vasoconstriction and reduction of neurogenic inflammation. Ergots act on 5-HT receptors to produce vasoconstriction.

Medication	Indication	Prescribing considerations	Side effect/adverse effects
Triptans sumatriptan (Imitrex), rizatriptan (Maxalt), zolmitriptan (Zomig), frovatriptan (Frova)	Acute migraine treatment	• Cardiac evaluation prior to administration in persons with risk factors for coronary artery disease • Contraindicated in history of stroke or arrhythmia • Cautious use in elderly • Multiple drug interactions	• Side effects: dizziness, malaise, and elevated blood pressure • Adverse effects: cardiac events, pain or pressure in chest/neck/throat/jaw
Ergots dihydroergotamine (Migranal), ergotamine (Cafergot)	Acute migraine and cluster headache treatment	• Contraindicated in angina, peripheral vascular disease, and pregnancy • Multiple drug interactions • ergotamine can result in dependence and rebound headaches • dihydroergotamine is for severe migraine cases only • **Black box warning**: do not give with macrolide antibiotics, 3A4 inhibitors, or protease inhibitors because of risk of peripheral ischemia	• Side effects: nausea, vomiting, transient tachycardia, and bradycardia • Adverse effects: chest pain, muscle pain, and seizures

Table 4.11.3 Headache Medications

Medications Used in the Treatment of Substance Abuse

Certain medications may be useful in the treatment of substance abuse of nicotine, opioids, and alcohol.

Medication	Mechanism of action and indication	Prescribing considerations	Side effects/adverse effects
bupropion hydrochloride (Zyban)	• Not clearly understood for nicotine withdrawal, bupropion inhibits the reuptake of dopamine, norepinephrine, and serotonin in the central nervous system • Nicotine withdrawal with smoking cessation	• Contraindicated in seizure disorders, anorexia nervosa, and bulimia • Do not use if abrupt discontinuation of antiepileptic drugs, barbiturates, benzodiazepines, or alcohol • Monitor for suicidal ideations	• Side effects: dry mouth, nausea, insomnia, dizziness, abdominal pain, agitation, palpitations, sweating, myalgia, anorexia, urinary frequency, rash • Adverse effects: seizures
varenicline (Chantix)	• Blocks and agonizes alpha-4-beta-2 nicotinic acetylcholine receptors • Decreases cravings for nicotine during smoking cessation	• Encourage patients to set quit date and start med 1 week prior to quit date • Initial treatment is for 12 weeks and medication is available in a starting pack (increasing dose) and continuing pack (consistent dose) • Caution if history of seizures, mental illness, CV disease, or alcohol use	• Side effects: photosensitivity, abnormal dreams, fatigue, headache, insomnia, appetite changes • Adverse effects: suicidal ideation, change in behavior, depression, MI, renal failure, CVA, hypokalemia, arrhythmias

Table 4.11.4 Medications for Substance Abuse Treatment

Medication	Mechanism of action and indication	Prescribing considerations	Side effects/adverse effects
disulfiram (Antabuse)	• Blocks the oxidation of alcohol at the acetaldehyde stage, resulting in significantly uncomfortable symptoms if alcohol is consumed • Used for post-withdrawal treatment of alcoholism	• Do not administer if alcohol consumed within prior 12 hours • Contraindicated in coronary occlusion and severe myocardial disease	• Side effects: drowsiness, fatigue, headache, rash • Adverse effects: optic neuritis, hepatitis, liver failure
methadone (Methadose, Dolophine)	• Binds to opiate receptors in the central nervous system, altering pain perception and response • Used for detoxification and maintenance of opioid addiction treatment	• Avoid concomitant use with cytochrome 450P inhibitors, benzodiazepines, and CNS depressants • Schedule C-II • Multiple drug interactions	• Side effects: cardiac arrhythmias, agitation, confusion, headache, GI upset • Adverse effects: dependence, respiratory depression, prolonged Q-T interval, seizure, severe hypotension
naltrexone (Vivitrol)	• Competitive antagonist at opioid receptor sites and modifies the hypothalamus-pituitary-adrenal axis to suppress alcohol consumption • Used for the treatment of alcohol and opioid dependence	• Do not start until off other opioids for 7 days, if fails naloxone challenge, or if urine positive for opioids • Monitor for suicidal ideation	• Side effects: syncope, headache, insomnia, dizziness, GI upset • Adverse effects: eosinophilic pneumonia, suicidal thoughts

Table 4.11.4 Medications for Substance Abuse Treatment (Continued)

Education

- Bupropion and varenicline may be taken for one week prior to smoking cessation
- Do not consume alcohol or medications containing alcohol while taking disulfiram
- Methadone should not be stopped abruptly
- Treatment for addiction is multidisciplinary; encourage patients to keep follow-up appointments for counseling and support groups

Medications Used with Neurodegenerative Disorders

Neurodegenerative disorders such as Parkinson's disease (PD), Alzheimer's disease, amyotrophic lateral sclerosis (ALS), and Huntington's disease may not be cured, but medications may palliate the symptoms, prolong survival, and slow progression of the disease.

Medication	Mechanism of action and indication	Prescribing considerations	Side effects/adverse effects
Dopamine agonists pramipexole (Mirapex), ropinirole (Requip), rotigotine (Neupro)	• Stimulates dopamine receptors to treat motor features of PD • Used if early Parkinson's disease and sleep-related movement disorders	May delay the need to use levodopa in early PD	• Side effects: orthostatic hypotension, sleepiness, confusion, nausea, vomiting, hallucinations • Adverse effects: sleep attacks
carbidopa-levodopa (Sinemet)	• carbidopa inhibits the breakdown of levodopa (a metabolic precursor of dopamine), allowing conversion to dopamine by striatal enzymes • Used for bradykinetic symptoms of PD	Start with small (partial tablet) doses and titrate upwards as tolerated	• Side effects: nausea, somnolence, dizziness, headache • Adverse effects: dyskinesia, dystonia, elevated homocysteine levels associated with increased hip fracture risk
Acetylcholinesterase inhibitors donepezil (Aricept), galantamine (Razadyne), rivastigmine (Exelon)	• Inhibits acetylcholinesterase, resulting in a modest decrease in the rate of cognitive decline • Used for Alzheimer disease	• Use with caution in cardiac conduction disorders, seizure disorder, hepatic or renal impairment, PUD, COPD, and asthma • When converting to extended release, the evening immediate release dose should be taken; then start extended release dose the next morning (same total dose per day)	• Side effects: bradycardia, tremors, nausea, diarrhea, vomiting, anorexia, muscle cramps • Adverse effects: CNS depression, SJS
NMDA receptor antagonist memantine (Namenda)	• Antagonizes NMDA receptors, resulting in a modest decrease in the rate of cognitive decline • Used for moderate to severe Alzheimer's disease	Use with caution in cardiovascular disease, seizure disorder, hepatic or renal impairment	• Side effects: confusion, agitation, and restlessness • Adverse effects: prolonged Q-T interval
riluzole (Rilutek)	• Inhibits glutamate release and blocks sodium channels to prolong survival in ALS • Used for ALS	• Use with caution in hepatic impairment • Monitor LFTs in the first 3 months	• Side effects: nausea, weakness • Adverse effects: angioedema, anaphylaxis, cardiac failure, arrhythmia, CNS depression, neutropenia
tetrabenazine (Xenazine)	• Inhibits human vesicular monoamine transporter type 2, to improve movement disorders • Used for Huntington chorea	• Contraindicated in hepatic impairment • Multiple drug interactions • Monitor closely for signs of depression	• Side effects: sedation, fatigue, nausea, upper respiratory infection • Adverse effects: depression, suicidal ideation, extrapyramidal reactions

Table 4.11.5 Medications for Neurogenerative Disorders

Education

- Do not stop dopamine agonists or levodopa preparations abruptly, as akinetic crisis may occur
- Take levodopa with a meal or snack to decrease incidence of nausea
- Medications for Alzheimer disease will not cure it, but may lessen the rate of cognitive decline
- Take riluzole at the same time daily, one hour before or two hours after a meal
- When taking tetrabenazine, use caution when performing actions requiring mental alertness

Takeaways

- Many medications for neurological disorders have interactions with multiple other drugs.
- Antiepileptics, barbiturates, benzodiazepines, methadone, dopamine agonists, and levodopa preparations should not be stopped abruptly.

LESSON 12: OTC MEDICATIONS

Learning Objectives

■ Understand the action, indications, contraindications, side effects, and interactions of common over-the-counter (OTC) medications

■ Develop a teaching strategy for discussing various OTC medications with patients

Note: the tables below offer truncated drug profiles and do not cover all medications in each category. For complete drug information, consult a medication manual.

An OTC medication can be purchased by the public without having a prescription and has been deemed safe to use by the Food and Drug Administration (FDA) without seeing a healthcare provider. There are approximately 80 classes of OTC medications. With the rising cost of healthcare, patients are more likely to self-treat with OTC meds prior to seeking care. It is imperative to question OTC and herbal medication use when taking a medication history.

The following classes of OTC medications are frequently encountered in family practice:

- Analgesics/antipyretics
- Cold and sinus medications: antihistamines, decongestants, antitussives, expectorants, and nasal steroids
- Gastrointestinal medications: antidiarrheals, antiflatulants, antinausea, antireflux, and anti-constipation meds
- Genitourinary/gynecological medications: antifungal, urinary analgesics
- Antiparasitic: lice preparations, pinworm treatment
- Topical medications: acne preparations (*see the remaining topical medications in Chapter 16, Lesson 2*)

Pro Tip

Ginkgo, ginger, and garlic can increase bleeding risk by interacting with antiplatelet drugs to inhibit platelet aggregation and fibrinolysis, whereas ginseng reduces the anticoagulant effect of warfarin, increasing the patient's risk for a clotting event.

A thorough review of medical diagnoses, prescription, and OTC medications, as well as all supplements, is absolutely critical.

Analgesics/Antipyretics

NSAIDs—Salicylates

Mechanism of Action

Salicylates inhibit cyclooxygenase, which is required to synthesize prostaglandins and metabolites of arachidonic acid in the central nervous system and peripheral nervous system. Prostaglandins and metabolites of arachidonic acid work in the inflammatory response, cause fever, and increase the response of pain receptors.

NSAIDs—Nonacetylated Salicylates

Mechanism of Action

Nonacetylated salicylates have the same action as salicylates, except there is little to no effect on platelet aggregation.

Other—Acetaminophen

Mechanism of Action

Acetaminophen inhibits synthesis of prostaglandins, primarily in the central nervous system. Because of its limited action in the peripheral nervous system, acetaminophen does not cause gastric irritation, renal failure, or Reye syndrome, or alter platelet aggregation.

Examples	Indications	Prescription considerations	Side effects/adverse effects
salicylate aspirin (ASA)	Fever (adults only), pain, inflammation	• Used for cardiac risk reduction because it suppresses platelet aggregation • Caution when prescribing other NSAIDs and steroids	• Side effects: nausea, vomiting • Adverse effects: gastrointestinal bleeding, kidney failure, increased risk of bleeding
nonacetylated salicylate ibuprofen (Advil, Motrin) naproxen sodium (Aleve)	Fever, pain, inflammation	• Caution when prescribing other NSAIDs and steroids • Do not use in infants <6 months of age	• Side effects: nausea, vomiting • Adverse effects: gastrointestinal bleeding, kidney failure
acetaminophen (Tylenol)	Fever, pain	• Can prescribe other NSAIDs when a patient takes acetaminophen • Adults should not exceed 3000 mg daily • Safe for use during pregnancy	• Side effects: nausea, headache, rash • Adverse effects: liver failure

Table 4.12.1 NSAIDs

Education

- Emphasize that many OTC medications fall into this class and not to take more than one type of OTC pain reliever or fever reducer
- Teach your patient signs of gastrointestinal bleeding (dark/tarry stool, nausea, vomiting, new heartburn) and to report these immediately

- Teach parents not to give aspirin to children with a fever because of the risk of Reye syndrome
- Avoid alcohol while taking acetaminophen
- Patients with a history of MI or CVA should avoid nonacetylated salicylates

Cold and Sinus Medications

Antihistamines (1st and 2nd Generation)

Mechanism of Action
- **1st generation antihistamines:** nonselectively antagonize central and peripheral histamine H1 receptors
- **2nd generation antihistamines:** selectively antagonize peripheral histamine H1 receptors

Decongestants

Mechanism of Action
Decongestants stimulate alpha 1-adrenergic receptors and cause vasoconstriction.

Antitussives

Mechanism of Action
Antitussive medications suppress the cough center in the medulla.

Expectorants

Mechanism of Action
Expectorants decrease the viscosity of secretions in the respiratory tract and increase those secretions.

Nasal Corticosteroids

Mechanism of Action
Nasal corticosteroids inhibit inflammatory cytokines.

Examples	Indications	Prescription considerations	Side effects/adverse effects
Antihistamines • **1st generation:** diphenhydramine (Benadryl), chlorpheniramine • **2nd generation:** fexofenadine (Allegra), cetirizine (Zyrtec), loratadine (Claritin)	Allergic rhinitis, runny nose, allergic reaction	• Risk of drowsiness with 1st generation; caution when prescribing medications that can worsen this effect • Safe for use during pregnancy (2nd generation preferred in breastfeeding) • Patients with renal impairment should use with caution (2nd generation)	• Side effects: drowsiness (1st gen), dry mucous membranes (1st and 2nd gen) • Adverse effects: increased intraocular pressure, urinary retention (1st gen)

Table 4.12.2 Cold and Sinus Medications

Examples	Indications	Prescription considerations	Side effects/adverse effects
Decongestants phenylephrine (Sudafed PE Congestion), pseudoephedrine (Sudafed Congestion)	Nasal congestion	• Contraindicated with MAO inhibitors • pseudoephedrine is an ingredient used in making methamphetamine; the Combat Methamphetamine Epidemic Act of 2005 limits the amount of pseudoephedrine a person can buy in a day and within 30 days • Use with caution with the following: HTN, glaucoma, PBH, renal impairment, seizure disorder	• Side effects: CNS stimulation, insomnia, headache • Adverse effects: elevated HR, BP
Antitussives dextromethorphan (Robitussin Lingering Cold, Long Acting Cough)	Cough	• Contraindicated with MAO inhibitors • When taken in quantities greater than recommended and by alternate routes, it can cause slurred speech, hallucinations, and disassociation (similar to PCP and ketamine); abuse potential • Serotonin syndrome potential with SSRIs/SNRIs or triptans • Safe to use during pregnancy	• Side effects: nausea, dizziness, fatigue, drowsiness • Adverse effects: serotonin syndrome, abuse potential
Expectorants guaifenesin (Mucinex)	Cough	Safe to use during pregnancy	• Side effects: nausea, vomiting, rash • Adverse effects: nephrolithiasis
Nasal corticosteroids • fluticasone propionate (Flonase) • triamcinolone (Nasacort) • budesonide (Rhinocort)	Allergic rhinitis	• Avoid use if exposure to measles, varicella, or tuberculosis • Avoid with nasal septal ulcers, nasal surgery, or nasal trauma d/t delayed wound healing • Caution if cataracts, increased intraocular pressure, or glaucoma	• Side effects: headache, epistaxis, cough, nasal or oral candidiasis, nasal burning/irritation/ulcer • Adverse effects: glaucoma, cataracts, adrenal suppression, immunosuppression (all with long-term use); pediatric patients: Cushing syndrome, reduction of growth velocity with long-term use

Table 4.12.2 Cold and Sinus Medications (Continued)

Education

- Many OTC cold and sinus medications contain multiple ingredients; choose one cold and sinus remedy and do not mix with others
- If hypertensive, avoid any decongestants and multi-symptom cold and sinus medications
- The FDA recommends avoiding decongestant and antihistamine use in children <2 years old, and recommends using cough/cold medicine products cautiously in children >2 years of age
- Advise parents of adolescents of potential for abuse of dextromethorphan

Gastrointestinal Medications

Antidiarrheal Medications

Mechanism of Action
- **Loperamide:** binds to opiate receptors of gut wall to inhibit peristalsis
- **Bismuth subsalicylate:** absorbs fluids and electrolytes via intestinal wall (antisecretory action) and inhibits prostaglandin action to decrease intestinal wall inflammation

Examples	Prescription considerations	Side effects/adverse effects
loperamide (Imodium)	• Advise against use with bloody or infectious diarrhea • Not for use in children <2 years of age • Avoid higher than recommended dose d/t risk of serious cardiac events	• Side effects: fatigue, dizziness, constipation, nausea, abdominal cramps • Adverse effects: paralytic ileus, urinary retention
bismuth subsalicylate (Pepto-Bismol)	• Advise against use with bloody diarrhea or history of ulcer • Do not use in febrile children (risk of Reye syndrome) • Stop use if abdominal pain worsens • Consult provider if diarrhea lasts >2 days	Adverse effects: black hairy tongue, GI bleeding

Table 4.12.3 Antidiarrheal Medications

Antinausea Medication

Mechanism of Action
Depresses labyrinthine function, diminishes vestibular stimulation, and competes with H1 receptors in GI and respiratory tracts and blood vessels.

Examples	Prescription considerations	Side effects/adverse effects
dimenhydrinate (Dramamine)	Use with caution in lactating women and older adults	Side effects: decreased mental alertness, drowsiness, urinary retention, blurry vision

Table 4.12.4 Antinausea Medication

Antireflux Medications

Mechanism of Action

- **H2-receptor antagonist (H2RA):** selectively antagonizes histamine H2 receptor (located on parietal cells of stomach), suppressing gastric acid secretion; histamine is the primary mediator of the basal rate of acid release during non-feeding periods; blocking acid releases during the night, which is especially important and is the rationale for the dosing of H2RAs at bedtime

- **Proton pump inhibitor (PPI):** inhibits hydrogen potassium ATPase (gastric acid production) and suppresses gastric acid secretion; PPIs may also be used in combination with antibiotics for the treatment of *H. pylori*

- **Antacids:** alkaline substances that neutralize acids by raising the pH to approximately 7.5 and inhibiting conversion of pepsinogen to pepsin; differ in acid neutralizing capacity (ANC), duration, and onset; these have largely been replaced by PPI and H2RA

  - **Calcium carbonate:** high ANC, rapid onset, long duration

  - **Aluminum hydroxide:** low ANC, slow onset, long duration

  - **Magnesium hydroxide:** high ANC, rapid onset, long duration

  - **Sodium bicarbonate:** low ANC, rapid onset, short duration

Examples	Prescription considerations	Side effects/adverse effects
H2 blockers • cimetidine (Tagamet) • famotidine (Pepcid) • ranitidine (Zantac)	• If taken long-term, monitor CBC, creatinine, B12 • Can interfere with the absorption of some medications and B12	• Side effects: headache, diarrhea, dizziness, nausea, vomiting, confusion, rash, increased ALT/AST, vitamin B12 deficiency • Adverse effects: aplastic anemia, neutropenia, thrombocytopenia, agranulocytosis, hallucinations, psychosis
PPI • omeprazole (Prilosec) • esomeprazole (Nexium)	• If taken long-term, monitor magnesium level, B12 • Controversy exists over appropriateness of long-term use • Can interfere with the absorption of some medications and B12	• Side effects: headache, nausea, vomiting, diarrhea, low B12 • Adverse effects: hypomagnesemia, pancreatitis, blood dyscrasias, fractures, Stevens-Johnson syndrome
Antacids • calcium carbonate: $CaCO_3$ (TUMS) • aluminum hydroxide: $Al(OH)_3$ (Gaviscon ES) • magnesium hydroxide: $Mg(OH)_2$ (Milk of Magnesia); also used as a laxative • sodium bicarbonate: $NaCO_2$ (Alka Seltzer—sodium bicarb in combo with citric acid)	• Calcium carbonate can worsen or precipitate nephrolithiasis • OTC preparations often in combination of antacids • Can impair absorption of co-administered medications • Check electrolytes with long-term use	Side effects: • calcium carbonate: nausea, constipation • aluminum hydroxide: constipation, abdominal pain, hypophosphatemia • magnesium hydroxide: diarrhea, abdominal pain, nausea • sodium bicarbonate: diarrhea, edema, nausea, vomiting, hypernatremia Adverse effects: • calcium carbonate: hypercalcemia, hypophosphatemia, dehydration, renal impairment • aluminum hydroxide: aluminum intoxication, osteomalacia, encephalopathy • magnesium hydroxide: hypermagnesemia • sodium bicarbonate: CHF exacerbation, seizures, metabolic alkalosis

Table 4.12.5 Antireflux Medications

Anti-Constipation Medications

Mechanism of Action

- **Bulk-forming laxatives:** increase stool bulk by increasing water absorption, thereby increasing peristalsis
- **Lubricant laxatives:** soften and lubricate stool facilitating passage
- **Osmotic laxatives:** stool retains water, which softens stool; swelling of stool increases peristalsis
- **Stimulant laxatives:** stimulate peristalsis
- **Stool softeners:** increase water and electrolyte secretion into intestine
- **Enema:** increases fluid in the large intestine, leading to stool evacuation

Examples	Prescription considerations	Side effects/adverse effects
Bulk-forming laxatives • methylcellulose (Citrucel) • psyllium (Metamucil)	Contraindicated if acute abdomen or bowel obstruction, impaction	• Side effects: nausea, diarrhea, abdominal cramps; psyllium (constipation, bronchospasm) • Adverse effects: none reported
Lubricant laxatives mineral oil: PO or enema	Contraindicated if acute abdomen	• Side effects: nausea, vomiting, abdominal cramps, rectal pruritis, abdominal cramps • Adverse effects: none reported
Osmotic laxatives • magnesium citrate • magnesium hydroxide (Milk of Magnesia, Pedia-Lax chewable tablet) • polyethylene glycol 3350 (Miralax)	• Contraindicated if acute abdomen • Caution if obstruction or with prescription meds that can affect fluid and electrolyte balance	• Side effects: abdominal cramping, diarrhea • Adverse effects: electrolyte disturbances, dehydration, hypotension, laxative dependence; magnesium hydroxide can cause hypermagnesemia
Stimulant laxatives • bisacodyl: PO or suppository (Dulcolax) • sennosides (Senokot)	• Contraindicated if acute abdomen • Caution if gastroenteritis, rectal bleeding, obstruction • Caution with prescription meds than can affect fluid and electrolyte balance	• Side effects: nausea, vomiting, abdominal cramps, abdominal distention, flatulence • Adverse effects: electrolyte disturbance, laxative dependence, laxative abuse
Stool softener docusate sodium (Dulcolax, Colace)	• Contraindicated if acute abdomen • Caution if obstruction, impaction	• Side effects: diarrhea, abdominal cramps • Adverse effects: none reported
sodium phosphate enema (Fleet)	• Do not use >1 enema per 24 hours • Use pedi-fleet for age 5–11 years, 1/2 pedi-fleet age 2–4 years • Do not use in children <2 years of age	• Side effects: bloating, abdominal pain • Adverse effects: fluid and electrolyte imbalances, kidney or heart damage (typically in overdose or patients with underlying kidney dysfunction/CHF), allergic reaction

Table 4.12.6 Laxatives

Pro Tip

Bulk-forming laxatives are first-line treatment for constipation: they are not systemically absorbed and are typically well-tolerated.

CHAPTER 4 | **PHARMACOLOGY OVERVIEW**

Antiflatulant Medications

Mechanism of Action
Antiflatulant medications change the surface tension of gas bubbles in the GI tract.

Examples	Prescription considerations	Side effects/adverse effects
simethicone (Gas-X)	Contraindicated if GI obstruction or perforation	• Side effects: diarrhea, nausea • Adverse effects: none reported

Table 4.12.7 Antiflatulent Medications

Antiparasitic Medications

Mechanism of Action
Oral antiparasitic medications cause paralysis of the worm by acting as a neuromuscular blockade.

Examples	Indication	Prescription considerations	Side effects/adverse effects
pyrantel (Pin-X)	Pinworm infection	• Dose may be repeated in 2 weeks • All family members should be treated	• Side effects: nausea, vomiting, headache, abdominal cramps, diarrhea, anorexia • Adverse effects: none reported

Table 4.12.8 Antiparasitic Medications

Education
- Advise to seek medical care for prolonged use of antacids
- Discuss laxative abuse potential with parents of adolescents that are high-risk for eating disorders
- Educate about normal bowel function to prevent overuse of laxatives
- Inform of potential for dependence on laxatives if long-term use

Topical Medications

Acne Preparations

Mechanism of Action
- **Benzoyl peroxide:** keratinolytic and bactericidal against *Propionibacterium acnes*
- **Salicylic acid (0.5%–2%):** decreases formation of keratin (keratinolytic)

Examples	Indications	Prescription considerations	Side effects/adverse effects
• salicylic acid (Aveeno Clear complexion, Clearasil products) • benzoyl peroxide (Oxy 10)	Acne (salicylic acid and benzoyl peroxide)	Used for mild to moderate acne	• Side effects: irritation, photosensitivity, burning, peeling, itching • Adverse effects: metabolic and respiratory alkalosis, CNS toxicity (salicylic acid)

Table 4.12.9 Topical Medications

Education

- Do not use an occlusive dressing over a topical steroid because of increased absorption; OTC steroids should not be used long term
- Remind patients it is important to report all medications including topical agents

Urinary Analgesic

Mechanism of Action

Phenazopyridine causes local analgesia of the urinary tract when excreted in the urine.

Examples	Indications	Prescription considerations	Side effects/adverse effects
phenazopyridine (AZO Urinary Pain Relief, Uristat)	Dysuria	• Do not use with glomerulonephritis, renal, or hepatic impairment • Will cause nitrate-positive results on urinalysis	• Side effects: headache, pruritis, rash, nausea, anemia, dyspepsia, staining of contact lenses • Adverse effects: anaphylaxis, methemoglobinemia

Table 4.12.10 Urinary Analgesic

Education

- Phenazopyridine will turn urine orange and can possibly stain contact lenses (rare)
- Do not use phenazopyridine for more than 2–3 days

Takeaways

- In addition to knowing all medications a patient is taking (prescription and OTC), it is important to inquire about herbal medications (tablet, teas, etc.).
- Teach patients to read the active ingredient list.
- Many OTC medications have a combination of active ingredients; caution patients about using these medications.

LESSON 13: PRESCRIPTION WRITING

Learning Objectives

- Understand the rules associated with prescribing controlled substances
- Identify the uses and significance of a DEA number
- Recognize and understand the current pregnancy and lactation categories

How to Write a Prescription

Every great nurse knows the "Five Rights" of medication administration: *Patient, Medication, Dose, Route,* and *Time.* Some nurses have added two more "rights," *Reason* and *Documentation,* to preserve and promote patient safety. As a nurse practitioner with prescription writing privileges, use these collective seven "rights" to not only guide the process, but also to evaluate and complete your proposed treatment plan. The steps to writing a prescription are as follows:

Step 1: Chart Review

- Patient's age
- Patient's allergies, with consideration toward possible cross-sensitivities
- Any medical conditions or current medications that may impair or accelerate the absorption of certain medications leading to either a subclinical or toxic effect
- Any medical conditions that put the patient at higher risk for adverse side effects
- If female, the patient's pregnancy or breastfeeding status

Step 2: Write Your Prescription

Include the following:

- Date
- Patient's full name and date of birth (DOB)
- Medication name (generic preferred; must indicate if brand name is to be dispensed)
- Medication strength
- Dosage form
- Directions and implications for use
- Quantity of medication to be dispensed
- Number of refills authorized (if any)

Note: prescriptions may only be typed or written in ink or indelible pencil.

M. Smith, FNP

123 Clinic Street

Anytown, Any State 00000

(555) 555-5555

Jane Doe, DOB: __/__/__

Date: __/__/__

Macrobid 100 mg—1 tablet PO BID × 5 days.

Signature: _____

Quantity: 10   Refills: 0

Step 3: Review Your Treatment Plan

After writing each prescription, review the "seven rights" and confirm that you have written it for the appropriate reason.

> **Pro Tip**
>
> Electronic Medical Record (EMR) systems often allow for more than one patient chart to be open at the same time. Always double-check the name on the chart before signing off on orders; it is very easy to accidentally document on the wrong patient!

Step 4: Sign Your Prescription

- Paper prescriptions for noncontrolled substances may be stamped or signed in ink or indelible pencil
- Prescriptions for noncontrolled substances that are written using EMRs may either be printed, signed, and handed to the patient, or "e-scribed" and electronically signed

Step 5: Document Clearly

Communicate your exam findings and plan through documentation. If a medication or treatment plan needs adjustment, a colleague should be able to do so based on the original plan of care.

Step 6: Follow Up

Not every patient who is prescribed a medication requires follow-up, but many do. This can be achieved through another office visit, a telephone call, or a plan for the patient to notify you if the desired effect is not achieved.

Controlled Substances

Prescriptions of controlled substances are regulated by the United States Drug Enforcement Administration (DEA). The rules are very specific and are designed to protect both the patient and the prescriber. To be valid, a controlled substance must be issued by a registered practitioner providing routine care for a legitimate medical purpose.

When writing a prescription for a controlled substance apply the following rules:

- Prescriptions should include the patient's address, as well as the prescriber's address and DEA number
- A prescription must be physically (not electronically) signed by the prescriber on the same day as it is written
- A person in your office may be designated to prepare your prescription; however, you are the only one allowed to sign it
- Individual states may have additional conditions that must be met for a prescription to be valid; it is up to you to make sure you are following both the federal guidelines and those specific to your state of licensure

Controlled substances are organized into five schedules, or categories, which identify them as being highly addictive or having the potential to lead to abuse based on national statistics. There are further specific rules for prescribing each category of medication.

DEA drug schedule	Definitions *Examples*	Rules for prescribing
I	"Drugs with no currently accepted medical use and a high potential for abuse" *Illegal drugs*	
II	"Drugs with a high potential for abuse, with use potentially leading to severe psychological or physical dependence" *Narcotics, CNS stimulants, medications with <15 mg hydrocodone per dosage unit*	• Must be a written prescription (Rx) with the exception of emergency situations, during which a verbal order may be used • No time limit for when an Rx must be filed after it is signed • There is no federal limit to the quantity of medication that may be prescribed; however, most states limit the quantity to 30 days of treatment • Refills are prohibited; however, you may write up to three separate prescriptions, which would cover up to 90 days of treatment; each prescription should include the earliest date that it may be filled • Rx may be faxed to the pharmacy, but the original Rx must be presented to the pharmacist before the medication is dispensed; 3 exceptions to this rule: (1) narcotics that require compounding for administration via parenteral, IV, SQ, IM, or intraspinal routes, (2) prescriptions for residents living in long-term care facilities, (3) narcotics for patients in a hospice program that is certified and/or paid for by Medicare, or licensed by the individual state • An Rx may be called in to the pharmacy in an emergency; quantity is restricted to the exact amount needed to treat the emergency only; you must submit a signed Rx to the pharmacist within 7 days of the verbal order, and the pharmacy should notify the DEA if it is not received
III	"Drugs with a moderate to low potential for physical and psychological dependence" *Anabolic steroids, butalbital, ketamine, testosterone, medications with less than 90 mg of codeine per dosage unit*	• May be written, faxed, or called in to the pharmacy • May be refilled via written, faxed, or oral communication • Refills are allowed. For schedules III and IV, a new Rx is required after 5 refills or 6 months of treatment
IV	"Drugs with a low potential for abuse and low risk of dependence" *Zolpidem, benzodiazepines, tramadol*	
V	"Drugs with lower potential for abuse than Schedule IV and consist of preparations containing limited quantities of certain narcotics" *Lomotil, Lyrica, liquid medications with <200 mg of codeine per 100 mg*	

Table 4.13.1 DEA Drug Schedules

www.deadiversion.usdoj.gov

Federal DEA Numbers

Outpatient Use

If you desire the ability to prescribe controlled substances, you must first apply for a DEA number or be exempt from registration by regulation. The application Form 224 can be found here: **https://apps.deadiversion.usdoj.gov/webforms/jsp/regapps/common/newAppLogin.jsp**. There is a nonrefundable application fee. Certain states require a second controlled substance license in addition to a DEA number. Please refer to the DEA website for an up-to-date list.

Inpatient Orders

Federal regulations do not require DEA registration for mid-level providers who write inpatient medical orders, as long as the provider is an employee or agent of the hospital. If the provider will be prescribing controlled substances for the discharged patient, DEA registration is required.

Special Populations: Pregnant and Breastfeeding Women

Pregnancy and Lactation Categories

The FDA has recently developed a new way of communicating pregnancy and lactation risk that will replace the existing system of pregnancy categories by 2020 for all medications except for over-the-counter (OTC) drugs. Furthermore, it includes women during labor and delivery under the population of "Pregnancy," changes the name of the category for "Nursing Mothers" to "Lactation," and adds a new category called "Females and Males of Reproductive Potential." Different from the current letter system (A, B, C, D, and X), the new system will include a risk summary for each medication that will specifically denote whether or not the medication has systemic absorption. If a medication does have systemic absorption, the summary will include a statement identifying whether the risk is based on animal or human data.

FDA Pregnancy Categories and Significance until 2020

FDA pregnancy category	Significance
A	• Safe for pregnancy • Human studies show no harm to fetuses
B	• Generally considered safe for pregnancy • Animal studies show no harm • There may not be adequate human studies available to determine risk
C	• Clinician must make an educated decision about whether or not to prescribe this medication • Harm has been noted in animal studies • There are not adequate human studies to prove safety • Benefit may outweigh harm
D	• Generally considered to be unsafe for pregnancy • Harm has been noted in human studies • Benefit may outweigh harm
X	• Unsafe for pregnancy • Known to cause birth defects • Harm outweighs benefits

Table 4.13.2 Current FDA Pregnancy Categories

Digital Resource

Mother to Baby—a service of the Organization of Teratology Information Specialists—creates lists of medications usable during pregnancy and lactation. This information is geared to be provided to patients and is available here: **http://mothertobaby.org/fact-sheets-parent**.

Dr. Thomas W. Hale's book *Medications and Mother's Milk* is a commonly used reference for breastfeeding women. The book's lactation categories are part of regular terminology used to communicate lactation safety.

Dr. Hale's Lactation Categories

Category	Significance
L1	**Safest** • Appears to be no increase in adverse effects • Controlled studies show absence of risk to the infant/possibility of harm unlikely • Not orally bioavailable
L2	**Safer** • Studied in a limited number of breastfeeding women, yet appears to have no increase in adverse effects • Evidence of a related risk associated with the medication is minimal
L3	**Moderately safe** • Absence of controlled studies in breastfeeding women/potential for adverse effects to infant possible • Controlled studies show minimal untoward effects • Benefit must outweigh possible risk
L4	**Possibly hazardous** Evidence of risk exists; however, benefit can outweigh the risk (grave illness or life-threatening situation where safer drugs cannot be used/are ineffective)
L5	**Contraindicated** • Documented risk to the infant • Medication has a significant risk of harm • Risk outweighs any benefit

Table 4.13.3 Dr. Hale's Lactation Categories

App Alert

LactMed is a free mobile app created by the National Institute of Health to aid in the safe prescription of medication to breastfeeding women. The app provides detailed information (if available) on the levels of medication found in both mothers and their breast milk, as well as the potential effects such medication may have on a nursing infant.

Takeaways

- When writing a prescription, consider the "seven rights"; ensure the prescription is written for the appropriate reason.

- DEA guidelines regarding controlled substances are designed to protect both the patient and the prescriber; know the drug schedules.

- When prescribing medications for the pregnant/lactating woman, care must be taken that the drug will pose the least amount of harm to the infant; be aware of the pregnancy and lactation categories.

PRACTICE QUESTIONS

Select the ONE best answer.

Lesson 1: Pharmacology Basics

1. All of the following may affect a drug's absorption except:

   A. Size of the drug molecule

   B. Food in the gut

   C. Available surface area

   D. P450 enzyme system

2. The primary means of medication excretion is through:

   A. The liver

   B. The kidneys

   C. Exhaled air

   D. Sweat from pores

3. Which of the following describes an agonist?

   A. A chemical that has a harder time crossing the blood–brain barrier

   B. A chemical that binds to a receptor and stimulates cellular activity

   C. A chemical that binds to a receptor and blocks or inhibits cellular activity

   D. A chemical that has a longer half-life than a competing chemical

4. Chirality refers to:

   A. The shape of the medication molecule

   B. The shape of a drug receptor

   C. A drug that blocks a matching receptor

   D. A drug that shows affinity for certain receptors

5. The P450 enzyme system affects the way medications are metabolized. Which of the following is an example of the P450 system in action?

   A. The ease that a medication is bound by plasma binding proteins

   B. A bigger molecule having a harder time crossing membranes

   C. Grapefruit juice interacting with a medication's metabolism

   D. The need to lower the dose of a medication because of poor kidney function

Lesson 2: Anti-Infectives

6. An 88-year-old male is being treated for complicated pyelonephritis with gentamicin IM daily. His wife called the office to report that he didn't hear his alarm clock go off this morning. In addition, when their granddaughter called earlier that day, he had to hand the phone to his wife because he couldn't understand what she was saying. Based on this information, you are most concerned about which possible serious adverse effect of gentamicin?

   A. Dementia

   B. Hepatotoxicity

   C. Xerophthalmia

   D. Ototoxicity

7. A 56-year-old male presents to the office as a new patient. When reviewing his medical history you notice "medication-induced tendonitis with subsequent tendon rupture" listed under past problems. Even though he cannot remember the medication, you know that it is a serious adverse effect of which of the following drugs?

   A. ceftriaxone (Rocephin)

   B. ciprofloxacin (Cipro)

   C. darifenacin (Enablex)

   D. phenazopyridine (Pyridium)

8. A 33-year-old female presents to the office with complaints of urinary urgency, frequency, pressure, and dysuria. You would like to prescribe nitrofurantoin (Macrobid) 100 mg PO BID × 5 days for her uncomplicated UTI. Which medical information would cause you to choose a different antibiotic?

   A. She reports bright orange urine after taking Pyridium earlier today

   B. She sometimes takes diphenhydramine to sleep at night

   C. She has a history of an allergic reaction to amoxicillin

   D. She is currently 39 weeks pregnant

9. Edith L. is a 36-year-old pregnant woman who presents at the clinic with symptoms of fever, chills, and body aches. Symptoms started last night, and she tests positive for influenza A. Which of the following would you prescribe?

   A. oseltamivir (Tamiflu)

   B. zanamivir (Relenza)

   C. peramivir (Rapivab)

   D. amantadine (Symmetrel)

10. Phillip R. is a 42-year-old male who presents to the clinic with recurrent genital herpes. Which of the following is recommended for the treatment of genital herpes in this individual?

    A. ganciclovir (Zirgan)

    B. atazanavir (Reyataz)

    C. valacyclovir (Valtrex)

    D. ribavirin (Virazole)

11. Lucas M. is a 65-year-old male who presents with elevated liver enzymes, and further testing indicates he has hepatitis C (HCV). All of the following are true of pharmacologic treatment of HCV except:

    A. Test all patients for evidence of current or prior hepatitis B virus (HBV) infection before initiating treatment with HCV direct acting antivirals

    B. Hepatitis C treatment is generally swift, simple, and straightforward

    C. The most common initial treatments are combination medications based on the genotype of the virus

    D. Patients should be evaluated for co-infection with HIV and the presence of cirrhosis

Lesson 3: Antineoplastics

12. Which is not a mechanism of action of chemotherapy?

    A. Ensuring the RNA inside a cancer cell is unchanged

    B. Cell apoptosis due DNA damage

    C. Destruction of checkpoint proteins

    D. Intervention at some point in the cell life cycle of DNA replication

13. Jennifer P. is a 58-year-old female being treated with cisplatin for breast cancer. The nurse practitioner knows that part of the management plan should include frequent testing of which lab test?

    A. Serum glucose

    B. Complete blood count (CBC)

    C. Urinalysis

    D. Uric acid

14. The following patients are being seen in the oncology clinic: Melissa F., who is receiving whole brain irradiation for metastatic breast cancer; Jason S., who is receiving interferon for Kaposi sarcoma; and Sandra M., who is receiving treatment with cyclophosphamide for ovarian cancer. The nurse practitioner knows that these three patients are at risk for which common side effect?

    A. Increased energy prior to treatment

    B. Insomnia

    C. Tachycardia

    D. Oral candidiasis

15. Which of the following is a chemotherapeutic (anticancer) dosing principle?

    A. Drugs should be administered at low doses but with increased frequency

    B. Drugs are more beneficial if major toxicities are nonoverlapping

    C. Drugs should be administered infrequently to minimize side effects

    D. Drugs are rarely effective in combination

16. Which of the following is an antineoplastic drug that is also used to treat psoriasis and rheumatoid arthritis?

    A. methotrexate (Trexall)

    B. mercaptopurine (Purixan)

    C. allopurinol (Zyloprim)

    D. procarbazine (Matulane)

Lesson 4: Cardiovascular

17. While performing patient education about drug-food interactions, the nurse practitioner cautions a patient to avoid grapefruit juice because he takes which of the following medications?

    A. lisinopril (Zestril)

    B. verapamil (Calan)

    C. warfarin (Coumadin)

    D. timolol (Timoptic)

18. Mrs. K. comes to the clinic because she has experienced nausea, vomiting, and diarrhea for three days. She has lost two pounds. Her medications include rosuvastatin, lisinopril, vitamin D, digoxin, and zolpidem. Which lab is most critical for the nurse practitioner to draw?

    A. Lipid profile

    B. Urinalysis

    C. Vitamin D level

    D. Digoxin level

19. Daria is a 27-year-old female who is being started on propranolol for migraine prophylaxis. In addition, she is taking metformin and glipizide for diabetes. It is important to include what information when teaching her about this new medication?

    A. Signs and symptoms of low blood sugar may not be as apparent

    B. It is okay to stop the propranolol if her migraines don't improve

    C. If a rash occurs, it is a minor side effect and should go away

    D. She should expect her total cholesterol and LDL levels to improve

20. Which patient is a candidate for warfarin (Coumadin) following a diagnosis of DVT?

    A. 45-year-old on irbesartan and fluvastatin

    B. 34-year-old with coffee ground emesis

    C. 18-year-old who is 36 weeks pregnant

    D. 29-year-old female with von Willebrand disease

21. Which calcium channel blocker has little to no effect on conduction through the SA and AV nodes?

    A. procainamide (Pronestyl)

    B. verapamil (Calan)

    C. amlodipine (Norvasc)

    D. diltiazem (Cardizem)

Lesson 5: Respiratory

22. The nurse practitioner is seeing a patient for an acute exacerbation of asthma. The patient reports increasing shortness of breath and wheezing the last two days. He ran out of his albuterol inhaler and has been using his grandmother's inhaler (formoterol) with no improvement. What is the best rationale for the ineffectiveness of the formoterol?

    A. His grandmother may have used all of the medicine in her inhaler

    B. formoterol is a long-acting beta agonist and is not effective for acute symptoms

    C. formoterol is an inhaled corticosteroid and is not effective for acute symptoms

    D. He is not using the inhaler correctly

23. Which medication has the following mechanism of action: decreases inflammation and mucus production and causes bronchodilation by selectively binding leukotriene receptors?

    A. zafirlukast (Accolate)

    B. omalizumab (Xolair)

    C. ciclesonide (Alvesco)

    D. cromolyn sodium (Intal)

24. Which medication would cause concern prior to prescribing ipratropium bromide (Atrovent)?

    A. albuterol (Proair)

    B. fluoxetine (Prozac)

    C. montelukast (Singulair)

    D. tamsulosin (Flomax)

25. Kayla complains of pain on her tongue and a white coating to her tongue. She is diagnosed with oral candidiasis. The nurse practitioner knows this diagnosis is a complication of which medication?

    A. metoprolol tartrate (Lopressor)

    B. mometasone (Asmanex)

    C. lamotrigine (Lamictal)

    D. colchicine (Colcrys)

Lesson 6: Endocrine

26. In order to cover meals eaten within 30–60 minutes, which type of insulin should be prescribed by the nurse practitioner?

    A. Intermediate-acting insulin

    B. Long-acting insulin

    C. Rapid-acting insulin

    D. Short-acting insulin

27. A patient has recently been diagnosed with hyperthyroidism. Which medication will the nurse practitioner prescribe?

    A. hydrocortisone (Cortef)

    B. levothyroxine (Levoxyl)

    C. methimazole (Tapazole)

    D. metformin (Glucophage)

28. What is the mechanism of action of sulfonylureas used for type 2 diabetes?

    A. Decrease hepatic production of glucose

    B. Enhance insulin secretion by binding to pancreatic beta cell receptor sites

    C. Mimic endogenous insulin by binding to cell wall receptors

    D. Stimulate insulin secretion in a short-acting manner

29. The nurse practitioner is caring for a patient with Addison disease with low aldosterone levels. Which medication will the nurse practitioner prescribe for aldosterone replacement?

    A. cortisone (Cortone)

    B. fludrocortisone (Florinef)

    C. hydrocortisone (Cortef)

    D. prednisone (Deltasone)

30. Which type of insulin should be prescribed specifically to cover insulin needs for about half the day or overnight?

A. Intermediate-acting insulin
B. Long-acting insulin
C. Rapid-acting insulin
D. Short-acting insulin

Lesson 7: Eye and Ear

31. The nurse practitioner is prescribing antipyrine and benzocaine for a child with otitis externa. Which is the correct prescription?

A. Fill affected ear canal and repeat daily
B. 2 drops to affected ear canal twice daily
C. 2 drops to affected ear canal 4 times daily
D. Fill affected ear canal, repeat every 2 hours as needed

32. Which medication should be discontinued if eye pain or irritation occurs?

A. cyclosporin
B. ocular lubricants
C. brimonidine
D. gentamicin

33. For which of the following medications is the patient required to keep the eyes closed for 2–3 minutes without blinking or squinting?

A. cyclosporin (Restasis)
B. brimonidine (Alphagan)
C. pilocarpine (Salagen)
D. carbachol (Miostat)

34. Which next step should be included in the instructions following the administration of carbamide peroxide?

A. Keep the eyes closed for 2–3 minutes
B. Wait 15 minutes prior to inserting contact lenses
C. Gently irrigate the ear canal with warm water
D. Make sure vision is clear before driving

Lesson 8: GI

35. The nurse practitioner is prescribing medication for a patient with gastroesophageal reflux disease (GERD). Which of the following medication classes would be an inappropriate choice?

A. Antacids
B. Antispasmodics
C. H2 blockers
D. Proton pump inhibitors

36. A child has recently been diagnosed with giardiasis. Which of the following medications will the nurse practitioner prescribe?

A. ivermectin (Stromectal)
B. mesalamine (Apriso)
C. metoclopramide (Reglan)
D. metronidazole (Flagyl)

37. Which of the following medications may cause hypohidrosis?

A. lactulose (Cephulac)
B. atropine/diphenoxylate (Lomotil)
C. arlex (Sorbitol)
D. cimetadine (Tagamet)

38. The nurse practitioner is caring for an 18-month-old who has had vomiting and diarrhea for one day. Which of the following antiemetics should the nurse practitioner avoid prescribing?

A. chlorpromazine (Thorazine)
B. metoclopramide (Reglan)
C. ondansetron (Zofran)
D. promethazine (Phenergan)

39. A patient has been diagnosed with irritable bowel syndrome (IBS) by the nurse practitioner. Which medication is the nurse practitioner likely to prescribe?

    A. cimetidine (Tagamet)

    B. dexamethasone (Decadron)

    C. dicyclomine (Bentyl)

    D. infliximab (Remicade)

40. Which meal choice will the nurse practitioner recommend for the patient to have when taking a dose of ivermectin?

    A. Baked lean chicken and asparagus

    B. Grilled whitefish and broccoli

    C. Pork chop with baked potato and butter

    D. Vegetable salad with lemon juice

Lesson 9: GYN/GU

41. A 75-year-old man presents to the office with complaints of blurry vision, urinary retention, dry mouth, and constipation. Based on these symptoms, you know he is most likely experiencing an adverse reaction to which of the following?

    A. nifedipine (Procardia)

    B. baby aspirin (Bayer low dose)

    C. solifenacin (VESIcare)

    D. omega-3 fish oil

42. An 18-year-old female presents to the office for insertion of the Skyla LNG IUD. As you prepare for the procedure, which information in her chart would cause you to reschedule her appointment for a later date?

    A. She was recently diagnosed with a right-sided ovarian cyst

    B. She is currently being treated for pelvic inflammatory disease

    C. She has poorly controlled type 1 diabetes mellitus

    D. She takes amphetamine/dextroamphetamine for attention deficit disorder

43. A 33-year-old presents to the office with the desire to start combined oral contraceptives. This method is contraindicated if which of the following is part of her health history?

    A. First-degree relative with breast cancer

    B. Gestational hypertension during her second pregnancy

    C. Smoking five cigarettes per day

    D. Factor V Leiden

44. Which statement is true regarding the use of backup contraception following the initial start of combined oral contraceptives (COC)?

    A. Backup contraception should be used for the first seven days of the menstrual cycle after a Sunday start

    B. Backup contraception is not needed with the quick start method

    C. Backup contraception is needed for the first full menstrual cycle following the first day start method

    D. Backup contraception should be used for the first 14 days of the menstrual cycle with the Sunday start method

45. Which complaint would not be of concern in a patient newly started on norethindrone/ethinyl estradiol?

    A. Headache

    B. Abdominal pain

    C. Diplopia

    D. Irregular bleeding

Lesson 10: MS/Analgesic

46. The nurse practitioner (NP) is evaluating a teenager who reports having taken 42 extra-strength acetaminophen (Tylenol) caplets. What will the NP order as an antidote?

    A. magnesium sulfate (Epsom salt)

    B. calcium gluconate (Kalcinate)

    C. acetylsalicylic acid (Aspirin)

    D. acetylcysteine (Mucomyst)

47. Which of the following medications is least likely to be associated with Stevens-Johnson syndrome?

    A. acetaminophen (Tylenol)

    B. allopurinol (Zyloprim)

    C. morphine (Roxanol)

    D. naproxen (Anaprox)

48. A patient has had repeat attacks of gout over a one- to two-year period. Which medication should the nurse practitioner choose for long-term treatment for this patient?

    A. ibupofen (Motrin)

    B. allopurinol (Zyloprim)

    C. hydrocortisone (Cortef)

    D. colchicine (Colcrys)

49. The nurse practitioner has just diagnosed a patient with mild rheumatoid arthritis. Which medication will the nurse practitioner likely prescribe?

    A. Corticosteroid

    B. Disease-modifying anti-rheumatic drug (DMARD)

    C. Nonsteroidal anti-inflammatory drug (NSAID)

    D. Opioid

50. Which testing is needed prior to initiation of biologic response modifiers for rheumatoid arthritis?

    A. Complete blood count

    B. Chest x-ray

    C. Hepatitis B and C

    D. All of the above

51. For the adult patient, what is the maximum amount of acetaminophen that can be taken per day?

    A. 1 gram

    B. 2 grams

    C. 4 grams

    D. 5 grams

Lesson 11: Neurologic

52. Regarding benzodiazepines, which of the following is true?

    A. They provide sedative effects

    B. They produce general anesthesia

    C. They have analgesic actions

    D. They require weeks for an effect

53. What is sumatriptan used for?

    A. Treatment of a severe headache

    B. Prophylaxis of migraine headaches

    C. Acute treatment of a migraine headache

    D. Acute treatment of a tension headache

54. The nurse practitioner is caring for a 28-year-old woman with myoclonic seizures that are well controlled on valproic acid. The woman states that she would like to become pregnant in the next year. What should the NP consider regarding the woman's anticonvulsant medication?

    A. Continue the present therapy

    B. Consider changing to lamotrigine

    C. Decrease the valproic acid dose

    D. Add a second anticonvulsant

55. In Alzheimer's disease, donepezil is used to increase which chemical in the brain?

    A. Serotonin

    B. Norepinephrine

    C. Dopamine

    D. Acetylcholine

56. Which of the following medications is the only one FDA-approved for the management of amyotrophic lateral sclerosis (ALS)?

    A. pramipexole (Mirapex)

    B. riluzole (Rilutek)

    C. tetrabenazine (Xenazine)

    D. topiramate (Topamax)

Lesson 12: OTC Medications

57. Opal calls the clinic to ask for advice about OTC medications. She is complaining of runny nose and sneezing with no other symptoms. Past medical history is remarkable for hypertension. You would intervene if you overheard the office nurse tell her which of the following?

    A. "You may take an over-the-counter antihistamine like diphenhydramine or loratadine."

    B. "If your symptoms don't improve in 7 to 10 days, or if they get worse, come into the clinic."

    C. "You can take any of the over-the-counter cold remedies."

    D. "Be sure to wash your hands after sneezing or blowing your nose."

58. A 5-month-old infant is diagnosed with influenza A. Her mother asks for information about keeping her fever down. Based on your knowledge of OTC antipyretics, which of the following statements by the nurse practitioner is best?

    A. "You may use acetaminophen for her fever."

    B. "You may use aspirin for her fever."

    C. "You may use ibuprofen for her fever."

    D. "You may use a combination of acetaminophen and ibuprofen for her fever."

59. A patient that has been taking ranitidine and omeprazole for 2 years is at risk of _____ deficiency?

    A. potassium

    B. vitamin C

    C. calcium

    D. vitamin B12

60. A patient with LLQ abdominal pain, fever, nausea, vomiting, and diarrhea presents to the primary care clinic. Your initial workup includes a urinalysis and CBC with differential. The patient wants symptomatic relief while awaiting a diagnosis. Which medication would be contraindicated?

    A. acetaminophen (Tylenol)

    B. ibuprofen (Advil)

    C. loperamide (Imodium A-D)

    D. promethazine (Phenergan)

Lesson 13: Prescription Writing

61. The "Five Rights" of medication administration can help the nurse practitioner remember how to safely write a prescription. It is prudent to remember which additional two "rights" to ensure best prescribing practices?

    A. Pharmacy and location

    B. Rationale and documentation

    C. Nurse practitioner and patient's addresses

    D. Response and follow-up

62. Which of the following is true about Schedule II controlled substances?

    A. A prescription may only be called into the pharmacy in the event of an emergency

    B. They are highly addictive, and currently do not have any medical use

    C. Refills may be written, faxed, or called in to the pharmacy

    D. The patient will need a new prescription after five refills or six months

63. According to the rule for prescribing scheduled medications, refills for schedule IV drugs such as lorazepam:

    A. Are allowed, and a new Rx is needed after one year of treatment

    B. Are allowed, and a new RX is needed after three months of treatment

    C. Are allowed, and a new RX is needed after six months of treatment

    D. Are not allowed

64. The FDA is in the process of eliminating the pregnancy categories (A, B, C, D, and X) and replacing them with a new labeling system. All of the following are benefits of the new system, except:

    A. It will include information for females and males of reproductive potential, pregnancy, and lactation

    B. It will summarize the specific risks associated with each medication

    C. The organization will be much simpler than using the five categories

    D. If a medication is absorbed systemically, it will state whether the information is based on animal or human studies

ANSWERS AND EXPLANATIONS

Lesson 1: Pharmacology Basics

1. D

The P450 enzyme system **(D)** affects the metabolism of the drug, not absorption. Size of the drug molecule (A), food in the gut (B), and the available surface area (C) all influence the drug's absorption.

2. B

The kidneys **(B)** are the primary means of medication excretion. The liver (A) is involved in metabolism. Exhaled air (C) and sweat from pores (D) are possible means for excretion, but they are not the primary means.

3. B

A chemical that binds to a receptor and stimulates cellular activity **(B)** describes an agonist. A chemical that has a harder time crossing the blood–brain barrier (A) describes a factor in absorption. A chemical that has a longer half-life than a competing chemical (C) describes an antagonist. A chemical that has a longer half-life than a competing chemical (D) may influence a decision on dose or frequency but does not describe an agonist.

4. A

Chirality refers to the shape of the medication molecule **(A)**. The shape of a drug receptor (B) will affect which medication will attach to it, but it is not the definition of chirality. A drug that blocks a matching receptor (C) describes an antagonist. A drug that shows affinity for certain receptors (D) describes an agonist.

5. C

Grapefruit juice interacting with a medication's metabolism **(C)** is an example of the P450 enzyme system in action. The ease that a medication is bound by plasma binding proteins (A) relates to distribution. A bigger molecule having a harder time crossing membranes (B) relates to absorption. The need to lower the dose of a medication because of poor kidney function (D) relates to excretion, not metabolism.

Lesson 2: Anti-Infectives

6. D

Ototoxicity **(D)** is a serious side effect of gentamicin that is more likely to occur in patients with limited renal function, including the elderly. Dementia (A) is not an adverse effect of gentamicin, although confusion can be. Hepatotoxicity (B) is not an adverse effect. Xerophthalmia (C), otherwise known as dry eye, is a common adverse effect; however, it is not more serious than ototoxicity.

7. B

Ciprofloxacin **(B)**, a fluoroquinolone, has a black box warning that tendon rupture can occur when taking this medication. Ceftriaxone (A), darifenacin (C), and Pyridium (D) do not have this adverse effect.

8. D

Women who are pregnant and close to delivery **(D)** should not be prescribed nitrofurantoin due to the risk of hemolytic anemia of the newborn. Orange urine is expected after taking Pyridium (A). There are no known negative drug interactions between nitrofurantoin and diphenhydramine (B). There are no known cross-sensitivity reactions between penicillins and nitrofurantoin (C).

9. A

Oseltamivir **(A)** is recommended for both Influenza A and B. Zanamivir (B) is recommended for the early treatment of influenza in people seven years of age and older, and for the prevention of influenza in people five years of age and older. Peramivir (C) is recommended for the early treatment of influenza in people two years of age and older. However, neither zanamivir or peramivir have been as well-studied in pregnant women as oseltamivir, which has been found safe and effective. They are therefore not recommended for a pregnant woman. Amantadine (D) is no longer recommended for the treatment of influenza due to increased resistance.

10. C

Both acyclovir and valacyclovir **(C)** are drugs of choice for treatment of initial and recurrent episodes of genital herpes or herpes zoster. Start therapy at the earliest sign of recurrent episodes of genital herpes or herpes zoster. Ganciclovir (A) is used in the treatment of cytomegalovirus. Atazanavir (B) is used to treat HIV. Ribavirin (D) is used to treat RSV or chronic HCV.

11. B

The idea that hepatitis C treatment is generally swift, simple, and straightforward **(B)** is not true regarding the treatment of HCV. All patients should be tested for evidence of current or prior HBV (A) before treatment is started. Combination medications (C) are used initially in the treatment of HCV. That patients should be evaluated for co-infection with HIV and for cirrhosis (D) is a true statement.

Lesson 3: Antineoplastics

12. A

Chemotherapy does not leave the RNA inside of a cancer cell unchanged **(A)**. They damage the DNA to the point that the cell must go through apoptosis (B), destroy checkpoint proteins (C), or interfere with the process of DNA replication (D).

13. B

Cisplatin is an alkylating agent that is made from platinum. Known side effects are myelosuppression and reduction in red and white blood cells. Therefore, CBC **(B)** should be monitored closely. Serum glucose (A) levels should be monitored if the treatment plan included steroids. It would not be prudent to obtain frequent urinalysis (C), as UTI is not a concern, or uric acid (D) levels, as the patent is not at risk for gout.

14. D

Oral candidiasis **(D)** is a common side effect of all chemotherapeutic agents. Kaposi sarcoma is seen in patients with AIDS, indicating immunocompromise. Increased energy prior to treatment (A) is not seen with cyclophosphamide or interferon; radiation therapy commonly causes fatigue. Insomnia (B) can be a side effect but it is not common. Tachycardia (C) is not typically seen as a side effect of cyclophosphamide, interferon, or radiation therapy.

15. C

Chemotherapeutic drugs should be administered infrequently as possible to maximize dose intensity, limit tumor regrowth, and minimize side effects **(C)**. They are not administered at low doses (A), but rather the maximum dose possible. Whether major toxicities overlap (B) has no effect on whether the drug is beneficial. Chemotherapy is often given in combination (D) to maximize effectiveness.

16. A

Methotrexate **(A)** is a chemotherapy agent used to treat acute lymphoblastic leukemia (ALL), osteosarcoma, non-Hodgkin lymphoma (NHL), and other cancers. It is also an immune system suppressant used to treat autoimmune disorders like rheumatoid arthritis and psoriasis. Mercaptopurine (B) is used to treat ALL, as well as Crohn's disease. Allopurinol (C) is a uric acid reducer used to treat gout and sometimes kidney stones. Procarbazine (D) is typically used to treat Hodgkin lymphoma.

Lesson 4: Cardiovascular

17. B

Grapefruit juice can interact with verapamil **(B)**, which is a calcium channel blocker. Grapefruit juice is problematic with statins, amiodarone, and CCBs. There is no interaction between grapefruit juice and lisinopril (A), warfarin (C), or timolol (D).

18. D

It is most critical to draw a digoxin level **(D)**, as nausea, vomiting, and diarrhea can all be signs of digoxin toxicity. A lipid profile (A) and vitamin D level (C) would not be critical labs to draw on this patient at this time. A urinalysis (B) would be beneficial to determine hydration status; however, it is more important to know if she has digoxin toxicity.

19. A

It is important to include information that signs and symptoms of low blood sugar may not be as apparent **(A)**. Beta-blockers can mask the signs of hypoglycemia. Beta-blockers should not be stopped abruptly (B). Erythema multiforme and Stevens-Johnson syndrome are serious adverse reactions of beta-blockers. Rashes should be reported (C). Beta-blockers can increase total cholesterol and LDL (D).

20. A

The 45-year-old on irbesartan and fluvastatin **(A)** is a candidate for anticoagulant therapy. A 34-year-old with coffee ground emesis (B) likely has a GI bleed and is not a candidate. Warfarin is contraindicated in pregnancy (C). A-29-year-old with von Willebrand disease (D) has a bleeding disorder and thus is not a candidate.

21. C

Amlodipine **(C)**, which is a dihydropyridine CCB, has little to no effect on conduction through the SA and AV node. Procainamide (A) is not a CCB. Verapamil (B) is a phenylalkylamine, and diltiazem (D) is a benzothiazepine CCB. Both have a large effect on conduction through the SA and AV node.

Lesson 5: Respiratory

22. B

The formoterol is ineffective because it is a long-acting beta agonist **(B)**. It is possible that his grandmother may have used all of the medication (A); however, the medication would still be ineffective because it is not for acute symptoms. Formoterol is not an inhaled corticosteroid (C). It is possible that he's not using the inhaler correctly (D); however, the medication would still be ineffective for acute symptoms.

23. A

The mechanism of action described in the question refers to a leukotriene receptor antagonist, and zafirlukast **(A)** is in this class. Omalizumab (B) is an anti-IgE medication. Ciclesonide (C) is an inhaled corticosteroid. Cromolyn sodium (D) is a mast cell stabilizer.

24. D

Flomax **(D)** would be a cause for concern if prescribing ipratropium bromide. Ipratropium bromide is an anticholinergic medication and can cause urinary retention. Flomax is used for treatment of benign prostatic hypertrophy (BPH) and ipratropium should be used cautiously in patients with BPH because of the risk of urinary retention. There is no interaction between medication or diagnosis associated with medication for albuterol (A), fluoxetine (B), or montelukast (C).

25. B

Oral candidiasis is a complication of mometasone **(B)**, an inhaled corticosteroid. Patients should be taught to rinse their mouth out after use to prevent this complication. Metoprolol tartrate (A) is a beta-blocker and is not associated with oral candidiasis. Lamotrigine (C) is used to treat seizure disorders and bipolar depression and is not associated with oral candidiasis; neither is colchicine (D), an anti-gout medication.

Lesson 6: Endocrine

26. D

Short-acting insulin (regular) **(D)** has an onset of action in 30–60 minutes, making it the best choice for meal coverage. Intermediate-acting insulin (A) has on onset of action in 1–2 hours. Long-acting insulin (B) has an onset of action in 1.5–2 hours. Rapid-acting insulin (C) has an onset of action in 5–15 minutes; it is used to rapidly decrease blood glucose levels.

27. C

Methimazole **(C)** inhibits iodine absorption, resulting in reduced thyroid hormone synthesis, and thus is used in the treatment of hyperthyroidism. Hydrocortisone (A) is used for cortisol replacement in Addison disease. Levothyroxine (B) is a synthetic thyroid hormone used as replacement therapy in hypothyroidism. Metformin (D) is a biguanide used for the treatment of elevated glucose in those patients with insulin resistance and type 2 diabetes mellitus.

28. B

Sulfonylureas enhance insulin secretion by binding to pancreatic beta cell receptor sites **(B)** in individuals with some pancreatic beta cell activity still present. Biguanides decrease hepatic production of glucose (A). Exogenous insulins mimic endogenous insulin by binding to cell wall receptors (C). Non-sulfonylurea secretagogues stimulate insulin secretion in a short-acting manner (D).

29. B

Fludrocortisone **(B)** is prescribed for aldosterone replacement. Cortisone (A), hydrocortisone (C), and prednisone (D) are used for cortisol replacement.

30. A

Intermediate-acting insulin **(A)** has a duration of more than 12 hours, enabling it to provide coverage for about half the day or overnight. Long-acting insulin (B) has a duration of 12–24 hours. Rapid-acting insulin (C) has a duration of about 4–6 hours; it is used to rapidly decrease blood glucose levels. Short-acting insulin (regular) (D) has a duration of about 6–8 hours.

Lesson 7: Eye and Ear

31. D

The correct prescription for this anesthetic, pain-reducing medication is to fill the affected ear canal and repeat every 2 hours as needed **(D)**. Using once daily (A) is insufficient for pain management. Using only 2 drops (B and C) will not provide the numbing required for pain relief.

32. B

Ocular lubricants **(B)** should be discontinued if eye pain, visual changes, redness, or eye irritation occurs. Expected side effects of burning or eye irritation with cyclosporin (A) may occur, as may burning or itching with brimonidine (C). Side effects of burning or irritation may occur with gentamicin (D).

33. A

With cyclosporin **(A)**, the patient should keep the eyes closed for 2–3 minutes without blinking or squinting after administration. This is not a required instruction with brimonidine (B), pilocarpine (C), or carbachol (D).

34. C

Carbamide peroxide is a cerumenolytic, and should be followed with warm water irrigation **(C)** in order to dislodge the impacted cerumen. Keeping the eyes closed for 2–3 minutes (A) should follow cyclosporin administration. Waiting 15 minutes to insert contact lenses (B) should occur following brimonidine administration. Making sure vision is clear prior to driving (D) is an instruction that should be given with pilocarpine prescription.

Lesson 8: GI

35. B

Antispasmodics **(B)** are used to treat irritable bowel syndrome, not GERD. Medications commonly used to treat GERD include antacids (A), H2 blockers (C), and proton pump inhibitors (D).

36. D

Metronidazole **(D)** is an antibiotic with antiprotozoal action (*Giardia* is a protozoa). Ivermectin (A) is an anthelmintic used to treat worm infestation. Mesalamine (B) is an anti-inflammatory agent used to treat ulcerative colitis. Metoclopramide (C) is an antiemetic.

37. B

The atropine component in Lomotil **(B)** is responsible for causing hypohidrosis. As anti-constipation medications, both Cephulac (A) and Sorbitol (C) may cause dehydration, but not hypohidrosis. Tagamet (D) is an antiemetic, and does not cause hypohidrosis.

38. D

Promethazine **(D)** is contraindicated for use in children less than 2 years of age. Chlorpromazine (A) should not be used in infants less than 6 months of age. Metoclopramide (B) should not be used in neonates. Ondansetron (C) should be avoided in patients at risk for prolonged QT interval.

39. C

Dicyclomine **(C)** is an antispasmodic with anticholinergic action, which is helpful in the management of IBS. Cimetidine (A) is used in the treatment of gastroesophageal reflux disease. Dexamethasone (B), a corticosteroid, may be used as an adjuvant for treatment of emesis. Infliximab (D), a monoclonal antibody, is used to treat ulcerative colitis.

40. C

The pork chop with baked potato and butter **(C)** is a high-fat meal. Taking ivermectin with fatty food increases its bioavailability. Baked lean chicken and asparagus (A), grilled whitefish and broccoli (B), and vegetable salad with lemon juice (D) are all low-fat meal choices.

Lesson 9: GYN/GU

41. C

Solifenacin **(C)** is an anticholinergic medication, which can cause the adverse effects the patient is experiencing. Nifedipine (A), a calcium channel blocker; baby aspirin (B), a salicylate; and omega-3 fish oil (D), a supplement, do not have these adverse effects.

42. B

Current pelvic inflammatory disease **(B)** is a contraindication to IUD insertion. Ovarian cysts (A), type 1 diabetes mellitus (C), and amphetamine/dextroamphetamine (D) are not contraindications for placement.

43. D

Factor V Leiden **(D)** is classified as U.S. MEC category 4 (unacceptable health risk) and is therefore a contraindication. Family history of breast cancer (A) is not considered to be a risk. Hypertension during pregnancy (B) is classified as U.S. MEC category 2 (benefits outweigh risks). Smoking five cigarettes per day (C) is classified as category 2 in a patient less than 35 years of age.

44. A

Backup contraception should be used for first seven days of the menstrual cycle **(A)** following a Sunday start and, contrary to (B), used with the quick start method. Backup contraception is not needed with the first day start method (C). Backup contraception is needed for 7 days, not 14 (D), following the Sunday start method.

45. D

Irregular bleeding **(D)** could be an expected finding after newly starting COCs. Complaints concerning ACHES would prompt further workup for possible thrombosis. Headache (A), abdominal pain (B), and diplopia (C) are part of the ACHES acronym.

Lesson 10: MS/Analgesic

46. D

Acetylcysteine **(D)** is the antidote for acetaminophen. Magnesium sulfate (A) is an electrolyte useful for preeclampsia and gestational hypertension. Calcium gluconate (B) is the antidote for magnesium sulfate. Acetylsalicylic acid (C) is the chemical name for aspirin.

47. C

Opioids **(C)** are not known to be likely causes of Stevens-Johnson syndrome. In contrast, acetaminophen (A), allopurinol (B), and NSAIDs (D) are associated with the development of this rare but serious adverse effect.

48. B

Allopurinol **(B)** reduces uric acid production and is used for the long-term treatment of gout. NSAIDs (A) and corticosteroids (C) are used to acutely decrease inflammation associated with gout. Colchicine (D) also reduces inflammation and is most effective if started at the first signs of a gout attack.

49. C

NSAIDs **(C)** are most often prescribed for mild cases of rheumatoid arthritis. Corticosteroids (A) are useful as chronic adjunctive therapy in patients with severe disease that is not well controlled on NSAIDs and DMARDs. DMARDs (B) are used in severe cases of rheumatoid arthritis. Opioids (D), while having an analgesic effect, do not have an anti-inflammatory effect and should be reserved for cases of moderate to severe pain.

50. D

Due to the immunosuppression resulting from the use of biologic response modifiers (TNF inhibitors and non-TNF agents), all of the screenings **(D)** must occur prior to initiation of treatment. In addition to CBC (A), a chest x-ray (B), and determination of hepatitis B and C status (D), immunizations should also be updated.

51. C

4 grams **(C)** is the maximum recommended adult daily dose of acetaminophen. 1 gram (A) is the maximum recommended adult single dose of acetaminophen. 2 grams (B) is less than the recommended daily adult dose, and 5 grams (D) is more than the recommended daily adult dose.

Lesson 11: Neurologic

52. A

All benzodiazepines have some sedative effects **(A)**, and some of them are used for sleep disorder treatment. They do not produce general anesthesia (B). While benzodiazepines help to decrease the anxiety associated with pain, they do not have analgesic actions (C). Benzodiazepines do not require weeks to have an effect (D).

53. C

An acute migraine headache **(C)** may be treated with sumatriptan. Severe headache treatment (A) may include NSAIDs and opioids. Prophylaxis of migraines (B) may be achieved with beta-blockers, tricyclic antidepressants, or topiramate. Combinations of NSAIDs, opioids, and caffeine may be used for acute treatment of tension headaches (D).

54. B

Valproic acid is a poor choice in women of child-bearing age, as it may have a detrimental effect on the fetus; thus, changing to lamotrigine **(B)** would be appropriate. Continuing the valproic acid (A) would be inappropriate in light of the possibility of pregnancy. Valproic acid should be discontinued with the possibility of pregnancy, not have its dosage decreased (C). Adding a second anticonvulsant (D) is unnecessary, as her seizures have been well-controlled.

55. D

Cholinesterase inhibitors, such as donepezil, work to increase the amount of acetylcholine **(D)** in the brain. They do not increase serotonin (A), norepinephrine (B), or dopamine (C).

56. B

Riluzole **(B)** is the only FDA-approved agent to manage ALS. It is used to delay the progression of the disease and postpone the need for ventilator support. Pramipexole (A) is an antiparkinsonian agent. Tetrabenazine (C) is used to palliate the movement disorder of Huntington disease. Topiramate (D) is an anticonvulsant.

Lesson 12: OTC Medications

57. C

Many OTC cold remedies **(C)** contain multiple ingredients, including decongestants. Decongestants are contraindicated in HTN. The patient in the scenario is exhibiting signs of allergic rhinitis or the common cold, so she would benefit from an antihistamine (A). A viral infection can take 7–10 days (B) to resolve. Symptoms lasting longer than that may be related to bacterial infection or unresolved allergic rhinitis. Proper handwashing (D) is key to preventing the spread of infection in this patient.

58. A

Acetaminophen **(A)** is appropriate to use for all-age infants for fever reduction. Aspirin (B) is not an appropriate medication to use for fever reduction in children because its use increases the risk of Reye syndrome. Ibuprofen (C) is appropriate to use for fever reduction in infants six months and older. Acetaminophen is appropriate, but ibuprofen is not (D).

59. D

Long-term use of H2 receptor blockers (ranitidine) and PPI (omeprazole) increases the risk of B12 deficiency **(D)**. These medications do not increase the risk of potassium (A), vitamin C (B), or calcium (C) deficiency.

60. C

This patient is exhibiting signs of acute abdomen. Loperamide **(C)** is contraindicated in cases of acute abdomen. Acetaminophen (A) is not contraindicated and could be used as a fever reducer. Ibuprofen (B) is not contraindicated and could be used as a fever reducer, although acetaminophen would be preferred as ibuprofen may worsen nausea. Promethazine (D) would be beneficial to prevent nausea and vomiting and subsequent fluid deficit.

Lesson 13: Prescription Writing

61. B

Rationale and documentation **(B)** are the two extra "rights" that will help to ensure that you have prescribed the medication for the right reason and that your visit note supports your decision to prescribe it. Sending the medication to the correct pharmacy and location (A) are certainly important; however, they are not considered to be part of the "rights." The nurse practitioner and patient's addresses (C) are only required for controlled substances and are not considered to be part of the "rights." Evaluating the patient's response and creating a follow-up plan (D) are integral parts of comprehensive patient care. They will often be your next steps after going through all seven "rights."

62. A

A Schedule II controlled substance prescription may be called in to the pharmacy, but only in the event of an emergency **(A)**. Schedule I substances are considered to be highly addictive and have no current medical use (B). Schedule III substances may have refills written, faxed, or called in to the pharmacy (C), and the patient will need a new prescription after five refills or six months (D). Refills are prohibited with Schedule II substances.

63. C

Refills are allowed for schedule IV drugs; a new Rx is required after five refills or six months of treatment **(C)**.

64. C

The new FDA labeling has been created in large part because the five categories (A, B, C, D, and X) were thought to be too simple **(C)**, which many clinicians found confusing. Therefore, to communicate each medication's risk more clearly, the new labeling will summarize the risk (B) of each medication, specifying whether or not there is systemic absorption, and if so, documenting whether the information is based on animal or human studies (D). The summaries will include information for females and males of reproductive potential, pregnancy, and lactation (A).

PART TWO

Body Systems

CHAPTER 5

Eyes, Ears, Nose, Mouth, and Throat

LESSON 1: EYES

Learning Objectives
- Identify clinical manifestations of eye disorders
- Choose and interpret laboratory/diagnostic testing used for disorders of the eye and vision
- Differentiate appropriate treatment and referrals related to disorders of the eye and vision

Any patient presenting with an issue related to the eye(s) should also have their vision assessed. Accurate assessment and diagnosis are critical for the preservation of vision in many cases. In addition, the FNP must be aware of conditions that require prompt referral to the ophthalmologist.

Definitions
- **Blepharitis:** inflammation of the eyelid
- **Cataract:** progressive opaqueness of the lens resulting in blurred vision
- **Chalazion:** benign painless nodule inside the eyelid
- **Conjunctivitis:** inflammation or infection of the conjunctivae
- **Dacryocystitis:** infection of the lacrimal sac
- **Hordeolum:** acute focal infection involving eyelid glands (a stye)
- **Hyphema:** pooling of blood inside the anterior chamber of the eye
- **Intraocular pressure:** pressure of fluid inside the eye
- **Keratitis:** corneal inflammation
- **Uveitis:** inflammation of the uvea

> **DANGER SIGN** When hyphema is noted on an ophthalmoscopic exam, refer the patient to ophthalmology immediately for evaluation and treatment, which may include limited activity, head of bed elevation, steroid and/or dilating ophthalmic drops, and monitoring of intraocular pressure. In some cases, surgery is necessary.

Assessment

Note history of recent viral illness. Determine history of chronic disease such as hypertension, diabetes mellitus, collagen vascular or rheumatic disease, multiple sclerosis, or allergic rhinitis.

> **DANGER SIGN** Rapid onset of vision loss ALWAYS requires prompt referral to the ophthalmologist.

Review of Systems

- **Constitutional:** fever
- **Eyes:** history of scratching eye or getting something in it, trauma to eye
- **Skin:** lesions on nose or face

> **DANGER SIGN** A fixed and dilated pupil is a sign of subarachnoid hemorrhage. REFER IMMEDIATELY!

> **Pro Tip**
> For the ophthalmoscopic exam, use the right hand to assess the right eye and the left hand to assess the left eye. Note that arteries are narrower than veins and brighter red in color.

Diagnosis

Conjunctivitis

Red eyes and drainage are the hallmarks of conjunctivitis. Conjunctivitis may be either viral, bacterial, or allergic in nature.

Type	Subjective findings	Objective findings
Viral	Tearing, sensation of foreign body, possible URI symptoms, photophobia, impaired vision; may start with one eye and progress to other	Clear discharge, reddened conjunctivae, preauricular or submandibular lymphadenopathy
Bacterial	Burning, stinging, or gritty sensation to eyes; crusted eyelids upon awakening	Reddened conjunctivae, eyelid swelling, copious purulent or mucopurulent drainage, positive gram stain if gonorrhea suspected, positive culture if chlamydia suspected (neonates)
Allergic	Bilateral itchy, watery eyes; seasonal symptoms; often history of allergic rhinitis	Edema of lids, no vision change, bilateral hyperemia of eyes

Table 5.1.1 Distinguishing Conjunctivitis

Corneal, Iris, and Lens Disorders

Disorder	Subjective findings	Objective findings
Cataract (may be congenital or related to disease, medication, or trauma)	Starbursts with lights, glare with night driving	Dark opacity in media of eye with ophthalmoscope; absence of red reflex in newborn
Corneal abrasion (history of scratching eye)	Reduced vision, tearing	Normal pupil, abrasion fluoresces with Wood's lamp/fluorescein exam
Corneal foreign body (history of getting something in the eye)	Possible reduced vision, tearing	Normal pupil, possible visible foreign body
Iritis/uveitis (may occur with collagen vascular or rheumatoid disease, diabetes, eye trauma, or Lyme disease)	Photophobia	Affected pupil smaller, circumlimbal flush, possible reduced visual acuity
Keratitis (may be herpes simplex or herpes zoster)	Reduced vision with either, foreign body sensation with herpes simplex	Decreased visual acuity, tearing with herpes simplex, dendrite fluorescein pattern with Wood's lamp exam, facial lesions along nerve distribution (herpes zoster—on tip of nose indicates ocular involvement)

Table 5.1.2 Distinguishing Corneal, Iris, and Lens Disorders

Dacryocystitis

The patient may complain of eye pain. Note redness, edema, tearing, possible fever, and purulent eye discharge expressed from lacrimal duct.

Dry Eyes

Dry eyes are often age-related, though other risk factors include history of Lasik surgery, being a postmenopausal female, having arthritis, or taking diuretics or chemotherapeutic agents. The patient will complain of the eye feeling dry or gritty.

Eyelid Disorders

Disorder	Subjective findings	Objective findings
Blepharitis (excess shedding of skin cells blocking oil glands)	Burning, itching, tearing, dry eye, photophobia	Erythema or edema of lid margin, dryness, scaling, or flaking
Chalazion (chronic lipogranulomatous inflammation of meibomian gland)	Tearing, feels like foreign body in eye	Red or gray subconjunctival mass; possible preauricular lymphadenopathy; if infected, painful eyelid edema
Hordeolum (stye) (infection of the eyelid glands, more common in children)	Eye tenderness	Purulent discharge, redness and edema of lid with localized area, possible preauricular lymphadenopathy; pointing may be seen on eyelid eversion

Table 5.1.3 Distinguishing Eyelid Disorders

Glaucoma

Type	Subjective findings	Objective findings
Acute angle closure (aqueous fluid doesn't drain due to blockage of anterior chamber angle by the iris)	Reduced visual acuity	Avoid pupil, clouded cornea, increased intraocular pressure
Open angle (trabecular network not draining aqueous fluid, angle is open—can be congenital or steroid-induced)	Usually without symptoms, painless, peripheral vision loss over time	Increased intraocular pressure, optic nerve cupping

Table 5.1.4 Comparison Chart: Glaucoma

Macular Degeneration

Type	Causes	Loss of central vision
Wet	Genetic, smoking, macular blood vessel proliferation	Sudden
Dry	Genetic, age-related (>65 years old)	Gradual

Table 5.1.5 Comparison Chart: Macular Degeneration

Optic Neuritis

With inflammation of the optic nerve, the patient may exhibit these clinical manifestations:

- History of multiple sclerosis or recent viral illness
- Eye pain
- Central scotoma
- Decreased color vision
- Affected eye decreased pupillary reaction
- Papillitis

Retinal Detachment

May occur with diabetes, trauma, family history, a retinal tear, or high myopia. Characterized by new onset of flashing lights or floaters, or patient may describe a curtain coming down over vision.

Plan

Diagnosis	Treatment	Patient education	Refer to ophthalmologist
Allergic conjunctivitis	• Topical antihistamine drops (not recommended for children <3 years old): azelastine HCl (Optivar), olopatadine HCl 0.1% (Patanol), or olopatadine HCl 0.2% (Patanol); OR mast cell stabilizer (patients >4 years old), cromolyn sodium • Artificial tears may also be helpful • Some patients may benefit from an oral antihistamine • In severe atopic keratoconjunctivitis, ketorolac tromethamine (Acular)	• Good handwashing • Cool compresses several times a day • Clean eyes inner to outer canthus with clean moist warm cloth • Discard all eye makeup	

Table 5.1.6 Treatment and Referral Plan of Disorders of the Eye

Diagnosis	Treatment	Patient education	Refer to ophthalmologist
Bacterial conjunctivitis	Antibiotic eye drops for 5–7 days	Same as allergic conjunctivitis	
Blepharitis	Bacitracin or erythromycin ointment only if needed	• Warm compresses twice daily for 10 minutes, followed by lid scrub (pads available over the counter) • Mindful handwashing • Lubricant eye drops	
Chalazion	Warm compresses for 15 minutes, 4 times a day	Mindful handwashing	If nonresponsive to therapy
Corneal abrasion	Antibiotic drops or ointment	Return for re-evaluation if needed	
Corneal foreign body	• Anesthetic eye drops and remove foreign body with sterile cotton swab (if trained) • Antibiotic eye drops or ointment		If foreign body difficult to remove or rust ring present or globe perforated
Dacrocystitis	• Adults: oral dicloxacillin or erythromycin Infants: antibiotic eye drops	• Discard all eye makeup • Warm/moist compresses at least four times daily • Good handwashing	If recurrent due to infantile dacryostenosis
Dry eyes	• Artificial tears may help • Cyclosporine (Restasis) eye drops may be used to increase tear production		If punctal plug evaluation
Glaucoma (open angle)	Eye drops (beta-blockers, prostaglandin analogues, alpha$_2$ agonist, carbonic anhydrase inhibitors); CAI available in PO form	Comply with follow-up appointment schedule	
Hordeolum	Sulfacetamide sodium (Sulamyd) 10% ointment, polymyxin B sulfate and bacitracin zinc (Polysporin) ophthalmic ointment, or sulfacetamide sodium (Sulamyd) 10% ophthalmic drops	• Good handwashing • Discard all eye makeup	
Iritis/Uveitis	Treat underlying disease		For possible steroid eye drops to reduce inflammation
Keratitis	• Artificial tears/lubricant • Antiviral medications such as valacyclovir (Valtrex) • Steroids contraindicated		Assessment of ocular involvement
Macular degeneration (dry)	No treatment available		
Macular degeneration (wet)		Smoking cessation	For treatment
Viral conjunctivitis	Artificial tears if needed	Same as allergic conjunctivitis	

Table 5.1.6 Treatment and Referral Plan of Disorders of the Eye (Continued)

Always Refer
- **Apparent refractive errors:** for further evaluation and vision correction
- **Cataract:** for lens removal and implant insertion
- **Glaucoma (acute angle closure):** for immediate evaluation
- **Macular degeneration (wet):** for treatment
- **Optic neuritis:** for systemic steroids
- **Papilledema:** indicates increased intracranial pressure
- **Retinal detachment:** for immediate dilated eye exam
- **Retinopathy (whether diabetic or hypertensive):** for evaluation and treatment

Takeaways
- Prescribe antibiotics only for disorders likely to be bacterial in nature, such as bacterial conjunctivitis, dacryocystitis, and possibly hordeolum.
- Cool compresses are helpful in conjunctivitis, while warm compresses should be used for blepharitis and dacryocystitis.
- Prescribe valacyclovir in confirmed herpes keratitis.

LESSON 2: EARS

Learning Objectives
- Identify clinical manifestations of ear disorders
- Choose and interpret laboratory/diagnostic testing used for disorders of the ear and hearing
- Differentiate appropriate treatment and referrals related to disorders of the ear and hearing

Many patients presenting with an issue related to the ear(s) may also have an issue with hearing and balance.

Definitions
- **Audiogram:** graph showing pure-tone hearing results
- **BPPV:** benign paroxysmal positional vertigo
- **Conductive hearing loss:** hearing loss occurring due to disruption of sound through the middle ear
- **Otalgia:** ear pain
- **Otorrhea:** ear drainage
- **Pneumatic otoscopy:** maneuver used to determine tympanic membrane mobility achieved by gently squeezing and releasing the otoscope bulb to pressure changes
- **Sensorineural hearing loss:** hearing loss caused by hair cell damage in cochlea or along auditory pathway
- **Tinnitus:** ringing in the ear
- **Tympanogram:** graphic representing relationship between the air pressure in the ear canal and the movement of the tympanic membrane
- **Vertigo:** feeling as if the individual or the environment is rotating

Assessment

Determine incidence and frequency of previous ear infections. Explore the patient's history for risk factors such as:

- Day care attendance, secondhand smoke, supine bottle feeding, pacifier use (otitis media)
- Recent viral illness (otitis media, BPPV)
- Head injury (BPPV)
- Increasing age (BPPV, hearing loss)
- Cerumen impaction, prematurity, childhood meningitis or mumps, aminoglycoside receipt (hearing loss)
- Swimming, excess cerumen removal (otitis externa)

Subjective

Symptoms

- Spinning sensation
- Tinnitus
- Hearing loss
- Balance disturbance
- Aural pressure
- Otalgia
- Irritability

> **Pro Tip: Ear Pain in the Preverbal Child**
>
> In the infant or preverbal child, signs of acute otitis media include fussiness, irritability, crying inconsolably (especially when lying down), batting/tugging at the ears, and rolling the head from side to side.
>
> Note: These behaviors may also occur with teething or otitis media with effusion (OME), or may just be a habit.

Review of Systems

- **Constitutional:** fever, anorexia, lethargy, difficulty sleeping
- **EENT:** nasal drainage
- **Resp:** antecedent or concurrent upper respiratory infection symptoms
- **Neuro:** vertigo, balance disturbance

> **Pro Tip: Straightening the Ear Canal**
>
> To appropriately visualize the tympanic membrane or instill ear drops:
>
> - In the young child (<3 years of age), pull the earlobe down and back
> - In the older child (>3 years of age), pull the pinna up and back

Objective

- **HEENT:** pain when the tragus is touched, otorrhea, ear edema, edema/erythema of the ear canal, immobile tympanic membrane (TM), red/bulging TM, nasal drainage, cervical lymphadenopathy, results of audiogram and/or tympanometry showing tympanic membrane immobility
- **CV:** auscultate for cardiac bruit (vertigo)
- **Neuro:** positive Dix-Hallpike maneuver (BPPV)

> **DANGER SIGN** If clear or pale yellow drainage is coming from the ear, check the fluid for the presence of glucose—if positive, the drainage is likely cerebrospinal fluid leakage.

Diagnosis

Hearing loss:

- Negative Rinne test (bone conduction lasts longer than air conduction) indicates conductive hearing loss
- Weber test: sound heard louder in affected ear indicates conductive hearing loss; sound heard louder in unaffected ear indicates sensorineural hearing loss
- Remove impacted cerumen if it is the cause for hearing loss (conductive)

> **DANGER SIGN** Do not attempt cerumen removal when a tympanic perforation is suspected.

	Benign paroxysmal positional vertigo	Ménière's disease
Sudden onset	Yes	Yes
Vertigo	Yes	Yes
Balance disturbance	No	Yes
Length of episode	Last seconds to minutes	20 minutes to 24 hours
Nausea and vomiting	Yes	Maybe
Hearing loss	May be present	Increased (sensorineural)
Tinnitus	May be present	Increased
Aural fullness	May be present	Yes—pressure

Table 5.2.1 Comparison of Vestibular Disorders

Otitis

	Acute otitis media (AOM)	Otitis media with effusion (OME)	Otitis externa (OE)
Definition	Acute infectious process of middle ear with rapid onset pain, fever	Fluid collection in middle ear without pain or fever (chronic OME ≥3 months)	Infection and inflammation of skin of external ear canal
Upper respiratory infection	Frequently precedes	Can be concurrent	Not related
Fever	Acute onset	No	Possible
Otalgia	Acute onset, may be severe	No, sensation of fullness rather than pain (popping)	Significant, particularly with tragus palpation; also may itch or feel like canal is full
Ear canal	Normal	Normal	Red, edematous, possibly too swollen to allow visualization of TM
Tympanic membrane	Moderate to severe bulging or mild bulging with ear pain; immobile as demonstrated by pneumatic otoscopy or tympanometry; intense erythema; visible greenish or yellow pus behind TM; bullae may be present on the TM (bullous myringitis)	Dull, opaque, with retraction; if non-opaque, fluid level or air bubble seen; poor mobility or immobile as demonstrated by pneumatic otoscopy or tympanometry	Normal if visualization possible
Otorrhea	New onset in absence of OE (perforated TM)	No	White or colored drainage in canal
Cervical lymphadenopathy	Usually	Not usually	Possibly
Cause	Viral pathogens, *S. pneumoniae, H. influenzae, M. catarrhalis*	Recurrent URI, eustachian tube dysfunction, allergy, adenoid hypertrophy	*P. aeruginosa, Candida, Aspergillus*, other bacteria/fungi

Table 5.2.2 Differentiating Otitis

> **DANGER SIGN** Malignant otitis externa is a potentially life-threatening infection usually caused by *Pseudomonas aeruginosa*. It most often occurs in elderly patients with diabetes or patients with HIV infection who present with extraordinary otalgia and otorrhea, with granulation tissue in the external canal. Refer for intravenous antibiotic treatment.

Plan

Disorder	Treatment	Patient education	Referral
Acute otitis media	• In adults and children for whom antibiotics will be prescribed, use amoxicillin (high dose) if no antibiotics in past month • If antibiotics taken in past month use amoxicillin-clavulanate or cefprozil, cefuroxime axetil (Ceftin), Cefdinir (Omnicef), or cefpodoxime (Vantin) • In penicillin allergy (not IgE-mediated), use a cephalosporin • In IgE-mediated penicillin allergy, use azithromycin (Zithromax), sulfamethoxazole-trimethoprim (Bactrim), or clarithromycin (Biaxin) (there is a high failure rate with the last 3 antibiotics) • *Table 5.2.4* details treatment recommendations for children • Fever and pain management with acetaminophen or ibuprofen • Benzocaine (Auralgan) otic drops if ear pain is severe • In children, follow up in 3 weeks to determine resolution or presence of OME	• Warm or cool compress may help with pain • Return for re-evaluation if not improving within 48–72 hours • If antibiotics prescribed, finish entire course	If treatment failure with second- or third-line drug, recurrent AOM episodes, signs of intracranial or intratemporal complications
BPPV	• Bedrest during an acute episode of vertigo • Canalith reposition procedure (Epley maneuver) • Vestibular suppressant medications are not recommended	• After the Epley procedure, wear soft cervical collar for two days • Avoid sleeping on affected ear • Avoid hyperextension of neck to look upwards	Refer to physician if symptoms not improved in 2–4 weeks
Hearing loss			Refer to otolaryngology and/or audiology for further evaluation and possible augmentation
Ménière's disease	Diuretics may help with the vertigo, but do not impact hearing loss	Avoid episode triggers by limiting sodium intake (2–3 g daily), caffeine, alcohol, nicotine, and stress	Refer to otolaryngology for long-term management and evaluation of hearing
Otitis externa	• Analgesics and warm compress for pain • Placement of a wick if needed, antibiotic or antifungal otic drops	After resolution, "dry ears" precautions to avoid further episodes	Granulation in ear canal (malignant otitis externa)
Otitis media with effusion	• Watchful waiting (antihistamines, decongestants, antibiotics, and corticosteroids are not recommended, as they have not been proven to hasten the resolution of OME) • Recheck children every 4 weeks • Monitor hearing and language development in young child	Do not prop bottle nor allow supine bottle-feeding	• Refer for hearing evaluation if OME lasts >12 weeks • Refer to otolaryngology if hearing is impaired

Table 5.2.3 Treatment and Referral Plan for Disorders of the Ears

Age	Certain diagnosis of AOM: signs & symptoms	Treatment
<6 months	Unilateral or bilateral AOM	Antibiotics
6 months to 2 years	Bilateral AOM	Antibiotics
6 months to 2 years	Unilateral AOM with severe illness[a] OR otorrhea	Antibiotics
6 months to 2 years	Unilateral AOM without either severe illness[a] or otorrhea	Antibiotics or observation[b]
>2 years	Unilateral AOM with severe illness[a] OR otorrhea	Antibiotics
>2 years	Unilateral AOM without either severe illness[a] or otorrhea	Antibiotics or observation[b]

[a]Severe illness is defined as temperature 102.2°F (39°C) or higher or moderate to severe otalgia or otalgia for at least 48 hours. Non-severe illness is defined as mild otalgia for <48 hours and fever 102.2°F (<39°C).

[b]Observation is appropriate when follow-up can be ensured in order that antibiotic therapy may begin if the child fails to improve or worsens within 48–72 hours.

Table 5.2.4 Treatment of Acute Otitis Media

Adapted from Lieberthal, A.S., Carroll, A.E., Chonmaitree, T., Ganiats, T.G., Hoberman, A. Jackson, M., ... Tunkel, D.E. (2013). Clinical Practice Guideline: The diagnosis and management of acute otitis media. *Pediatrics, 131*(3), e964 e999.

Takeaways

- Bed rest is needed during an acute episode of vertigo.
- Ascertain surety of acute otitis media diagnosis prior to prescribing antibiotics.
- Otitis media with effusion may follow AOM; if it persists longer than 12 weeks, refer patient to otolaryngology.

LESSON 3: NOSE

Learning Objectives
- Identify clinical manifestations of nose disorders
- Choose and interpret laboratory/diagnostic testing used for nose disorders
- Differentiate appropriate treatment and referrals related to nose disorders

When patients present with nasal and sinus complaints, the ears and throat should also be appropriately examined.

Definitions
- **Dennie Morgan lines:** a fold or line in the skin below the lower eyelid
- **Epistaxis:** bleeding from the nose
- **Rhinitis:** inflammation of the nasal mucous membranes
- **Rhinorrhea:** significant volume of mucosal fluid in the nasal cavity (runny nose)
- **Sinusitis:** inflammation of the paranasal sinus's mucous membranes

Assessment

Subjective

Ask about exposure to others with similar symptoms. Determine if season of the year has an impact on the symptoms. Note if the patient has a history of hypertension or arteriosclerosis.

Symptoms

- Nasal congestion
- Sneezing
- Rhinorrhea (clear or colored)
- Cough
- Bloody nose

> **DANGER SIGN** If clear or pale yellow drainage is coming from the nose (in the absence of nasal congestion or a cold, and particularly following a head injury), check the fluid for the presence of glucose. If positive, the drainage is likely cerebrospinal fluid leakage.

Review of Systems

- **Resp:** wheezing, rhonchi, transmitted upper airway congestion

> **Pro Tip**
> Palpate the sinuses in patients with a nasal complaint, keeping in mind that the frontal sinuses are not well-developed until about 8 years of age.

Diagnosis

Epistaxis

The diagnosis is based upon the clinical presentation of nasal bleeding. Note amount of blood loss. A traumatic area may be seen within the nose. Ensure no nasal foreign body present.

Allergic Rhinitis and Acute Bacterial Rhinosinusitis

Disorder	Subjective findings	Objective findings	Other distinguishing factors
Allergic rhinitis (may be seasonal or perennial, dependent upon patient's allergies)	Nasal congestion and itchiness, postnasal drip, sore throat, itchy eyes, dry mouth, headache	Clear rhinorrhea, cough, tearing, eye puffiness, Dennie Morgan lines, allergic shiners, allergic salute, pale blue and boggy nasal mucosa, cobblestone pharynx, halitosis, possibly eczematous rash	Eosinophils present on Wright's stain of nasal secretions, positive allergy skin test or radioallergosorbent test (RAST), eosinophilia on complete blood count
Acute bacterial rhinosinusitis (symptoms present >10 days or worsening after initial improvement if <10 days [double worsening])	Green or yellow nasal discharge (thick), fever, sore throat, face pain, headache, toothache, can't smell (anosmia), fatigue, snoring/ mouth breathing	Cough (possibly chronic) that is worse when lying down, periorbital edema, halitosis, nasal quality to speech, erythematous pharynx, pain upon sinus palpation	Diagnosis usually made via history and physical examination, though sinus x-rays may reveal air-fluid levels; CT scan only for suspected chronic sinusitis

Table 5.3.1 Distinguishing Diagnostic Factors for Allergic Rhinitis and Acute Bacterial Rhinosinusitis

Plan

Disorder	Treatment	Patient education	Referral
Epistaxis	• Apply pressure to front of nose for up to 20 minutes while sitting in an upright position to avoid aspiration • Hold ice pack to the nose for vasoconstriction • After traumatic area scabs, and as preventative, apply nasal moisturizing gel • May cauterize anterior bleeding with silver nitrate stic	• Avoid forceful nose blowing • Use a humidifier or water-based lubricant to keep nasal mucosa from drying out • Hold pressure as described while sitting upright if bleeding recurs	If posterior bleed, refer to otolaryngologist (ENT) immediately; also refer for recurrent cases to ENT and to hematology for further evaluation of possible bleeding disorder
Allergic rhinitis	• Prescribe steroid nasal sprays to prevent allergic rhinitis (leukotriene modifiers or mast cell stabilizers may also be used) • Recommend saline spray for liquefaction of nasal secretions • Use antihistamines for rescue therapy	• Avoid forceful nose blowing • Maintain environmental control of allergens • Use Neti pot daily to cleanse nasal mucosa	Refer if non-responsive to therapy, severe symptoms, or for immunotherapy evaluation
Acute bacterial rhinosinusitis	• First-line treatment is amoxicillin-clavulanate (Augmentin), second-line treatment is doxycycline (Vibramycin); in the beta-lactam allergic, use clindamycin (Cleocin) plus cefpodoxime (Vantin), or in adults only levofloxacin (Levaquin) or moxifloxacin (Avelox) • Steroid sprays may be used to decrease nasal inflammation • Oral and nasal decongestants are not recommended, as their use has not been shown to have influence on patient outcomes. When nasal decongestants are used longer than 4 days, rhinitis medicamentosa (rebound rhinitis) may occur	• Avoid smoking and secondhand smoke • Use a room humidifier to liquefy secretions • Ibuprofen or acetaminophen may help facial pain • Take entire prescribed course of antibiotics even when feeling better	Refer if patient is not improving on antibiotic, has an anatomic abnormality, visual, or neurologic problem, or if allergy evaluation needed

Table 5.3.2 Treatment and Referral Plan for Disorders of the Nose

Takeaways

- Forceful nose blowing should be avoided.
- If recurrent epistaxis occurs, may need hematology referral.
- Allergic rhinitis and acute bacterial sinusitis benefit from liquefying nasal secretions.

LESSON 4: MOUTH

Learning Objectives

- ■ Identify clinical manifestations of disorders of the mouth
- ■ Choose and interpret laboratory/diagnostic testing used in mouth disorders
- ■ Differentiate appropriate treatment and referrals related to disorders of the mouth

Stomatitis may have an infectious cause, and pain is a presenting feature common to many of the mouth disorders. The presence of pain may affect the patient's ability to properly eat and drink, resulting in the possibility of dehydration, so palliation becomes important.

Definitions

- **Avulsion:** pulled or torn away (as in a tooth)
- **Cheilitis:** cracks on the lips
- **Cheilosis:** cracking in the corners of the lips (also termed "angular cheilitis")
- **Plaque:** sticky deposit or localized abnormal patch
- **Stomatitis:** inflammation of the oral mucous membranes
- **Ulcer:** loss of tissue surface integrity with necrosis of epithelial tissue

Assessment

History

- Day care attendance
- Cigarette smoking or smokeless tobacco use
- Alcohol use
- History of cancer or immunosuppression
- Use of chemotherapy, immunosuppressive drugs, or antibiotics

Subjective

Symptoms
- Oral or pharyngeal lesions
- Pain
- Fever
- Decreased appetite, difficulty with food/fluid intake

Review of Systems
- **Constitutional:** vitamin deficiency
- **EENT:** difficult swallowing, mouth trauma
- **Skin:** skin lesions
- **Endo:** uncontrolled diabetes, hormonal changes
- **Hematologic/lymphatic:** lymph node swelling or pain

Objective

- **HEENT:** inspect lips (lesions, cheilitis, or cheilosis); tongue (ulcerations, plaques, fissures, or discolorations); palate and entire oral mucosa (erythema, lesions, or discoloration); gums for erythema, edema (dental abscess), bleeding (tooth avulsion), and red plaques under dentures (candidiasis); palpate cervical lymph nodes to determine swelling or pain
- **Skin:** inspect skin for lesions, vesicles, ulcerations

> **Pro Tip**
> A map-like appearance to the surface and sides of the tongue resulting from irregular, red smooth patches that change positions is a benign condition called geographic tongue or migratory glossitis.

> **DANGER SIGN** Quickly progressive swelling of the lips, tongue, and uvula may be angio-edema related to medication use (such as an ACE inhibitor). Discontinue the offending medication and document the allergy.

Diagnosis

Most mouth lesions are diagnosed based on history or physical examination.

Disorder	Fever	Lesion description	Associated findings	Length of illness
Aphthous ulcers (canker sores)	Absent	Shallow, painful, round or oval ulcers on a gray-colored base	None	10–14 days; outbreaks reoccur, becoming less frequent in adulthood
Behçet syndrome	Absent	Similar to aphthous ulcers	Genital ulcerations	1–3 weeks
Herpes stomatitis	Children may present with fever with initial eruption	Intraoral vesicular lesions/erosions on an erythematous base	With recurrent outbreaks, may have prodromal tingling or burning; young children may drool	7–14 days; outbreaks reoccur
Oral candidiasis	Possible	White plaques or patches on tongue, buccal mucosa, palate or oropharynx—erythema without plaques under dentures	Beefy red tongue, angular cheilitis (cheilosis), difficulty sucking (infants), anorexia; infants may have associated diaper rash	Usually requires treatment for resolution

Table 5.4.1 Differentiating Oral Lesions

Disorder	Fever	Lesion description	Associated findings	Length of illness
Oral cancer	Typically absent	Relatively painless plaques, erosions, ulcer, or patches that persist	Immobile, nontender lymph nodes	Persistent
Herpangina	Usually high for several days	Red vesicles on palate and posterior pharyngeal structures, eventual ulceration	Headache or neck pain	3–7 days
Hand, foot, and mouth disease	Usually high	Red vesicles in oropharynx, eventual ulceration	Hand and foot maculopapular rash evolves to vesicles which ulcerate	1–2 weeks
Leukoplakia	Absent	Flat white patches/plaques on oral mucosa	History of smokeless tobacco use	Can recur or progress; usually benign, but may be precursor to oral cancer
Hairy leukoplakia	Absent	White patches on tongue or oral mucosa with a corrugated or hairy appearance	Associated with Epstein-Barr virus and HIV infection	Persists, but may resolve with immune system improvement
Koplik spots	Typically present	Small white spots, possibly red base—on buccal mucosa	Measles (rubeola) vaccine-naïve, maculopapular rash, malaise, cold symptoms	12–72 hours

Table 5.4.1 Differentiating Oral Lesions (Continued)

The diagnosis of candidiasis may be confirmed with a KOH prep of a plaque scraping that, if positive, shows budding yeast. HSV-1 infection may be confirmed with a Tzanck smear showing multinucleated giant cells. In Behçet syndrome, a positive pathergy test is helpful in reaching the diagnosis. Significant edema and erythema in the gum surrounding a tooth or teeth may indicate a dental abscess. An avulsed tooth will leave an opening in the gum at that location.

Disorder	Causative agent
Aphthous ulcers	Probably infectious, not clearly identified
Behçet syndrome	Neutrophilic inflammatory disorder
Herpes stomatitis	Herpes simplex virus type 1 (HSV-1)
Oral candidiasis	Candida albicans, or other candida strains
Oral cancer	Increased incidence with alcohol and tobacco use, HPV 16
Herpangina	Coxsackievirus
Hand, foot, and mouth disease	Coxsackievirus
Leukoplakia	Not identified
Koplik spots	Measles virus

Table 5.4.2 Etiology of Oral Lesions

> **DANGER SIGN** A patient with possible Ludwig angina (an apparent infection of the sub-mandibular area) is at risk for airway compromise. Refer to the hospital for intravenous antibiotics and potential airway management (tracheostomy may be needed).

Plan

Treatment

As most oral lesions are accompanied by pain, attempt to provide pain relief and promote hydration.

Disorder	Treatment
Aphthous ulcers	Numbing gels may help with the discomfort
Behçet syndrome	Colchicine (Colcrys, Mitigare) or numerous immunosuppressive medications
Herpes stomatitis	Acyclovir (Zovirax) for 1 week, begun within 3 days of outbreak, may limit severity of lesions
Oral candidiasis	Nystatin suspension (Mycostatin, Bio-Statin) or clotrimazole (Mycelex) troche
Herpangina, and hand, foot, and mouth disease	Supportive care
Leukoplakia	No treatment needed; monitor for progression
Koplik spots	Supportive care for measles

Table 5.4.3 Treatment of Oral Lesions

Education

Acetaminophen may provide some relief of discomfort and fever. Additionally, "magic mouthwash" (various mixtures are used) swished and spit out every 2 hours may be helpful. Reducing pain is important to improve oral intake and avoid dehydration. Additionally, avoidance of hot, spicy, or salty foods, as well as hard or sharp foods, may be helpful. Encourage cold foods, ice, and popsicles. Utilize a soft toothbrush to brush teeth.

Referral

Refer patients with the following:

- **Suspected oral cancer:** to the oncology team for biopsy and potential diagnosis/treatment
- **Dental abscess:** may prescribe antibiotics prior to appointment with dentist
- **Avulsed permanent tooth:** after gently rinsing, place back in socket if able or place tooth in saliva, milk, or special culture material, and refer to dentist (pediatric dentist if a child)

Takeaways

- Patients with oral lesions are often in pain; ensure discomfort relief and promotion of hydration.
- Diagnosis of most oral lesions is made based upon clinical presentation.
- Oral candidiasis requires treatment with an antifungal agent.
- Herpes stomatitis may be limited in severity if acyclovir is begun with three days of outbreak initiation.
- Refer patients with suspected oral cancer, dental abscess, or avulsed permanent tooth.

LESSON 5: THROAT

Learning Objectives
- Identify clinical manifestations of disorders of the throat
- Choose and interpret laboratory/diagnostic testing for throat disorders
- Differentiate appropriate treatment and referrals related to disorders of the throat

Many disorders of the throat are infectious, with most being viral in nature. If determined to be bacterial, anti-infective medications are warranted. Pain is a presenting feature common to many of these disorders.

Pro Tip
Younger children's tonsils are ordinarily larger than those of older children or adults.

Definitions
- **Epiglottitis:** inflammation of the epiglottis, most commonly with Haemophilus influenzae type B
- **Kissing tonsils:** tonsils greater than 4+, touching; can result in airway compromise; more common in younger children
- **Odynophagia:** difficulty swallowing
- **Pharyngitis:** inflammation of the oropharynx
- **Scarlatiniform rash:** red, fine, sandpaper-like rash; characteristic of scarlet fever
- **Trismus:** reduced opening of the jaw, commonly referred to as "lockjaw"

Assessment

History
Ask about infectious exposures.

Subjective

Symptoms
- Sore or scratchy throat
- Fever
- Malaise, fatigue
- Headache

> **DANGER SIGN** Sudden onset of fever, dysphagia, drooling, muffled voice accompanied by very ill appearance, stridor, forward sitting or tripod position, and respiratory distress without cough may indicate epiglottitis (most frequently in the 2–8-year-old child, though can occur at any age). Do not attempt to reposition patient or to visualize throat. Send/refer immediately to the nearest emergency department for potential emergent airway maintenance.

Review of Systems

- **Constitutional:** anorexia
- **EENT:** snoring, pain with swallowing
- **GI:** abdominal pain, nausea/vomiting
- **GU:** decreased urine output
- **MS:** achiness
- **Skin:** rash, particularly on abdomen/trunk
- **Neuro:** headache
- **Hematologic/lymphatic:** painful or swollen cervical lymph nodes

Objective

- **HEENT:** note exudate or erythema in the mouth, pharynx, tonsils, or petechiae on the palate or gums; tongue may be red; determine airway patency; note tender anterior cervical nodes (consistent with strep A infection), tender posterior cervical nodes or generalized lymphadenopathy (consistent with mononucleosis); assess for nuchal rigidity; note lack of common cold signs (watery eyes, coryza, rhinitis)
- **CV:** auscultate heart, listen for murmur (suggestive of rheumatic fever post pharyngitis); measure blood pressure
- **Resp:** auscultate lungs (pneumonia or pleural effusion can occur with mononuleosis; stridor may be present with epiglottitis)
- **GI:** percuss liver and spleen; palpate for organomegaly or costovertebral angle tenderness
- **Skin:** observe for scarlatiniform rash on abdomen, with possible coalescing in skin folds; in infants, inspect for redness around anus

> **DANGER SIGN** Peritonsillar abscess is identified by fever, severe throat pain, odynophagia, cervical adenopathy, trismus, and unilateral bulging in posterior palatine area, which may quickly result in airway obstruction. Immediately refer to otolaryngology for incision and drainage!

Diagnosis

When a patient presents with a sore throat, it is important to distinguish between pharyngitis/tonsillitis and infectious mononucleosis. The vast majority of cases of pharyngitis/tonsillitis are viral in nature, and when bacterial, group A streptococcus is the most common bacterial cause. Appropriately treat group A strep to avoid complications such as rheumatic fever (*see Chapter 17, Lesson 3*) and acute glomerulonephritis (*see Chapter 9, Lesson 1*). Scarlet fever is diagnosed in the patient positive for group A strep, with presence of scarlatiniform rash. Infectious mononucleosis results from infection with Epstein-Barr virus.

Clinical manifestation	Pharyngitis/tonsillitis	Infectious mononucleosis
Sore throat	Present	Present
Pharyngeal or tonsillar exudate	May be present	May be present
Cervical lymphadenopathy	Usually anterior	Usually posterior or generalized
Headache	Common	Common
Scarletinaform rash	With scarlet fever	Not present
Fatigue	Present	Pronounced
Malaise	Present	Pronounced
Hepatosplenomegaly	Not present	May be present
Abdominal pain	Possible	Especially in younger children

Table 5.5.1 Clinical Manifestations Used in Diagnosis

Laboratory testing may be helpful in the differential diagnosis for the patient presenting with pharyngitis/tonsillitis. The Centor criteria may be used to determine when a patient needs neither laboratory testing nor antibiotic therapy (hence predictive of viral infection). The Centor criteria are:

1. Fever by history
2. Absence of cough
3. Tonsillar exudate
4. Tender anterior cervical adenopathy

In adults, viral infection is likely in patients with zero, one, or two of the criteria. If the patient is age 3 to 14 years old, that age counts as one positive criterion as well.

The gold standard for documenting the presence of *Streptococcus pyogenes* is the throat culture, yet cultures require 24–48 hours to obtain a result. The rapid antigen detection test (RADT or rapid strep test) may be obtained in the office, provides results within 10 minutes, and is extremely sensitive and specific for group A strep.

In the patient suspected of having infectious mononucleosis, the heterophile antibody test (Mono spot) may be ordered. The test is usually positive at two to six weeks after infection with Epstein-Barr virus begins, so it may be negative early in the course of infectious mononucleosis. It is also much less sensitive in infants and young children. When the heterophile antibody test is negative, testing for EBV antibodies may then be warranted. A complete blood count with differential may reveal atypical lymphocytes and lymphocytosis in the patient with mononucleosis.

Plan

Treatment

Viral pharyngitis/tonsillitis requires only supportive care. For documented group A, C, or G strep infection, in addition to supportive care prescribe one of the following:

- Penicillin V potassium (PenVK) 250 mg 4 times a day or 500 mg twice daily (adolescents and adults) or 250 mg 2–3 times daily (children) for 10 days
- Amoxicillin 50 mg/kg once daily or 25 mg/kg twice daily for 10 days (children)
- Pencillin G benzathine 600,000 units (patients less than 27 kg) or 1,200,000 units (patients greater than 27 kg) intramuscularly times 1 dose

In the penicillin-allergic patient, prescribe cephalexin, cefadroxil, azithromycin, clarithromycin, or clindamycin. Other bacteria may be determined by throat culture requiring antibiotic treatment:

- *Fusobacterium necrophorum:* prescribe clindamycin or amoxicillin-clavulanate (Augmentin)
- *Neisseria gonorrhoeae:* prescribe ceftriaxone (Rocephin) intramuscularly plus azithromycin (Zithromax) orally

For the patient with recurrent bacterial pharyngitis, options include clindamycin, penicillin V potassium with rifampin, amoxicillin-clavulanic acid, or penicillin G benzathine with rifampin.

Antiviral medications are not prescribed in viral pharyngitis/tonsillitis and infectious mononucleosis.

Education

Supportive care for pharyngitis/tonsillitis includes warm or cool fluids to soothe the throat, lozenges, and avoidance of salty or spicy foods. Use acetaminophen or other NSAIDs to ease fever and pain (avoid aspirin use in children). Increase fluid intake. If antibiotics are prescribed, complete the entire course of medication. Notify the nurse practitioner if swallowing or breathing becomes difficult due to the sore throat.

For mononucleosis, follow the same instructions for pharyngitis/tonsillitis in relation to palliation of sore throat. In addition, rest in bed, gradually returning to the normal activity level. Fatigue may last for several weeks. Avoid physical activity (especially contact sports) until cleared by the nurse practitioner. If severe pain in the upper left abdomen occurs (splenic rupture), seek medical attention immediately. If antibiotics are prescribed for a concomitant bacterial infection, a rash may follow their use.

Referrals

Consult physician if dysphagia or dyspnea present. Refer patients with:

- **Recurrent tonsillitis**, and those with large tonsils who snore (possible obstructive sleep apnea), to the otolaryngologist for evaluation for tonsillectomy
- **Suspected epiglottitis:** immediate referral to the nearest emergency room for appropriate airway management
- **Peritonsillar abscess:** immediate referral to otolaryngology for incision and drainage

Takeaways

- Supportive care related to hydration and throat pain palliation is important in both pharyngitis/tonsillitis and infectious mononucleosis.
- Use the Centor criteria to determine need for rapid antigen detection testing for pharyngitis/tonsillitis.
- Prescribe antibiotics for pharyngitis only in documented cases of bacterial infection.
- Perform skillful abdominal assessment and order appropriate imaging studies in the patient with mononucleosis to determine extent of hepatosplenomegaly.

PRACTICE QUESTIONS

Select the ONE best answer.

Lesson 1: Eyes

1. Fluorescein stain and a Wood's lamp are useful in diagnosing which disorders?

    A. Corneal abrasions and herpes keratitis

    B. Glaucoma and allergic conjunctivitis

    C. Herpes keratitis and bacterial conjunctivitis

    D. Corneal abrasions and glaucoma

2. Which of the following sets of clinical manifestations is consistent with acute angle-closure glaucoma?

    A. Gradual increase in intraocular pressure resulting in eye pain

    B. Sudden increase in intraocular pressure without eye pain

    C. Gradual increase in intraocular pressure without eye pain

    D. Sudden increase in intraocular pressure with eye pain

3. Which of the following is not a symptom of herpes keratitis?

    A. Eye pain

    B. Photophobia

    C. Seeing halos

    D. Blurred vision

4. The NP is assessing a young child and notes a 2 mm pustule on the left lower eyelid margin accompanied by erythema, swelling, and a small amount of purulent discharge. This finding is most consistent with which condition?

    A. Blepharitis

    B. Chalazion

    C. Conjunctivitis

    D. Hordeolum

5. What should the NP prescribe for acute dacryocystitis?

    A. Antiviral medication

    B. Dacryocystorhinostomy

    C. Antimicrobial medication

    D. Cold compresses

6. What is a key diagnostic finding in open-angle glaucoma?

    A. Papilledema

    B. Increased intraocular pressure

    C. Eye pain

    D. Sluggish pupils

Lesson 2: Ears

7. Which of the following would the NP use to determine hearing loss?

    A. Audiogram

    B. Tympanogram

    C. Pneumatic otoscopy

    D. Computed tomography

8. In a child with otitis media with effusion (OME), which characteristic will the tympanic membrane have upon otoscopic examination?

    A. Erythematous

    B. Bulging

    C. Retracted

    D. Vascular in appearance

9. When educating a patient with Ménière disease about prevention of episodes, the NP teaches the patient to restrict all of the following except:

    A. Sodium

    B. Nicotine

    C. Fluid intake

    D. Caffeine

10. Of the following measures, which is recommended for preventing otitis media?

    A. Allowing supine bottle feeding

    B. Avoiding secondhand smoke

    C. Placing in a day care setting

    D. Allowing pacifier use

11. The NP has diagnosed an older adult patient with benign paroxysmal positional vertigo (BPPV). Which of the following tests aids in diagnosis?

    A. Positive Epley maneuver

    B. Pneumatic otoscopy

    C. Computed tomography

    D. Positive Dix-Hallpike test

12. Which of the following objective findings would be consistent with the diagnosis of otitis externa?

    A. Bullae on the tympanic membrane

    B. Red, bulging tympanic membrane

    C. Increased pain with tragus palpation

    D. Tympanic membrane immobility

Lesson 3: Nose

13. Which of the following is not a preventive measure for epistaxis?

    A. Using a water-based lubricant in the nares

    B. Not taking hot showers

    C. Avoiding forceful nose blowing

    D. Using a humidifier

14. The NP has diagnosed a patient with allergic rhinitis. What diagnostic testing would be appropriate?

    A. Blood chemistries

    B. Computed tomography of the sinuses

    C. Radioallergosorbent testing

    D. Plain x-ray films of the sinuses

15. Which medication is considered first-line treatment for acute bacterial rhinosinusitis?

    A. doxycycline (Monodox)

    B. levofloxacin (Levaquin)

    C. amoxicillin-clavulanate (Augmentin)

    D. moxifloxacin (Avalox)

16. In the patient diagnosed with allergic rhinitis, which medication would be used as rescue therapy?

    A. Oral antihistamines

    B. Corticosteroid nasal spray

    C. Mast cell stabilizers

    D. Leukotriene modifiers

17. Which finding is most consistent with the diagnosis of acute bacterial rhinosinusitis?

    A. Upper respiratory symptoms lasting less than 7 days

    B. Mild tenderness and fullness with sinus palpation

    C. Upper respiratory symptoms lasting longer than 10 days

    D. Thick nasal drainage that has become discolored

Lesson 4: Mouth

18. How is herpes stomatitis differentiated on physical examination?

    A. Large white patches or plaques on tongue

    B. Round ulcers on a gray base in oral cavity

    C. Ulcerations on an erythematous base

    D. Small white spots on buccal mucosa

19. Which diagnostic test is most appropriate for confirming the diagnosis of oral candidiasis?

    A. Bacterial culture and sensitivity

    B. KOH prep

    C. Positive pathergy test

    D. Tzanck smear

20. The NP is evaluating a patient with a 2-day history of fever, poor appetite, and mouth pain. The NP notes red vesicles inside the mouth. Which additional assessment is most important for the determining the patient's diagnosis?

    A. Assess for a sandpaper-like rash on the abdomen

    B. Observe the hands and feet for erythematous lesions

    C. Palpate lymph nodes for swelling, determining if tender

    D. Inspect genital area for presence of ulcerations

21. The NP is caring for a 6-year-old who had one of his front (permanent) teeth kicked out. The child is crying hysterically. In addition to referring the child to a pediatric dentist immediately, what should be done with the avulsed tooth?

    A. Place it in a container of milk

    B. Put the tooth in ice or water

    C. Allow the child to hold the tooth in his mouth

    D. Scrub the tooth vigorously to disinfect it

22. What do Koplik spots occur with?

    A. Leukoplakia

    B. Rubella

    C. Rubeola

    D. Behçet syndrome

23. The NP is caring for a patient who describes recent stress in her life and presents with a recurrent mouth lesion. The lesion came up again 2 days ago, is on the interior lip border, is ulcerative and painful, and has an erythematous base. What is the medication treatment of choice for this patient?

    A. colchicine (Colcrys)

    B. amoxicillin (Amoxil)

    C. acyclovir (Zovirax)

    D. mycostatin (Nystatin)

Lesson 5: Throat

24. Which of the following describes a peritonsillar abscess?

    A. Inflammation of the tonsils

    B. Decreased blood supply to the tonsils

    C. Autoimmune destruction of the tonsils

    D. Palpable collection of pus around the tonsils

25. Of the following treatments, which is not included in the plan for strep pharyngitis?

    A. throat lozenges

    B. ibuprofen (Motrin)

    C. prednisone (Deltazone)

    D. penicillin V (PenVK)

26. Which of the following is not a common manifestation of infectious mononucleosis?

    A. Paroxysmal coughing

    B. Fatigue

    C. Sore throat

    D. Lymphadenopathy

27. Group A strep pharyngitis may result in which of the following?

    A. Rheumatic fever, Kawasaki syndrome, acute glomerulonephritis

    B. Scarlet fever, acute glomerulonephritis, hemolytic uremic syndrome

    C. Hemolytic uremic syndrome, rheumatic fever, scarlet fever

    D. Rheumatic fever, acute glomerulonephritis, scarlet fever

28. When treating infectious mononucleosis, the NP should recommend which of the following?

    A. Antibiotics, analgesics, fluids, rest

    B. Antivirals, analgesics, fluids, rest

    C. Fever and pain reduction, fluids, rest

    D. Allow sports participation, fluids, analgesics

29. Which laboratory tests are appropriate for evaluating a patient with suspected mononucleosis?

    A. Complete blood count (CBC), heterophile antibody test

    B. Rapid antigen detection test, complete blood count (CBC)

    C. Only a heterophile antibody test is necessary

    D. Lymphocyte count, rapid plasma reagin test

30. Which common findings should the NP monitor for in a patient diagnosed with infectious mononucleosis?

    A. Hepatomegaly, splenomegaly, heart failure

    B. Hepatomegaly, lymphocytosis, splenomegaly

    C. Heart failure, lymphocytosis, hepatomegaly

    D. Renal failure, hepatomegaly, splenomegaly

31. Which statement is true concerning pharyngitis?

    A. All sore throats require antibiotic treatment

    B. Most cases of pharyngitis are bacterial in nature

    C. Most cases of pharyngitis are viral in nature

    D. Empiric treatment of pharyngitis is important

32. The NP is caring for a 10-year-old with a sore throat and rash. Which test should be ordered to verify the most common cause of bacterial pharyngitis?

    A. Anti-streptolysin O

    B. Heterophile antibody test

    C. Rapid antigen detection test

    D. Rapid plasma reagin

ANSWERS AND EXPLANATIONS

Lesson 1: Eyes

1.   A
Wood's lamp visualization of fluorescein staining is helpful in the diagnosis of corneal abrasions and herpes keratitis **(A)**. The yellow stain may reveal a scratch on the cornea (abrasion) or dendrite pattern (keratitis). Fluorescein and the Wood's lamp are not used in the diagnosis of conjunctivitis (B and C) or glaucoma (B and D).

2.   D
A sudden increase in intraocular pressure with eye pain **(D)** occurs with acute angle closure glaucoma. The increase in intraocular pressure is not gradual (A and C), nor is there absence of eye pain (B and C).

3.   C
Seeing halos **(C)** does not occur with herpes keratitis. Eye pain (A), photophobia (B), and blurred vision (D) are all symptoms of herpes keratitis.

4.   D
A hordeolum **(D)**, more commonly called a stye, is caused by a bacterial infection on the lid margin. Localized redness, edema, and purulence will occur. Blepharitis (A), inflammation of the eyelid margins, results in burning/itching/tearing with erythema/edema of the lid margin and dryness or flaking, not purulence. Chalazion (B) may be distinguished from hordeolum by its lack of purulence. Conjuncitivis (C) is inflammation of the conjunctivae.

5.   C
An appropriate treatment for acute dacryocystitis is antibiotics **(C)**. Acute dacryocystitis is caused by bacterial buildup in the lacrimal duct, so antiviral medication (A) is inappropriate. Chronic dacryocystitis may benefit from the procedure dacryocystorhinostomy (B); it is not a first-line treatment for acute dacryocystitis. Warm, not cold, compresses (D) may also be helpful.

6.   B
Open-angle glaucoma is characterized by a gradual increase in intraocular pressure **(B)**. Papilledema (A) is an indication of increased intracranial pressure. Open-angle glaucoma is not accompanied by eye pain (C), nor does it affect pupillary reactivity (D).

Lesson 2: Ears

7.   A
The audiogram **(A)** is a graphic representation of pure-tone hearing response and is useful in the determination of hearing loss. Tympanography (B) and pneumatic otoscopy (C) are utilized to evaluate tympanic membrane movement. Computed tomography (D) does not determine hearing loss.

8.   C
In otitis media with effusion, the tympanic membrane (TM) appears to be retracted **(C)**. An erythematous (A), bulging (B) TM occurs with acute otitis media. Increased vascular appearance (D) of the TM is not associated with OME.

9.   C
It is not necessary to restrict fluid intake **(C)** to avoid an episode of Ménière disease. Excessive salt intake (A), nicotine (B), and caffeine (D) should be restricted in an attempt to avoid triggering future episodes of vertigo.

10.   B
Secondhand smoke exposure **(B)** is a risk factor for the development of otitis media and should be avoided. Supine bottle feeding (A), day care attendance (C), and pacifier use (D) past early infancy are also risk factors—not preventive measures.

11.   D
A positive Dix-Hallpike test **(D)** is diagnostic of BPPV. The Epley maneuver (A) is a treatment for BPPV. Pneumatic otoscopy (B) is used to evaluate tympanic membrane mobility. Computed tomography (C) is not necessary for the diagnosis of BPPV.

12.   C
Increased pain with tragus palpation **(C)** is present due to the inflamed ear canal. Bullae on the tympanic membrane (A) is associated with myringitis. With acute otitis media, the tympanic membrane may be erythematous and bulging (B). The tympanic membrane is immobile (D) in acute otitis media and otitis media with effusion.

Lesson 3: Nose

13. B

Hot showers **(B)** aren't related to the occurrence of epistaxis; in fact, showers may assist with moistening the nasal mucosa and can be used as a form of relief. Using a water-based lubricant in the nares (A) (especially in a dry environment), avoiding forceful nose blowing (C), and using a humidifier (D) are all measures to help prevent epistaxis.

14. C

Radioallergosorbent testing (RAST) **(C)** is appropriate for the determination of the patient's allergies. Blood chemistries (A) are not needed. Computed tomography (B) and plain x-rays (D) would be appropriate for chronic and acute sinusitis respectively.

15. C

Amoxicillin-clavulanate **(C)** is recommended as the first-line medication for empiric treatment of acute bacterial rhinosinusitis. Doxycycline (A) is indicated as second-line. Levofloxacin (B) and moxifloxacin (D) are recommended for those with beta-lactam allergy.

16. A

Using oral antihistamines **(A)** serves as a rescue therapy (to inactivate formed inflammatory mediators), rather than a controller type therapy. Corticosteroid nasal spray (B), mast cell stabilizers (C), and leukotriene modifiers (D) may all be used for controller therapy (prevention of the allergic response).

17. C

Acute bacterial rhinosinusitis is considered in the patient with upper respiratory-like symptoms lasting longer than 10 days **(C)** and that have persisted or worsened. Viral upper respiratory infections tend to last 5–7 days (A). Mild tenderness and fullness with sinus palpation (B) may occur with a viral URI. Discolored nasal drainage (D) is not a quality indicator of viral vs. bacterial infection.

Lesson 4: Mouth

18. C

Ulcers with an erythematous base **(C)** are consistent with herpes stomatitis. Large white patches or plaques on the tongue (A) are associated with oral candidiasis or leukoplakia. Ulcerations on a gray base (B) occur with aphthous ulcers. Small white spots on the buccal mucosa, possibly with mild erythema present (D) are Koplik spots and are distinctively indicative of rubeola (measles).

19. B

Candida is a fungus and is appropriately identified with KOH prep **(B)**. The other choices are incorrect. Most infectious agents resulting in oral lesions are viral in nature, so a bacterial culture and sensitivity test (A) would not be appropriate. The positive pathergy test (C) is useful in Behçet syndrome, while the Tzanck smear (D) is used to identify herpes stomatitis.

20. B

The history and physical examination is suggestive of coxsackievirus infection, which would be herpangina if only the mouth is involved, and hand, foot, and mouth disease if lesions are also present on the hands and/or feet **(B)**. A sandpaper-like abdominal rash (A) occurs with streptococcal type A infections. Lymph node swelling (C) is common with oral cancer (painless mouth lesions). The history of fever is inconsistent with Behçet syndrome in which genital ulcerations also occur (D).

21. A

Placing the tooth in milk **(A)**, saliva, or special culture media would be appropriate. Placing the tooth in ice or water (B) is inappropriate. The child is too distraught to safely hold the tooth in his mouth (C). The tooth should be gently rinsed, not vigorously scrubbed (D).

22. C

Koplik spots are pathognomonic for rubeola (measles) **(C)**. They do not occur with leukoplakia (benign white patch condition) (A), rubella (German measles) (B), or Behçet syndrome (D), a neutrophilic inflammatory disorder.

23. C

The clinical manifestations are indicative of a herpes simplex outbreak. Acyclovir **(C)** may be used to lessen the severity of a herpes stomatitis, if started within three days of the outbreak. Behçet syndrome may be treated with the anti-gout medication colchicine (A). Most other infectious oral lesions are viral in nature, thus using an antibiotic (B) would be inappropriate. Nystatin (D) is an antifungal agent appropriate for the treatment of oral candidiasis.

Lesson 5: Throat

24. D

Peritonsillar abscess, a complication of tonsillitis (A), is defined as a collection of pus around the tonsils **(D)**. It is most often caused by group A streptococcus, may result in airway obstruction, and requires immediate referral to otolaryngology for incision and drainage. Decreased blood supply (B) and autoimmune destruction (C) may be eliminated.

25. C

Corticosteroids such as prednisone **(C)** are not used to treat strep throat. Relief of throat pain may be achieved through the use of lozenges (A) or analgesics (B). The antibiotic treatment of choice is penicillin (D), with macrolides or cephalosporins used in the penicillin-allergic.

26. A

Paroxysmal coughing **(A)** is not a common finding in infectious mononucleosis. The classic triad of presenting manifestations of mononucleosis are fatigue (B), sore throat (C), and posterior cervical lymphadenopathy (D).

27. D

Scarlet fever is defined as strep pharyngitis accompanied by a scarlatiniform rash, which coalesces in the folds of the skin, and facial flushing. Acute glomerulonephritis and rheumatic fever can both be complications of non-fully treated group A strep infection **(D)**. Kawasaki syndrome (A) is an acute febrile illness usually occurring in early childhood resulting in vasculitis; it is possibly infectious in nature but also thought to have genetic and/or autoimmune components. Hemolytic uremic syndrome (B and C) is a renal complication of infection with shiga toxin–producing Escherichia coli.

28. C

Recommending fluids, rest, and analgesics **(C)** to reduce pain and fever is appropriate. Mononucleosis is caused by the Epstein-Barr virus, so antibiotics (A) are inappropriate and antivirals (B) are not recommended. Mono may result in organomegaly; if so, contact sports are prohibited (D) until hepatosplenomegaly resolves.

29. A

A CBC may reveal atypical lymphocytes and lymphocytosis; the heterophile antibody test becomes positive about two weeks after infection **(A)**. The rapid antigen test (B) is for the determination of the presence of group A strep, not Epstein-Barr virus. The heterophile antibody test (C) may not become positive until two weeks after infection, so if performed early and mononucleosis is ruled out based on that result, the diagnosis could be incorrect. The rapid plasma regain test (D) is for determination of syphilis infection, not Epstein-Barr virus.

30. B

Infectious mononucleosis most often results in lymphocytosis and hepatosplenomegaly **(B)**. Heart failure (A and C) and renal failure (D) are not common complications of mononucleosis.

31. C

Viral causes account for most cases of pharyngitis **(C)**, with fewer cases actually caused by a bacteria (B), most often group A streptococcus. As such, antibiotic treatment (A) should be reserved for documented bacterial infection and not prescribed empirically (D).

32. C

The rapid antigen detection test **(C)**, commonly called a rapid strep test, is highly specific and sensitive for determining group A strep infection. The anti-streptolysin O test (A) is used for identification of past group A beta-hemolytic streptococcal infections and can be eliminated. Eliminate heterophile antibody test (B), as it used for determining Epstein-Barr virus infection. Eliminate rapid plasma reagin (D), as it is used for confirmation of syphilis (not the most common cause of pharyngitis).

CHAPTER 6

Respiratory

LESSON 1: ASTHMA

Learning Objectives
- Predict patients at risk for asthma and identify expected findings related to a diagnosis of asthma
- Determine the severity of asthma
- Apply the stepwise approach to asthma management across the life span

Asthma is a recurrent, partially or completely reversible airway obstruction, pulmonary inflammation, and bronchial hyperresponsiveness. It results in decreased oxygenation and air trapping. Remodeling of the airways can occur over time. There are various causes of asthma, and often the cause is multifactorial.

Assessment

Subjective

Symptoms
Ascertain if there is a history of recurrent wheezing and coughing, chest tightness, or difficulty breathing. If these symptoms are present, consider when they started, how long they have been occurring, their frequency and severity, whether there are aggravating and/or alleviating factors, and if the symptoms are worse at night. In addition, other symptoms to inquire about include the following:

- Fever, weight loss or gain, night sweats
- Runny nose, congestion, sore throat, ear pain
- Chest pain, palpitations
- Coughing, wheezing, shortness of breath
- Nausea, vomiting, heartburn, or reflux
- Rashes

ROS
Genetic factors, allergens, viral infection, stress, exercise, and hard crying or laughing can trigger asthma.

History

- **PMH:** frequent lung infections, seasonal or chronic allergies, atopic dermatitis, exposure to possible lung irritants, difficulty breathing, wheezing or chest tightness, frequent ER visits or hospitalizations for lung infections, history of GERD

- **PSH:** ENT or lung surgery

- **FH:** asthma, atopic disease, or eczema

- **SH:** smoking or exposure to secondhand smoke

If the patient is a child, inquire about prematurity, respiratory complications after delivery, inability to keep up with peers when playing, and age-appropriate growth and development.

Objective

- **Vital Signs:** increased respiratory rate and decreased SpO_2

- **HEENT:** ears—effusion, edema and/or erythema; nose—visualize the nasal cavity condition of turbinates, presence of polyps, edema and/or erythema of nasal mucosa, drainage; oropharynx—erythema, injection and/or edema, post-nasal drainage

- **Neck:** cervical, pre- or post-auricular lymphadenopathy

- **Resp:** respiratory distress, use of accessory muscles, retraction of nares or intercostal muscles, adventitious lung sounds, presence of prolonged expiration, and decreased or absent sounds

- **CV:** elevated heart rate or blood pressure suggestive of distress, presence of cardiac murmurs

- **Skin:** erythematous, pruritic, patchy rash to antecubital or popliteal fossa

Diagnosis

Making the diagnosis of asthma is best achieved by a thorough history, physical, and diagnostic testing. Diagnostic testing may include a chest x-ray (CXR) and spirometry. A CXR is not necessary in diagnosis but may be helpful to rule out differential diagnoses, such as infection. In the presence of asthma, the CXR may reveal air trapping.

Spirometry is the gold standard for diagnosing asthma and should be ordered on all patients over the age of 5. When doing spirometry, a baseline is obtained and then the patient is given a short acting beta agonist; spirometry is repeated 10–15 minutes later. An increase in FEV1 >200mL and >12% from the baseline can be attributed to the medication and indicates reversibility of airflow obstruction, thus confirming a diagnosis of asthma. Peak expiratory flow rate is limited and less reliable in making the diagnosis of asthma; it is more useful for monitoring asthma and determining risk for exacerbation.

Once the diagnosis of asthma is made, the severity must be determined. There are six key questions to ask to aid in this process:

1. How often do symptoms occur in a week/month?
2. How often in a week/month is the patient awakened at night by their symptoms?
3. Is the patient's ability to perform normal activities impaired?
4. What are the patient's spirometry results?
5. How often in a week/day is a short-acting beta agonist used?
6. How often in a year has the patient been given tapered steroids to control exacerbations?

Digital Resource

Asthma Quick Care Reference: A guide to diagnosing and managing asthma can be accessed here: **www.nhlbi.nih.gov/files/docs/guidelines/asthma_qrg.pdf**.

Plan

Treatment

Treatment of asthma is based on its severity. The goal of treatment is to prevent permanent lung changes and to minimize risk and impairment. Treatment should include:

- Modification of potential triggers such as allergens and cigarette smoke
- Control of comorbid conditions such as allergic rhinitis, allergic sinusitis, sleep apnea, allergic bronchopulmonary aspergillosis, obesity, stress, depression, and GERD

Medications frequently used to treat asthma include short-acting beta agonist (SABA), anticholinergics, inhaled corticosteroids (ICS), combination inhaled corticosteroids and long-acting beta agonist (LABA), leukotriene receptor antagonist, methylxanthines, cromolyn sodium, nedocromil, immunomodulators, and systemic corticosteroids. Medications are chosen using the stepwise approach, which is dependent on patient age and severity of asthma.

Patients with asthma need frequent follow-up to determine effectiveness of treatment and need for additional interventions. There may be a need for a step up or a step down in therapy depending on the symptoms and severity of asthma.

Education

Teach patients to monitor their peak flow rate to determine if they are beginning to have airway obstruction prior to symptoms and if they are at risk of an exacerbation. Patients should have an asthma action plan based on their daily peak flow and symptoms. The plan will specify which medications to take and what to do if their peak flow and/or symptoms are worsening.

Referral

Refer patients to an asthma specialist if they have atypical symptoms, or symptoms that are refractory to lifestyle changes and stepwise approach to treatment.

> **DANGER SIGN** Status asthmaticus (SA) is an emergent situation requiring immediate transfer to ER. The patient experiencing SA is rapidly deteriorating (tachypnea, low SpO_2, wheezing to decreased breath sounds, use of intercostal muscles, nasal flaring, change in LOC, confusion, difficulty speaking, tachycardia, diaphoresis) and may require intubation and mechanical ventilation if airflow obstruction cannot be reversed.

Takeaways

- Asthma is a disease characterized by reversible airflow obstruction.
- Spirometry is the gold standard for diagnosis and should be performed on patients 5 years of age and older suspected of having asthma.
- Spirometry is suggestive of asthma if the FEV1 increases >200 mL or greater than 12% of baseline value after the administration of SABA.
- Treatment is based on a stepwise approach and based on the severity of asthma.

LESSON 2: COUGH/BRONCHITIS

Learning Objectives
- Identify potential causes of cough and acute bronchitis
- Differentiate acute bronchitis from other infectious conditions
- Select the appropriate treatment measures for acute bronchitis

Cough is one of the most common presenting symptoms in adults who seek treatment in ambulatory care. Acute bronchitis is defined as inflammation of the trachea, bronchi, and bronchioles. It is a transient infection, lasting anywhere from 3–6 weeks. An increase in the frequency and severity of acute bronchitis is seen with cigarette smoking.

Assessment

Subjective

A persistent cough, one that lasts longer than 10–14 days, is the most commonly reported complaint of acute bronchitis and may be the only symptom. The cough is initially dry, but may progress to productive with sputum that is yellow, green, or clear. Other symptoms are variable and may include:

- Low-grade fever, less than 101°F (38.3°C)
- Fatigue, malaise
- Occasional dyspnea or wheezing, especially with exertion
- Headache
- Substernal chest discomfort or burning pain

It is important to gather a thorough history to assist with ruling out other causes of cough, such as medication use (ACE inhibitors), smoking, environmental allergies, and gastroesophageal reflux.

Objective

The physical examination in a patient with acute bronchitis is usually unremarkable. They are afebrile, with lungs that are clear to auscultation and resonant to percussion. Occasionally, wheezing or crackles that clear with coughing may be present.

Diagnosis

It is important to distinguish acute bronchitis from the other most common causes of cough.

Differential Diagnosis

Differential diagnosis	Characteristics
Common cold	Duration of ~7–10 days, rhinorrhea, nasal congestion
Pneumonia	Tachycardia, tachypnea, fever, rales/crackles, rhonchi or wheezes, decreased breath sounds
Gastroesophageal reflux	Cough occurs at night
Allergic rhinitis	Post nasal drip, nasal congestion, sneezing, rhinorrhea

Table 6.2.1 Common Differential Diagnosis for Cough

Additional differential diagnoses for cough: **asthma, influenza, pertussis, tuberculosis, cystic fibrosis, medication side effect, and COPD**

Diagnosis of acute bronchitis is based on clinical presentation. The causative pathogen implicated in the majority of cases is viral. Sputum culture is not recommended since most cases are viral, though if a bacterial pathogen is suspected, sputum cultures may prove helpful in identifying the causative organism. If clinical suspicion for tuberculosis or other pulmonary processes exists, a chest radiograph may be ordered to rule in or out alternate differentials. The chest x-ray will be normal in a patient with acute bronchitis.

Plan

Treatment

Since most cases of acute bronchitis are viral, treatment is focused on managing the patient's symptoms. Rest, increased fluid intake, use of a humidifier, and smoking cessation are included in the treatment plan.

For pharmacological management, antitussives (e.g., codeine, dextromethorphan) are often prescribed for patients 6 years of age and older for short-term symptomatic relief from the persistent cough. Bronchodilators may be beneficial in patients with wheezing and a history of lung disease. NSAIDs may help with constitutional symptoms. Treatment with antimicrobials is not recommended in patients with uncomplicated acute bronchitis. If a bacterial infection is suspected, the choice of antimicrobial should be selected based on the offending organism. Mucolytics/expectorants are used in patients with lung disease, such as COPD, but are not used routinely in uncomplicated cases of acute bronchitis. The use of corticosteroids for acute bronchitis is controversial and generally not recommended.

Education

Patients who present with acute bronchitis are often expecting to be given a prescription. It is important to take the time to explain the reasoning behind the avoidance of using antimicrobial agents. Overprescribing antimicrobial agents leads to medication resistance. Since an overwhelming majority of cases of acute bronchitis are caused by viruses, the use of antimicrobials would prove to be ineffective and potentially harmful.

Referral

If the cough persists longer than six weeks, referral to a specialist should be made.

Takeaways

- Viruses are the most common cause of acute bronchitis.
- Other common causes of cough include medication side effects, smoking, environmental allergies, pneumonia, URI, reflux, pertussis, and TB.
- A persistent cough, one last lasting longer than two weeks and as long as six weeks, is typically the only presenting symptom of acute bronchitis.
- The disease is self-limiting and will resolve without definitive care, thus the focus of treatment is on symptom management.
- Antimicrobial therapy is not recommended unless there is a clear bacterial source.

LESSON 3: COPD

Learning Objectives

■ Recognize modifiable risk factors for COPD and identify key indicators for considering a diagnosis of COPD

■ Accurately assess and stage severity of COPD condition based upon clinical features and spirometry results

■ Identify secondary prevention measures critical to COPD management

■ Select appropriate pharmacologic treatment therapy reflective of COPD severity

Chronic obstructive pulmonary disease (COPD) has been cited as one of the most important public health challenges worldwide. COPD is characterized by progressive airflow limitations, gas exchange abnormalities, and hypersecretion of mucus usually induced by significant exposure to noxious particles or gases. Symptoms may not be fully reversible post-treatment.

COPD is caused by a combination of small airway disease, parenchymal destruction, and mucus hypersecretion. The abnormal changes of COPD are variable and are typically subdivided into emphysema or chronic bronchitis.

- **Emphysema:** permanent abnormal enlargement or destruction of air spaces distal to the terminal bronchioles, including alveolar ducts, alveolar sacs, and alveoli

- **Chronic bronchitis:** clinically defined as a chronic productive cough for 3 consecutive months each year for 2 consecutive years, with other causes excluded

Assessment

Subjective

The most defining characteristic of COPD is chronic and progressive dyspnea. The occurrence of chronic cough or sputum production is variable, with only 30% of COPD patients presenting with a productive cough. Consider COPD and initiate spirometry if any of these indicators are present in an individual 40 years and older with risk factors:

- Dyspnea: progressive, worsens with exercise, or persistent
- Cough: intermittent and/or unproductive
- Sputum production
- Wheezing, chest tightness
- Recurrent lower respiratory tract infections

Independently, these indicators are not diagnostic for COPD, though presence of multiple key indicators increases the likelihood of a COPD diagnosis.

Risk factors for COPD	
Tobacco smoke	Substantial increase in likelihood occurs with >40 pack-years history
Indoor and outdoor air pollution	Influenced by socioeconomic status
Occupational exposures	Including organic/inorganic airborne particles, chemical agents, and fumes
Genetic factors	i.e., genetic deficiency of alpha-1 antitrypsin
Age and gender	Greater prevalence among women and adults >45 years
Lung growth and development	Impaired maturity during gestation, poor nutrition, and/or recurrent childhood infections

Table 6.3.1 Risk Factors for COPD

Due to the potential costs and lack of evidence of benefit, screening in asymptomatic individuals at increased risk is not recommended by the American College of Physicians (ACP), Global Initiative for Chronic Obstructive Lung Disease (GOLD), and the U.S. Preventative Services Task Force.

In addition to exploration of current symptoms and risk factors, it is critical to assess:

- **Presence of comorbidities:** particularly depression and anxiety, which are common in COPD and are associated with increased risk of exacerbations
- **Impact of disease on patient's life:** including impact on activities of daily living, employment, and sense of well-being

Objective

Physical Examination

Physiologic changes incurred with airflow limitation and inflammatory remodeling typically do not emerge as physical signs until profound impairment of lung function occurs. As a result, absence of physical signs such as increased AP diameter, weight loss, accessory muscle use, and tachypnea does not exclude the diagnosis.

Spirometry

Spirometry is the most reliable and objective mechanism for measurement of airflow limitation. When performed properly, its pre- and post-bronchodilator measurements include the volume of air forcibly exhaled from point of maximal inspiration (forced vital capacity, FVC) and the volume of air exhaled during the first second of this maneuver (forced expiratory volume in one second, FEV_1). The ratio of these two measurements (FEV_1/FVC) is calculated; a ratio of less than 0.7 confirms persistent airflow obstruction.

Diagnosis

According to the GOLD Guidelines, the diagnosis of COPD is established by a post-bronchodilator $FEV_1/FVC < 0.70$ (<70%) spirometry measurement among individuals with appropriate symptoms and significant exposure to noxious agents.

Classification of the severity of airflow limitation in COPD patients is based upon post-bronchodilator FEV_1 measurements.

In patients with $FEV_1/FVC < 0.70$:		
GOLD 1	Mild	$FEV_1 > 80\%$ predicted
GOLD 2	Moderate	$50\% \leq FEV_1 < 80\%$ predicted
GOLD 3	Severe	$30\% \leq FEV_1 < 50\%$ predicted
GOLD 4	Very Severe	$FEV_1 < 30\%$ predicted

Table 6.3.2 Classification of Airflow Limitation Severity in COPD

A validated questionnaire can determine both the severity of cough and activity limitations and the effectiveness of medical interventions, and can be found at:

1. The Modified Medical Research Council dyspnea scale (mMRC) **http://copd.about.com/od/copdbasics/a/ MMRCdyspneascale.htm** or
2. The COPD Assessment Test (CAT) **www.catesonline.org**

The GOLD Combined Assessment considers questionnaire results in combination with number of exacerbations per year and degree of airflow obstruction to classify patients with COPD into one of four categories.

Risk group	GOLD spirometric classification	Exacerbations per year	mMRC score	CAT score
A (low risk, fewer symptoms)	GOLD 1 or 2	≤1	0 or 1	<10
B (low risk, more symptoms)	GOLD 1 or 2	≤1	≥2	≥10
C (high risk, fewer symptoms)	GOLD 3 or 4	≥2	0 or 1	<10
D (high risk, more symptoms)	GOLD 3 or 4	≥2	≥2	≥10

Table 6.3.3 GOLD Combined Assessment of COPD

Plan

Treatment

Treatment plans for COPD should include interventions that will reduce the number of and minimize the impact of symptoms and reduce future exacerbations and adverse health events.

Critical to the treatment plan is the assessment of airflow limitation and characterization of a patient's symptoms. These measurements guide both preventative and pharmacologic interventions, but also assist in determining a COPD patient's risk for exacerbation.

Encourage all COPD patients to receive an annual influenza vaccine and counsel them on the appropriateness of pneumococcal vaccination. PCV13 and PPSV23 are recommended for all patients 65 years of age or older, according to the Advisory Committee on Immunization Practices (ACIP) recommendations. PPSV23 is recommended for younger COPD patients with significant comorbidities, such as chronic heart or lung disease, and has been shown to reduce the incidence of community-acquired pneumonia in COPD patients with a FEV_1 <40% predicted.

As a patient's condition progresses to moderate to severe COPD, periodic evaluations for hypoxemia should be performed to assess the need for long-term oxygen therapy. The administration of oxygen in patients with severe chronic resting arterial hypoxemia has been proven to increase survival. Severe resting hypoxemia is characterized as PaO_2 of 55 mm Hg or less, or an oxygen saturation of 88% or less. Measurements for hypoxemia should occur after the patient has been breathing room air for 30 minutes or via arterial blood gas levels. Goals for oxygen therapy include a minimum use of 15 hours per day to achieve a target oxygen saturation level of 88%–92%, or a PaO_2 level greater than 60 mmHg.

Pharmacologic Therapy

Patient group	Initial therapy	Secondary agent(s)	Escalation/ de-escalation strategies
Group A (lower risk, fewer symptoms)	SABA (albuterol, Ventolin HFA) *or* add SAMA (ipratropium, Atrovent)	Try alternative class of bronchodilator *or* LABA (salmeterol, Serevent)	• Continue if symptomatic benefit achieved
Group B (low risk, more symptoms)	LABA (salmeterol, Serevent) *or* LAMA (tiotropium, Spiriva) For those with severe symptoms, start with use of 2 bronchodilators	SABA + LABA *or* LABA + LAMA	• LABA should be scheduled dosing with option to use SABA as scheduled or PRN
Group C (high risk, fewer symptoms)	LAMA (tiotropium, Spiriva)	LAMA + LABA *or* LABA + ICS (fluticasone, Flovent)	• ICS can increase risk for developing pneumonia
Group D (high risk, more symptoms)	LAMA + LABA *or* LABA + ICS *or* LAMA only (if LABA contraindicated)	LAMA + LABA + ICS	• Consider roflumilast (Daliresp) in chronic bronchitis and FEV_1 <50% predicted • Consider macrolide in former smokers

Table 6.3.4 GOLD Pharmacologic Therapy for Stable COPD

Refer to Chapter 4, Lesson 5, for more information regarding bronchodilators, beta$_2$-agonists, anti-muscarinics, methylxanthines, inhaled corticosteroids (ICS), oral glucocorticoids, and phosphodiesterase-4 (PDE4) inhibitors.

Education

Since 80% of all cases are related directly to tobacco use, encourage interventions supporting smoking cessation, including pharmacotherapy such as bupropion (Zyban) and varenicline (Chantix), OTC nicotine replacement products, structure support groups, and/or clinician counseling. COPD patients also benefit from education on avoidance of secondhand smoke, minimizing exposure to allergens and air pollution, and maintaining good hygiene, as well as advice on hydration, nutrition, exercise training, and pulmonary rehabilitation.

COPD Exacerbations

COPD exacerbations are characterized by an acute worsening of respiratory symptoms. These changes are typically associated with increased airway inflammation, increased mucus production, and worsening of air trapping. Common symptoms of an acute exacerbation include increased dyspnea and increased sputum purulence and volume, accompanied by marked cough and/or wheeze.

Indications for Hospital or Emergency Room Assessment

- Severe symptoms or worsening of resting dyspnea, tachypnea, abnormal oxygen saturation, confusion, drowsiness
- Onset of new physical signs (e.g., cyanosis, peripheral edema, weight loss)
- Failure of exacerbation to respond to initial pharmacologic management

- Existence of serious comorbidities (e.g., heart failure, diabetes, cardiac arrhythmias)
- Lack of or minimal home support

Management of Non-Life-Threatening Exacerbations

- Assess severity of symptoms, obtain blood gases and chest x-rays as appropriate
- Bronchodilators:
  - Increase dose and/or frequency of SABA
  - Consider adding SAMA (e.g., ipratropium bromide)
  - Use spacers or nebulizers as appropriate
- Consider use of oral corticosteroids; limit duration of therapy to 5–7 days
- Consider oral antibiotics when signs of bacterial infection are present
  - Sputum culture will help confirm appropriate antimicrobial therapy
  - Limit duration of therapy to 5–7 days
  - Recent studies suggest azithromycin (250 mg/day or 500 mg, 3 times per week) or erythromycin (500 mg twice per day) for 1 year in patients susceptible to exacerbations; reduce risk of exacerbations compared to usual stable COPD pharmacologic management
  - No data beyond 1-year demonstrating efficacy or safety of chronic antibiotic use to reduce COPD exacerbations
- Monitor fluid balance
- Assess and treat associated comorbidities (i.e., heart failure, arrhythmias)

Takeaways

- Tobacco use is the greatest and most modifiable risk factor for the development of COPD. Patients can greatly benefit from provider counseling and pharmacologic intervention.
- Spirometry results confirm COPD diagnosis and classification of disease severity, which guides practitioners in the formulation of treatment plans aimed at controlling symptoms and reducing risk for future exacerbations.
- Future exacerbation risks can also be mitigated by patient education on triggers and risk factors, as well as through preventative interventions such as influenza and pneumonia vaccines.

LESSON 4: LUNG CANCER

Learning Objectives
- Identify the clinical presentation typical of late-stage lung cancer
- Identify patients at high risk for developing lung cancer and discuss screening measures
- Select the appropriate tests to diagnose lung cancer
- Discuss treatment options for lung cancer

Lung cancer is the foremost cause of mortality from malignancy in the U.S. The single most significant risk factor for developing lung cancer is cigarette smoking, which accounts for approximately 90% of cases. Secondhand exposure to cigarette smoke and environmental pollutants are associated with an increased risk. Early detection is imperative, as mortality rates dramatically increase once metastasis occurs. Unfortunately, 75% or more of lung cancer cases are symptomatic at the time of diagnosis, indicating advanced disease.

Assessment

Subjective

Typical presentation occurs in older males, late in disease progression. Clinical findings are dependent on the location of the tumor and involvement of nodes and other organs. Presenting symptoms are often vague, such as:

- Generalized fatigue
- Weight loss
- Decreased appetite
- Fever

The most common early complaint is a dry "smoker's cough," which may occasionally be productive and accompanied by:

- Dyspnea
- Chest pressure
- Hemoptysis
- Hoarseness

A diagnostic clue may be discovered when gathering a patient's history if they report frequent or persistent upper or lower respiratory infections unresponsive to treatment.

Objective

In smokers, the presence of adventitious lung sounds is likely; yet in many patients, the physical exam may be unremarkable, since the majority of cases are diagnosed once the cancer has metastasized. They may present with symptoms in the organs most at risk for metastasis of lung cancer—bones, liver, brain, lymph nodes, spinal cord, and adrenal glands. Signs of advanced disease include:

- Lymphadenopathy
- Hepatomegaly
- Spinal cord compression (weakness, numbness, pain)
- Neurological symptoms

Diagnosis

While a chest radiograph is not diagnostic in itself and in fact may be negative, abnormalities indicate the need for additional workup with either an MRI or CT scan. Definitive diagnosis requires cytologic or histologic evidence, which is typically obtained via bronchoscopy with biopsy.

Screening guidelines are available from the American College of Chest Physicians (ACCP), the National Comprehensive Cancer Network (NCCN), and the U.S. Preventative Services Task Force (USPSTF).

ACCP	NCCN	USPSTF
Annual LDCT for current smokers aged 55–74 w/ smoking history of at least 30 pack-years; former smokers of same age who have quit within last 15 years with same smoking history	Annual LDCT for current smokers aged >50 with smoking history of at least 20 pack-years with at least one additional risk factor	Annual LDCT for current smokers aged 55–80 with 30 pack-year history or have quit within the last 15 yrs

Table 6.4.1 Screening Guidelines for Lung Cancer

Differential Diagnosis

Differential diagnoses for lung cancer: **pneumonia, lung abscess, bronchitis, tuberculosis**

Pro Tip: Cancer Staging

Staging is based on the TNM system from the *American Joint Committee on Cancer (AJCC), 7th edition.* The 8th edition has been published and will be implemented starting January 1, 2018.

(T) Tumor: the size of the primary tumor

(N) Nodes: if the cancer has spread to regional lymph nodes

(M) Metastasis: if the cancer has metastasized to other organs in the body

https://cancerstaging.org/About/news/Pages/Implementation-of-AJCC-8th-Edition-Cancer-Staging-System.aspx

There are also various apps that can assist with cancer staging; most are disease-specific (lung cancer, breast cancer, etc.) and can be found by searching the app store on your mobile device.

Plan

Treatment

If caught early, definitive treatment such as surgery is more effective. Since the majority of lung cancers are not diagnosed at an early stage, only 25% of patients are candidates for surgery at the time of diagnosis. Thus, chemotherapy and radiation are the mainstays of treatment. Smoking cessation is essential, and patients should be encouraged to avoid exposure to pollutants. Despite treatment, prognosis for patients with lung cancer is poor.

App Alert

When caring for cancer patients, selected ASCO Clinical Practice Guidelines (including expert recommendations, algorithms, and calculators) can be searched using a free app. You can access this link in order to download: **www.asco.org/practice-guidelines/quality-guidelines/guidelines**.

Education

A realistic assessment of the patient's prognosis and quality of life and the pros and cons of therapy, pain control, and palliative/hospice care should be performed with the participation of both the patient and their family.

Takeaways

- Typical presentation occurs late in the disease with symptoms such as cough, fatigue, anorexia, weight loss, chest discomfort, dyspnea, and hemoptysis.
- The recommended screening for patients at high risk for lung cancer consists of an annual low-dose CT scan.
- Definitive diagnosis requires cytologic or histologic evidence.
- Chemotherapy and radiation are the mainstays of treatment.

LESSON 5: PNEUMONIA

> **Learning Objectives**
> - Predict patients at risk for pneumonia
> - Identify proper indication of the PPSV vaccine for pneumonia prevention
> - Identify clinical presentation, signs and symptoms, and diagnostic criteria consistent with pneumonia
> - Determine appropriate treatment, care, and referral of patients diagnosed with pneumonia

Pneumonia is a pulmonary infection that includes the parenchyma, alveolar spaces, and/or interstitial tissue and is commonly classified as community acquired (CAP) or nosocomial. Pulmonary infection is often bacterial in nature, most specifically *Streptococcus pneumoniae*. A few infections are viral-based, and in the immunocompromised patient, fungi may be the causative agent.

Assessment

Patients with recent URI, immunosuppression, and comorbidities (such as asthma, COPD, or alcoholism) are at increased risk for pneumonia. Other risk factors include exposure/access to day care centers, convalescent homes, infected persons with pneumonia, firsthand or secondhand smoke exposure, and use of antibiotics (penicillin, cephalosporin, macrolide, or quinolone) within the last 90 days.

A history of exposure (e.g., travel, animal, occupational, and environmental) can be helpful in determining possible etiologies:

- Exposure to air-conditioning or water systems: Legionella species
- Exposure to overcrowded areas (e.g., school dorms, homeless shelters, jails): *S. pneumoniae, Mycobacteria, Mycoplasma, Chlamydophila*
- Exposure to animals: cats, cattle, sheep, goats: *C. burnetii, B. anthracis*; turkeys, chickens, ducks or other birds *C. psittaci*; rabbits, rodents: *F. tularensis, Y. pestis*

A productive cough is the most consistent presenting symptom, though not diagnostic. Sputum may be rust-colored (*S. pneumoniae*), green (*Pseudomonas, Haemophilus*), yellow, or red (*Klebsiella*), and may be foul-smelling and bad-tasting (anaerobic infections). Other physical findings vary (*see Table 6.5.1*).

Symptoms may include but are not limited to: fever, weight loss or gain, night sweats, fatigue; presence of wheezing or other adventitious breath sounds, dyspnea, tachypnea, sneezing, ear pain; chest pain/pleuritic chest pain, palpitations; nausea, vomiting, heartburn or reflux; and rashes.

Diagnosis

S. pneumococcus is the most common causative organism, regardless of host. Three aspects are of priority in the management of pneumonia:

- Determining the presence of bacteria
- Assessing the severity of disease at presentation
- Identifying the causative agent

Diagnostic testing plays an important role, as results will significantly alter empiric therapy and treatment decisions. Testing may include a CXR and SpO_2. Infiltrate observed on CXR is the gold standard for diagnosis of pneumonia. History, duration of symptoms, and current symptoms and severity may help to rule out differential diagnosis such as upper respiratory infection.

Use of the CURB-65 is helpful in determining severity of symptoms and predicting mortality in patients with CAP. Using the CURB-65 score (pneumonia severity index), one point is assigned for each feature:

- C: confusion of new onset
- U: urea ≥7mmol/L (BUN >19 mg/dL)
- R: respiratory rate ≥30 per minute
- B: blood pressure <90 mmHg systolic or <60 mmHg diastolic
- 65: age ≥65 years

A score of 0–1 indicates low severity and management takes place in the community. Scores of 2 indicate moderate severity, and one should consider hospital admission. Scores of 3–5 indicate high-severity; management involves inpatient care with consideration for admission to an intensive care unit. About one-third of patients with CAP require hospital admission.

Additional lab work may not assist in diagnosis but can help to determine severity of illness and management decisions. Obtain serum chemistry panel, ABG, and CBC with differential. Leukocytosis with a left shift is common in any bacterial infection. Leukopenia may indicate impending sepsis.

	Drug-resistant *Strep* pneumonia	Atypical pathogens
At-risk populations	• Age >65 years • Immunocompromised • Patients with comorbidities • Exposure to day care and long-term care facilities • Antibiotic use within the last 90 days • Alcohol	• Young adults, otherwise healthy • Non-smokers • Community outbreak
Symptoms	• Abrupt onset with fever, chills, cough, pleuritic chest pain, rust-colored sputum • Older patients exhibit fewer symptoms (confusion, absence of fever)	Cough, low-grade fever, chills, headache, malaise, rash, joint aches, arrhythmias
Diagnosis	CXR is gold standard for diagnosis	CXR is gold standard for diagnosis

Table 6.5.1 Community-Acquired Pneumonia: At-Risk Populations, Symptoms, and Diagnosis

Plan

Treatment

Almost all decisions regarding management of pneumonia are based on the severity of symptoms. An initial management decision is that of hospitalization (or not), and second is the selection of antibiotics.

Infectious Disease Society of America (IDSA) and American Thoracic Society (ATS) 2007 Guidelines for Treatment of Pneumonia
- For most patients who are previously healthy, with no antibiotic exposure in the last 90 days and no drug-resistant *S. pneumoniae (DRSP)* suspected (*S. pneumoniae* and atypical pathogens):
  - Macrolide
  - Doxycycline
- For patients with suspected DRSP:
  - Respiratory fluoroquinolones
  - Pregnant patients: high-dose amoxicillin

- For patients with pathogens producing beta lactamase (*H. influenzae*):
  - Beta-lactam (cephalosporins, penicillins) plus macrolide or doxycycline

Treatment may also include bronchodilators (nebulizers) for bronchospasm, supplemental oxygen for dyspnea, and fluid replacement in patients with hypotension and/or tachycardia (or conversely, diuretics as needed, analgesics, and/or antipyretics).

Follow-up CXR:

- Routine, not mandatory if patient is responding appropriately
- Follow up in 7–12 weeks after treatment if patient is 40 years of age or older or is a smoker, to confirm resolution of pneumonia

Referral

Patients with CAP may sometimes require hospitalization. Patients with a CURB-65 score of 3 or more are at high risk of death and require urgent hospital admission.

Pneumococcal Vaccine Guidelines

Pneumococcal polysaccharide vaccination: PCV13, PPSV23

- PPSV23 (Pneumovax)
  - Adults 19–64 years who are at increased risk of pneumococcal disease (asthma, COPD, cardiovascular disease, etc.)
- PCV13 (Prevnar), then PPSV23 (in 1 year)
  - All adults 65 years of age or older
  - Aged 19–64 with asplenia, immunocompromised conditions, CSF leaks, cochlear implants, plus an additional PPSV23

Refer to Chapter 3, Lesson 4, for more information.

Takeaways

- Initial management of pneumonia is with empirical antibiotics.
- The CURB-65 score is used to assess disease severity and guide management.
- Vaccination is indicated in patients over 65 years or with disease or immunosuppression.

LESSON 6: PULMONARY EMBOLISM

Learning Objectives
- Define pulmonary embolism and differentiate between an embolism and an embolus
- Identify risk factors for developing a pulmonary embolism
- Discuss the clinical findings in a patient with a pulmonary embolism
- Select the gold standard of care for diagnosing a pulmonary embolism
- Discuss treatment options for pulmonary embolism

A pulmonary embolism (PE) is not a disease, rather it is a complication of underlying venous thrombosis. It occurs when an embolus made of blood, solid, liquid, or gaseous material travels to the lung via the venous system and lodges in the pulmonary arterial circulation, blocking blood flow. The extent of injury is determined by the size of the embolus. Examples of embolic material are fat, air, tumor fragments, amniotic fluid, and septic debris.

> **Pro Tip**
> - Virchow's triad is comprised of venous stasis, vessel wall injury, and hypercoagulability
> - Factors that place an individual at risk for venous stasis include DVTs in LE/pelvis, CHF, dehydration, prolonged immobility, obesity, and advanced age
> - Surgery, trauma, and bone fractures lead to vessel wall injury
> - Malignancies, pregnancy, certain medications, and genetic conditions (such as Factor V Leiden, prothrombin gene mutation, and elevated levels of homocysteine) can all lead to hypercoagulability

Assessment

Dyspnea is the most common presenting symptom in a patient with a PE and may be the patient's only symptom. Abrupt shortness of breath, pleuritic chest pain, and hypoxia comprise the classic triad of presentation. Severity ranges from sudden hemodynamic collapse to progressive, worsening dyspnea.

Risk factors for developing a PE include Virchow's triad, certain genetic conditions, and a previous history of PE.

Subjective	Objective	Vital sign changes
Dyspnea, chest pain, anxiety, feeling of impending doom	Hypoxia, rales, hemoptysis, syncope, wheezing, altered LOC, flank or abdominal pain, increased work of breathing, accentuated 2nd heart sound, decreased cardiac output, diaphoresis	Tachycardia, tachypnea, hypertension followed by hypotension, fever

Table 6.6.1 Signs and Symptoms of a Pulmonary Embolism

Diagnosis

Pulmonary emboli are frequently missed and misdiagnosed. Diagnostic testing is done on patients who are symptomatic, with a high suspicion of PE. Routine chemistries are not generally helpful. An ABG is recommended to assess hypoxemia and acute respiratory alkalosis. A coagulation workup may reveal clotting abnormalities. ECG usually shows sinus tachycardia and nonspecific changes. Chest radiographs are not routinely recommended as a diagnostic tool, as they are nonspecific; however, they may be used to rule out other differential diagnoses.

The gold standard for diagnosing a pulmonary embolism is a multidetector-row computed tomography angiography (MDCTA). If MDCTA is not available, the criterion standard is pulmonary angiography. A ventilation-perfusion (V/Q) scan may be done if the CT scan is not available or contraindicated. Venous doppler studies may show DVTs in the lower extremities.

Plan

Treatment

In patients with a suspected pulmonary embolism, treatment with anticoagulants should begin immediately with either low-molecular-weight heparin (LMWH) or fondaparinux (Arixtra). A direct thrombin inhibitor or factor Xa inhibitor may be used as an alternative. Warfarin therapy should also be started in conjunction with one of the above and titrated to achieve an INR of 2–3. Anticoagulant therapy should be continued for at least 3 months, then reassessed.

For patients with acute PE accompanied by hypotension/shock, thrombolytic therapy using alteplase (Activase or tPA) or reteplase (Retavase) may be considered if the patient is not at high risk for bleeding. If fibrinolysis is contraindicated or ineffective, surgical or catheter embolectomy may be considered. Ideally, vena cava filters should not be used in patients who have experienced a PE, and are only indicated under very specific circumstances.

Supportive care includes the use of supplemental oxygen, compression stockings, and early ambulation.

Education

Instruct patients on the importance of adherence to anticoagulation therapy and routine follow-up care. Counsel them on potential food/medication interactions and potential complications of therapy. Warfarin therapy requires lab monitoring. Patient teaching should include the signs/symptoms of DVTs/PEs and what to do if they begin to experience them.

Takeaways

- Pulmonary embolism is a must-not-miss diagnosis, and should be suspected if a patient presents with severe dyspnea and no clear cause. Typical presentation includes sudden onset dyspnea that gets progressively worse, pleuritic chest pain, and hypoxia.
- The gold standard for diagnosing a PE is a multidetector-row computed tomography angiography (MDCTA), though a CT angiography may be used if MDCTA is not available.
- Treatment of pulmonary emboli includes the use of anticoagulants, thrombolytics, embolectomy, and supportive care.

LESSON 7: TUBERCULOSIS

Learning Objectives

- Identify the organism that causes tuberculosis and understand how it is transmitted
- Identify persons most at risk for acquiring active pulmonary tuberculosis
- Diagnose active and latent tuberculosis
- Order the correct treatment for an active tuberculosis infection

Pulmonary tuberculosis (TB) is a prevalent, chronic infectious disease caused primarily by *Mycobacterium tuberculosis*, a gram-positive, acid-fast bacillus that is transmitted via aerosolized droplets. The occurrence of TB worldwide is high, with the highest incidence occurring in developing nations, persons living in poor/overcrowded conditions, the homeless, illegal drug users, and minorities. Individuals infected with HIV are particularly susceptible to acquiring TB and have a high mortality rate from the disease.

Once exposed to the droplets, an individual may develop either a primary TB infection (if their immune system fails to contain the organism) or a latent TB infection (LTBI). In LTBI, the disease may either lie dormant indefinitely or reactivate and cause active disease.

Mycobacterium tuberculosis that exists outside of the lungs is referred to as extrapulmonary or disseminated TB. Extrapulmonary TB can occur as part of a primary infection or serve as the site of a reactivation. It tends to affect lymph nodes, kidneys, bones, meninges, and GI tract. Miliary tuberculosis is a clinical condition in which the bacterium has been disseminated via the vascular system throughout the lungs or body. Similar to extrapulmonary TB, miliary TB can occur as a part of the primary infection or due to the reactivation of latent TB. It is characterized by the multiplicity of tiny pulmonary nodules on a chest x-ray that appear similar to millet seeds, and can be fatal if left untreated.

Definitions

- **Latent tuberculosis infection (LTBI):** confirmed *Mycobacterium tuberculosis* in an asymptomatic patient with no histologic evidence of active disease and with negative diagnostic imaging.
- **Bacille Calmette-Guérin vaccine (BCG):** a TB vaccination used in endemic areas outside of the U.S.

> **Pro Tip**
> LTBI is not the same as active TB and is not contagious.

Assessment

Subjective

During the early stage of TB, patients are usually asymptomatic. Symptoms develop as the disease progresses. Common symptoms include:

- Diurnal fever
- Night sweats
- A dry or productive cough (frank hemoptysis is rare)
- Pleuritic chest pain (less common)
- Dyspnea (late sign)
- Anorexia, weight loss, malaise (late signs)

The patient should be asked about recent travel, close contact with persons with known active disease or the symptoms listed above, current living situation, recent incarceration, and illicit drug use.

Objective

As the disease progresses, the patient may appear chronically ill. Auscultation of the lungs may reveal apical rales and positive whispered pectoriloquy. Though the chest examination is most often normal, tactile fremitus may be increased over the consolidated area with a dullness heard on percussion. Atypical presentation is common in immunocompromised persons.

Diagnosis

The Mantoux tuberculin skin test (TST) is the most commonly used screening method of identifying individuals with active disease or a history of prior exposure. Erythema is common and not an indication of a positive result. The guidelines for determining a positive TST varies based on the patient and clinical situation, as shown in the table below. Prior BCG vaccination does not usually affect the interpretation of the test, though it may rarely produce a false-positive result. The TST is not without limitations: a low sensitivity in persons who are immunocompromised and results subject to reader bias. In light of these limitations, the QuantiFERON-TB blood test is increasingly being used in place of the TST. It requires one visit, with results available within 24 hours, and it is more sensitive in immunocompromised patients.

Induration of ≥5 mm	Induration of ≥10 mm	Induration of ≥15 mm
• Recent close contact with a person infected with tuberculosis (TB) • Persons with evidence of inactive (latent) disease • Patients infected with HIV • Patients who are immunocompromised • Organ transplant recipients • Patients with chronic fibrotic changes on chest x-ray consistent with a prior history of tuberculosis (TB)	• Healthcare workers • Recent immigrants from high-risk areas • IV drug users • High-risk minorities • Residents and employees of high-risk settings (nursing homes, prisons, etc.) • Persons with medical conditions that place them at high risk (DM, cancer, ESRD) • Children <4 years old	Any person in all populations

Table 6.7.1 Interpretation of Mantoux Tuberculin Skin Test Results

If a TST or QuantiFERON-TB test is positive, order a chest x-ray to either rule in or out a diagnosis of active TB. The x-ray may show a pulmonary mass or consolidation, infiltrates, or cavitation. Obtain a sputum sample and send for acid-fast bacilli smear and culture if TB is suspected. Culture results are diagnostic of TB; however, they take 3–8 weeks to result. If TB is highly suspected, treatment should be initiated while the culture results are pending.

Differential Diagnosis

Differential diagnoses for TB: **pneumonia, malignancy, pleurisy, histoplasmosis, COPD, tularemia, sarcoidosis**

Digital Resource

Refer to the Centers for Disease Control and Prevention (CDC) for more information about tuberculosis: **www.cdc.gov/tb/default.htm**.

Plan

Treatment

For patients with latent tuberculosis, pharmacological treatment using isoniazid PO for 6–9 months should be considered to prevent conversion to active disease. For active pulmonary tuberculosis, combination therapy is recommended using isoniazid, rifampin, and pyrazinamide for two months, and isoniazid and rifampin for an additional four months. Liver toxicity is a potential risk of therapy, particularly in the elderly, so draw baseline liver function tests prior to the start of therapy. Following completion of drug therapy, monitor patient for evidence of recurrence for one year.

Education

Close contacts of persons with active disease should be monitored for signs of TB.

Referral

Refer the patient to a pulmonary specialist upon diagnosis of TB. Since multidrug-resistant TB is a very real concern, consultation with local TB health experts to determine local resistance patterns is recommended. Report active disease cases to state and local health departments.

Takeaways

- Pulmonary tuberculosis is caused by *Mycobacterium tuberculosis* and is transmitted via aerosolized droplets.
- TST, QuantiFERON-TB blood test, and chest x-ray screen for TB. Sputum culture is diagnostic.
- Treatment for active pulmonary tuberculosis consists of a multidrug regimen that includes isoniazid, rifampin, and pyrazinamide.

LESSON 8: UPPER RESPIRATORY INFECTION

Learning Objectives

■ Appropriately diagnose patients that present with symptoms of upper respiratory infection (URI)

■ Prescribe an appropriate treatment plan for a URI

■ Display an understanding of potential complications of a URI and how to treat complications

Upper respiratory infection is defined as inflammation of the mucosa of the upper respiratory tract (nose, sinuses, pharynx) caused by a virus, bacteria, or fungus. The common cold is a URI in its mildest form. Typically, the cause of a URI is a virus (e.g., rhinovirus, coronavirus, adenovirus, or enterovirus). This illness is usually self-limiting and lasts approximately 7–10 days. The goal of therapy is aimed at minimizing symptoms and preventing complications.

Assessment

Subjective

Symptoms of a URI may include runny nose, nasal congestion, and/or sneezing. Question patients about severity, length of symptoms, and treatments used. In addition, the patient may complain of fever, fatigue, chills, sweats, ear pain, sore throat, mouth pain, tooth pain, facial pain/pressure/fullness, cough—productive/nonproductive, shortness of breath, wheezing, abdominal pain, nausea, vomiting, diarrhea, myalgia, or rash. If these complaints are present, consider differential diagnosis or complications (symptoms more than 7–10 days).

The patient's past medical history, surgical history, and social history should be reviewed to determine if they are at a greater risk of a bacterial infection and/or a complication.

- **PMH:** prematurity, recurrent otitis media, frequent hospitalizations for lower respiratory tract infections, asthma, allergic rhinitis, a congenital defect that would impair the upper respiratory system, frequent sinusitis, bronchitis, pneumonia, COPD, high-risk sexual behavior, a diagnosis or medications that would impair an individual's immune system, recent antibiotic use
- **PSH:** tonsillectomy, adenoidectomy, myringotomy with tympanostomy tube placement, sinus surgery, lung surgery
- **FH:** asthma
- **SH:** smoking or exposure to secondhand smoke, travel outside of the U.S.

Objective

- **Vital signs:** Are there any abnormalities such as elevated temp, HR, BP, RR, decreased BP, RR, or SPO_2? Is the patient experiencing any pain?
- **HEENT:**
  - Ears: ear pinna pain on manipulation; erythema, edema, or drainage of external auditory canal; tympanic membrane erythema/injection, edema, drainage; dulling of the light reflex; presence of tympanostomy tubes or serous fluid behind the tympanic membrane

- – Nose: rhinorrhea, nasal mucosa erythema and/or edema, nasal polyps, turbinates pale and boggy or erythematous
- – Mouth/throat: ulcerations, exudate, erythema or injection of mucosa/pharynx, enlarged tonsils (if present), post nasal drainage
- **Sinuses:** pain with percussion and poor trans illumination of frontal and maxillary sinuses
- **Neck:** lymphadenopathy pre/post auricular and anterior and posterior cervical chain (shotty, diffuse or focal, mobile, fixed)
- **CV:** presence of murmurs
- **Resp:** respiratory distress, wheezes, rhonchi or rales on auscultation
- **Skin:** rash-maculopapular, lacy and reticular, "sandpaper"

Diagnosis

URI is usually a transient illness, but it can lead to complications and/or secondary bacterial infection. Diagnostic testing that could be done for prolonged or worsening symptoms includes rapid strep test, RSV test in infants and small children, rapid influenza test, monospot, complete blood count with differential, throat culture, and a chest x-ray (CXR). Choosing the appropriate testing depends on the symptoms and the severity of those symptoms.

> **Pro Tip**
> If a diagnostic test will not change the treatment plan, then it is not prudent to perform the test in question.

The diagnosis of URI encompasses several other diagnoses: common cold, viral pharyngitis, viral sinusitis, laryngotracheitis (croup), and laryngitis. Complications include bacterial sinusitis, bacterial pharyngitis/tonsillitis, otitis media, lower respiratory tract infection, asthma or COPD exacerbation, pneumonia, and epiglottitis.

Symptom	Differential diagnosis/complication
Ear pain	Otitis media, otitis externa (*see Chapter 5, Lesson 2*)
Sore throat	Epiglottitis, pharyngitis, tonsillitis, infectious mononucleosis (*see Chapter 5, Lesson 5*)
Headache	Sinusitis (*see Chapter 5, Lesson 3*), influenza
Malaise	Sinusitis, infectious mononucleosis, influenza
Fever	Viral/bacterial infection
Facial pain/pressure	Sinusitis, abscessed tooth
Cough	Pertussis, bronchiolitis, bronchitis (*see Chapter 6, Lesson 2*), pneumonia (*see Chapter 6, Lesson 5*), asthma (*see Chapter 6, Lesson 1*), or COPD exacerbation (*see Chapter 6, Lesson 3*)

Table 6.8.1 Differential Diagnosis/Complication

Plan

Treatment

The goal of treating a URI is to minimize symptoms. Since the pathogen is usually a virus, antibiotics are of little to no value. Medications that are commonly used to treat symptoms include decongestants, antihistamines, antipyretics, and antitussives. Over-the-counter cough and cold medications are contraindicated in those under 4 years of age; treat with nasal saline and a bulb syringe for nasal congestion. If a patient is diagnosed with influenza, an antiviral such as oseltamivir (Tamiflu) can be prescribed if started within 48 hours of symptoms to minimize the severity and lessen the duration of influenza. Nasal saline rinses and nasal steroids can provide some relief from congestion when decongestants are contraindicated (e.g., HTN). The patient should be instructed to rest, eat a well-balanced diet, and drink hydrating liquids.

If symptoms last longer than 7–10 days, then the pathogen causing the URI is most likely bacterial in nature and the patient should be treated with antibiotics. The antibiotic of choice depends on the type of infection. See individual chapter for treatment information (referenced in Table 6.8.1) and refer to the appropriate pharmacology lessons (*see Chapter 4*).

Education

Many patients request antibiotics for URIs, despite efforts to inform the public regarding antibiotic resistance and the need to properly utilize antibiotics. Educate the patient regarding the reason for not prescribing antibiotics and discuss options for symptom control. In addition, educate regarding potential complications and when to seek further medical attention. It is important to give the patient expectations regarding the natural course of a URI.

Referral

Referral for a URI is typically not necessary unless there are persistent complications. Refer to an otolaryngologist and work up for immunocompromise if a patient is frequently diagnosed with URIs. Keep in mind that frequent URIs are common in the pediatric population. Immediately refer patients that are showing signs of distress and worsening complications to the ER or for hospitalization.

Takeaways

- URI is a mild, self-limiting illness.
- Illness lasting longer than 7–10 days may indicate a complication or a secondary bacterial infection.
- The goal of treatment of a URI is to minimize symptoms and prevent complications.
- Treatment of a complication depends on the diagnosis and the common pathogen of that particular diagnosis.

PRACTICE QUESTIONS

Select the ONE best answer.

Lesson 1: Asthma

1. Manny is a 45-year-old male who comes to your clinic complaining of shortness of breath since starting his new job at a saw mill. He smokes one pack per day and states he had asthma when he was younger but "grew out of it." Which objective finding is most suggestive of a diagnosis of asthma?

   A. Productive cough noted during exam, respiratory rate of 16, and wheezing on auscultation of posterior left upper lobe

   B. Pale, boggy nasal turbinates, clear air fluid level behind bilateral tympanic membranes, barrel chest, FEV_1 <80% predicted, and FEV_1 increased 5% after administration of albuterol

   C. SpO_2 = 94%, heart rate of 88, and bilateral wheezes on auscultation

   D. Dry cough noted during exam, SpO_2 = 95%, FEV_1 <80% predicted, and FEV_1 increased 15% after administration of albuterol

2. An 18-year-old male patient presents for routine follow-up on asthma that was diagnosed at age 6. The current medication regimen includes fluticasone (Flovent) 44 mcg/actuation 2 puffs BID inhaled with albuterol (ProAir FHA) as a rescue inhaler. The patient tells you he uses fluticasone daily as prescribed, and he has used the albuterol inhaler twice daily for the last month. What would be your plan of care for this patient using a stepwise approach?

   A. Add montelukast (Singulair) to his current regimen

   B. Change fluticasone (Flovent) to 110 mcg/actuation, 2 puffs BID

   C. Have patient keep track of peak flow measurements and return to clinic for follow-up in 1 week

   D. Refer to a pulmonologist

3. Which of following is correct regarding diagnosing asthma in a 2-year-old?

   A. Spirometry is unreliable in patients under the age of 5

   B. Patients under 4 years old cannot be diagnosed with asthma

   C. Eczema is not seen concomitantly with asthma

   D. If on exam the patient is not wheezing, then asthma is unlikely

4. Tara is a 35-year-old patient newly diagnosed with asthma. PMH includes seasonal allergies. Social history includes previous 1 pack-per-day smoker for 10 years. She has a history of coughing and wheezing during the spring and fall, but she attributes this to smoking. She stopped smoking 2 years ago, and the coughing and wheezing have not resolved. She admits she sleeps poorly 3–4 nights out of the week because of coughing. She is unable to walk for exercise as much as she would like because she gets short of breath. She also has coughing and wheezing every morning when she wakes up. You are waiting on her spirometry results. How would you classify her asthma based on the information you have been given in her history?

   A. Moderate

   B. Intermittent

   C. Severe

   D. Mild

Lesson 2: Cough/Bronchitis

5. The cough associated with acute bronchitis typically lasts:

   A. 2 weeks

   B. 3 weeks

   C. 4 weeks

   D. 6 weeks

6. Diagnosis of acute bronchitis is made by:

   A. Clinical presentation

   B. Chest x-ray

   C. Sputum culture

   D. White blood cell count (WBC)

7. A 28-year-old male presents to the clinic with a 15-day history of cough that started out dry, but has progressed to productive, with occasional orange-yellow sputum. He denies fever, chills, dyspnea, or nasal congestion, but complains of a burning sensation in his chest when he coughs. The physical exam is unremarkable. As part of his treatment, the nurse practitioner prescribes:

   A. A macrolide antibiotic, such as azithromycin, for 10 days

   B. Rest, increased intake of fluids, and use of a humidifier

   C. An antitussive, rest, and use of an air purifier

   D. An antihistamine, an antitussive, and increased intake of fluids

8. Persistent cough is the most common presenting symptom in adults in ambulatory care. It is important for the nurse practitioner to distinguish the difference between acute bronchitis and other common causes of cough. All of the following are differentials for acute bronchitis except:

   A. Upper respiratory infection

   B. Pharyngitis

   C. Pneumonia

   D. Allergic rhinitis

Lesson 3: COPD

9. While discussing the need for immunizations with a 54-year-old diabetic man with chronic obstructive pulmonary disease (COPD), you would recommend which of the following?

   A. Inactivated influenza vaccine

   B. PPSV23 pneumococcal vaccine

   C. PCV13 pneumococcal vaccine

   D. Annual Td vaccination

10. A COPD patient with a GOLD spirometric classification of 2, with a self-report of 3 exacerbations in the past year and CAT score of 12 would be characterized as which risk group?

    A. Group A

    B. Group B

    C. Group C

    D. Group D

11. According to GOLD, pharmacologic treatment regimen should be guided by:

    A. Severity of symptoms

    B. Abnormal findings on chest radiograph

    C. Impaired FEV_1 measurement on spirometry

    D. Immunization status

12. All of the following induce a bronchodilation response except:

    A. Fluticasone HFA

    B. Albuterol HFA

    C. Tiotropium HFA

    D. Theophylline

Lesson 4: Lung Cancer

13. According to the guidelines by the American College of Chest Physicians (ACCP), annual screening with low-dose computed tomography (LDCT) for lung cancer should occur in which of the following patient populations?

    A. Current smokers aged 50 and older with at least a 20 pack-year smoking history

    B. Current smokers aged 55–74 years with at least a 30 pack-year smoking history

    C. Former smokers aged 55–74 years with at least a 30 pack-year smoking history who have quit within the past 20 years

    D. Current smokers aged 50 and older with at least a 20 pack-year smoking history and at least one additional risk factor

14. A 72-year-old male has just been diagnosed with lung cancer. Which of the following recommendations should be made by the nurse practitioner as part of his immediate treatment plan?

    A. Morphine IVP for pain control

    B. Chest x-ray every three months

    C. Smoking cessation

    D. Serial CT scans every 3 months to monitor the size of the tumor

15. Presenting symptoms of lung cancer may include all of the following except:

    A. Wheezing

    B. Dyspnea

    C. Chest discomfort

    D. Anorexia

16. Which of the following diagnostic tests provides a definitive diagnosis for lung cancer?

    A. MRI

    B. CT scan

    C. Chest x-ray

    D. Cytology

Lesson 5: Pneumonia

17. Risk factors for infection with DRSP include all of the following except:

    A. Comorbidities

    B. Systemic antibiotic use in the last 90 days

    C. Non-smoking

    D. Age >65

18. What is the appropriate treatment of community-acquired pneumonia in a 52-year-old male who has a dry cough, fatigue, no recent antimicrobial use, and no comorbidity? The patient currently takes no routine medications.

    A. amoxicillin (Amoxil)

    B. clarithromycin (Biaxin)

    C. levofloxacin (Levaquin)

    D. ceftriaxone (Rocephin)

19. A 65-year-old female with congestive heart failure and diabetes mellitus presents with productive cough, fever, and dyspnea. Which diagnosis is most likely?

    A. Asthma exacerbation

    B. Acute bronchitis

    C. Influenza

    D. Pneumonia

20. A previously healthy 68-year-old patient presents with a 4-day history of productive cough, temperature of 101.5 F, BP 115/80, pulse 90, and respiratory rate of 25. Physical examination shows the patient to be alert and oriented, with diminished breath sounds in the RLL. BUN is 16 and WBC is elevated. On CXR, the RLL demonstrates infiltrates. Which of the following is true?

A. According to CURB-65, this patient has a score of 1 and can be treated as an outpatient

B. According to CURB-65, this patient has a score of 2 and can be treated as an outpatient

C. According to CURB-65, this patient has a score of 3 and can be treated as an outpatient with a combination of antibiotics rather than a single-agent regimen

D. According to CURB-65, this patient has a score of 4 and hospitalization is needed

Lesson 6: Pulmonary Embolus

21. A 53-year-old male presents to the clinic with a chief complaint of sudden onset shortness of breath and non-radiating chest pain that he describes as sharp and substernal. He rates it 6/10. His vital signs are: T 100.5 F, HR 119, RR 21, BP 152/90. Upon exam, he appears anxious and you note an accentuated second heart sound and rales. The FNP suspects which of the following diagnoses?

A. Acute myocardial infarction

B. Pneumothorax

C. Pleurisy

D. Pulmonary embolism

22. A patient presents with acute onset of dyspnea, pleuritic chest pain, and hypoxia. No clear cause can be determined by clinical examination. General chemistries are normal and a chest x-ray is negative. The FNP suspects a pulmonary embolism and will order which of the following diagnostic tests to confirm the diagnosis?

A. Multidetector-row computed tomography angiography

B. Coagulation studies

C. V/Q scan

D. D-dimer

23. A 68-year-old female has been diagnosed with a pulmonary embolism. The FNP places the patient on anticoagulant therapy using which of the following preferred medications?

A. alteplase (Activase)

B. fondaparinux (Arixtra)

C. streptokinase (Streptase)

D. heparin sodium (Heparin)

24. Following a pulmonary embolism diagnosis, anti-coagulant therapy should be continued for _____ month(s) and then reevaluated.

A. one

B. two

C. three

D. six

25. Risk factors for developing a pulmonary embolism including Virchow's triad, genetics, and a previous history of a pulmonary embolism. Which three conditions comprise Virchow's triad?

A. Prolonged immobility, hypercoagulability, and venous stasis

B. Hypercoagulability, vessel wall injury, and venous stasis

C. Trauma, venous stasis, and peripheral vascular disease

D. Vessel wall injury, dehydration, and Factor V Leiden

26. A 49-year-old male presents with a pulmonary embolism. The NP would expect to find which clinical symptoms upon assessment of this patient?

A. Lower extremity edema, stridor, hypotension

B. Crackles, S4 gallop, bradycardia

C. Rales, accentuated second heart sound, wheezing

D. Hemoptysis, hypotension, diminished heart sounds

Lesson 7: Tuberculosis

27. A female healthcare worker presents to employee health for her annual tuberculin skin test (TST). Her previous results have been negative. When she returns 48 hours later, the results show 10 mm of induration surrounded by erythema. She is asymptomatic and her chest x-ray is normal. The most appropriate management is to:

    A. Prescribe isoniazid for a duration of 9 months to prevent conversion to active disease

    B. Repeat the Mantoux tuberculin skin test in 3 months

    C. Monitor for signs of active disease and perform a repeat chest x-ray in one year

    D. Prescribe isoniazid, rifampin, and pyrazinamide for a duration of 9 months

28. A 43-year-old female with HIV has just been diagnosed with active pulmonary tuberculosis (TB). She has a 19-year-old daughter that lives with her and has been caring for her. Which of the following actions should be taken with regard to the patient's daughter?

    A. Because of her age, TB prophylaxis is contraindicated, even if she has a positive TST

    B. If her TST is positive, but her chest x-ray is negative and she displays no clinical symptoms, no further evaluation or treatment is indicated

    C. She should receive TB prophylaxis if her TST is ≥5 mm induration

    D. She should be treated for active pulmonary TB with a multidrug regimen

29. Ninety percent of patients are asymptomatic at the time of primary tuberculosis (TB) infection. As the disease progresses, clinical findings include all of the following except:

    A. Night sweats

    B. Dyspnea

    C. Diurnal fever

    D. Dry cough

Lesson 8: Upper Respiratory Infection

30. Paige is a 35-year-old female who calls the primary care clinic about a sneeze, runny nose, and cough. She wants to know if she should come into the clinic. The most important question to ask the patient is:

    A. "Do you smoke?"

    B. "How long have you had the symptoms?"

    C. "Have you traveled out of the country recently?"

    D. "Are you running a fever?"

31. An 18-year-old patient complaining of a two-day history of fever, running nose, nasal congestion, and a sore throat is suspected of having a URI. All of the following will be included in the appropriate diagnostic workup except:

    A. Chest x-ray

    B. Rapid strep test

    C. Rapid influenza test

    D. Throat culture

32. You receive a callback from the mother of a 5-year-old patient seen in clinic yesterday by another provider. The mother is requesting antibiotics. She states her child is not getting better and that the other provider did nothing to help her child. Prior to getting on the phone with the mother, you look through the patient's chart for which piece of information?

    A. Patient's height and weight at most recent visit

    B. Mother's history of calling the clinic

    C. Patient's allergy list

    D. Patient's diagnosis and treatment plan from most recent visit

33. All of the following are appropriate treatments in a patient diagnosed with a URI except:

    A. oxymetazoline 0.05% nasal (Afrin)

    B. theophylline 300 mg (Theo-Dur)

    C. loratadine 10 mg (Claritin)

    D. dextromethorphan 10 mg (Robitussin)

ANSWERS AND EXPLANATIONS

Lesson 1: Asthma

1. D

FEV_1 increased 15% after administration of albuterol **(D)** is most suggestive of asthma. An improvement in FEV_1 12% indicates reversible airway obstruction, which is a hallmark of asthma. Choices (A) and (C) are possible findings in a patient with asthma, but you can see these findings in other disease processes as well. An improvement in FEV_1 of 5% (B) is not great enough to indicate reversible airway obstruction.

2. B

Changing fluticasone to 110 mcg/actuation, 2 puffs BID **(B)** is the next step to follow as part of a stepwise approach, because this patient is not well-controlled on their current plan. The next step would be to add a medium dose of inhaled corticosteroid. Adding montelukast (A) is not the next step when using the stepwise approach. It would be important for the patient to keep track of peak flow measurements (C), but a change is needed in the treatment plan, as the patient is not experiencing good asthma control. If this patient were having severe, atypical symptoms or not responding to usual treatment, pulmonology referral (D) would be appropriate.

3. A

Spirometry is not ordered on children under the age of 5 because the results are unreliable **(A)**. Choices (B), (C), and (D) are incorrect as patients under 4 years of age can be diagnosed with asthma, eczema is often seen in patients that have asthma, and the absence of wheezing does not rule out the diagnosis of asthma.

4. A

This patient has nightly symptoms greater than 1/week, but not nightly, and activity is somewhat limited. She is having daily symptoms. These three items are in the category of moderate asthma **(A)**. Intermittent asthma (B) is characterized by symptoms 2 or fewer days per week, nighttime awakenings 2 or fewer times per month, and no interference in daily activities. Severe asthma (C) is characterized by symptoms throughout the day, nighttime awakenings often 7 times a week, and extreme limitation in daily activities. Mild asthma (D) is characterized by symptoms greater than 2 times per week but not every day, nighttime awakenings 3–4 times per month, and minor interference in daily activities.

Lesson 2: Cough/Bronchitis

5. B

The typical duration of the cough associated with acute bronchitis lasts 3 weeks **(B)**. In some cases, it can last 4–6 weeks, though that is uncommon.

6. A

Diagnosis of acute bronchitis is made by clinical presentation **(A)**. A chest x-ray (B) will be normal. Sputum cultures (C) are only helpful if a bacterial pathogen is suspected and is not routinely ordered. The WBC (D) will be normal.

7. B

Treatment for acute bronchitis includes rest, increased intake of fluids, and the use of a humidifier **(B)**. An antibiotic (A) would be appropriate only if the patient displayed signs/symptoms of a bacterial infection. Antitussives (C) and antihistamines (D) are not recommended.

8. B

Cough is not associated with pharyngitis **(B)**. URI (A), pneumonia (C), and allergic rhinitis (D) are all common causes of persistent cough and should be considered in the differential for acute bronchitis.

Lesson 3: COPD

9. B

For COPD patients <65 years of age with significant comorbidities, the Advisory Committee on Immunization Practices (ACIP) recommends administration of PPSV23 pneumococcal vaccination **(B)**. Inactivated, rather than activated, influenza vaccination (A) is recommended for those with a potentially weakened immune system. PCV13 pneumococcal vaccine (C) is recommended for patients over the age of 65. For all individuals, Td vaccination (D) is recommended every 10 years.

10. D

Despite the GOLD spirometric classification of 2, a COPD patient with a self-report of ≥2 exacerbations in the past year and CAT score of ≥10 is characterized as risk group D **(D)**. The Global Initiative for Chronic Obstructive Lung Disease (GOLD) in the setting of conflicting information recommends using the higher-risk category to characterize condition and formulate treatment and management plan.

11. A

The "GOLD Diagnosis, Management, and Prevention of COPD, 2017" report emphasizes effective management and reflects an individualized assessment of symptom severity **(A)** and future risk of exacerbation to create a customized treatment involving pharmacologic and non-pharmacologic interventions. Abnormal findings on chest radiograph (B) are not specific to the narrowing of the airway found in COPD. Impaired FEV1 (C) is used to classify the severity of airflow limitation, not necessarily treatment. Immunization status (D) reflects risk for airway infections, but is not specific to the treatment of COPD.

12. A

Fluticasone HFA **(A)** is a type of inhaled corticosteroid; it possesses an anti-inflammatory mechanism of action rather than working as a bronchodilator. Choices (B), (C), and (D) involve activity that antagonizes bronchoconstriction or promotes bronchodilation.

Lesson 4: Lung Cancer

13. B

The ACCN guidelines for screening of high-risk individuals for lung cancer includes an annual LDCT for current smokers aged 55–74 with at least a 30 pack-year smoking history, as well as former smokers of the same age and smoking history who have quit within the last 15 years **(B)**. Option (D) is the NCCN's guideline for screening of high-risk patients. Choice (A) is incorrect due to wrong age (50 rather than 55 and no upper limit cutoff) and wrong pack-year history (20 rather than 30). Choice (C) is incorrect as it should be smokers who quit within the past 15 years, not 20 years.

14. C

Smoking cessation **(C)** is essential in the treatment of lung cancer and is the immediate priority. Pain control (A) is important in the treatment of lung cancer and may be achieved using various modalities. A PO formulation is more likely to be prescribed, over IVP. Due to the risk of radiation exposure, x-rays (B) and serial CT scans (D) are not recommended.

15. A

Typical presentation for lung cancer occurs late in the disease when patients become symptomatic. Wheezing **(A)** is not typically seen with lung cancer, but is a common symptom of asthma. Common symptoms include dyspnea (B), chest discomfort (C), and anorexia (D).

16. D

Definitive diagnosis of lung cancer can only be made using cytologic or histologic evidence **(D)**. Diagnostic imaging such as MRIs (A), CT scans (B), and x-rays (C) are often used during the initial workup and for monitoring purposes following diagnosis.

Lesson 5: Pneumonia

17. C

A non-smoking **(C)** patient is at greater risk for an atypical pathogen. Risk factors for infection with DRSP include patients with comorbidities (A), antibiotic use within the last 90 days (B), >65 years of age (D), immunosuppression, alcohol use, and exposure to day care and long-term care facilities.

18. B

For patients who are previously healthy, with no antibiotic exposure in the last 90 days and where DRSP is not suspected, a macrolide **(B)** is the ideal treatment. Amoxicillin (A) may be used for patients who are pregnant. Levofloxacin (C) is a respiratory fluoroquinolone and would be used for the patient with suspected DRSP. Rocephin (D) is a cephalosporin and is used for the patient with pathogens producing beta lactamase, such as *H. influenza.*

19. D

Given the patient's age, presence of multiple comorbidities, and respiratory symptoms including productive cough and dyspnea, this patient likely has pneumonia **(D)**. Asthma exacerbation (A) is not as likely, given stated comorbidities and productive cough; symptoms would include dyspnea, chest pain, cough, and wheezing. Acute bronchitis (B) and influenza (C) may present with a productive cough, but also present with fatigue, wheezing, rhinorrhea, and/or pharyngitis.

20. A

Diagnosis of pneumonia is based on positive CXR and symptoms including, but not limited to: cough, fever, tachypnea, and adventitious breath sounds. The CURB-65 score indicates severity of symptoms of pneumonia. One point is given for confusion, urea >7 mmol/L, respiratory rate >30/min, SBP <90 or DBP <60, age >65 years. This patient has a CURB-65 score of 1 **(A)** and can be treated as an outpatient. Scores of 2–5 indicate increasing severity, and hospitalization should be considered with a score of 2; hospitalization is required for a score of 3–5.

Lesson 6: Pulmonary Embolus

21. D

The patient is displaying signs of a pulmonary embolism **(D)**. In an acute MI (A), rales are not typically heard and fever isn't usually present. Rales, accentuated second heart sound, and fever aren't typical of a pneumothorax (B). The chest pain associated with pleurisy (C) is worse with deep breathing and characterized as "stabbing."

22. A

A MDCTA **(A)** is the gold standard test used to diagnose a pulmonary embolism. Coagulation studies (B) are part of the workup after diagnosis. A V/Q scan (C) may be done if a MDCTA is contraindicated or unavailable. D-dimer (D) can help confirm but is not used as a diagnostic test for pulmonary embolism.

23. B

The preferred anticoagulants are low-molecular-weight heparin or fondaparinux **(B)**. Alteplase (A) and streptokinase (C) are thrombolytics. Heparin (D) is not the preferred anticoagulant.

24. C

Anticoagulant therapy should be continued for at least three months **(C)** following a diagnosis of pulmonary embolism.

25. B

Virchow's triad is comprised of hypercoagulability, vessel wall injury, and venous stasis **(B)**.

26. C

The FNP should expect to find rales, an accentuated second heart sound, and wheezing **(C)**. Lower extremity edema (A) may be present with a DVT, but stridor is not seen with PE and hypertension occurs prior to hypotension. While an S4 gallop (B) may be present, crackles are not usually heard with a PE and tachycardia. Hemoptysis (D) may be present, but hypotension and diminished heart sounds are not.

Lesson 7: Tuberculosis

27. A

A TST result of $\geq$10 mm is considered positive in a healthcare worker. TB prophylaxis requires treatment with isoniazid for 9 months to prevent conversion to active disease **(A)**. There is no need to repeat the TST in 3 months (B), as the result will once again be positive. Monitoring for signs of active disease (C) is appropriate, but treatment should begin immediately to prevent conversion to active disease. A full multidrug regimen (D) is not required when no clinical signs of active disease are present.

28. C

A positive TST is $\geq$5 mm in persons in close contact with a person diagnosed with active disease and the daughter should receive TB prophylaxis **(C)**. Her age is not a contraindication to TB prophylaxis (A). If her TST is positive (B), she should receive TB prophylaxis with isoniazid for 9 months to prevent conversion to active disease. With no clinical symptoms or positive chest x-ray, there is no need to treat her with a full multidrug regimen (D).

29. B

Dyspnea is rarely reported unless the disease is extensive **(B)**. Night sweats (A), fever (C), and a dry cough (D) are common symptoms of progressive TB disease.

Lesson 8: Upper Respiratory Infection

30. B

The priority question is, "How long have you had the symptoms?" **(B)**. If the patient has been symptomatic for 7–10 days, they should be seen because of possibility of bacterial infection and/or a complication. Other pertinent questions related to the history would be if the patient is experiencing SOB or wheezing or has a history of asthma, COPD, or other respiratory comorbid conditions. (A) and (C) would be appropriate questions to ask, but not the most important. A patient can run a fever with a URI (D), but a fever does not correspond to the severity of an illness.

31. A

This patient is showing classic symptoms of a URI; a CXR **(A)** would not be a cost-effective, prudent diagnostic test to perform in this patient. There are no signs this patient is experiencing a complication or more severe illness. Choices (B), (C), and (D) are all appropriate diagnostic tests to perform, and could change the treatment plan if any of the tests were positive.

32. D

You need to know the patient's diagnosis and treatment plan **(D)** prior to talking with the mother to appropriately discuss the patient and make recommendations. You do not need the information in (A), (B), or (C) to discuss the patient with the mother.

33. B

Theophylline **(B)**, a xanthine derivative, is not appropriate for a URI. It may be used, although rarely, to treat asthma. Oxymetazoline (A), loratadine (C), and dextromethorphan (D) may all be appropriately prescribed.

CHAPTER 7

Cardiovascular

LESSON 1: ACUTE MI

Learning Objectives
- Identify the risk factors that can lead to Acute Coronary Syndrome (ACS)
- Determine clinical manifestations representative of ACS
- Define diagnostic test and appropriate treatment options

Coronary artery disease (CAD) is the single largest killer of American men and women in all ethnic groups. CAD is a broad term that includes chronic stable angina and acute coronary syndrome (ACS). Under the umbrella of ACS is myocardial infarction (MI) and unstable angina. ACS is usually a result of atherosclerosis creating ischemia of the myocardium.

Non-atherosclerotic etiologies include emboli and mechanical obstruction (e.g., chest trauma, aortic dissection, arteritis, DIC, cocaine or IV drug use, aortic stenosis, and hypertrophic cardiomyopathy).

Modifiable	Nonmodifiable
• Smoking • High blood pressure • High cholesterol • Diabetes • Physical inactivity • Being overweight or obese • Excessive alcohol intake • Illicit drug use • Excessive stress	• Age • Gender • Family history of heart disease

Table 7.1.1 ACS Risk Factors

Definitions
- **Stable angina:** predictable chest discomfort that occurs with moderate to prolonged exertion and results if lack of oxygen supply is temporary and reversible
- **Unstable angina:** unpredictable chest pain or discomfort that occurs at rest or with exertion and causes severe activity limitation; a serious indicator of an impending myocardial infarction
- **Myocardial infarction:** occurs when myocardial tissue is abruptly and severely deprived of oxygen; when blood flow is quickly reduced by 80–90%, ischemia develops
- **STEMI:** ST elevation MI; full thickness necrosis of the myocardium caused by total occlusion of the artery (traditional manifestation)
- **NSTEMI:** non-ST elevation MI; partial thickness necrosis of the myocardium caused by subtotal occlusion of the artery (common in women)

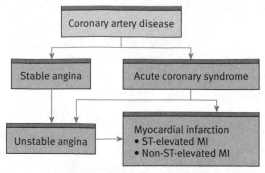

Figure 7.1.1 Defining CAD

Assessment

Subjective

Symptoms

Clinical consequences will depend on the size and location of the infarct. Onset of symptoms with an MI can be abrupt and intense. However, a more common presentation includes symptoms that start slowly and persist for hours, days, or weeks before a myocardial infarction. Symptoms include:

- Chest pain or discomfort, which may be described as severe pressure, tightness, heaviness, or fullness
- Pain or discomfort in one or both arms, the jaw, neck, back, or stomach (indigestion or epigastric pain)
- Shortness of breath/dyspnea
- Cough
- Dizziness or lightheadedness
- Nausea and vomiting
- Diaphoresis

DANGER SIGN

Women: extreme fatigue and epigastric discomfort are usually the initial symptoms of MI in women; may also experience shortness of breath or dyspnea with or without chest discomfort

Older adults: indigestion and shortness of breath or dyspnea may be the only symptoms; major manifestation of MI in people >80 years of age may be disorientation or acute confusion

Diabetics: due to diabetic neuropathy, diabetic patients do not have the typical "chest pain"; instead, chest pain is presented as midscapular, jaw, lip, and gum pain

---

History

These conditions place a patient at greater risk of MI:

- **PMH:** previous MI, HTN, CAD, hyperlipidemia, angina, clotting disorder, thromboembolism, PVD, endocarditis, arteritis, aortic stenosis, hypertrophic cardiomyopathy, abdominal aortic aneurysm
- **PSH:** percutaneous coronary intervention (PCI), CABG, angiography
- **FH:** CAD, MI, sudden cardiac death, HTN

- **SH:** diet high in saturated or trans fats, high intake of refined carbohydrates, sedentary lifestyle, smoking, alcohol use, illicit drug use, stress
- **Medications:** phosphodiesterase-5 inhibitors

Objective

The following are suggestive of an MI:

- **LOC/mental status:** disorientation, confusion
- **VS:** hypotension, tachycardia or bradycardia, tachypnea, hypoxemia
- **Resp:** respiratory distress, rales, crackles, wheezing, use of accessory muscles
- **CV:** S3 or S4, mitral regurgitation murmur, chest discomfort reproduced by palpation, displaced PMI, jugular vein distention, arrhythmias
- **GI:** vomiting
- **Skin:** pallor, diaphoresis, cold/clammy extremities, decreased capillary refill

Diagnosis

Diagnostic Tests	
Blood tests	• Troponin • CK-MB • Myoglobin • CMP • CBC • CRP • Clotting studies (fibrinogen, PT, APTT, INR, homocysteine) • ABG
Imaging studies	• 12-lead ECG • Echocardiogram • Cardiac catheterization (angiography) • Chest x-ray

Table 7.1.2

ECG Abnormalities
Myocardium localization based on ECG abnormalities
Inferior wall: II, III, aVF
Lateral wall: I, aVL, V4 through V6
Anteroseptal: V1 through V3
Anterolateral: V1 through V6
Right ventricular: RV4, RV5
Posterior wall: R/S ratio greater than 1 in V1 and V2, and T-wave changes in V1, V8, and V9

Table 7.1.3

For further information related to ECG/arrhythmias, refer to Chapter 7, Lesson 2.

Plan

Treatment

> **DANGER SIGN** In an outpatient setting, dial 911 if you suspect your patient might be experiencing a myocardial infarction. Early diagnosis and treatment is vital. Delay in treatment can lead to death.
>
> - Assess ABCs and vital signs
> - Aspirin four 81 mg tabs (or one 325 mg tab)
> - Sublingual nitroglycerin (if available)
> - Oxygen (if available)

Medications: Post MI
• Aspirin: 325 mg PO daily maintenance
• Clopidogrel 75 mg PO daily maintenance **OR** prasugrel 10 mg PO daily maintenance
• Nitrates may be needed for angina
• Beta-blockers initiated within 24 hrs
• ACE inhibitors
• ARB (if intolerant to ACE inhibitors)
• Calcium channel blockers (if intolerant to beta-blockers)
• Statins
• Stool softeners
• Oxygen 2–4 L/min (titrate to keep sat >90)
• Antiarrhythmics as needed

Table 7.1.4

Education

Lifestyle modifications include maintaining a normal weight (BMI 18.5–24.9), heart-healthy diet including cholesterol management (total <200, HDL >40–60, LDL <100, triglycerides <150), sodium reduction (1500–2300 mg/day), physical activity (30 minutes of moderate for 5 days, 25 minutes of vigorous 3 days per week; for BP lowering, 40 minutes of moderate-to-vigorous 3–4 times per week), alcohol intake within normal limits for gender and age, and smoking cessation. It is also important for patients to keep blood pressure and blood sugar under control.

Referral

- Cardiologist
- Cardiac rehabilitation

Takeaways

- Women, older adults, and diabetics may have an atypical MI presentation.
- Early diagnosis with cardiac enzymes and ECG is of utmost importance.
- Health promotion and risk reduction are important components of care.

LESSON 2: ARRHYTHMIAS

Learning Objectives
- Apply systematic approach to assessing a 12-lead ECG
- Understand the role of ECG interpretation in determining arrhythmias
- Recognize arrhythmias commonly seen in practice, and be able to adequately diagnose and manage those arrhythmias

Cardiac arrhythmias can vary from benign to life threatening. It is necessary to be able to identify a patient whose complaints might be related to a cardiac arrhythmia. Arrhythmias that might be encountered in practice include sinus arrhythmia, premature atrial (PAC) or ventricular beats (PVC), sinus bradycardia, sinus tachycardia, atrial fibrillation (A-fib), atrial flutter (A-flutter), supraventricular tachycardia (SVT), and atrioventricular (AV) blocks.

Definitions
- **Bradycardia:** rate less than 60 beats per minute (BPM)
- **Tachycardia:** rate greater than 100 BPM
- **Axis:** pattern of electrical conduction through the heart
- **Ectopic beat:** a cardiac beat in an abnormal place
- **Proarrhythmia:** new arrhythmia that occurs often from initiating antiarrhythmic medications

ECG Interpretation

The 12-lead ECG can be used to determine heart rhythm, ischemia, infarction, altered conduction patterns, and enlargement of the heart. It is a "snapshot" of the heart from 12 different angles.

I (Lateral)	aVR	V1 (Septal)	V4 (Anterior)
II (Inferior)	aVL (Lateral)	V2 (Septal)	V5 (Lateral)
III (Inferior)	aVF (Inferior)	V3 (Anterior)	V6 (Lateral)
II (some ECG machines add a longer view of Lead II to the bottom of the ECG)			

Table 7.2.1 12-Lead ECG Schematic

The QRS complex in a normal ECG follows a predictable pattern of polarity. It should either be positioned upright (primarily above the baseline), down (primarily below the baseline), or can be either depending on the lead. An alteration in this polarity can mean there is a shift in the axis or the leads are placed incorrectly. Normal polarity should be as follows:

- **Upright:** I, II, III, aFV, V5 and V6
- **Down:** aVR, V1, V2
- **Can be either:** aVL
- **Biphasic (half up and half down):** V3 and V4

A systematic approach to interpreting a 12-lead ECG includes the following steps:

1. Determine the rate, rhythm, and presence of ectopic beats. Is the rate tachycardic, bradycardic, or normal? Is the rhythm normal sinus or something else?

   – **Bradyarrhythmias:** sinus bradycardia, junctional rhythms, AV blocks

   – **Tachyarrhythmias:** sinus tachycardia, atrial fibrillation, atrial flutter, supraventricular tachycardia, ventricular tachycardia

2. Determine the axis and if there is axis deviation. The axis shifts toward increased muscle mass or bundle branch blockages and shifts away from an area of infarction or a hemiblock. To determine axis, look at lead I and lead aVF and the polarity of the QRS complexes in these leads.

   – **Normal axis:** I-upright, aVF-upright

   – **Left axis deviation:** I-upright, aVF-down

   – **Right axis deviation:** I-down, aVF-upright

   – **Extreme axis:** I-down, aVF-down

3. Determine intervals:

   – PR Interval

   – QRS interval

   – QT interval

4. **P wave:** do they all look the same? Is there one P wave for every QRS?

5. **QRS complex:** is it wide? Is there increased voltage (hypertrophy)? Are Q waves present (normal in I, aVL, V4–V6)?

6. **ST Segment and T-wave:** is the ST segment depressed (ischemia) or elevated (injury)? Are T-waves inverted? T-wave is upright in I, II, V3–V6, and inverted in aVR. If T-wave is tall and peaked, consider hyperkalemia.

7. Are the abnormals present in more than 1 lead? Are the abnormals present in leads that represent the same area of the heart? (*See Table 7.2.1*)

8. Interpret the ECG based on the above information and determine course of action based on interpretation and patient's symptoms.

Assessment

Subjective

The health history can give clues about possible causes of symptoms and whether symptoms are related to a cardiac cause. There are potential modifiable causes of cardiac arrhythmias (medications, social habits/addictions), and it is important to ascertain if these are present.

- **PMH:** syncope or near syncope, exercise intolerance, medications that can cause possible arrhythmia or prolonged QT (antiarrhythmics, macrolide and fluoroquinolone antibiotics, antifungals, antihistamines, antidepressants, antipsychotics, triptans, diuretics, bronchodilators), congenital heart disease, sarcoidosis (AV blocks), amyloidosis, or Lyme disease (AV blocks)

- **PSH:** past cardiac surgery, placement of pacemaker or implantable defibrillator, previous cardioversion or resynchronization

- **FH:** history of arrhythmias, CVA, MI, pacemaker, hypertrophic cardiomyopathy, dilated cardiomyopathy, long QT syndrome, Brugada syndrome

- **SH:** smoking, caffeine consumption, exercise (patients that are highly conditioned often have sinus bradycardia), drug use (cocaine and other central nervous system stimulants)

Symptoms

Patients may complain of a variety of symptoms depending on the arrhythmia. Complaints can include fatigue, weakness, palpitations, skipped beat(s), shortness of breath, dyspnea on exertion, syncope or near syncope, dizziness, chest and neck pain/discomfort, anxiety, and edema. The symptoms can be related to the arrhythmia directly or the hemodynamic changes that occur because of the arrhythmia.

Objective

If the heart rate is elevated, slow, or irregular, a cardiac arrhythmia may be occurring at the time of the exam. Other data can determine if there is a potential noncardiac cause of symptoms. If an arrhythmia is present, data can tell if the patient is tolerating the arrhythmia.

- **Vital signs:** tachycardia, bradycardia, hypertensive, hypotensive, tachypnea; SpO_2 may be unreliable when an arrhythmia is present
- **Neck:** JVD
- **CV:** irregular heart rate, presence of murmurs or extra heart sounds, weak and/or irregular pulses, pedal edema
- **Resp:** crackles or rales—possible pulmonary edema, dyspnea on exertion, shortness of breath
- **Skin:** pale, diaphoretic

Diagnosis

The main tool that is used to initially diagnose an arrhythmia is the ECG. It can often be determined whether a complaint is related to a cardiac cause, whether a life-threatening or non-life-threatening arrhythmia is present, and whether further evaluation or emergency treatment is needed. Since the 12-lead ECG gives a picture of the rhythm at the time it was taken, it's possible that a transient arrhythmia might not be detected. For patients with a normal ECG in whom a cardiac cause is suspected, a diagnosis can be made with a 24–48 hour Holter monitor, event monitor, mobile telemetry, or implantable loop recorder. Educate patients to document any symptoms they have while wearing these monitors so that these can be correlated with their heart rhythm. Labs to check for other identifiable causes include CBC/diff, electrolytes, thyroid stimulating hormone, and B-type natriuretic peptide. A chest x-ray can show cardiomegaly.

Plan

Treatment

The treatment is based on the type of arrhythmia and the associated symptoms. For asymptomatic patients with sinus arrhythmia and occasional ectopic beats with no previous cardiac history, there is no treatment. Reassure these patients. The goal of treatment for other arrhythmias is to treat underlying causes, change and maintain sinus rhythm, prevent thrombosis and embolization, or slow the ventricular rate if persistent A-fib/A-flutter. For patients that need antiarrhythmic medication, these medications should be started with cardiology consultation. Many antiarrhythmics can cause proarrhythmias, and patients need close monitoring with inpatient or outpatient telemetry when starting them.

- **Frequent and/or symptomatic PACs:** limit or eliminate triggers (smoking, alcohol, caffeine); metoprolol tartrate or other antiarrhythmic agents; possible ablation
- **Frequent and/or symptomatic PVCs:** limit or eliminate triggers (alcohol, caffeine, illicit drugs); treat sleep apnea; beta-blockers and calcium channel blockers commonly used; may need antiarrhythmic agents and ablation
- **Symptomatic bradycardia:** consider medications as a cause (beta-blockers, diltiazem, verapamil, amiodarone, clonidine, lithium, amitriptyline) and withhold if possible; refer to specialist to evaluate for possible sick sinus syndrome, pacemaker insertion

- **A-fib/A-flutter:** rate control with beta-blockers, verapamil, and diltiazem; digoxin is used if heart failure and a decreased ejection fraction is present; amiodarone is used when other meds are ineffective; cardioversion for A-fib can return the rhythm to sinus and is indicated in certain circumstances; anticoagulation may be necessary prior to cardioversion and for sustained A-fib/A-flutter to prevent thrombosis and emboli; for A-flutter, radio-frequency ablation has a high success rate

- **Sinus tachycardia:** eliminate possible causes (alcohol, tobacco, caffeine, stimulants); treat underlying causes (infection, hyperthyroidism, hypovolemia, hypotension); ST is often the only ECG change seen with pulmonary embolism (emergent transfer if other symptoms suggest PE, *see Chapter 6, Lesson 6*); ST with no cause can be treated with metoprolol tartrate, metoprolol succinate, or catheter ablation

- **First- and second-degree type I AV block:** remove or change possible offending medications (digoxin, beta-blockers, verapamil, diltiazem), if possible; often no treatment, just reassurance; if symptomatic, patients should be referred; if unstable, emergency transport

- **Second-degree type II AV block:** consider possible causes, and if stable, transfer with pacing pads in place (can progress to third-degree AV block); if unstable, treat according to ACLS protocol and transfer immediately

- **SVT:** if stable, vagal maneuvers or carotid sinus massage to restore to normal sinus rhythm; if unstable or maneuvers/massage ineffective, follow ACLS protocol

Education

Counsel patients to limit caffeine and alcohol consumption. Educate regarding smoking cessation. It is important to stress medication adherence and not to stop medications abruptly.

Referrals

An arrhythmia that is symptomatic needs immediate referral and/or emergency treatment. A patient with a life-threatening arrhythmia needs emergency support with ACLS protocol until ER transport arrives. If a patient needs an antiarrhythmic medication, this should be done in consultation with a cardiologist. Interventional cardiac procedures require cardiology referral.

Takeaways

- If lead aVR is upright, the limb leads have been switched. Correct and rerun ECG.
- Often the patient's complaint and physical exam findings are related to the hemodynamic consequences of an arrhythmia.
- For all cardiac arrhythmias, if the patient is symptomatic, they require treatment. If they are unstable, they require emergency support.
- Any of the mentioned arrhythmias can be seen in the presence of acute MI, and the patient should always be questioned about related symptoms of a MI.

LESSON 3: CHEST PAIN

> **Learning Objectives**
> - Determine the key components of a thorough chest pain assessment
> - Describe "danger signs" that may indicate a life-threatening condition that needs prompt intervention
> - Identify the diagnostic tests that are useful in determining chest pain etiology

Chest pain is not something to be taken lightly, especially since it can be related to a cardiac condition. Chest pain can also have respiratory, musculoskeletal, neurologic, GI, and psychogenic etiologies. Some of these conditions can be serious and life-threatening. Other causes may include shingles, anemia, depression, panic disorder, and anxiety.

Assessment and Diagnosis

Subjective

It can be difficult to distinguish chest pain due to a heart problem from other types of chest pain. A thorough pain assessment is key.

- **Onset:** when the pain began, initial episode, repeat episode
- **Location:** central, lateral, axillary, substernal, epigastric, left- vs. right-sided
- **Quality:** dull, aching, sharp, crushing, pressure, stabbing, sharp, heaviness, fullness, burning, pins/needles, tingling, electrical, cramping
- **Timing/setting:** length of pain episodes, intermittent, constant, time of day, related to temperature changes, exertional, at rest, during sleep, daytime, nighttime, after meals
- **Severity:** intensity on scale of 0–10 or visual analogue scale
- **Radiation:** to anterior chest, ribs, shoulders, arms, neck, jaw, abdomen
- **Aggravating factors:** exertion, lying on the left side, palpation, inspiration
- **Alleviating factors:** rest, leaning forward, eating, vomiting, medications (NSAIDs, ASA, acetaminophen, antacids, NTG)
- **Associated symptoms:** dyspnea, shortness of breath, diaphoresis, palpitations, cough, nausea, vomiting, lightheadedness, hemoptysis, trouble swallowing, sour taste in the mouth

History should include identifying factors that may pose a risk for complications or suggest an etiology other than cardiovascular chest pain.

- **PMH:** angina, MI, HTN, CAD (including associated risk factors), clotting disorder, thromboembolism, endocarditis, arteritis, aortic stenosis, cardiomyopathy, abdominal aortic aneurysm, peripheral vascular disease, pneumonia, TB, bronchitis, emphysema, URI, PUD, GERD, gallstones, pancreatitis, anxiety, cancer
- **PSH:** percutaneous coronary intervention (PCI), CABG, angiography
- **FH:** CAD, MI, sudden cardiac death, HTN, asthma
- **SH:** diet high in saturated or trans fats, high intake of refined carbohydrates, sedentary lifestyle, smoking, alcohol use, illicit drug use (cocaine, methamphetamines, heroine), stress
- **Medications:** phosphodiesterase-5 inhibitors
- **Allergies:** seasonal, medications, food, animals

> **DANGER SIGN: CHEST PAIN RED FLAGS**
>
> The following may indicate a life-threatening condition:
>
> - Abnormal vital signs: bradycardia, tachycardia, hypotension or hypertension, tachypnea, hypoxemia, fever
> - Pallor, diaphoresis, chills, malaise
> - Use of accessory muscles
> - Absent breath sounds on one side
> - Asymmetric breath sounds
> - Tracheal deviation
> - Pulsus paradoxus
> - New heart murmur
> - Pericardial friction rub
> - Increased pain with inspiration or with lying on the left side
> - Pain relieved by leaning forward

Cause	Common pain description	Location/ radiation	Associated symptoms	Objective findings	Diagnosis
Acute coronary syndrome (angina, MI)	Pressure, heaviness, squeezing, crushing, tightness; may be precipitated by activity or occur at rest; may be relieved by rest or nitrates	Sub- or retro-sternal, left-sided, epigastric; can radiate to teeth, jaw, neck, one or both arms or shoulders; can be poorly localized pain	Indigestion, nausea, vomiting, dizziness, flushing, diaphoresis, palpitations, dyspnea	Hypotension, arrhythmia, tachypnea, S3 or S4, hypoxemia, pallor, diaphoresis	ECG, troponin, CKMB, myoglobin, echocardiogram, cardiac catheterization
Congestive heart failure	Angina-like	Sub- or retro-sternal	Anxiety, fatigue, cough, pink frothy sputum, shortness of breath, orthopnea, paroxysmal nocturnal dyspnea, abdominal distention, weight gain, nocturia, decreased functional capacity, cold/clammy extremities	Hypotension, tachypnea, hypoxemia, respiratory distress, rales, crackles, rhonchi, wheezing, diminished breath sounds, use of accessory muscles, displaced PMI, jugular vein distention, arrhythmias, S3 gallop, S4, murmur, heaves/ lift, cyanosis, ascites, lower extremity swelling	ECG, chest x-ray, BNP, ABG, CMP, CBC, echocardiogram

Table 7.3.1 Chest Pain Differentiation and Diagnosis

Cause	Common pain description	Location/ radiation	Associated symptoms	Objective findings	Diagnosis
Pericarditis	Constant soreness or sudden sharp and stabbing pain; worse when lying down and relieved by sitting forward; aggravated by deep inspiration; not usually made worse by exertion; unresponsive to nitrates	Substernal, can radiate to the trapezius	Fever, dry cough, muscle, and joint aches	Tachycardia, pleural friction rub, S3, S4	ESR, CRP, chest x-ray, blood culture, CBC, ECG
Pulmonary embolism	Pleuritic, sharp, stabbing pain worsening with deep breaths	Chest, back, shoulder, or upper abdomen	Feeling of impending doom, anxiety, apprehension, dyspnea, hemoptysis, cough, calf tenderness (DVT)	Cyanosis, tachypnea, pleural friction rub, tachycardia, wheeze, rales, distended neck veins, S3	Chest CT, ABG, fibrinogen, D-dimer, PT/PTT, CBC, ECG, chest x-ray, echocardiogram, VQ scan, pulmonary angiogram
Asthma	Tightness	Chest, back	Wheezing, dyspnea, cough (worse at night), chest tightness	Wheezing, diminished breath sounds, prolonged expiration, pulsus paradoxus, tachycardia, hypoxia, cyanosis, tachypnea, accessory muscle use, clubbing	Peak flow, spirometry, pulmonary function tests (PFT), ABG, allergy testing, CBC, immunoglobulins, chest x-ray
Pneumothorax	Acute/sudden and sharp	Lateral region of the chest, referred pain to shoulder	Acute dyspnea, cough	Diminished or absent breath sounds, asymmetry of respirations, decreased fremitus, hyperresonance to percussion, subcutaneous emphysema, tracheal deviation, respiratory distress, cyanosis, tachycardia, hypotension, altered mental status	Chest x-ray, ABG, CBC

Table 7.3.1 Chest Pain Differentiation and Diagnosis (Continued)

Cause	Common pain description	Location/ radiation	Associated symptoms	Objective findings	Diagnosis
Pneumonia	Sharp or stabbing pain associated with cough	Mostly generalized to one side of chest, but can have upper abdominal pain	Cough, fever, dyspnea, chills, sputum, myalgia, malaise	Crackles, rhonchi, decreased breath sounds, friction rub, dullness to percussion, tachypnea, tachycardia, cyanosis, altered mental status	Sputum culture, blood culture, CBC, CMP, ABG, chest x-ray
GERD	Burning sensation with eating large meals reproduced with lying down and relieved with sitting up; angina-like	Retrosternal, abdominal pain	Cough, regurgitation of food, hoarseness, dysphagia, weight loss, early satiety	Loss of dental enamel, anemia	Barium swallow, pH monitoring, esophageal manometry, CBC, endoscopy
Cholecystitis/ cholelithiasis	Sudden onset of pain that crescendos and can last for up to 20 minutes, usually after eating a fatty meal; biliary colic	Epigastrium or right upper abdomen that can radiate to right intrascapular region, shoulder, or back	Nausea, vomiting, anorexia, fever, chills, pruritis, clay-colored stools, steatorrhea	Murphy sign, local tenderness, hepatomegaly, jaundice, abdominal distention	CBC, ESR, CRP, ALT, AST, bilirubin, blood culture, amylase, lipase, ultrasound, x-ray, HIDA scan, CT scan, ERCP, MRCP
Pancreatitis	Sudden dull, boring, steady pain unrelieved by lying supine; leaning forward or the fetal position may ease pain	Epigastrium or periumbilical pain radiating to back	Nausea, vomiting, anorexia, fever	Hypotension, shock, jaundice, ileus, pleural effusion, Grey Turner sign, Cullen sign, hyperglycemia	CBC, CMP, ESR, CRP, ALT, AST, bilirubin, blood culture, amylase, lipase, abdominal ultrasound, abdominal and chest x-ray, CT scan, MRI, ERCP
Costochondritis	Sharp, pleuritic-type pain worsens with deep breathing, palpation, or movement; chest tightness	Area from 2nd through 5th intercostal spaces; can radiate to arm	Chest tightness, warmth at area of the pain	Rib tenderness	Complete and thorough history and physical
Trauma/strain	Sharp pain with movement, stretching, or pushing movements of the arms; pain reproducible with palpation	Area around the strained muscle, sternum, or ribs	Muscle spasm, crepitation, swelling, loss of strength	Chest tenderness to palpation, swelling, bruising	Chest x-ray, CT, MRI

Table 7.3.1 Chest Pain Differentiation and Diagnosis (Continued)

Cause	Common pain description	Location/ radiation	Associated symptoms	Objective findings	Diagnosis
Anxiety	Sharp, tight	Chest	Palpitations, dizziness, diaphoresis, shaking, choking sensation, restlessness, fatigue, irritability, difficulty concentrating, sleep disturbances, headache, backache	Tachycardia, diaphoresis	Complete and thorough history and physical, psychologic testing

Table 7.3.1 Chest Pain Differentiation and Diagnosis (Continued)

Possible follow-up testing:

- ECG
- CT (CT for coronary calcium score)
- MRI/PET scan
- Stress test
- Cardiac catheterization
- Pulmonary function test

Plan

Treatment

Treatment will vary, depending on the underlying cause of the chest pain. Since it can be difficult to distinguish chest pain due to a heart problem from other types of chest pain, have the patient seek medical attention promptly.

Time is crucial when dealing with cardiac chest pain. The following should be performed immediately: vital signs, ECG, continuous cardiac monitoring, IV access and labs including CMP, CBC, and cardiac enzymes. Perform percutaneous coronary intervention (PCI), if indicated, preferably within 90 minutes of arrival with MI symptom onset 12 hours.

A tension pneumothorax is a medical emergency. Be alert for diminished or absent breath sounds on the affected side, asymmetry of respirations, tracheal deviation, respiratory distress, cyanosis, pallor, weak and rapid pulse, hypotension, neck vein distention, and altered mental status. The following should be performed immediately: vital signs, chest x-ray, ABG, ECG, continuous cardiac monitoring, IV access and labs including CMP, CBC, and cardiac enzymes. Perform decompression via chest tube insertion as soon as possible.

Referral

Referral will vary depending on the underlying cause of the chest pain, but can include a consult with one of the following:

- Cardiologist
- Pulmonologist
- Gastroenterologist
- Neurologist

- Pain management
- Spine specialist
- Oncologist

Takeaways

- A thorough pain assessment is key to identifying the underlying cause.
- Be aware of the "red flags," as they may indicate a life-threatening condition that needs prompt intervention.

LESSON 4: CONGESTIVE HEART FAILURE

Learning Objectives
- ■ Define the risk factors for congestive heart failure (CHF)
- ■ Determine clinical manifestations representative of CHF
- ■ Identify diagnostic test and appropriate treatment options

Congestive heart failure (CHF) is a syndrome in which the heart is unable to sufficiently pump the amount of oxygenated blood needed to meet metabolic requirements of the body. It is a principle complication of heart disease, especially hypertension, coronary artery disease (CAD), and cardiomyopathy.

Definitions

- **Systolic failure:** ventricle loses ability to generate enough pressure to eject blood forward (most common cause of CHF)
- **Diastolic failure:** ventricles unable to fill and relax (commonly caused by hypertension)
- **Orthopnea:** dyspnea at rest in the recumbent position
- **Paroxysmal nocturnal dyspnea:** sudden awakening with a feeling of breathlessness 2–5 hours after falling asleep
- **Hepatojugular reflux:** distension of the neck veins precipitated by the maneuver of firm pressure over the liver
- **Ejection fraction (EF):** the fraction of outbound blood pumped from the heart with each heartbeat (normal 50–75%)

Assessment

CHF is the most common reason for hospitalization in adults older than 65 years of age. Risk factors include:

- **Age:** primarily a disease of the elderly (>65 years of age)
- **Ethnicity:** African Americans (related to the higher incidence of hypertension, diabetes, and CAD)
- **CAD associated:** obesity, sedentary lifestyle, smoking, alcohol use, high cholesterol, diabetes
- **Stress:** physical, emotional, or environmental

Cardiac	Respiratory	Renal	Endocrine
CAD MI Cardiomyopathy • Alcoholism • Viral (i.e., HIV) • Muscular dystrophy • Amyloidosis • Pregnancy Valvular disorders • Aortic stenosis • Aortic regurgitation • Rheumatic heart disease Arrhythmia • Atrial fibrillation • Ventricular tachycardia	• COPD • Pulmonary hypertension • Sleep apnea • ARDS	• Acute renal failure • Chronic renal failure • Renal artery stenosis	• Diabetes • Hyperthyroidism • Thyrotoxicosis • SIADH • Cushing disease • Pheochromocytoma

Table 7.4.1 CHF Risk Factors

Other contributing factors include conditions that can lead to inappropriate sodium and/or fluid loss as well as volume overload, congenital heart defects, anemia, drugs (NSAIDs; oral hypoglycemics drugs like rosiglitazone [Avandia] and pioglitazone [Actos]; negative inotropes [beta-blockers, IV amiodarone]); chemotherapy, and noncompliance with therapy for associated conditions.

Subjective

Symptoms

- Anxiety, decreased attention span, easily fatigued
- Chest pain
- Dyspnea, cough, pink frothy sputum
- Sleeping with multiple pillows or upright in a recliner
- Shoes fit more tightly, or shoes or socks may leave indentations on swollen feet
- May have removed their rings because of swelling in their fingers and hands
- Increased thirst, anorexia, nausea, vomiting, bloating, increased size of abdomen, right upper quadrant pain
- Weight gain
- Frequent awakening at night to urinate (nocturia)
- Decreased functional capacity (unable to walk one block or up one flight of stairs without stopping) and weakness
- Cool, cold, or clammy extremities

History may include:

- **PMH:** MI, HTN, CAD, hyperlipidemia, DM, endocarditis, myocarditis, pericarditis, valvular disorders, cardiomyopathy, supraventricular tachycardia, thyroid disease, AIDS, anorexia nervosa, scleroderma, amyloidosis, sarcoidosis
- **PSH:** CABG, angiography, PCI

- **FH:** CAD, MI, sudden cardiac death, HTN, cardiomyopathy
- **SH:** diet high in saturated or trans fats, high intake of refined carbohydrates, sedentary lifestyle, smoking, alcohol use, illicit drug use, stress
- **Medications:** antineoplastic drugs, iron-chelating agents, ephedra, cobalt, anabolic steroids, chloroquine, clozapine, amphetamine, methylphenidate, and catecholamines

Objective

- **LOC/mental status:** disorientation, confusion, lethargy, restlessness
- **VS:** hypotension, hypertension, orthostatic changes, tachycardia, tachypnea, hypoxemia
- **Resp:** respiratory distress, rales, crackles, wheezing, use of accessory muscles
- **CV:** S3 gallop, S4, murmur, heaves/lift, displaced PMI, jugular vein distention, arrhythmias
- **GI:** positive hepatojugular reflex, hepatomegaly, splenomegaly, ascites, increased weight
- **Skin:** peripheral edema, pallor, diaphoresis, cold/clammy extremities, decreased capillary refill, dusky appearance

Left-sided heart failure	Right-sided heart failure
• Restlessness • Confusion • Dyspnea on exertion (DOE) • PND • Orthopnea • Tachypnea • Cough • Wheezing • Crackles • Pink frothy sputum • Tachycardia • Cyanosis	• Fatigue • Difficulty breathing • Jugular vein distention • Ascites • Anorexia • GI distress • Hepatomegaly • Splenomegaly • Peripheral edema

Table 7.4.2 Left- vs. Right-Sided Heart Failure

Right-sided HF in the absence of left-sided HF is usually the result of pulmonary problems such as chronic obstructive pulmonary disease (COPD) or pulmonary hypertension. One-sided failure eventually leads to biventricular failure.

Diagnosis

The primary goal is to determine the underlying cause. Brain natriuretic peptide (BNP) or B-type natriuretic peptide is a useful marker of ventricular dysfunction. It is a cardiac neurohormone secreted by the ventricles of the heart in response to excessive stretching of cardiomyocytes.

CHF Diagnostic Tests	
Labs	BNP
	CMP
	CBC
	LFT
	ABG
	Cardiac enzymes (troponin, CK-MB, myoglobin)
	BUN/creatinine
	Thyroid function tests
	Hemoglobin A1c
	Urinalysis
Imaging	Echocardiogram
	ECG
	CXR
	CT or MRI
Procedures	Pulmonary function test (PFT)
	Cardiac catheterization
	Stress test

Table 7.4.3

Heart Failure Classification

New York Heart Association: Symptom-Based Classification

Class	Symptoms
I	No limitation of physical activity. Ordinary physical activity does not cause symptoms of heart failure.
II	Slight limitation of physical activity. Comfortable at rest. Ordinary physical activity results in symptoms of heart failure.
III	Marked limitation of physical activity. Comfortable at rest. Less than ordinary activity causes symptoms of heart failure.
IV	Unable to carry on any physical activity without symptoms of heart failure or symptoms of heart failure at rest.

Table 7.4.4 NYHA Functional Classification

Yancy, C.W., Jessup, M., Bozkurt, B., Butler, J., Casey, D.E., Drazner, M.H., … Wilkoff, B.L. (2013). 2013 ACCF/AHA guideline for the management of heart failure: Executive summary: A report of the American College of Cardiology Foundation/American Heart Association Task Force on practice guidelines. *Circulation, 128*(16), 1810-1852. doi: 10.1161/CIR.0b013e31829e8807

American College of Cardiology/American Heart Association: Stage-Based Classification

Class	Objective assessment
A	At high risk for heart failure. No objective evidence of cardiovascular disease. No symptoms and no limitation in ordinary physical activity.
B	Structural cardiovascular disease without signs and symptoms of heart failure.
C	Structural cardiovascular disease with prior or current signs and symptoms of heart failure.
D	Objective evidence of severe cardiovascular disease. Severe limitations. Experiences symptoms even while at rest.

Table 7.4.5 ACC/AHA Classification

Yancy, C.W., Jessup, M., Bozkurt, B., Butler, J., Casey, D.E., Drazner, M.H., ... Wilkoff, B.L. (2013). 2013 ACCF/AHA guideline for the management of heart failure: Executive summary: A report of the American College of Cardiology Foundation/American Heart Association Task Force on practice guidelines. *Circulation, 128*(16), 1810-1852. doi: 10.1161/CIR.0b013e31829e8807

Plan

Treatment

Heart failure should be treated immediately. Initial stabilization may require inpatient care in severe cases. Search for underlying correctable conditions and eliminate contributing factors when possible. The goal is to reduce preload, afterload, and inhibition of renin and the sympathetic nervous system. Treatment of heart failure is based on the stage. Medication management may include:

- ACE inhibitors or ARBs
- Diuretics
- Beta-blockers
- Digoxin
- Anticoagulation for those with atrial fibrillation

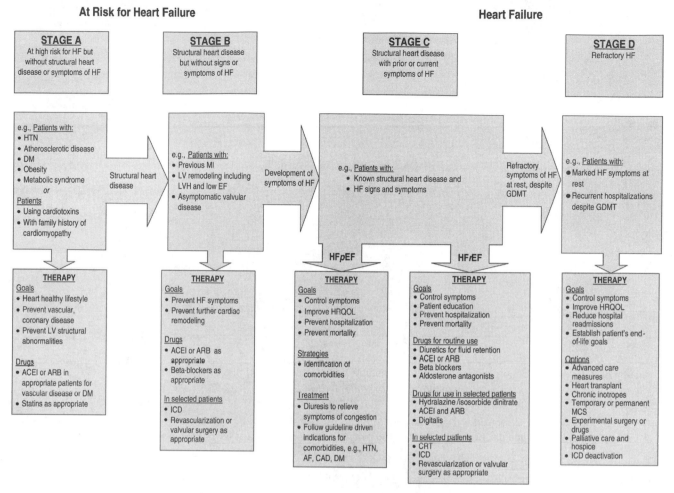

Figure 7.4.1 HF Treatment Recommendations by Stage

General measures may include:

- Supplemental oxygen
- Antiembolism stockings
- Sodium restriction

Education

Instruct on lifestyle modifications including maintaining a normal weight (BMI 18.5–24.9); heart-healthy diet including cholesterol management (total <200, HDL >40–60, LDL <100, tri <150) and sodium reduction (1500–2300 mg/day); increasing physical activity (30 min moderate for 5 times per week, 25 min of vigorous 3 times per week, for BP-lowering, 40 min moderate to vigorous 3–4 times per week); alcohol intake within normal limits for gender and age; and smoking cessation. It is also imperative for patients to have good control of HTN, high cholesterol, and DM. Also instruct on the following:

- Daily weight
- Tracking fluid intake
- Report rapid weight gain and respiratory difficulty
- Stress management
- Flu and pneumonia vaccine

Referral

- Cardiologist
- Cardiac rehabilitation
- Dietician

Takeaways

- It is imperative to manage comorbid conditions including HTN, high cholesterol, and DM.
- Know how to differentiate right-sided vs. left-sided heart failure.
- Health promotion and risk reduction are important components of care.

LESSON 5: ENDOCARDITIS

Learning Objectives

- Understand the major risk factors for endocarditis
- Determine how endocarditis is diagnosed and identify the associated symptoms
- Discuss when prophylaxis should be used for the prevention of infective endocarditis

Infective endocarditis (IE), also referred to as bacterial endocarditis, results when bacteria or fungi enter the blood-stream and settle on the endocardial surface of the heart, heart valve(s), or blood vessel. IE is relatively uncommon. Non-infective endocarditis is the result of inflammation of endocardium (lining of heart and valves) without signs of bacteria or fungi, such as a when a sterile thrombus forms on a valve. Focus on care of adults as IE is rare in children unless they have an unrepaired ventricular septal defect or complex congenital heart disease.

Definitions

- **Transthoracic echocardiogram (TTE):** most common type of echocardiogram; an ultrasound transducer is applied to the chest wall in order to visualize the cardiac chambers, valves, and heart muscle
- **Transesophageal echocardiogram (TEE):** long, soft ultrasound probe is inserted into the esophagus in order to capture more detailed images of heart; a topical anesthetic for the throat such as lidocaine/benzocaine spray and IV sedation may be given; patients may complain of sore throat; risk of bleeding and/or perforation

Assessment

Review of Systems

Preexisting structural heart abnormalities account for 75% of patients with endocarditis: a cardiac history is vital. Mitral valve prolapse and aortic valve disease are the most common predisposing lesions for IE in adults. It is important to note that when endocarditis results from injection drug use, less than half of these patients have an existing heart abnormality.

Patients at high risk for IE include:

- History of rheumatic valvular disease
- Mitral and/or aortic valve disease
- Prosthetic valve replacement
- Unrepaired congenital heart lesions such as VSD, PDA, tetralogy of fallot, etc.

- IV drug users
- Post-op organ transplant patients (cardiac, liver, and kidney)
- Poor dental hygiene
- Long-term hemodialysis
- Diabetes mellitus
- Immunosuppressed patients

Subjective and Objective Findings

Signs and Symptoms of Endocarditis	
Generalized	Fever, chills, fatigue, night sweats, headache, myalgia, arthralgia, nausea, vomiting, anorexia, weight loss
HEENT	Petechiae on mucous membranes, Roth spots (retinal hemorrhages)
Resp	Dyspnea, cough, hemoptysis
CV	Tachypnea, edema, chest pain, change in heart sounds (murmur)
GI/GU	Abdominal pain
Skin	Nontender macular or nodular hemorrhagic lesions on the palms or soles (Janeway lesions), or painful lesions on fingers and toes (Osler nodes), splinter hemorrhages on nail beds

Table 7.5.1

The "textbook" findings on physical exam are rare, as endocarditis symptoms vary between patients. Injection drug users often present differently, as they tend to have right-sided infections of the tricuspid valve. Other symptoms include fever and multiple pulmonary infiltrates on x-ray.

Emboli to different regions of the body may occur. These include spleen (may have referred pain from back to shoulder), kidney (flank pain, blood in urine), lungs (dyspnea, chest pain), or central nervous system (changes in neuro status). These are all signs of a medical emergency; patient should be referred to the emergency department.

Diagnosis

- Obtain three blood cultures in 24 hours, at least 1 hour apart
    - *Viridans streptococci* are the most common bacterial agents in native valve infections and in non-injection drug abusers. The cure rate of streptococcal IE is about 90%
    - In injection drug users, *Staphylococci aureus* is the most common cause. *S. aureus* often leads to mitral or aortic valve involvement and has frequent complications. Many sources note about a 40% chance of death when infection is widespread
- Other lab findings may include anemia and an increased erythrocyte sedimentation rate

Echocardiography is a key component in both the diagnosis and management of IE. The overall goal of echocardiography is to determine presence, location, and size of vegetation. A TTE is recommended. However, if a patient has a prosthetic valve, begin with TEE. TTE is inadequate in about 20% of patients due to obesity, COPD, and chest-wall deformities; TEE would be required. Furthermore, TEE should be performed if initial TTE is negative and there remains an ongoing suspicion of IE.

Plan

Treatment

It is difficult for white blood cells to travel to the heart valves due to poor blood supply to the valves themselves. Thus, white blood cells lack an effective means to fight the infection, and long-term antimicrobial therapy is needed. The antibiotic used is based on the organism identified from positive blood cultures. Streptococcal endocarditis may be treated with a 2-week course of penicillin G and gentamicin. If resistant to penicillin, vancomycin is a viable option and therapy increases to 4–6 weeks. Antibiotic regimens vary per region, and often combination therapies are needed due to drug resistance issues.

CHF and hemodynamic compromise are strong indicators that surgery will be needed to repair or replace damaged valves. Other indicators for surgery include persistent vegetation after antimicrobial therapy or embolic neurologic complications.

In right-sided IE, surgery is usually needed due to persistent vegetation. Many of these patients are injection drug users that may continuously reintroduce bacteria into their system; thus, infection is difficult to treat.

TTE should be performed once antimicrobial therapy or surgery has been completed to establish a new baseline.

Education

Patients should be reminded of the signs and symptoms of IE (fever, chills, dyspnea) and advised to seek medical treatment immediately if these occur. Patients should undergo a thorough dental exam and be treated for any oral infections. Stress the importance of ongoing good dental hygiene.

Many non-critically ill patients will go home on antibiotic therapy. They will often have a central line in place, so teaching about antibiotic therapy and central line care will be needed.

Once home, patients should inform their dentist and all other healthcare providers regarding their history of endocarditis. In patients with high cardiac risk such as a history of IE, antibiotic prophylaxis is recommended for **all** dental, oral, or respiratory tract procedures. Unlike in the past, the majority of heart conditions (i.e., mitral valve prolapse, coronary artery disease, atrial septal defects that have been closed more than 6 months) no longer require antibiotic prophylaxis.

High-risk cardiac conditions	Treatment regimens
Prosthetic cardiac valve	Antibiotics should be administered once as a single dose 30–60 minutes prior to procedure
History of IE	
Congenital heart disease (CHD) no longer requires prophylaxis unless your patient has the following conditions: • Unrepaired cyanotic congenital heart disease • Repaired CHD, during the first 6 months after the procedure • Repaired CHD with residual defects	Standard general prophylaxis: amoxicillin: adult dose 2 g PO Allergic to penicillin: clindamycin: adult dose 600 mg PO azithromycin: adult dose 500 mg PO Unable to take oral medication: ampicillin: adult dose 2 g IV/IM clindamycin: adult dose 600 mg IV/IM
Heart transplant recipients with underlying valve disease	

Table 7.5.2 Antibiotic Prophylaxis for IE

The following dental procedures do not require prophylaxis for IE:

- Routine anesthesia injections to non-infected tissue
- Dental x-rays
- Placement of removable orthodontic or prosthodontic devices
- Adjustment of orthodontic devices
- Bleeding from trauma to the lips or oral mucosa

Referral

IE is potentially lethal. Refer to a cardiologist and infectious disease specialist for a detailed treatment plan. Referral to a drug rehab program should be provided for those patients who acquire IE through injection drug use. Perform a dental exam on both inpatient and outpatient patients with IE. If embolic events result, refer to an appropriate specialist, such as a neurologist or nephrologist, for specific needs.

Takeaways

- IE is rare but can prove lethal if not treated. Early signs are fever, chills, night sweats, anorexia; later signs often include embolic-related symptoms.
- Multiple blood cultures within a 24-hour period, 1 hour apart, are needed to diagnose IE, along with a baseline TTE and/or TEE.

LESSON 6: HYPERLIPIDEMIA

Learning Objectives
- Identify patients who are candidates for hyperlipidemia therapy
- Discuss methods used to achieve lower LDL and triglyceride levels
- Examine recommendations for monitoring statin therapy

Hyperlipidemia refers to elevated cholesterol and triglyceride levels due to too many lipids (fat cells) in the blood. Elevated levels may increase your patient's risk of developing atherosclerotic cardiovascular disease (ASCVD). The decision to lower lipids is made on an individual patient basis, and there are guidelines in place to assess risk. These guidelines were set forth by the American College of Cardiology (ACC) and American Heart Association (AHA) and are based on the existence of ASCVD and/or other risk factors that may increase the risk of ASCVD.

Definitions

- **ASCVD:** condition caused by plaque accumulation in the arteries that can lead to events such as myocardial infarction (MI), angina, stroke, transient ischemic attack (TIA), peripheral arterial disease (PAD), and other problems
- **Primary prevention:** refers to methods used to prevent or delay the initial onset of ASCVD
- **Secondary prevention:** refers to methods used to treat known ASCVD and to prevent recurrent events or worsening of disease processes

Assessment

Subjective

Symptoms

Patients with hyperlipidemia are generally asymptomatic. ROS may reveal weight gain or anorexia. The U.S. Preventative Task Force (USPTF) recommends the following screening recommendations:

- Start screening at age 35 in men and age 45 in women if no known risk factors exist
- If ASCVD exists or risk factors for ASCVD exist (DM, FH of ASCVD, FH of hyperlipidemia, tobacco use, etc.), then screening should start at age 20–35 in men and age 20 in women

History

Health history elements that are pertinent to hyperlipidemia include:

- **PMH:** acute coronary syndrome, MI, angina, stoke, TIA, PAD, DM, nephrotic syndrome, chronic renal failure, biliary obstruction, and hypothyroidism
- **FH:** ASCVD or hyperlipidemia in a first-degree relative
- **SH:** diet high in saturated fats or trans fats, high intake of refined carbohydrates (may elevate triglycerides), excessive alcohol intake, weight gain, anorexia
- **Medications:** steroids, amiodarone, cyclosporine, estrogens, glucocorticoids, bile acid sequestrants, protease inhibitors, aromatase inhibitors, beta-blockers (not carvedilol), thiazide diuretics (all may cause elevated LDL or triglyceride levels)

> **DANGER SIGNS** Pregnancy and statins: if the patient is pregnant, LDL and triglyceride levels may rise, yet statins are contraindicated during pregnancy because of potential teratogenic effects. From known data, the risks outweigh the benefits.

Objective

Total cholesterol: high total cholesterol increases patient's risk of ASCVD, but treatment is based on LDL levels.

- Total cholesterol <200 mg/dL is **normal**
- Total cholesterol of 200–239 mg/dL is **borderline high**
- Total cholesterol ≥240 mg/dL is **very high**

LDL cholesterol (*primary target of therapy*): although general goals are listed below, optimal targets for LDL cholesterol level depend on whether the patient has known ASCVD or not. If a patient has no known ASCVD, then intensity of therapy for lowering cholesterol (primarily LDL with statins) depends on the patient's risk of developing ASCVD. The ACC/AHA have developed a risk calculator that utilizes standard cardiac risk factors to determine a patient's 10-year risk for a cardiovascular event (*see App alert for link*).

- LDL <100 mg/dL is **optimal**
- LDL of 100–129 mg/dL is **above optimal**
- LDL 130–159 mg/dL is **borderline high**
- LDL 160–189 mg/dL is **high**
- LDL ≥190 mg/dL is **very high**

Triglycerides: very high triglycerides increase risk for ASCVD, however little evidence shows that treating borderline or high levels improves outcomes.

- Triglyceride <150 mg/dL is normal
- Triglycerides 150–199 mg/dL is borderline high
- Triglycerides 200–499 mg/dL is high
- Triglycerides >500 mg/dL is very high

HDL cholesterol: elevated levels of HDL actually lower risk of ASCVD. There are no treatments for increasing HDL that help to reduce ASCVD.

- HDL ≤40 mg/dL is low
- HDL >60 mg/dL is high

Diagnosis

A standard lipid panel, including a measurement of total cholesterol, LDL, HDL, and triglycerides, is drawn to test for hyperlipidemia.

PLAN

Treatment of LDL

Lifestyle changes are the cornerstone of initial therapy to reduce lipid levels: heart-healthy diet, regular exercise, smoking cessation, and maintenance of a healthy weight. Unfortunately, lifestyle changes alone account for only a 5–10% reduction of LDL levels.

Again, optimal LDL goals depend on risk factors present. The outdated method of treat-to-goal therapy has several flaws; specifically, clinical trials do not indicate what the target should be. Use the maximum tolerated statin intensity to reduce ASCVD.

Recommendations from ACC/AHA focus on four major groups that may benefit from statin therapy.

- Patients with clinical ASCVD
- Patients with primary LDL >190 mg/dL
- Patients 40–79 years of age who have DM with LDL 70–189 mg/dL
- Patients without ASCVD or DM who are 40–75 years of age with LDL 70–189 mg/DL and an estimated 10-year ASCVD risk of 7.5% or higher

Patients who have known ASCVD or are at high risk for CV events (>7.5% in 10 years) should be given high-intensity statin therapy regardless of LDL level.

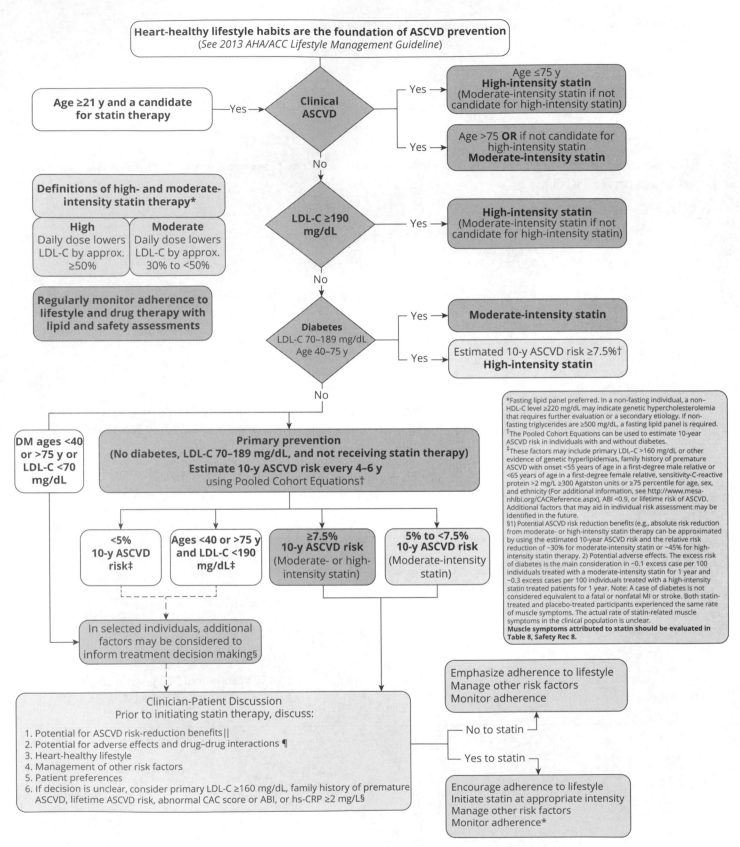

Figure 7.6.1 Recommendations in Statin Therapy for Prevention of ASCVD

Patient risk factors and 10-year risk can be calculated with the Pooled Cohort Risk equation.

> **App Alert**
>
> Both the ACC and AHA provide the Pooled Cohort equation (risk calculator) via apps. You can also go to **http://my.americanheart.org/cvriskcalculator**.

High-intensity statins	Moderate-intensity statins	Low-intensity statins
Daily dose lowers LDL by approximately >50%	Daily dose lowers LDL by approximately 30–50%	Daily dose lowers LDL by <30%
atorvastatin, 40–80 mg rosuvastatin, 20–40 mg	atorvastatin, 10–20 mg rosuvastatin, 5–10 mg simvastatin, 20–40 mg pravastatin, 40–80 mg lovastatin, 40 mg	simvastatin, 10 mg pravastatin, 10–20 mg lovastatin, 20 mg

Table 7.6.1 Statin Intensity Groups of Commonly Used Statins

Stone et al, 2014

Monitoring Statin Therapy

Once an abnormal initial fasting lipid panel is obtained, perform the following:

- Determine patient's ASCVD status and assign appropriate statin therapy
- Check a baseline measurement of hepatic aminotransferase levels (AST and ALT) prior to initiating statin therapy
- Obtain a CMP and lipids 6 weeks after initiation of therapy to monitor for liver toxicity and compliance. Statin therapy should be discontinued if AST and/or ALT levels are three times the upper limits of normal (ULN)
- Schedule a return visit every 3–12 months as clinically indicated. At each visit, monitor for new onset DM and adverse effects
- Patients who have had previous statin intolerance or muscle disorders are more likely to experience side effects. So are those patients with hepatic or renal issues
- Therefore, it is a good idea to inquire about prior or current muscle symptoms before starting statins
- If mild adverse effects are noted, patient should be given a lower dose of an alternative statin until no adverse effects have been identified
- If muscle symptoms are severe, promptly discontinue and address possibility of rhabdomyolysis by evaluating CK, creatinine, and urinalysis

> **DANGER SIGNS** Discontinue statin therapy if liver enzymes (AST and/or ALT) are 3 times the ULN.

Treatment of Hypertriglyceridemia

Although not the primary target of lipid therapy, triglycerides are treated as priority if levels are greater than 500 mg/dL. In these cases, the goal is to reduce risk of acute pancreatitis.

- Fibrates are the drug of choice, as they can significantly lower triglycerides (40–60%) and raise HDL. It is appropriate to mix fibrates with a statin if mixed dyslipidemia is present (again, overall goal is to treat LDL first). Statins alone may reduce triglycerides by 20–40%. Fibrates are contraindicated with gallstones or severe renal or hepatic disease

- Niacin may lower triglycerides levels by 20–30%. Although not as potent, it can raise HDL more effectively. Flushing is a common side effect, and these drugs should be avoided with gout or hyperglycemia

- Fish oil has been shown to lower triglycerides by 20–50%. Side effects are minimal but may include a GI upset or fishy aftertaste

Referral

Patients with diagnosed ASCVD or who present with several risk factors for ASCVD should be evaluated by a cardiologist for their specific condition as needed. Referral is particularly important for patients with diagnosed familial hyperlipidemia or severely elevated lipids as advanced treatment is required.

Takeaways

- Hyperlipidemia is a condition that may increase your risk of ASCVD.

- Primary prevention of hyperlipidemia requires the use of the Pooled Cohort equation to determine a patient's risk of developing ASCVD.

- Secondary prevention of hyperlipidemia is defined by the ACC/AHA guidelines.

- Treatment of elevated triglycerides alone should be reserved for very high levels. Initial treatment should be with fibrates.

LESSON 7: HYPERTENSION

Learning Objectives
- Understand when to diagnose a patient with hypertension
- Identify when to evaluate for secondary hypertension
- Individualize appropriate treatment plans

Hypertension (HTN) is the cause of significant mortality and morbidity. Early diagnosis and treatment are essential to prevent complications and disability. It is important to distinguish between primary and secondary HTN and to treat secondary causes.

Definitions

- **Hypertensive emergency:** Diastolic blood pressure (DBP) >120 with acute end organ damage (headache, nausea/vomiting, chest pain, altered mental status)

- **Hypertensive urgency:** DBP >120 and asymptomatic

- **White coat HTN:** BP elevated >140/90 in the office setting, but <140/90 out of the office

- **Masked HTN:** BP <140/90 in the office, but elevated >140/90 out of the office

- **Nocturnal HTN:** BP >140/90 at night, while patient is sleeping

Assessment

Subjective

Symptoms

Hypertension is called the "silent killer" because there are often no symptoms and a patient may go years without it being discovered. If blood pressure is extremely elevated or has been chronic and undiagnosed, symptoms may be present. Patients have vital signs checked at the beginning of most exams, so oftentimes hypertension is discovered on a visit for an unrelated complaint. With the popularity of home blood pressure monitors, the chief complaint may be elevated home readings.

Symptoms related to secondary hypertension may include vision changes, headache, anxiety, changes in urination (frequency, quantity), nocturia, peripheral edema, abdominal or back pain, chest pain, cough, or SOB.

- **PMH:** frequent elevated blood pressure readings, preeclampsia or elevated blood pressure in pregnancy, congenital heart or kidney malformations, depression, renal dysfunction, use of medications that can cause hypertension (decongestants, oral contraceptives, glucocorticoids, weight loss medications such as phentermine, cyclosporine, tricyclic and SSRI antidepressants, NSAIDs, stimulants like methylphenidate); current medical history to include advanced age, obesity, black ethnicity, hyperlipidemia, elevated sodium intake, a decreased number of nephrons, diabetes
- **PSH:** heart, lung, or renal surgery
- **FH:** HTN, MI, CVA, heart failure
- **SH:** inactivity, smoking, alcohol intake, illicit drug use (methamphetamine, cocaine), hostile or impatient personality trait

Objective

The exam should focus on checking for end organ damage, complications, (left ventricular hypertrophy, heart failure, myocardial infarction, cerebral vascular hemorrhage, chronic kidney disease, end stage renal disease) and possible secondary causes of HTN.

- **VS:** BP >140/90, elevated or decreased HR
- **HEENT:** eyes—decreased distant visual acuity, retinal hemorrhages, cotton wool spots, tortuous vessels
- **Neck:** JVD, carotid bruits
- **CV:** murmurs, cardiac rubs, peripheral pulses, peripheral edema (pitting or nonpitting), PMI shift to left
- **Resp:** crackles
- **GI:** abdominal pain on palpation, abdominal bruit
- **GU:** CVA tenderness, proteinuria, microalbuminuria
- **Skin:** smooth, shiny skin to lower extremities, decreased hair growth to lower extremities

> **Pro Tip**
> Ensure blood pressures are being taken with the appropriate size cuff. A cuff that is too small can result in a falsely elevated blood pressure, and the opposite with a cuff that is too large. Automatic blood pressure machines may not always give an accurate reading, and a manual blood pressure should be taken to confirm abnormal readings.

Diagnosis

There are two main schools of thought on screening frequency and diagnosis:

- Eighth Report of the National Committee on Prevention, Detection, Evaluation and Treatment of High Blood Pressure (JNC-8)
  - **http://jamanetwork.com/journals/jama/fullarticle/1791497**
- United States Preventative Services Task Force (USPSTF)
  - **www.uspreventiveservicestaskforce.org/Page/Document/RecommendationStatementFinal/high-blood-pressure-in-adults-screening**

JNC-8	USPSTF
Screen: Every 2 years in adults with normal blood pressure, yearly if prehypertension **Diagnosis:** Confirm elevated office blood pressure with repeat measurements taken on 2 different days. At least 2 separate measurements should be taken at each visit. May also confirm with ambulatory blood pressure monitoring (ABPM) or home blood pressure readings on a validated device. **Definitions:** Prehypertension: 120–139 systolic or 80–90 diastolic Stage I HTN: 140–159 systolic or 90–99 diastolic Stage II HTN: ≥160 systolic or 100 diastolic	**Screen:** Initially in all patients 18 and up **Re-screen:** Every 3–5 years age 18–39 with normal blood pressure and no risk factors; yearly in those >40 years old, those with high normal blood pressure, overweight, obese, and/or African Americans **Diagnosis:** If elevated blood pressure is found, it should be confirmed with 24-hour ABPM before diagnosis and treatment

Table 7.7.1 JNC-8 and USPSTF Screening and Diagnosis Recommendations

Make the diagnosis of HTN if the blood pressure is greater than 140/90 using the above criteria. If the blood pressure is greater than 180/110 on one occasion, HTN can be diagnosed without subsequent readings. Ambulatory blood pressure monitoring is an effective tool to use if there is concern regarding nocturnal HTN, white coat HTN, or masked HTN. Order the following labs: CBC, TSH, fasting lipids and glucose, urinalysis, electrolytes, and creatinine. An ECG should be performed. Consider an ECHO to check for left ventricular hypertrophy and urine microalbumin to check for renal compromise.

Differential Diagnosis

If the presentation of hypertension is unusual, check for these secondary causes: **primary renal disease, renovascular HTN, primary aldosteronism, Cushing disease, endocrine disorders (hyper/hypothyroidism, hyperparathyroidism), obstructive sleep apnea, pheochromocytoma**.

Plan

Treatment

All patients should be encouraged to make lifestyle changes regarding modifiable risk factors. Recommend a low sodium diet (less than 2400 mg of sodium daily), the DASH diet, increased activity and exercise (moderate to vigorous activity 3–4 days/week for 40 minutes at a time), and weight reduction.

Medications should be individualized. The goal of treatment is to decrease blood pressure to less than 140/90 if diabetic, chronic kidney disease, or less than 60 years old. If greater than 60 years old, the goal is less than 150/90. Caution should be taken in patients greater than 65 years old. Decreasing diastolic blood pressure to less than 55–60 in this age group increases the risk of CVA and MI.

Medication class	Indications	Medication considerations
Diuretics • hydrochlorothiazide, chlorthalidone (Thiazide) • potassium-sparing spironolactone, triamterene • loop-furosemide (Lasix)	• Heart failure, coronary artery disease, stroke, diabetes • Thiazide is usually considered to be a better choice than ACEI or BB as first-line monotherapy for African Americans	• Take med in the morning to prevent nocturia • Check potassium prior to starting and throughout therapy (hypokalemia should be treated and may need maintenance dose of potassium) • Potassium-sparing diuretics can increase potassium and can cause gynecomastia • Thiazides can increase uric acid level; caution with gout • Look for GFR <40
Calcium channel blockers • Dihydropyridines (DH): amlodipine (Norvasc) • Non-dihydropyridines (NDH): diltiazem ER, verapamil	African Americans, diabetes, coronary artery disease	• Can cause edema • DH have little to no negative effect on cardiac conduction and contraction • NDH have greater effect on cardiac conduction and contraction, less potent than DH
Angiotensin converting enzyme lisinopril, benazepril, ramipril	Diabetes, chronic kidney disease with proteinuria, heart failure, coronary artery disease, clinical coronary artery disease, stroke prevention	• Dry, hacking cough is a potential side effect; med should be changed to different class if this occurs • Angioedema can occur • Monitor potassium, risk of hyperkalemia
Angiotensin receptor blockers losartan, valsartan, olmesartan	Diabetes, chronic kidney disease with proteinuria, heart failure, post MI, clinical coronary heart disease	• Contraindicated in pregnancy • Obtain BUN/creatinine at baseline and monitor • Monitor potassium, risk of hyperkalemia
Beta-blockers carvedilol, labetalol **Selective beta 1 agonists** acebutolol, metoprolol succinate and tartrate, bisoprolol, betaxolol	Ischemic heart disease, heart failure with decreased ejection fraction	• Not recommended as first-line monotherapy unless indications present • With pregnancy, labetalol is first-line • Can alter glucose levels, mask symptoms of hypoglycemia, cause fatigue and decreased heart rate • Selective beta 1 safer with asthma, diabetics, COPD, and peripheral vascular disease
Central acting agents clonidine, methyldopa, guanfacine	Resistant hypertension (clonidine patch)	• clonidine can cause drowsiness

Table 7.7.2 Medications in HTN

Start patients on monotherapy, taking into account indications for certain classes. If blood pressure is greater than 160/100, dual therapy from 2 different classes will often be needed. Start on a low dose of the medication and titrate dose to blood pressure goal. If the goal is not reached on a maximum dose, add a medication from a different class. Follow up should be every 2–4 weeks until blood pressure is well-controlled and then follow up every 3–6 months.

Digital Resource

For an algorithm of the JNC-8 treatment guidelines: **www.nmhs.net/documents/27JNC8H TNGuidelinesBookBooklet.pdf**.

Education

Educate patients about modifiable risk factors. Specific information should be given about the DASH diet and weight reduction. Discuss smoking cessation and assist patients with this goal. Encourage decreased consumption of alcohol to a moderate intake. If the patient has comorbid conditions such as hyperlipidemia and diabetes, educate the patient about the importance of keeping these conditions under control. Medication education should include the importance of not skipping doses or running out of prescriptions and keeping regular follow-up appointments. Patients should avoid OTC cough and cold medications that contain decongestants and should exercise caution when taking OTC NSAIDs.

Referral

Refer to treatment patients who are refractory and those with hypertensive emergency and hypertensive urgency. If secondary hypertension is diagnosed, refer to the appropriate specialist based on the secondary diagnosis.

Takeaways

- Treating HTN can be challenging. If a patient is noncompliant with the medication regimen, discuss side effects (fatigue, impotence, etc.) and cost of medications. These are often the cause of noncompliance, and patients can be fearful to start a discussion about them.

- Do not treat with an ACE inhibitor and an ARB. These different classes should not be combined.

- When an antihypertensive medication is started, caution the patient to make position changes slowly to lessen the impact of orthostatic hypotension.

- Hypertension is never diagnosed based on measurements taken on one occasion, unless greater than 180/110.

- When choosing an antihypertensive medication, consider comorbidities and how medications can help or harm those comorbidities.

LESSON 8: MURMURS/VALVULAR DISORDERS

Learning Objectives
- Know landmarks for auscultating heart valves and recognize common murmurs and heart sounds
- Explore the signs and symptoms of valvular disorders
- Discuss treatments available for patients with heart valve disorders

Our heart valves are made up of complicated leaflets that ensure our blood flows in the right direction through the four heart chambers. Heart murmurs result from turbulent blood flow through the valves into our cardiac chambers and blood vessels. Congenital heart defects, age-related changes, infections, and other conditions (such as a myocardial infarction) that result in valve trauma may cause valves to not fully open or leak blood back into the heart chambers. It is essential to differentiate between benign and pathologic findings.

Definitions

- **S1:** first heart sound ("lub"); the sound of the mitral and tricuspid valves closing. If a systolic murmur is present, it will occur between S1 and S2 or immediately after the "lub" sound

- **S2:** second heart sound ("dub"); closure of aortic and pulmonic valves. If the pulmonic sound is louder than aortic sound at apex, suspect pulmonary hypertension. If S2 sound is split (two "dubs" noted), suspect pulmonary stenosis. S2 marks the end of systole; thus, diastolic murmurs occur between S2 and S1

- **S3:** third heart sound (often called a "ventricular gallop"). This is a low frequency vibration in early diastole that is often difficult to hear. Considered normal heart sound up to age 35–40. May indicate ventricular dysfunction (such as fluid overload) in older adults

- **S4:** fourth heart sound, heard in late diastole (thus it is actually heard shortly before the first heart sound, or S1). Also dull with a low frequency, it is heard best with the bell. May be present in individuals with coronary artery disease or chronic hypertension

- **Stenosis:** occurs when leaflets thicken, become stiff, or fuse together. This prevents the valve from fully opening

- **Regurgitation:** occurs when there is backflow and the valve does not close completely. Blood flows back into previous chamber of heart and does not move forward

---

Pro Tip

Where do I best auscultate valve sounds?

Try a mnemonic! (i.e., **A**ll **P**eople **E**njoy **T**ime **M**agazine)

- **Aortic valve:** right sternal border, 2nd intercostal space
- **Pulmonic valve:** left sternal border, 2nd intercostal space
- **Erb's point:** left 3rd intercoastal space, S2 sound heard best
- **Tricuspid valve:** left sternal border, 5th intercostal space
- **Mitral valve:** left midclavicular line, 5th intercostal space

---

Assessment

Subjective

Symptoms

The patient may complain of the following:

- Palpitations
- Dyspnea
- Angina
- Dizziness and/or syncope
- Heart failure symptoms

It is best to assess your patient in sitting, standing, and recumbent positions in a quiet location. Most sources recommend auscultating with both the bell and diaphragm of stethoscope. When listening to murmurs, note the frequency, intensity, quality, and duration. When grading murmurs, follow Levine's classification.

Grade	Quality and intensity of murmur
1	Very faint, only heard with special effort
2	Faint, but immediately audible when stethoscope placed on chest
3	Moderately loud but no palpable thrill
4	Very loud with palpable thrill
5	Extremely loud with palpable thrill and audible with one edge of the stethoscope touching the chest wall
6	So loud that it is audible with the stethoscope just removed from contact with the chest wall, palpable thrill

Table 7.8.1 Levine's Classification of Grading Systolic Murmurs

Walker et al, 1990

Objective

Murmur or heart sound	Objective findings	Additional findings	Causes
Aortic stenosis	Mid-systolic ejection murmur; ejection click may precede murmur (this is a high-pitched sound that occurs immediately after S1)	Syncope is common, associated aortic regurgitation may occur	Often damaged from congenital bicuspid valve. Later in life may be result from rheumatic fever or calcification of the valve
Aortic regurgitation (also known as aortic insufficiency)	A decrescendo, blowing diastolic murmur beginning immediately after S2 that extends into systole; may be difficult to hear	Best heard in sitting position or leaning forward	Commonly seen with bicuspid aortic valve (aortic valve should have 3 leaflets) or inflammatory conditions such as Marfan syndrome and ankylosing spondylitis. History of rheumatic fever or conditions leading to leaflet damage are risk factors
Mitral stenosis	Loud S1, then low-pitched rumbling diastolic murmur	Dyspnea and tachypnea are general signs	Primary cause is rheumatic fever, rare cases of congenital abnormalities
Mitral regurgitation	Grade 1–4/6 high-pitched pansystolic murmur that radiates to axilla	Tachypnea and atrial fibrillation are common, with significant MR	Often found with a history of rheumatic fever, coronary artery disease, mitral valve prolapse, or rupture of chordae tendineae. Slower onset is seen with calcification and endocarditis. Many people have no symptoms if MR is mild to moderate

Table 7.8.2 Common Heart Sounds and Associated Valve Disorder

Murphy & Lloyd, 2007

Murmur or heart sound	Objective findings	Additional findings	Causes
Mitral valve prolapse (most common cause of severe mitral regurgitation)	Mid-systolic click or systolic murmur (high-pitched, late peaking)	Occurs when mitral valve leaflet is deformed or "buckled"	Often associated with Marfan syndrome or thoracic skeletal abnormalities such as pectus excavatum. Most common heart valve problem
Atrial gallop	S4 sound occurs before S1	Not heard in healthy young individuals or in atrial fibrillation	May indicate acute myocardial infarction or systemic hypertension. Often present in patients with hypertrophic cardiomyopathy
Ventricular gallop	S3 sound occurs after S2	S3 sound is augmented during exercise and valsalva maneuvers	Normal finding in young adults or children. In older adults, suspect severe regurgitation or heart failure
Friction rub	Harsh, grating sound	Layers of tissue between pericardium and myocardium become inflamed	Pericarditis
Physiologic murmur (called Still murmur in childhood; has a "vibratory" or "musical" quality; may also be referred to as "innocent" or "functional" murmur)	Systolic murmurs; usually soft (<grade 2), short, and no clicks	Common at all ages (often confused with murmur of mitral regurgitation)	Related to increased blood flow or minor turbulence across aortic valve; no restrictions needed

Table 7.8.2 Common Heart Sounds and Associated Valve Disorder (Continued)

Murphy & Lloyd, 2007

> **DANGER SIGNS** Diastolic murmurs are considered pathologic. If detected, echocardiogram should be ordered immediately.
>
> Systolic murmurs may be pathologic if following signs are observed: the murmur is loud (>grade 3), long duration, opening snap or ejection click, and/or associated with loud S1 sound.

Diagnosis

To assess the morphology and severity of regurgitation or stenosis present, perform an echocardiogram. In addition, a chest x-ray or cardiac CT may be needed to check for cardiomyopathy, pulmonary edema, and/or overall heart appearance. An ECG will also be performed to check rate and rhythm. If signs and symptoms do not match with echo results, a cardiac catheterization may be needed to see if valve disease or other comorbidities exist.

Plan

Treatment

Patients who are hemodynamically unstable should seek rapid evaluation. IV fluids and vasodilators may be needed. However, most murmurs develop gradually and will require periodic monitoring to determine when treatment is needed. Medications to lower blood pressure and to prevent arrhythmia are often used in early prevention.

In severe mitral regurgitation, for example, surgery via repair or replacement may be needed if the patient is symptomatic. If your patient does receive a mechanical valve (made from metal), they will require lifelong treatment with blood thinners such as warfarin to prevent blood clots. Bioprosthetic valves (made from biologic materials such as a cow valve) generally do not require warfarin but often do not last as long. Those with mild mitral regurgitation should have an echocardiogram about every 3–5 years. While those with severe mitral regurgitation are seen every 6–12 months or sooner if symptomatic.

In aortic stenosis, patients may have very few symptoms at first, but once the valve becomes severely stenotic they may decline rapidly. Once diagnosed, aortic stenosis is not easily reversed with medications. If aortic stenosis becomes moderate to severe, surgery is often needed. Again, blood thinners and more frequent evaluations are needed once surgery and/or severe stenosis results.

App Alert

The American College of Cardiology provides an app titled, "ACC Guideline Clinical App," which includes clinical guidelines for the treatment of valvular heart disease.

In addition, the American College of Cardiology and American Heart Association updates treatment guidelines regularly with most recent valvular treatment guidelines, found here: **www.onlinejacc.org/content/70/2/252**.

Education

It is vital for patients to report signs and symptoms of worsening valvular disease. These include heart failure symptoms, dyspnea, syncope, and angina. There are no physical exercise restrictions for those that are asymptomatic with mild to moderate mitral regurgitation or aortic stenosis and have normal heart rhythms. Encourage patients to stay hydrated, engage in regular exercise, and maintain good dental hygiene. A patient may be on a low-sodium diet if they have heart failure symptoms. If surgery is performed to replace a valve, the patient is at future risk for infective endocarditis and will require antibiotic prophylaxis prior to dental, oral, or respiratory tract procedures (*see Chapter 7, Lesson 5*).

Referral

Patients will typically be followed by a cardiologist if they have a valvular disorder. If a congenital disorder exists, a pediatric cardiologist or adult structural heart specialist will collaborate in the care. In addition, regular dental follow-ups are required to prevent endocarditis.

Takeaways

- The nurse practitioner must differentiate normal S1 and S2 sounds with turbulent blood flow that results in systolic murmurs or diastolic murmurs (pathologic).
- When auscultating murmurs, note grade, intensity, and quality.
- Mitral valve prolapse is the most common valvular disorder. Valve replacement is common when a patient has severe regurgitation and is symptomatic.
- If patients receive a prosthetic or mechanical valve, they will require antibiotic prophylaxis for life to prevent infective endocarditis (*see Chapter 7, Lesson 5*).

LESSON 9: PERIPHERAL VASCULAR DISEASE

Learning Objectives

- Understand causes and types of peripheral vascular disease
- Recognize the diagnostic process and proper treatment of peripheral vascular disease
- Increase familiarity with obtaining ankle-brachial index
- Comprehend assessment, diagnosis, and treatment for deep venous thrombosis (DVT)

Peripheral vascular disease (PVD) describes diseased vasculature that occurs outside of the brain or heart. Oftentimes the term PVD and peripheral artery disease (PAD) are used interchangeably, but PVD encompasses arterial and venous disease, while PAD refers only to arterial disease. For the purpose of this lesson, PVD will be used. PVD will be discussed separately in terms of arterial disease and venous disease.

The most common cause of arterial disease is atherosclerosis. Venous disease, or chronic venous insufficiency (CVI), is caused by changes in the function of the venous system of the legs that occur from chronic elevations in venous pressure. Deep venous thrombosis (DVT) refers to thrombi in the deep veins of the pelvis or legs.

Definitions

- **Intermittent claudication ("to limp"):** pain in the buttock, thigh, or calf (unilateral or bilateral) with exercise or walking; pain relieved with rest
- **Rubor:** redness
- **Pallor:** paleness
- **Varicose veins:** large, engorged, dilated, and often twisted veins
- **Reticular veins:** medium sized, engorged veins; deeper under the skin; often appear blue or green on the thighs and behind the knees; often feeder vessels for telangiectasias
- **Telangiectasias:** dilation and/or engorgement of capillaries, "spider veins"

Assessment

Subjective

Symptoms

Many times PVD is asymptomatic and, as a result, is often under-diagnosed. The following table differentiates arterial from venous disease.

	Arterial	Venous
Defined	Decreased arterial blood flow to the lower extremities	Pooling of venous blood and diminished venous return
Symptoms	Intermittent claudication, atypical leg pain; altered sensation to lower extremities/feet; dependent rubor; pallor with elevation; thin, shiny skin to lower extremities; decreased hair growth to lower extremities; thick, brittle nails; coolness of lower extremity; ulcerations or poor healing wounds	Aching; heaviness in legs; fatigue; bilateral edema of feet and legs; if unilateral edema, suspect iliac vein obstruction by possible mass; altered sensation to lower extremities/feet (burning, tingling, or itching); presence of varicose veins, reticular veins, and/or telangiectasias; dry, flaking skin; brown pigmentation; poor healing wounds or ulcerations
Symptoms improve with:	Dependency	Elevation of legs and walking
Symptoms worsen with:	Elevation	Dependency and prolonged standing
Pain occurs with:	Activity and can occur at rest with advanced disease	At rest
Pain improves with:	Rest	Walking
Risk factors	Hypertension, diabetes, hyperlipidemia, smoking, leg trauma	Obesity, pregnancy, history of venous thrombosis, high estrogen states, prolonged standing, sedentary lifestyle, leg trauma (all are risk factors for DVT as well)

Table 7.9.1 Arterial vs. Venous Disease

Location of claudication can indicate location of arterial disease; symptoms occur distal to the diseased artery.

- **Buttock or hip claudication:** aortoiliac disease; can have decreased femoral pulses (unilateral or bilateral); additional symptoms with aortoiliac disease include hip or thigh weakness with exercise and erectile dysfunction
- **Thigh claudication:** common femoral artery disease, normal femoral pulses
- **Calf claudication:** pain in upper two-thirds from superficial femoral artery disease, pain in lower two-thirds from popliteal artery disease
- **Foot claudication:** tibial or peroneal artery (rare)
- **DVT:** unilateral leg pain, edema, warmth, and/or redness; if dyspnea or pleuritic chest pain is present, have a high index of suspicion for PE (*refer to Chapter 6, Lesson 6*)

**Arteries That Can Be Affected by
Peripheral Artery Disease (PAD)**

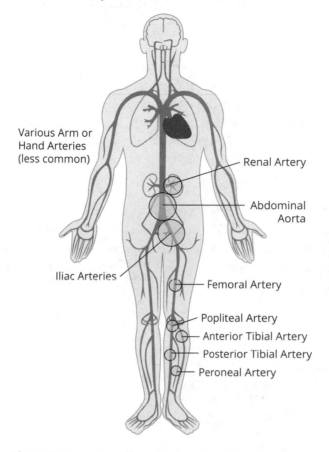

Various Arm or
Hand Arteries
(less common)

Renal Artery

Abdominal
Aorta

Iliac Arteries

Femoral Artery

Popliteal Artery

Anterior Tibial Artery

Posterior Tibial Artery

Peroneal Artery

Figure 7.9.1 Arteries Affected by Peripheral Vascular Disease

Review of Systems

For complaints of leg pain, it is important to ask the following (*see Table 7.9.1*):

1. Does pain occur at rest or with activity?

2. Does rest or activity improve or worsen pain?

3. If pain occurs with activity, how long into the activity or how far walking before pain occurs?

4. Does elevation improve or worsen symptoms?

5. Does dependency improve or worsen symptoms?

Advanced age is a risk factor for arterial and venous disease. After age 40, prevalence of arterial disease increases especially with diabetes, smoking, HTN, and hyperlipidemia.

- **PMH:** HTN, diabetes, hyperlipidemia, previous MI or CVA, poorly healing lower extremity wounds (arterial or venous), erectile dysfunction (arterial), recent trauma (DVT), current or recent use of oral contraceptives or hormone replacement therapy (DVT), current malignancy (DVT), thromboembolic disease (DVT), coagulation disorders (DVT), immobility greater than 3 days (DVT); inquire about risk factors (*see Table 7.9.1*)

- **PSH:** cardiac stent placement, open heart surgery, previous vascular surgery, recent surgery (DVT)

- **FH:** venous or arterial disease, hyperlipidemia (arterial)

- **SH:** smoking, recent prolonged travel greater than 8 hours (DVT)

Objective

- **VS:** elevated blood pressure (HTN is risk factor) or heart rate; check blood pressure in both arms
- **Neck:** presence of carotid bruits possibly indicating atherosclerosis/stenosis of carotid arteries, indicating wide-spread arterial disease
- **CV:** irregular elevated heart rate could indicate arrhythmia (A-fib increases risk of thromboembolism that could travel to lower limbs and cause ischemia); bilateral femoral, dorsalis pedis, and posterior tibial pulses (decreased in arterial disease and decreased distal to diseased artery); capillary refill (decreased-arterial); edema-bilateral (venous), unilateral (DVT); ankle-brachial index (arterial); bruits over involved artery possible; foot pallor with elevation (arterial); dusky toes or dependent rubor (arterial); bilateral calf circumference—measures below tibial tuberosity (DVT)
- **GI:** renal artery bruit (possible widespread arterial disease)
- **Neuro:** motor and sensory testing of lower extremities (decreased in arterial disease)
- **Skin:** condition of skin on lower extremities is tight, shiny skin (arterial); decreased hair (arterial); thickened nails (arterial); brown pigmentation (venous); thickened subcutaneous layer (venous); ulcerations or wounds (either); temperature of skin (cool—arterial, warm—DVT); presence of varicose veins, reticular veins, and/or telangiectasias (venous)

Diagnosis

Arterial disease: diagnosis of arterial disease is based on symptoms, risk factors, and physical exam. The ankle-brachial index (ABI) can confirm diagnosis:

- ABI ≤ 0.90 = peripheral artery disease
- ABI ≥ 0.90 + high suspicion of disease = perform post treadmill exercise ABI

Additional testing may include CBC/diff, metabolic panel, lipid panel, C-reactive protein, homocysteine, and lipoprotein A. Vascular testing can include pulse volume recordings, segmental pressures, and imaging with doppler. These tests can show the location and extent of arterial disease. Angiography may also be considered. Various grading systems are used to rank the severity of the arterial disease. The Fontaine scale is commonly used to grade the severity of arterial disease.

Stage	Symptoms
I	No symptoms
IIa	Mild claudication
IIb	Moderate to severe claudication
III	Ischemia at rest
IV	Gangrene or ulceration

Table 7.9.2 Fontaine Scale

Fontaine, R., Kim, M., & Kieny, R. (1954). Surgical treatment of peripheral circulation disorders [in German]. *Helvetica Chirurgica Acta, 21*(5–6), 499–533.

Venous disease: diagnosis is based on symptoms, physical exam, and duplex ultrasound. The ultrasound is useful to determine the nature and extent of venous reflux, which dictates treatment. A CT or MRI can be done for complex or advanced disease or for possible congenital etiology.

> **Pro Tip**
> The CEAP classification system is an acronym to classify the severity of venous disease. (C: clinical signs, E: etiology of venous disease, A: anatomy or location of venous disease, P: pathophysiology, whether obstruction or reflux).

DVT: diagnosis is based on symptoms, physical exam, Wells prediction score, D-dimer, and compression ultrasonography. The Wells prediction score divides the likelihood of having a DVT into 1 of 3 categories of probability: low, moderate, or high. If there is a history of previous DVT, add 1 additional point to the score. (0 or less = low probability, 1–2 = moderate probability, 3–8 = high probability). The Wells score may be less useful in primary care or the inpatient setting.

Characteristics	Points
Leg swollen in entirety	1
Presence of nonvaricose collateral superficial veins	1
Pitting edema greater in affected leg	1
Recent casting of leg or partial/complete paralysis	1
Tenderness localized to distribution of deep venous system	1
Active cancer or cancer within past 6 months or palliative care	1
Immobile for >3 days or major surgery within 4 weeks	1
Calf edema >3 cm when compared to unaffected leg	1
Differential diagnosis as likely or more likely than DVT	−2

Table 7.9.3 Wells Score to Predict Likelihood of DVT

Up-To-Date 2017

The D-dimer blood test has high sensitivity and low specificity for DVT and should be interpreted with extreme caution. It should never be used as the sole test for a DVT. It should be used with the Wells score and ultrasound/venous doppler. The D-dimer can be elevated in recent surgery, malignancy, pregnancy, sepsis, trauma, and renal failure, and should not be done in these patients. A patient that falls into this category in whom a DVT is suspected should be sent for ultrasound/venous doppler.

- Low Wells probability score and a negative moderate- or high-sensitivity D-dimer = no further testing
- Low Wells probability score and positive moderate- or high-sensitivity D-dimer = ultrasound
- Moderate Wells probability score and negative high-sensitivity D-dimer = no further testing
- Moderate Wells probability score and positive high-sensitivity D-dimer = ultrasound
- High Wells probability score = immediate ultrasound

Plan

Treatment

	Arterial disease	Venous disease	DVT
Modification of risk factors	• Weight reduction; control of hypertension, diabetes, and hyperlipidemia; smoking cessation • Moderate dose statins (regardless of LDL) and aspirin recommended for all patients	• Weight reduction, elevation of extremities, daily walking, ankle flexion exercises, and smoking cessation • Daily moisturization of lower extremities	Early ambulation
Symptomatic treatment	• Antiplatelet therapy: aspirin or clopidogrel (Plavix); ticagrelor (Brilinta) and vorapaxar (Zontivity) are used less frequently; cilostazol (Pletal) used for symptom relief, but contraindicated with heart failure • Supervised walking program: walking 30–45 minutes, 3 days a week for 12 weeks • Chronic or acute limb ischemia: start immediately on antiplatelet therapy and refer to a vascular specialist	• Knee-high graded compression stockings • ($\geq$20–30 mmHg at the ankle; 35–40 mmHg for more severe disease); must be followed for 3 months before determining effectiveness • Horse chestnut seed extract (300 mg/BID) has shown promise to decrease leg edema and volume • Ulceration with infection—culture and sensitivity and appropriate antibiotics • Ulceration without infection—compression dressing	• Proximal DVT (occurring in popliteal, femoral, or iliac veins) should be anticoagulated unless contraindicated (if contraindicated, then an inferior vena cava [IVC] filter may be placed) • Depending on the type of clot, thrombolysis or thrombectomy may be performed • Mixed reviews on whether a distal DVT should be anticoagulated • Start with low molecular weight heparin (Lovenox) subcutaneously every 12 hours for 4–7 days; warfarin (Coumadin) is typically started within 72 hours of enoxaparin to reach a therapeutic INR of 2–3; enoxaparin is anticoagulant of choice in pregnant women because warfarin crosses placenta • Other possible agents: rivaroxaban (Xarelto), apixaban (Eliquis), edoxaban (Savaysa), and dabigatran (Pradaxa)
Complications	• Acute limb ischemia—sudden decrease in limb perfusion, characterized by the 5 Ps: pain, pallor, paralysis, paresthesia, and pulselessness • Acute limb ischemia can be caused by thrombosis of an artery or previous bypass graft, arterial trauma, or a popliteal cyst and/or entrapment	Challenging wounds	PE, thrombotic stroke

Table 7.9.4 Treatment of Arterial, Venous Disease, and DVT

Education

In addition to the risk modification and treatment options above, patients need additional education. For the patient with arterial disease or DVT, advise about increased bleeding risk with antiplatelet therapy and the need to notify for increased bruising, bleeding, blood in stool, or dark, tarry stool. Encourage use of helmets and protective gear for activities in which injury is possible. Discourage from high-risk activities until after anticoagulation therapy is discontinued. Patients will typically be on anticoagulants from 3–12 months.

For patients with venous disease, teach to put on stockings first thing in the morning before getting out of bed and take them off at night while lying down.

Referral

Refer the patient with arterial disease with signs of acute or chronic limb ischemia or no improvement in pain despite intervention to a vascular specialist. Refer the patient with venous disease who has failed three months of conservative treatment to a vascular specialist. In addition, refer those with complicated wounds that are not responsive to treatment to either a plastic surgeon or wound care clinic.

Refer all patients with DVTs to a vascular specialist or treat in conjunction with a specialist. Refer pregnant patients to their obstetrician along with a vascular specialist for treatment.

Takeaways

- PVD is more common in males; CVI is more common in females.
- Identify whether a condition is arterial or venous based on history; the diagnosis and treatment becomes more obvious.
- Avoid using D-dimer as a standalone test to determine DVT.

PRACTICE QUESTIONS

Select the ONE best answer.

Lesson 1: Acute MI

1. Which of the following lab tests will be the most useful to determine if a patient is having an MI?

   A. Troponin

   B. Myoglobin

   C. CK-MB

   D. ESR

2. A patient who suffered a recent MI presents two weeks after undergoing revascularization via PTCA. He was prescribed metoprolol 25 mg PO BID but has developed dry mouth and erectile dysfunction. Which medication should be substituted due to beta-blocker intolerance?

   A. Calcium channel blocker

   B. ARB

   C. Anti-arrhythmic

   D. ACE inhibitor

3. An 85-year-old patient with a history of hypertension and hyperlipidemia presents to the office with his wife for a routine annual physical. She is concerned about her husband's risk for developing an MI and asks about warning signs. What do the patient and his spouse need to know?

   A. Patients over the age of 80 may present with atypical symptoms such as confusion and disorientation

   B. Extreme fatigue and epigastric discomfort are usually the initial symptoms of MI in men

   C. Assure the patient and his wife that he will not have an MI if he continues his daily aspirin

   D. Cough and gum pain are the classic symptoms of MI in older men

4. Therapeutic lifestyle changes are recommended for a patient who recently experienced an MI. What should be included as part of the plan?

   A. Decreasing sodium in the diet

   B. Cutting down to smoking half a pack of cigarettes a day

   C. Walking for 15 minutes once a week

   D. Lowering the amount of fiber consumed

5. On a routine visit, a 62-year-old female with type 1 DM presents to the office reporting chest pain unrelieved by rest, diaphoresis, and tachycardia. The ECG reveals changes in leads II, III, and aVF. What should the nurse practitioner do next?

   A. Call 911 immediately

   B. Repeat the ECG once the heart rate comes down

   C. Order an exercise stress test

   D. Order an anticoagulant

6. All of the following are non-atherosclerotic etiologies of MI except:

   A. Sarcoidosis

   B. Cocaine use

   C. Chest trauma

   D. Aortic stenosis

Lesson 2: Arrythmias

7. A.J. is a 22-year-old college student who complains of feeling his heart race. He states it is intermittent and has happened 3–4 times weekly for the last month. Each episode lasts 5–10 minutes. His vital signs are HR 92 and regular, BP 124/82, RR 16, SpO_2 99%, pain 0/10. Pertinent history would include all of the following except:

   A. Caffeine usage

   B. Prescription medications

   C. Sodium intake

   D. Illicit drug use

8. Appropriate next steps for a patient newly diagnosed with sinus bradycardia who is stable and without symptoms would include:

   A. Cardiology referral

   B. Preparing for immediate transport

   C. Giving atropine IV

   D. Tilt table test

9. On a 12-lead ECG, which leads normally exhibit upright QRS?

   A. I, II, AVR, AVF, V1, V2

   B. AVR, AVL, AVF, V1, V2, V5

   C. II, III, AVL, V1, V5, V6

   D. I, II, III, AVF, V5, V6

10. You are interpreting ECG findings in a 44-year-old male who complains of palpitations, cough, and peripheral edema. You notice that the QRS in lead I is upright, and in AVF it faces down. How would you describe the axis of this ECG?

    A. Extreme right axis deviation

    B. Left axis deviation

    C. Normal axis

    D. Right axis deviation

11. Tyler is a 68-year-old male who complains of fatigue and shortness of breath. He states his heart "feels funny." His exam shows HR 140 and irregular, BP 105/62, RR 18, SpO_2 98%, BMI 31. Medications include lisinopril 20 mg daily and tamsulosin 0.4 mg daily. A 12-lead ECG is obtained and the rhythm is atrial fibrillation. What would be your next course of action?

    A. Refer patient for a same-day ECHO

    B. Place transcutaneous pacing pads on patient

    C. Prepare the patient for immediate transport

    D. Refer to cardiology

Lesson 3: Chest Pain

12. The NP is performing a cardiovascular assessment on a 45-year-old female patient who complains of chest pain that worsens with deep breathing. While locating the PMI, the NP identifies pain with palpation of the 5th intercostal space. What should the NP do next?

    A. Order an NSAID to treat musculoskeletal pain

    B. Send the patient to the ER immediately

    C. Order an ECG

    D. Refer the patient to a cardiologist

13. An 80-year-old male comes into the office one week after discharge from the hospital after undergoing an ORIF for a hip fracture. He presents with tachypnea, anxiety, and sudden sharp, stabbing pain worsening with deep breaths. Which disorder is suspected?

    A. Pulmonary embolism

    B. Aortic stenosis

    C. Pneumonia

    D. Angina

14. The NP is performing a physical exam on a patient who reports sharp chest pain after being involved in a car accident. Which finding indicates a life-threatening condition?

    A. Tracheal deviation

    B. Shoulder pain

    C. Chest bruising

    D. Headache

15. Which of the following is most consistent with a patient who may be experiencing an MI?

    A. Chest pressure unrelieved by 3 doses of sublingual nitroglycerin

    B. Burning chest pain relieved by position change

    C. Chest tightness relieved by rest

    D. Aching chest pain relieved by ibuprofen

16. A 68-year-old male with a history of HTN and CAD presents to the office with progressive SOB and chest tightness. The NP notices a heart rate of 102 and a blood pressure of 95/78. Which diagnostic test will help the NP differentiate between a diagnosis of pneumonia vs. CHF?

    A. BNP

    B. CBC

    C. CMP

    D. ABG

17. Which of the following is likely to be reported by a patient experiencing chest pain related to pericarditis?

    A. Chest pain relieved by sitting forward

    B. Chest pain relieved by lying down

    C. Chest pain relieved by deep inspiration

    D. Chest pain relieved by rest

Lesson 4: Congestive Heart Failure

18. The NP is performing a physical exam on a 58-year-old male with a long-standing history of HTN and COPD. The NP detects JVD with HOB 60 degrees, an S3 gallop, and 2+ pitting pedal edema. What is the most likely diagnosis?

    A. Right-sided heart failure

    B. Biventricular failure

    C. Left-sided heart failure

    D. Diastolic failure

19. A patient suspected of having heart failure is sent for further diagnostic examination, including a blood test to assess BNP levels. What is the significance of the BNP level?

    A. BNP is secreted by the ventricles of the heart in response to excessive stretching of cardiomyocytes

    B. BNP elevations are only accurate in diagnosing diastolic dysfunction

    C. BNP is a good marker for differentiating between renal and pulmonary causes of dyspnea

    D. In decompensated heart failure, BNP levels decrease

20. During a routine follow-up appointment, an echocardiogram of a patient with a history of hypertension reveals left ventricular dysfunction and an ejection fraction of 45%. The patient denies weight gain, difficulty breathing, or shortness of breath and is currently taking atenolol to manage HTN. Based on this finding, which medication is likely to be initiated?

    A. ACE inhibitor

    B. ARB

    C. Calcium channel blocker

    D. Digitalis

21. A patient with a history of Stage C HF presents to the office for a routine follow-up. The patient is currently being managed on lisinopril (Zestril), digitalis (Lanoxin), and furosemide (Lasix). What should be included as part of the plan?

    A. Monitor potassium

    B. Discontinue digitalis (Lanoxin)

    C. Assess liver function

    D. ECG monthly

22. The NP sees a patient with a history of HF for a one-month follow-up. Digoxin was previously added to his regimen of enalapril and furosemide. AV heart block is present on the patient's ECG. Which of the following manifestations of digoxin toxicity is the patient most likely to report?

    A. Visual disturbances

    B. Constipation

    C. Polyphagia

    D. Hyperactivity

Lesson 5: Endocarditis

23. Which of the following objective findings does not result from embolic events related to infective endocarditis?

    A. Janeway lesions

    B. Osler nodes

    C. Impetigo

    D. Roth spots

24. A patient presents to the ER with fever, chills, and Roth spots and reports a history of rheumatic valvular disease. The nurse practitioner is suspicious of infective endocarditis. It is appropriate to order which of the following tests initially?

    A. Chest x-ray and lipid panel

    B. Blood culture and transthoracic echocardiogram

    C. Cardiac MRI and guaiac stool test

    D. Initial blood culture and cardiac stress test

25. Which of the following patients would be at greatest risk for infective endocarditis?

    A. 35-year-old patient who is a chronic injection drug user

    B. 49-year-old patient undergoing chemo treatments for stage II breast cancer

    C. 55-year-old patient who has coronary artery disease

    D. 64-year-old patient with chronic migraines

26. A 55-year-old female with a history of mitral valve prolapse is being discharged from the hospital and sent home with antibiotic therapy for infective endocarditis (IE). Which statement indicates an understanding of the patient's future prophylactic needs?

    A. "I will not require antibiotic prophylaxis after I have completed my current antibiotic therapy."

    B. "I will require antibiotic prophylaxis but only for the next 6 months after discharge."

    C. "I will only require antibiotic prophylaxis for dental procedures that require general anesthesia."

    D. "I will require antibiotic prophylaxis before all dental procedures with the exception of x-rays and minor orthodontic adjustments."

27. A 56-year-old female patient who is allergic to penicillin with a prosthetic heart valve is visiting her dentist to undergo a tooth implant. Which antibiotic is recommended at this time?

    A. doxycycline (Vibramycin)

    B. clindamycin (Cleocin)

    C. ampicillin (Amoxil)

    D. cefaclor (Ceclor)

28. An IV drug user is being treated for infective endocarditis (IE) and complains of dyspnea, chest pain, and lightheadedness. The nurse practitioner understands that these are common signs of which finding seen in IE?

    A. Splenic emboli event

    B. Myocardial infarction

    C. Pulmonary emboli event

    D. Renal emboli event

Lesson 6: Hyperlipidemia

29. A 45-year-old patient presents with no known risk factors for hyperlipidemia (HL), LDL 98 mg/dL, HDL 42 mg/dL, and triglycerides 720 mg/dL. The nurse practitioner should consider making which of the following statements?

    A. "The addition of a fibric acid such as fenofibrate is recommended at this time to lower your triglyceride levels."

    B. "We should recheck your levels in 4–6 weeks as triglyceride levels do fluctuate."

    C. "Your triglyceride levels are high, but we generally do not initiate drug therapy until levels are greater than 1000 mg/dL."

    D. "Your triglycerides levels are very high, but you are not at risk for acute pancreatitis at this time."

30. You examine a 56-year-old patient with type 2 DM who is at the office for follow-up 4 weeks after initiating statin therapy with atorvastatin. The patient states, "I have had mild aches and pains since starting this medication." The NP should perform which of the following actions?

    A. Discontinue statin use and initiate niacin treatment

    B. Discontinue statin and initiate a lower dose of different statin until adverse effects improve

    C. Encourage daily muscle strengthening exercises

    D. Explain to the patient that the addition of fenofibrate will help improve symptoms

31. A 61-year-old patient is being discharged from hospital after a recent MI and new onset DM. According to most recent guidelines, which treatment is an example of a high-intensity statin drug to initiate upon discharge?

    A. rosuvastatin 20 mg (Crestor)

    B. pravastatin 40 mg (Pravachol)

    C. simvastatin 10 mg (Zocor)

    D. lovastatin 20 mg (Mevacor)

32. A 45-year-old patient with known ASCVD prefers to forgo statin use and make lifestyle modifications. The nurse practitioner knows that the average LDL reduction with diet changes only is approximately:

    A. 1–3%

    B. 3–5%

    C. 5–10%

    D. 10–20%

Lesson 7: Hypertension

33. Which medication would be a first-line antihypertensive for a new hypertension diagnosis in a patient who is African American with a family history of diabetes?

    A. metoprolol tartrate (Toprol)

    B. clonidine transdermal patch (Catapres)

    C. chlorthalidone (Thalitone)

    D. benazepril (Lotensin)

34. A patient that is newly diagnosed with hypertension returns for their first follow-up after being on Lisinopril 10 mg daily for 1 month. If blood pressure is 152/94, what would be the next step?

    A. Increase the dosage

    B. Change to a different class

    C. Stop the medication and focus on lifestyle changes

    D. Workup for secondary hypertension

35. Which patient would not warrant a workup for secondary hypertension?

    A. 5-year-old with blood pressure greater than the 99th percentile for height with a positive family history of HTN

    B. 35-year-old with a 2-month history of BP 150/90s on amlodipine 10 mg daily and benazepril 40 mg daily; BP on follow-up in the office is 165/100 with repeat measurements

    C. 65-year-old with blood pressure 172/98 with right upper quadrant abdominal bruit

    D. 25-year-old female with BMI of 37 and a blood pressure of 145/98 one month after starting phentermine

36. Thomas is a 55-year-old with a history of diabetes and COPD. His medications include metformin (Glucophage) 500 mg BID, simvastatin (Zocor) 10 mg nightly, lisinopril/HCTZ (Zestoretic) 20/12.5 mg every AM and salmeterol (Serevent) 50 mg/dose 1 puff BID albuterol (ProAir HFA) 90 mcg/actuation prn, which he uses 2–3 times daily. He presents for follow-up on HTN. His home readings have been 145–155/92–105 for the last 3 months. What would be the next step in the treatment plan?

    A. Advise to start walking 45 mins/day, 5 days/week

    B. Increase lisinopril to 30 mg daily

    C. Increase the HCTZ to 25 mg daily and change to PM dosing

    D. Add carvedilol (Coreg) 6.25 mg daily and have patient follow up in 1 month

37. Patients with HTN should be educated regarding:

    A. Stopping smoking

    B. Decreasing alcohol intake to 3 drinks/day

    C. Exercising 60 mins/day, 6 days/week

    D. Avoiding over-the-counter guaifenesin

Lesson 8: Murmurs/Valvular Disorders

38. The nurse practitioner notes a grade 3 systolic murmur with an ejection click at the right sternal border. Which finding does the nurse practitioner expect to see in this patient?

    A. Pericarditis

    B. Mitral valve prolapse

    C. Aortic regurgitation

    D. Aortic stenosis

39. The nurse practitioner suspects mitral valve prolapse in a 62-year-old female patient complaining of shortness of breath and dizziness. Which test would the nurse practitioner order initially to confirm this diagnosis?

    A. Cardiac stress test

    B. Transthoracic echocardiogram

    C. Blood culture

    D. Cardiac catheterization

40. During an annual wellness check of an asymptomatic 22-year-old male patient, the nurse practitioner notes an S3 sound that is short in duration. Which statement should the nurse include in her teaching instructions to patient?

    A. "Please refrain from exercise at this time."

    B. "A prompt evaluation with a cardiologist is needed."

    C. "This is a normal variant and no further testing is required at this time."

    D. "A transthoracic echocardiogram will be ordered today."

41. A 42-year-old male presents to clinic complaining of fatigue and mild edema. Upon auscultation of his chest wall, the NP hears a loud systolic murmur, but it has no palpable thrill. Upon documentation, how would the nurse practitioner grade this murmur?

    A. Grade 1

    B. Grade 3

    C. Grade 4

    D. Grade 6

42. A 62-year-old patient with a history of mild aortic stenosis reports a recent episode of syncope and more frequent angina. Which action by the nurse practitioner is best?

    A. Obtain a chest x-ray to look for heart enlargement

    B. Explain to patient that this is a normal finding with aortic stenosis

    C. Obtain an echocardiogram and refer to a cardiologist

    D. Discuss the addition of nitroprusside for angina pain

43. A 55-year-old female patient with a history of mitral stenosis presents to your clinic for follow-up. The nurse practitioner may expect to see which finding in the patient's history?

    A. Rheumatoid arthritis

    B. Rheumatic fever

    C. Alopecia areata

    D. Graves disease

Lesson 9: Peripheral Vascular Disease

44. Which subjective and objective findings suggest an arterial cause of leg pain?

    A. Complaint of aching to legs that improves with elevation, varicose veins, and dependent rubor

    B. Dorsalis pedis and posterior tibial pulses 1+ bilaterally and right calf pain, warmth, and edema that started 2 days after driving from Michigan to Florida

    C. Pain in buttocks and thighs with walking, capillary refill greater than 5 secs, ABI = 0.80

    D. Bilateral leg edema that improves with elevation, legs with increased pigmentation and multiple telangiectasias

45. Esme is a 42-year-old hair dresser who complains of bilateral aching and swelling in her legs. The swelling and pain are worse at the end of the day. She is a nonsmoker. BMI is 32, HR 75, BP 126/84, RR 18, and SpO$_2$ 98%. She walks 45 minutes twice a week for exercise without difficulty. She has tried to change her shoes and add insoles to her shoes with no improvement. Proper treatment for this patient would include:

    A. Wearing graded compression socks of 20–30 mmHg for 3 months and then return for follow-up

    B. Starting an exercise program that includes walking to the point of pain, resting until pain resolves, and start walking once pain has resolved

    C. Referring to vascular surgery

    D. Taking an aspirin 325 mg daily

46. Initial diagnostic workup for a DVT includes:

    A. Obtaining a D-dimer

    B. Ordering a doppler ultrasound of the affected extremity

    C. Ordering a spiral CT of the chest

    D. Determining pretest probability

47. Rob is a 65-year-old with a 5-year history of bilateral lower leg arterial disease. BMI is 24, HR 75, BP 126/75, RR 18, and SpO$_2$ 99%. His medications include metoprolol tartrate (Lopressor) 50 mg BID and ASA 325 mg daily. He has smoked 1 pack-per-day for 20 years and drinks a six-pack of beers nightly. Fasting labs from one week ago: total cholesterol 250, triglycerides 176, LDL 180, HDL 30, and blood sugar 95. He presents for follow-up and lab review. Which of the following would not be included in the treatment plan?

    A. Atorvastatin (Lipitor) 20 mg every night

    B. Counseling regarding smoking cessation

    C. Hemoglobin A1C level

    D. Counseling regarding weight loss

48. Which of the following is not included in Wells criteria?

    A. Family history of DVT

    B. Swelling of the entire leg

    C. Recent cast of the leg

    D. Active cancer diagnosis

ANSWERS AND EXPLANATIONS

Lesson 1: Acute MI

1. A

There is no single ideal blood test to diagnose MI. Troponin **(A)** is the most sensitive and specific for MI and cardiac necrosis. Myoglobin (B) and CK-MB (C) are common laboratory tests that can be ordered (troponins T and I, creatine kinase-MB [CK-MB], and myoglobin). ESR (D) is used to evaluate things such as inflammatory conditions/autoimmune disorders, not an MI.

2. A

Calcium channel blockers **(A)** are utilized if a patient is intolerant to beta-blockers. Beta-blockers are initiated within 24 hours of an MI. ARBs (B) are utilized if intolerant to ACE inhibitors (D). An anti-arrhythmic (C) would not be an appropriate substitution for an antihypertensive.

3. A

The major manifestation of MI in people older than 80 years may be disorientation or acute confusion **(A)**. Extreme fatigue and epigastric discomfort (B) are usually the initial symptoms of MI in women. False reassurance (C) is not an appropriate answer. Diabetic patients do not have the typical "chest pain," instead, chest pain is presented as midscapular, jaw, lip, and gum pain (D).

4. A

Lifestyle modification includes sodium reduction (1500–2300 mg/day) **(A)**. Smoking cessation (B) is recommended, not cutting back on tobacco use. Walking for 15 minutes (C) is incorrect, as the patient should increase physical activity (30 min of moderate exercise for 5 days; 25 min of vigorous exercise 3× a week; for BP-lowering, 40 moderate to vigorous, 3–4× a week). A heart-healthy diet is recommended, which includes high fiber, not low fiber (D). Other modifications: maintaining a normal weight (BMI 18.5–24.9), cholesterol management (total <200, HDL >40–60, LDL <100, triglycerides <150), and alcohol intake within normal limits for gender and age.

5. A

ECG abnormalities in leads II, III, and aVF indicate an inferior wall MI. The NP should call 911 **(A)**, as the patient might be experiencing an MI. Early diagnosis and treatment are vital. Delay in treatment can lead to death. Repeating the ECG (B) is not appropriate, and changes will not resolve once tachycardia has subsided. If the patient was exhibiting signs of stable angina, a stress test (C) and consideration for initiating anticoagulation (D) would be appropriate.

6. A

Sarcoidosis **(A)** is an inflammatory disease that leads to the development of granulomas that alter the normal structure and function of certain organs, but mostly the lungs and lymph nodes. Non-atherosclerotic etiologies include emboli, mechanical obstruction (e.g., cocaine or IV drug use (B), chest trauma (C), aortic stenosis (D), aortic dissection, arteritis, DIC, and hypertrophic cardiomyopathy.

Lesson 2: Arrythmias

7. C

Sodium intake **(C)** would not be pertinent information to obtain in this young patient with normal blood pressure. It would be important to know caffeine usage (A), use of prescription medications (B), and illicit drug use (D). They all have the potential to cause accelerated heart rate and/or arrhythmia.

8. A

It would be appropriate to refer a patient to cardiology **(A)** if they have newly diagnosed asymptomatic bradycardia. Sick sinus syndrome needs to be ruled out in these patients. The patient is stable and without symptoms, so they would not need immediate transport (B) or atropine IV (C). A tilt table test (D) would not be an appropriate test in this patient.

9. D

On a normal ECG lead, the QRS complex on lead I, II, III, AVF, V5, and V6 **(D)** are normally upright. AVR, V1, and V2, included in both choices (A) and (B), and the QRS complex of V1 (C), face downward on a normal ECG.

10. B

Left axis deviation **(B)** is shown by QRS upright in lead I and facing downward in lead AVF. Extreme right axis (A) is shown when lead I and AVF are both facing downward. A normal axis (C) is shown when lead I and AVF are both facing upright. Right axis deviation (D) is shown when lead I is facing downward and AVF is facing downward.

11. C

This patient is unstable and needs to be prepared for transport **(C)**. A same day ECHO (A) would not benefit this patient. This patient needs to have his heart rhythm normalized and heart rate decreased quickly. Transcutaneous pacing pads (B) would not be used for atrial fibrillation. If this patient is referred to cardiology (D), their condition may continue to deteriorate before they are seen.

Lesson 3: Chest Pain

12. A

The patient is exhibiting signs and symptoms of costo-chondritis. These include sharp, pleuritic-type pain that worsens with deep breathing, palpation, or movement, and chest tightness typically located in the area of the 2nd through 5th intercostal spaces. Anti-inflammatories **(A)** are an appropriate treatment. Cardiac-related chest pain (angina, MI) would require emergent report to the ER (B), may warrant further testing like ECG (C) and blood tests, and a follow-up with a cardiologist (D).

13. A

Given the recent ORIF, the patient is at risk for problems related to immobility, including pulmonary embolism and pneumonia. The patient is exhibiting manifestations of pulmonary embolism **(A)**, which can include pleuritic, sharp, stabbing pain worsening with deep breathing, feeling of impending doom, anxiety, dyspnea, cyanosis, and tachypnea. Symptoms of aortic stenosis (B) can include dyspnea, angina, and syncope occurring on exertion; marked fatigue; and peripheral cyanosis. Pneumonic pain may present with chest pain, but will usually be accompanied by coughing, mucus production, fever, shortness of breath. Angina (D) is characterized as pressure, heaviness, squeezing, crushing, or tightness that may or may not be precipitated by activity or occur at rest, and can be poorly localized pain.

14. A

The presence of sharp chest pain and tracheal deviation **(A)** is a danger sign and indicates that the patient may be experiencing a tension pneumothorax. A tension pneumothorax is a medical emergency. The NP must be alert for diminished or absent breath sounds on the affected side, asymmetry of respirations, tracheal deviation, respiratory distress, cyanosis, pallor, weak and rapid pulse, hypotension, neck vein distention, and altered mental status. Shoulder pain (B) and chest bruising (C) can occur after an MVA due to the seat belt trauma along with headache (D); although these may require follow-up, these are not life threatening.

15. A

MI-related chest pain typically presents as pressure, heaviness, squeezing, crushing, and tightness that may be precipitated by activity or occur at rest, and may not be relieved by rest or nitrates **(A)**. Burning chest pain relieved by a position change (B) is indicative of heartburn. Chest tightness relieved by rest (C) is consistent with stable angina. Aching pain relieved by ibuprofen (D) is indicative of costochondritis.

16. A

Patients with both pneumonia and CHF can experience chest pain; respiratory symptoms including dyspnea, SOB, and tachypnea; as well as tachycardia and hypotension. BNP **(A)** will be elevated in a patient with CHF, whereas CBC (B), CMP (C), and ABG (D) can be abnormal with both conditions.

17. A

Patients with pericarditis typically present with constant substernal soreness or sudden sharp and stabbing pain, relieved by sitting forward **(A)**. Pain is worse when lying down, not relieved (B). Pain is aggravated by deep inspiration, not improved (C). Pain is not usually made worse by exertion (D).

Lesson 4: Congestive Heart Failure

18. A

The patient is presenting with classic signs of right-sided heart failure **(A)**. Biventricular failure (B), mixed diastolic and systolic failure, is often seen in patients with cardiomyopathy. These patients have extremely poor ejection fractions and diagnosis cannot be made on these presenting symptoms alone. Signs of left-sided heart failure (C) may include crackles, dyspnea, orthopnea, PND, and confusion. Diastolic failure (D), failure with preserved left ventricular function, occurs when the left ventricle can't relax adequately during diastole. Inadequate relaxation or stiffening prevents the ventricle from filling with sufficient blood to ensure an adequate cardiac output. This represents about 20–40% of HF and occurs primarily in older adults and women who have chronic HTN and CAD.

19. A

BNP (brain natriuretic peptide) will be elevated in patients with heart failure, as it's secreted by the ventricles of the heart in response to excessive stretching of cardiomyocytes **(A)**. BNP elevations are accurate in diagnosing diastolic dysfunction with the same effectiveness as in systolic dysfunction, making (B) an incorrect option. BNP is a good marker for differentiating between cardiac and pulmonary causes of dyspnea, not renal and pulmonary causes (C). BNP levels rise, not decline (D), in decompensated heart failure; as heart failure is treated, BNP levels will decline.

20. A

Angiotensin converting enzyme (ACE) inhibition **(A)** should be used in patients who are at risk for developing heart failure. These include patients with a history of atherosclerotic vascular disease, diabetes mellitus, or hypertension. Recommendations for patients with asymptomatic left ventricular systolic dysfunction and reduced EF include ACE inhibitors. In addition, ACE inhibitors should be used in patients with a reduced ejection fraction, whether or not they have experienced a myocardial infarction. ARBs (B) are reserved for patients who are unable to tolerate ACEs. Calcium channel blockers (C) are used to treat symptomatic HF. Digitalis (D) is used for the treatment of symptoms of HF and to enhance exercise tolerance, unless contraindicated in patients with symptomatic HF.

21. A

Monitoring potassium levels **(A)** in this patient takes priority. ACE inhibitors can increase potassium levels, putting the patient at risk for arrhythmias. Furosemide can decrease potassium levels. Hypokalemia puts the patient at risk for digoxin toxicity. For patients with Stage C HF (symptomatic left ventricular dysfunction), digitalis is used for the treatment of symptoms of HF, not discontinued (B), unless contraindicated. Renal function should be monitored with patients on ACE inhibitors, not liver function (C). ECGs (D) are not warranted monthly.

22. A

Patients with digoxin toxicity are likely to report nausea, vomiting, arrhythmias, and visual changes **(A)**. Diarrhea may also be found, not constipation (B). Patients can also report anorexia, not polyphagia (C). In addition, fatigue and malaise can be reported, not hyperactivity (D).

Lesson 5: Endocarditis

23. C

Impetigo **(C)** is a superficial infection not related to infective endocarditis. Janeway lesions (A) (nontender lesions on palms and soles), Osler nodes (B) (tender lesions on palms and soles), and Roth spots (D) (retinal hemorrhages) are all signs of embolic changes to the skin and eyes in a patient suffering from infective endocarditis.

24. B

Infective endocarditis is often a diagnosis of exclusion, but if the nurse practitioner is suspicious, it is appropriate to order a blood culture and echocardiogram **(B)**. Three blood cultures at least 1 hour apart should be gathered in the first 24 hours to confirm diagnosis. An echocardiogram is used to visualize vegetation. Cardiac MRI and chest x-ray may be ordered, but the lipid panel (A), guaiac stool test (C), and cardiac stress test (D) are not tests for infective endocarditis.

25. A

Infective endocarditis occurs when bacteria or fungi enter bloodstream, causing inflammation of the heart lining or valves. Injection drug users **(A)** are at high risk, as drugs and contaminates can enter into bloodstream and cause infections that are difficult for white blood cells to attack, such as near valves. Chemo treatments (B) may increase one's risk of thrombi and infection, but not endocarditis specifically. Coronary artery disease (C) alone and chronic migraines (D) are not risk factors for endocarditis.

26. D

Although AHA has decreased the need for antibiotic prophylaxis (it is no longer needed for most cardiac conditions), it is still recommended that patients who have previously had IE take antibiotic prophylaxis before all dental procedures **(D)**.

27. B

If a patient is allergic to penicillin, AHA recommends clindamycin **(B)** 600 mg PO 30–60 minutes prior to a dental procedure. Doxycycline (A) is a tetracycline and not the drug of choice for dental prophylaxis. Ampicillin (C) is a penicillin; the patient is allergic to penicillin. The patient may have a cross-sensitivity reaction with cefaclor (D), a cephalosporin drug, if allergic to penicillin.

28. C

Embolic events are commonly seen during infectious endocarditis. IV drug users often present with complaints of dyspnea, chest pain, and lightheadedness, suggesting pulmonary emboli events **(C)**. Spleen emboli (A) present with sharp abdominal pain that radiates to left side up to shoulder. It is not common for a myocardial infarction (B) to result from IE. Renal emboli (D) present with flank pain and abnormal urine results.

Lesson 6: Hyperlipidemia

29. A

According to the most recent guidelines, if a patient has no known risk factors (i.e., ASCVD, DM), you should initiate fenofibrate to achieve lower triglycerides **(A)** unless LDL goals have not been achieved. Treatment should be initiated; choices (B) and (C) are incorrect. Choice (D) is incorrect, as patients with a triglyceride level 500 mg/dL are at risk for acute pancreatitis.

30. B

It is appropriate to try lower dose of a different statin **(B)**, unless the symptoms are severe. Statin therapy has been shown to drastically reduce LDL and has better outcomes than niacin treatment (A). Muscle symptoms related to statin use often will not improve with daily strengthening exercises (C), and fenofibrates (D) are not indicated as a treatment. It is best to try a lower dose of different statin.

31. A

Rosuvastatin 20 mg **(A)** is an example of a high-intensity statin that is appropriate to administer to this patient, as they have known ASCVD. Pravastatin 40 mg (B) is considered a moderate-intensity statin, and both simvastatin 10 mg (C) and lovastatin 20 mg (D) are low-intensity drugs.

32. C

Diet changes alone only account for a 5–10% reduction in LDL levels **(C)**. The ACC/AHA recommends statin use to help lower LDL to optimal levels vs. diet alone. While both (A) and (C) may occur, the average reduction is slightly greater. This is why statin use is the mainstay of therapy, as a reduction of 10–20% seen in (D) is not likely to occur.

Lesson 7: Hypertension

33. C

Chlorthalidone **(C)** is a thiazide diuretic, which is preferred for African Americans. Metoprolol tartrate (A) is a beta-blocker, and there are no indications that it should be considered as first-line for this patient. A clonidine transdermal patch (B) is not first-line. Benazepril (D) is an ACE inhibitor. Thiazides are preferred over ACE inhibitors for African Americans.

34. A

Increasing the dosage **(A)** is the initial step if a patient isn't responding to therapy. Change to a different class (B) after the patient is at maximum dosage of the previous drug. Lifestyle changes (C) should be emphasized, but the medication should not be stopped. There are no indications that this patient's hypertension has secondary causes (D).

35. D

A 25-year-old with a BMI of 37 **(D)** is obese and is taking a medication that can increase BP. She should stop phentermine and try lifestyle modification. A 5-year-old (A) is prepubertal and requires a workup even though there is a positive family history. A 35-year-old (B) is on the maximum dose of 2 different classes of blood pressure medications, and blood pressure is increasing. HTN in presence of concerning physical findings like a right upper quadrant abdominal bruit (C) should be worked up for secondary hypertension. An abdominal bruit could indicate renal artery stenosis.

36. B

The lisinopril dose at 20 mg can be increased **(B)**, which would be preferable to adding a different class of medications. The patient is having to use their albuterol 2–3 times daily, so they would not tolerate a vigorous exercise plan (A). Changing the HCTZ dosing to PM (C) would cause the patient to have nocturia. The dosage should be maximized on their current meds before changing to a different class (D).

37. A

Smoking is a modifiable risk factor that can elevate blood pressure and increase morbidity and mortality in those with HTN **(A)**. Consumption of 3 alcoholic beverages daily (B) is excessive alcohol intake and can increase blood pressure. Patients should be counseled to exercise 3–4 days per week for 30–40 mins, making (C) incorrect. Guaifenesin is an antitussive medication and will not increase blood pressure (D).

Lesson 8: Murmurs/Valvular Disorders

38. D

The right sternal border is the best position to hear aortic heart sounds. A systolic murmur with an ejection click is a hallmark sign of aortic stenosis **(D)**. Pericarditis (A) will produce a harsh, grating sound on auscultation. A mitral valve prolapse (B) is not heard best in right sternal border, nor does it have an associated ejection click. In aortic regurgitation (C), a diastolic murmur would be heard.

39. B

The best way to visualize the heart valves and confirm mitral valve prolapse is via a transthoracic echocardiogram **(B)**. A stress test (A) and cardiac catheterization (D) may be needed to confirm heart enlargement or coronary involvement but would not be the initial choice. Blood cultures (C) would be needed if infective endocarditis is suspected.

40. C

An S3 sound may be heard in healthy young patients, **(C)**. No restrictions of activity (A) or further evaluation (B and D) are needed unless the patient reports symptoms or there are associated abnormal findings. Document the finding and follow-up with patient at the next wellness check.

41. B

Murmurs are generally graded using the Levine classification system. Grade 3 murmurs **(B)** are loud but do not have a palpable thrill. Grade 1 murmurs (A) are so faint that it may take several minutes to hear with stethoscope. Grade 4 (C) and 6 (D) murmurs are very loud and both have palpable thrill.

42. C

Aortic stenosis often progresses and can be dangerous if the valve becomes too narrow, thus requiring surgery. If the patient reports new symptoms, they should be referred to a cardiologist and undergo an echocardiogram **(C)** to look for worsening stenosis. A chest x-ray (A) may be obtained, but is not a priority. These are signs of worsening disease and not normal findings (B). The addition of a nitroprusside (D) may be needed, but the patient should be assessed first.

43. B

The majority of patients that develop mitral stenosis have a history of rheumatic fever **(B)**. Rheumatic fever generally develops 2–4 weeks after untreated strep throat or scarlet fever. An inflammatory disease that affects our joints and nervous system due to group A *Streptococcus* bacteria, rheumatic fever may also scar our heart valves and is the predominant cause of mitral stenosis. Rheumatoid arthritis (A), alopecia areata (C), and Graves disease (D) are all autoimmune diseases unrelated to mitral stenosis.

Lesson 9: Peripheral Vascular Disease

44. C

Pain in the buttocks and thighs with walking **(C)** can be a sign of arterial disease, as well as ABI <0.90. Complaint of aching in legs that improves with elevation and varicose veins (A) suggests venous disease; arterial disease pain would worsen with elevation. Dorsalis pedis and posterior tibial pulses 1+ (B) are decreased with arterial disease. Unilateral pain, warmth, and edema after prolonged driving suggest a DVT. Leg edema, increased pigmentation, and telangiectasias (D) are seen with venous disease.

45. A

The history suggests venous disease. Graded compression hose/socks **(A)** is an appropriate intervention and must be tried for 3 months before vascular interventions are an option. A graded exercise program (B) is appropriate for a patient with arterial disease. Referral to a vascular surgeon (C) is not appropriate at this time; noninvasive interventions should be tried first. A daily aspirin (D) might be an appropriate intervention for arterial disease.

46. D

Pretest probability **(D)** determines how to proceed with additional diagnostic testing. Obtaining a D-dimer (A) might be appropriate in combination with a doppler ultrasound of the affected extremity (B), but only after pretest probability is determined. A spiral CT of the chest (C) is done if a pulmonary embolism is suspected.

47. C

Hemoglobin A1C levels **(C)** are checked to determine diabetes control. While controlling diabetes is an important aspect of controlling arterial disease, nothing in the history indicates diabetes (e.g., both BMI and fasting blood sugar are normal). Arterial disease of the legs often indicates arterial disease throughout the body. This patient should be treated to modify cardiovascular risk factors, which includes controlling hyperlipidemia with atorvastatin (A) and smoking cessation (B). Counseling regarding weight loss (D) is important in reducing cardiovascular risk; however, this patient is not overweight or obese.

48. A

Wells criteria is used to determine probability of a DVT in a patient. Family history of DVT **(A)** is not a risk factor for a DVT. Swelling of the entire leg (B), recent casting of the leg (C), and an active diagnosis of cancer (D) are all risk factors for DVT and included in Wells criteria.

CHAPTER 8

Gastrointestinal

LESSON 1: ACUTE ABDOMEN

Learning Objectives
- Differentiate appendicitis, cholecystitis, pancreatitis, and diverticulitis
- Understand key diagnostic tools for each type of acute abdomen
- Effectively manage the patient presenting with an acute abdomen

Abdominal pain is a common complaint in primary and acute care. It is important to distinguish between abdominal pain that represents a self-limiting illness, a chronic condition, or an acute condition. Acute abdominal pain of an emergent nature requires immediate treatment and referral. Appendicitis, cholecystitis, pancreatitis, and diverticulitis can rapidly progress to rupture and/or peritonitis and require a rapid approach from assessment to treatment.

Definitions
- **Appendicitis:** acute inflammation of appendix caused most commonly by obstruction leading to infection, gangrene, and rupture if not treated
- **Cholecystitis:** acute or chronic inflammation of the gallbladder typically caused by cholelithiasis (gallstones); gallstones can cause inflammation and/or obstruction; gallbladder contracts against inflammation or obstructing stone, which causes pain
- **Pancreatitis:** inflammation of the pancreas most commonly caused by alcohol ingestion and biliary tract disease; other possible causes include medication, surgery, abdominal trauma, peptic ulcer, cancer, exposure to chemicals, and elevated triglycerides; acute pancreatitis can progress to organ failure
- **Diverticulitis:** inflammation or perforation of colonic diverticula (herniations of mucosa) that can cause bowel obstruction, perforation, abscess, or fistula
- **Peritoneal signs:** tests that indicate possible peritoneal inflammation
- **Cullen sign:** gray blue discoloration around umbilicus (sign of intra-abdominal bleeding)
- **Grey Turner sign:** bluish discoloration of flanks (sign of intra-abdominal bleeding)

Assessment

Subjective

Symptoms

	Appendicitis	Cholecystitis	Pancreatitis	Diverticulitis
Pain	• Right lower quadrant is classic, but may present with periumbilical pain early in the course which moves to RLQ • Pain can be located in other areas if appendix is retrocecal or malrotated	• Colicky, RUQ, and/or epigastric pain; can radiate to flank area and right shoulder • Pain after eating high-fat meal	Sudden, persistent, and severe epigastric, RUQ or LUQ pain; pain can radiate to the back	LLQ pain; can be relieved by defecation
Anorexia	Present	Present	May be present	May be present
Nausea and vomiting	Common, typically starts after abdominal pain	Nausea common, occasional vomiting	Nausea and vomiting	Nausea and vomiting
Bowel sounds	Irregular bowel sounds	Normal to hyperactive	Normal to hypoactive	Normal to hyperactive
Fever	Present	Absent	Present	Present (low-grade)
Atypical signs	Diarrhea, indigestion, malaise, flatulence	Jaundice (if biliary obstruction present)	Dyspnea, jaundice (if obstruction of biliary tract), tachycardia, Cullen sign, Grey Turner sign	Diarrhea
Pediatric considerations	Children often present atypical; may complain of above symptoms and abdominal pain with running, jumping, or coughing; right hip pain; limp or refusal to walk or move; lethargy; irritability; temperature instability; poor intake of fluids and/or food	Uncommon in children	Uncommon in children	Uncommon in children

Table 8.1.1 Symptoms with Acute Abdomen

Review of Systems

To rule out differential diagnoses, inquire about GU symptoms: dysuria, hematuria, urinary frequency or urgency, change in urinary stream, urinary hesitancy, pelvic pain, vaginal discharge or odor, and rectal pain. Items in the past medical history can guide decision making when ruling out differential diagnoses. PMH of GERD, alcohol intake, or frequent NSAID intake may indicate a gastric or duodenal ulcer and possible perforation (*see Chapter 8, Lesson 6*). A change in bowels, presence of blood in stool, or dark or tarry stools could indicate upper/lower GI bleed or malignancy. Constipation increases the risk of bowel obstruction, which also requires immediate intervention (*see Chapter 8,*

Lesson 4). A history that includes IBS, Crohn's disease, ulcerative colitis, renal calculi, frequent cystitis or pyelonephritis, pelvic inflammatory disease, or prostatitis increases the risk that a patient presenting with some of the symptoms of acute abdomen is experiencing a flare or recurrence of a previous diagnosis. Acute abdomen must still be ruled out as a priority. Past surgical history of an appendectomy or a cholecystectomy will allow for immediate rule out of appendicitis or cholecystitis. Diverticuli found on colonoscopy increase the risk of diverticulitis.

Objective

- **VS:** heart rate (increased with pain, fever, shock), blood pressure (increased with pain, decreased with shock), respiratory rate (increased with pain and fever), level of pain (use rating scale or faces), weight (overweight/obese females have increased risk of cholecystitis); see if patient shows signs of distress (crying, holding abdomen, difficulty walking)

- **Eyes:** sclera jaundiced (cholecystitis)

- **CV:** tachycardia, bradycardia, hypertension, hypotension, weak peripheral pulses

- **Resp:** shallow respirations (pain, abdominal distention)

- **GI:** abdomen size, bowel sounds, abdominal distention, tenderness or pain on palpation, guarding, occult blood in rectal exam (diverticulitis)

- **Peritoneal signs**

  1. **Psoas sign:** increased pain on lifting right thigh with a flexed knee against resistance of examiner's hand (appendicitis)

  2. **Obturator sign:** flex the right hip and knee passively and internally rotate the hip; pain in the right lower quadrant is positive (appendicitis)

  3. **Heel jar:** with a closed fist lightly pound on the right heel; pain in the right lower quadrant is positive (appendicitis)

  4. **Rovsing sign:** palpate the left lower quadrant, and patient has pain in the right lower quadrant (appendicitis)

  5. **McBurney point tenderness:** point located one-third the distance between a line drawn from umbilicus to right anterior superior iliac spine (appendicitis)

  6. **Murphy sign:** increased abdominal pain or catching breath on inspiration while palpating the right upper quadrant along the costal margin (cholecystitis)

  7. **Rebound tenderness:** palpate area of greatest pain with flat portion of hand; depress hand and hold for 30–60 seconds; remove hand, and increased pain is positive (generalized test for peritoneal inflammation, location of rebound, can give clues to diagnosis—see location of pain under symptoms)

- **GU:** suprapubic tenderness, flank or CVA tenderness (cystitis, pyelonephritis, renal calculi); if differential includes possible genital diagnosis, pelvic exam, or testicular/prostate exam

- **Skin:** jaundice (cholecystitis)

Diagnosis

Patients often present in atypical fashion with an acute abdomen. Blood work should include CBC/diff, CMP, amylase, lipase, stool for occult blood, stool studies, urinalysis, and urine pregnancy test for all female patients of reproductive age.

	Appendicitis	Cholecystitis	Pancreatitis	Diverticulitis
WBC	Elevated—left shift as appendicitis progresses	Elevated	Elevated	Elevated
Pertinent labs	Elevated bilirubin possible	Elevated liver function test	Elevated amylase (increases in 6–12 hrs and returns to normal in 3–5 days), lipase (increases in 4–8 hrs and returns to normal within 8–14 days). Possible to have elevated Hct, BUN, hypo or hyperglycemia, hypocalcemia	Possible stool for occult blood positive
Diagnostic testing and results	• CT scan of abdomen with contrast: enlarged appendix with occlusion of lumen, >6 mm; wall thickening, >2 mm; periappendiceal fat stranding; appendix wall enhanced; fluid collection in right lower quadrant (perforation) • Ultrasound (not as sensitive as CT): enlarged appendix, >6 mm MRI when CT contraindicated (pregnancy): appendix >7 mm	• RUQ ultrasound: gallstones • HIDA scan: positive for obstruction of common hepatic or cystic duct if gallbladder does not fill within 60 mins of administration of tracer	• Abdominal US: enlarged and hypoechoic pancreas • Abdominal CT with contrast: enlarged pancreas, heterogeneous enhancement with contrast • MRI with contrast: can be more sensitive in early disease but may not be readily available on emergent basis	CT: localized bowel wall thickening >4 mm. History of previous colonoscopy that revealed diverticulosis

Table 8.1.2 Results of Testing for Acute Abdomen

Pro Tip

Must meet two of these three characteristics to definitively diagnosis pancreatitis:

1. Acute onset of severe epigastric pain, often radiates to back
2. Elevated lipase and amylase to three times upper limit of normal
3. Positive imaging studies

Plan

Treatment

- **Appendicitis**

  - NPO, immediate surgical referral/hospitalization for appendectomy, pain control only after diagnosis is made, as pain medication can mask signs of peritonitis

  - Rarely treated with IV antibiotics and watchful waiting

  - Surgical referral of pediatric patients with a suspicion of appendicitis to determine if imaging is needed

- **Cholecystitis**

  - Acute pain control, keep NPO, IV hydration, refer to surgeon for cholecystectomy

  - Chronic pain control, monitor liver function, avoid offending high-fat foods, refer to gastroenterologist

- **Pancreatitis**

  - Hospitalization, IV hydration and antibiotics, enteral or parenteral feedings, pain control, close monitoring for organ failure

  - After discharge: treatment of cause, counseling for alcohol use, treatment of elevated triglycerides, alternative therapy if caused by medication

- **Diverticulitis**

  - Outpatient: clear liquids, pain control, antibiotics for 7–10 days: ciprofloxacin (Cipro) + metronidazole (Flagyl); levofloxacin (Levaquin) + metronidazole (Flagyl); sulfamethoxazole-trimethoprim (Bactrim) + metronidazole (Flagyl); amoxicillin-clavulanate (Augmentin) or moxifloxacin. Follow up in 2–3 days

  - Refer for inpatient treatment if criteria met (*see Pro Tip below*), worsening, or no improvement with outpatient therapy

  - Inpatient: NPO, pain control, IV antibiotics, surgery if unresponsive to treatment

> **Pro Tip: Criteria for Inpatient Treatment of Diverticulitis**
> - CT reveals complication (perforation, abscess, fistula, obstruction)
> - Signs of sepsis
> - Fever >102.5°F (39.2°C)
> - Severe abdominal pain or peritonitis
> - Immunocompromised
> - Unable to tolerate PO fluids
> - Significant elevation in WBC
> - Advanced age
> - Multiple comorbidities
> - Failed outpatient treatment

Education

- **Appendicitis:** post-op care—turn, cough, and deep breath; incentive spirometer; advance diet as tolerated because ileus is of concern; no driving or operating heavy machinery while taking pain medications; finish full course of antibiotics; monitor incision for infection; notify for fever, severe or worsening pain, or constipation

- **Cholecystitis:** avoid offending foods; post-op care if cholecystectomy done

- **Pancreatitis:** avoid alcohol and tobacco

- **Diverticulitis:** high-fiber foods; colonoscopy after symptoms resolved (6–8 weeks after resolution)

Takeaways

- Of the four types of acute abdomen discussed, appendicitis is the only one that occurs with frequency in children.

- CT scan with contrast, if not contraindicated, may be the best diagnostic tool if unsure of diagnosis.

- Appendicitis, cholecystitis, and pancreatitis require immediate referral for treatment. Diverticulitis may be treated on an outpatient basis.

LESSON 2: CROHN'S DISEASE & ULCERATIVE COLITIS

Learning Objectives

- ■ Define the characteristics of Crohn's disease and ulcerative colitis
- ■ Identify diagnostic criteria for Crohn's disease and ulcerative colitis
- ■ Select appropriate treatment options for Crohn's disease and ulcerative colitis

Crohn's disease (CD) can be described as chronic transmural inflammation of the gastrointestinal tract anywhere from the mouth to the perianal area. While CD can affect the GI tract anywhere along its length, it most commonly affects the ileum and the colon.

Ulcerative colitis (UC) is also an inflammatory disease affecting the GI tract, but the condition is confined to only the colon (beginning at the rectum). In terms of intestinal tissue layers, it affects only the mucosal layer of the colon.

Together, Crohn's disease and ulcerative colitis are known as "irritable bowel disease" or IBD. Note that "irritable bowel disease" and "irritable bowel syndrome" are not the same. (*See Lesson 9 for further explanation on the distinction between the two.*)

Risk factors are similar for CD and UC. First-degree relatives of IBD patients are up to 20 times more likely to suffer from IBD. A higher incidence of IBD is seen in Caucasians and people of Ashkenazi Jewish ancestry. Living in an industrialized nation or urban area increases one's risk.

	Crohn's disease	**Ulcerative colitis**
Age	Diagnosis peaks between ages 20–30 years old and around age 50	Usually develops before age 30
Gender	Affects men and women equally	Slightly more common in males
Smoking	More common among smokers	More common among non-smokers/ex-smokers

Table 8.2.1 Risk Factors of Crohn's Disease and Ulcerative Colitis

Assessment

Subjective

Fatigue and abdominal pain are common in patients with both Crohn's disease and ulcerative colitis. The patient with CD often reports colicky abdominal pain and relief with defecation. The patient with UC may report intermittent abdominal pain.

Objective

CD and UC symptoms include: (1) fever, (2) extra-intestinal involvement (eye inflammation, skin manifestations, arthritis, hypercoagulability [leading to potential thrombi], kidney stones [more common in CD than UC], pulmonary involvement, bone loss [due to malabsorption from the inflamed GI tract; chronic steroid use], and liver involvement [such as primary sclerosing cholangitis—inflammation of liver bile ducts]), (3) diarrhea (although more common with UC), (4) rectal bleeding, sometimes with mucus and pus (although more common with UC), and (5) weight loss. Both are characterized by periods of symptom remission and flares. The table below reflects common differences, though sufferers will not necessarily manifest all symptoms listed.

Symptom	Crohn's disease	Ulcerative colitis
GI tract involvement	Most patients have only partial involvement: • About 50% have only colon and ileum involvement • About 20% have only colon involvement	Typically involves only the colon (starting with the rectum) • Up to 50% have only rectal or rectosigmoid involvement • About 20% have inflammation along the entire length of the colon
GI lesions	Skip lesions (non-contiguous), inflammation of all tissue layers (as opposed to only the mucosal layer), and granulomas (seen on histological examination)	Continuous, even to the point of involving the entire large intestine (confined to the colonic mucosa [as opposed to all tissue layers])
Associated skin issues	Skin tags, perianal fissures (typically anterior or posterior) and/or abscesses, erythema nodosum, pyoderma gangrenosum	Erythema nodosum and pyoderma gangrenosum
Fibrosis and strictures	Fibrosis of the colon and sometimes strictures (narrowing)	Fibrosis is not common; strictures are possible but rare
Other	Sinus tracts and/or fistulas, anal fissures, aphthous ulcers/mouth ulcers	Tenesmus, fecal incontinence, anemia from chronic blood loss

Table 8.2.2 Objective Symptoms Crohn's Disease and Ulcerative Colitis

Pro Tip

• Arthritis is the most common extra-intestinal manifestation of IBD
• IBD patients are at increased risk for colorectal cancer
• Female UC patients should have regular Pap smears, as they are at increased risk for cervical dysplasia

Diagnosis

For UC, the classic sign is recurrent diarrhea (often with blood and/or mucus). Other key signs include cramping rectal pain and rectal urgency. Underlying infectious causes or carcinoma should be ruled out.

For Crohn's disease, onset may be insidious. A combination of crampy abdominal pain, fever, weight loss, and perianal manifestations (such as anal fissures) may point to Crohn's disease.

In up to 15% of patient cases—since CD and UC overlap in symptomology—the diagnosis is "indeterminate," meaning clinicians can state the patient has irritable bowel disease (IBD) but cannot determine which type.

Diagnostic Tests of Crohn's Disease and Ulcerative Colitis	
Crohn's disease	**Ulcerative colitis**
Stool examination for ova and parasites	Stool examination for ova and parasites
Stool specimen culture	Stool cultures (including for *C. diff*), testing for *Giardia*, and additional *E. coli* testing
CBC, electrolytes, glucose	CBC, electrolytes, albumin (albumin can serve as a negative marker, as it decreases during inflammatory episodes)
Kidney and liver function tests	STD testing including gonorrhea, herpes simplex virus, and syphilis (which can cause rectal inflammation)
ESR (shows inflammation)	ESR
CRP (shows inflammation)	CRP
Endoscopy/biopsy (can exclude other causes of tissue inflammation)	Endoscopy/biopsy
Serum iron and B12 (to assess blood loss, possibility of pernicious anemia)	
Colonoscopy/barium enema	
MRI (image perianal fistulas)	

Table 8.2.3

Differential Diagnosis

Differential diagnoses for CD/UC: **colitis (medication-related, infections, etc.), lactose intolerance, rectal ulcer, endometriosis, appendicitis, irritable bowel syndrome, carcinoma, diverticulitis**

> **Pro Tip**
>
> Granulomas are strongly indicative of Crohn's disease, but their absence does not exclude Crohn's: they may only be seen in about 10% of Crohn's cases.
>
> Signs that suggest Crohn's disease as opposed to UC include involvement of the small intestine, sparing of the rectum, or if anus involved, perianal signs like anal fissures, fistulas, and skin tags.

Plan

Treatment

Treatment for both CD and UC include lifestyle modifications, medications, and possibly surgical intervention.

- Lifestyle modifications: adequate hydration, diet adjustment, exercise, relaxation techniques
- Medications
  - Aminosalicylates: mesalamine (Pentasa), sulfasalazine (Azulfidine)
  - Corticosteroids
  - Antibiotics (including ciprofloxacin or metronidazole for Crohn's disease); antibiotics are not typically used for UC, as use can lead to *C. diff*
  - Immune modulators: azathioprine (Imuran), 6-mercaptopurine (Purinethol), methotrexate
  - Biologics: adalimumab (Humira), infliximab (Remicade)
- Surgical interventions
  - About 20% of UC patients will require colectomy; often proctocolectomy (removal of the colon and rectum) is performed since disease may recur in any remaining tissue
  - Crohn's disease patients may also require surgery such as bowel resection (to remove a diseased portion and anastomose the remaining portions)

Education

IBD patients should stay current with colon cancer and Pap screenings, as they can be at increased risk.

IBD patients should be vigilant for signs of anemia (from blood loss) and nutritional deficits (especially as some patients may avoid certain foods or experience reduced absorption of nutrients due to inflammation).

Complications of IBD

With acute complications, prompt hospitalization is necessary:

- Toxic megacolon (acute colitis with distention of the colon)
- Uncontrolled bleeding
- Abscess/perforation/strictures/fistula
- Malabsorption/malnutrition

Referral

A gastroenterology specialist should be involved in the care plan. Additional consultations/referrals may include hepatology and/or nephrology (if liver or kidney involvement), nutrition, and any other specialties associated with the extraintestinal IBD sites (such as ophthalmology for eye inflammation, dermatology for skin manifestations, etc.).

Takeaways

- IBD can manifest with extra-intestinal signs/symptoms such as bone loss, arthritis, kidney/liver involvement, and skin lesions, which require additional management. IBD patients are at increased risk for conditions such as cervical dysplasia and colon cancer, requiring vigilant screening.
- 50–75% of Crohn's disease and ulcerative colitis patients may require surgery at some point in their disease progression.
- Crohn's disease is characterized by transmural inflammation, skip lesions, and granulomas.
- UC is characterized by contiguous sites of inflammation in the mucosal tissue layer, tenesmus, and bloody diarrhea.

LESSON 3: COLORECTAL CANCER

Learning Objectives
- Identify the risk factors associated with developing colorectal cancer
- Discuss the signs and symptoms associated with colorectal cancer
- Discuss standard screening guidelines for colorectal cancer
- Identify the correct diagnostic method for average- vs. high-risk patients
- Identify when referral for further evaluation and/or treatment is needed

In the U.S., colorectal cancer is the third most common cancer in both sexes. African Americans have the highest rate of occurrence and mortality from the disease. Multiple factors have been identified that increase an individual's risk for developing the disease:

- Advancing age
- Chronic inflammatory bowel disease
- Family history of colorectal cancer
- Personal history of malignancy
- History of colon polyps
- Genetic factors: Lynch syndrome, familial adenomatous polyposis (FAP), MUTYH-associated polyposis (MAP) or Peutz-Jeghers syndrome contribute to a significantly elevated lifetime risk of developing colorectal cancer

Modifiable risk factors include:

- Smoking
- Alcohol consumption
- Sedentary lifestyle
- Obesity
- Diet: high in fat, red meat; low in fruits, vegetables, fiber, calcium

Definition
- **Tenesmus:** a sensation of incomplete defecation

Assessment

Subjective

Similar to lung cancer, patients with colon cancer are typically asymptomatic until the disease has progressed. The signs and symptoms also vary based on location of the tumor.

Right-sided colon cancer	Left-sided colon cancer
Vague, crampy abdominal pain	Constipation alternating w/diarrhea
Unexplained weight loss	Lower abdominal pain
Fatigue	Red blood in stool
Occult blood in the stool	Tenesmus
Iron-deficiency anemia	Change in stool caliber/character

Table 8.3.1 Symptoms of Colon Cancer by Location

Common complaints with rectal cancer include: tenesmus, bright red rectal bleeding, rectal pain, changes in stool shape and mucous discharge.

Objective

It is not uncommon for the physical exam to be unremarkable in patients with colorectal cancer. In advanced cases, physical examination may reveal abdominal tenderness, a palpable mass in the abdomen, lymphadenopathy, rectal mass, hepatomegaly, or macroscopic rectal bleeding. Masses are rarely palpable on rectal exam, thus digital rectal examinations are not recommended when evaluating for colorectal cancer.

Diagnosis

Since most cases of colon cancer are asymptomatic until the later stages of the disease, screening plays a vital role in detection. Screening methods include at-home testing of stool for occult blood via the guaiac-based fecal occult blood test (gFOBT) or fecal immunochemical test (FIT) annually. This is an effective method of early detection and, if positive, should be followed up with a colonoscopy. At-home stool DNA testing can also be done every three years to assess for DNA from cancerous tumors or polyps.

The most common screening method for colorectal cancer and the diagnostic method of choice in adults is a colonoscopy. Screening should start at age 50 and be repeated every 10 years if normal, with a gFOBT or FIT annually. Colonoscopies should continue until age 75. Screening beyond that, up to age 85, should be made on an individual basis depending on the person's risk factors and ability to withstand treatment should it be indicated.

If a colonoscopy is contraindicated, other screening methods are available, including flexible sigmoidoscopy, double barium contrast enema, and a CT colonography (virtual colonoscopy). Screening using one of these methods should start at age 50 and be repeated every 5 years, if normal.

Alternative screening schedules are recommended for individuals with an increased risk for developing colorectal cancer. These schedules include screening earlier and more frequently than the standard guidelines.

Screening methods for colon cancer	Frequency
Guaiac-based fecal occult blood test (gFOBT)	Annually
Fecal immunochemical testing (FIT)	Annually
Stool DNA testing	Every 3 years
Colonoscopy (diagnostic & screening method of choice)	Every 10 years
Flexible sigmoidoscopy	Every 5 years
Double barium contrast enema	Every 5 years
CT colonography	Every 5 years

Table 8.3.2 Screening Methods for Colon Cancer and Their Frequency

Additional workup may include a CBC to evaluate for iron-deficiency anemia, serum chemistries, liver, renal function tests, and a baseline CEA level.

Differential Diagnosis

Differential diagnoses for colorectal cancer: **diverticulitis, lymphoma, irritable bowel syndrome, inflammatory bowel disease, thrombosed hemorrhoids, appendicitis**

Plan

Treatment is dependent on the stage of the disease at diagnosis. Treatment often includes surgical resection. A variety of surgical resections can be performed, depending on the location and size of the tumor. Chemotherapy and radiation are also utilized, usually for more advanced disease. Long-term prognosis is dependent on the location, size of the tumor, metastasis at time of diagnosis, and overall health of the patient. Palliative care should be considered if metastasis is present at the time of diagnosis, as these patients have a poor prognosis. Screening will continue one year after treatment, often on a yearly basis.

Takeaways

- Risk factors associated with the development of colorectal cancer are multifaceted and include those that are modifiable and unmodifiable.
- Symptoms usually present late in the disease process and include abdominal pain, change in bowel habits, weight loss, fatigue, weakness, iron-deficiency anemia, and/or blood in the stool.
- A colonoscopy is the diagnostic method of choice. Screening guidelines recommend starting at age 50.
- Surgical resection is the mainstay of treatment for colorectal cancer in stages I–III.

LESSON 4: CONSTIPATION

Learning Objectives
- Define constipation
- Identify potential causes of constipation
- Recognize common symptoms of constipation
- Discuss diagnostic criteria and initial workup for constipation
- Develop a treatment plan for constipation using non-pharmacologic and pharmacologic methods

Constipation is a common complaint affecting every age group, especially children and the elderly. While most cases are acute, patients may develop chronic constipation if symptoms last more than 12 weeks. Although there is no one clinically accepted definition for constipation, it is usually defined as dry, hard stool that occurs less than three times per week.

The causes of constipation are often multifactorial and are classified as either primary and secondary.

Primary causes include:

- Idiopathic
- Functional
  - Slow or impaired colonic motility
  - Pelvic floor dysfunction

Secondary causes include:

- Dietary/lifestyle factors
  - Inadequate water, fiber intake
  - Increased intake of caffeine, alcohol, tea
  - Inadequate amount of physical activity
- Structural issues
  - Anal fissures
  - Hemorrhoids
  - Colonic strictures
  - Obstructing tumors
- Medications
  - Opioids
  - Antidepressants
  - Anticholinergics
  - Antacids
  - Iron
  - Sympathomimetics
  - Long-term laxative use
- Pregnancy
- Connective tissue disorders
  - Scleroderma
  - Amyloidosis
  - Mixed connective tissue disease
- Psychological disorders
  - Depression
  - Anxiety
  - Eating disorders

- Endocrine/metabolic disorders
  - Diabetes mellitus
  - Electrolyte imbalances
  - Hypothyroidism
- Neurologic disorders

  - Parkinson's disease
  - Multiple sclerosis
  - Cerebrovascular accident
  - Hirschsprung disease
  - Chagas disease
  - Spinal cord injury

Assessment

Subjective

Pertinent elements of the history include medication review, diet, activity/exercise, number of pregnancies (and noting if currently pregnant), and a detailed explanation of bowel movements.

Presentation may range from seemingly asymptomatic to severe. Patients may report infrequent, dry, hard, and/or lumpy stools. Abdominal pain, particularly in the left lower quadrant, bloating, and straining with defecation are often reported. Other symptoms include: cramping, malaise, rectal bleeding, hemorrhoids, rectal pain, tenesmus, increased flatulence, and low back pain.

Objective

Abdominal tenderness or distention may be present. Bowel sounds may be hyperactive. Hemorrhoids, anal fissure, or fecal impaction can be contributed to constipation. In severe cases, stool may be palpable during the abdominal exam.

A common assessment tool used to evaluate a patient's stool shape and quality is the Bristol Stool Scale. Patients can accurately describe their bowel movements by referring to the scale. It assists providers with determining how long the feces has been in the colon. Stool types 1 and 2 are indicative of constipation, are difficult to pass, and may require straining; types 3 and 4 are considered normal, healthy stool; types 5, 6, and 7 are loose, liquid stools that reflect diarrhea and may be difficult to control the urge to pass.

Bristol Stool Chart

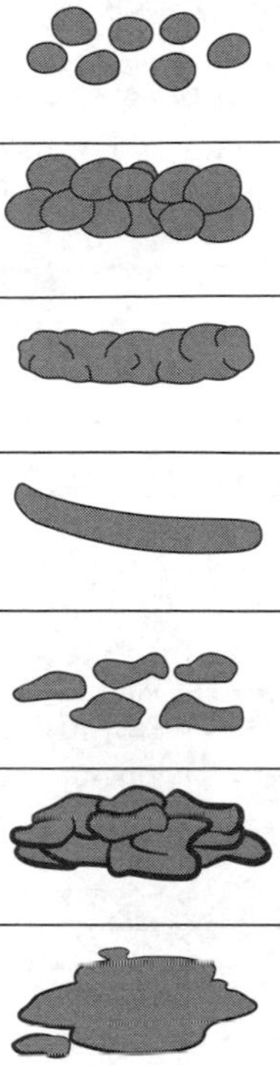

Type 1		Separate hard lumps, like nuts (hard to pass)
Type 2		Sausage-shaped but lumpy
Type 3		Like a sausage but with cracks on its surface
Type 4		Like a sausage or snake, smooth and soft
Type 5		Soft blobs with clear-cut edges (passed easily)
Type 6		Fluffy pieces with ragged edges, a mushy stool
Type 7		Watery, no solid pieces; entirely liquid

Figure 8.4.1

Diagnosis

The Rome III criteria is frequently used as the standard for diagnosis. Patients must not meet the criteria for IBS, and loose stools must rarely be present without the use of laxatives. At least two of the following symptoms must be present for at least 12 weeks:

- Less than three bowel movements per week
- Forced bowel movements
- Tenesmus
- Irregularly shaped, firm, dry stool
- Feeling of anorectal blockage

Initial workup for acute constipation includes gFOBT to test for blood, abdominal x-ray to assess for an obstruction, CBC to assess for anemia and infection, CMP to exclude electrolyte imbalance, and TSH to rule out hypothyroidism. Further workup may include colonoscopy, colonic transit study, defecography, or anorectal manometry.

Differential Diagnosis

Differential diagnoses for constipation: **colon cancer, IBS, diverticulosis, bowel obstruction, endocrine disorder, metabolic disorder, neurological disorder, psychological disorder, connective tissue disorder**

Plan

Treatment

Initial management should focus on lifestyle factors, as most cases of acute constipation will respond to these changes. Dietary changes, such as increasing water intake to at least eight cups a day and increasing dietary fiber to 20–35 g/day, should be implemented. Decreasing caffeine, alcohol, tea, and dairy products have proven beneficial. Physical activity can increase the colonic motility and improve symptoms.

If lifestyle factors are ineffective, pharmacologic methods are often employed.

Medication	Examples	Recommended use
Bulk-forming agents	fiber, psyllium, methylcellulose	Long-term, inexpensive, safe
Emollient stool softeners	docusate (Colace)	Easy to use, short-term use only, loses effectiveness with time
Osmotic laxatives	polyethylene glycol (Miralax), lactulose, sorbitol	Easy to use, effective, inexpensive, approved for long-term use (though safety over decades undetermined)
Stimulant laxatives	senna (Senokot), bisacodyl	Short-term use only
Saline laxatives	magnesium hydroxide, citrate, or sulfate	Short-term use only, may cause electrolyte imbalance
Lubricant laxatives	enemas, mineral oil	Short-term use only, gentler than other laxatives
Laxatives, other	plecanatide (Trulance), linaclotide (Linzess), lubiprostone (Amitiza)	Long-term use for chronic idiopathic constipation

Table 8.4.1 Pharmacologic Treatment of Constipation

If an impaction is present, manual removal is required. For patients with pelvic floor dysfunction, biofeedback may be helpful.

Education

Focus on the importance of lifestyle changes, specifically diet and physical activity. Recommend that water and fiber intake be increased, while caffeine and dairy be decreased. Physical activity, such as frequent, brisk walking, has been shown to improve symptoms.

Referral

Refer the patient for GI workup if unresponsive to lifestyle changes and short-term medical management. For psych, metabolic, endocrine, and connective-tissue etiologies, refer to appropriate specialties for further workup.

Takeaways

- Constipation is generally defined as hard, lumpy stool that occurs less than three times per week.
- Treatment should focus on diet and exercise prior to implementing pharmacologic measures.
- Most medications used to treat constipation are for short-term use only.

LESSON 5: GASTROENTERITIS

Learning Objectives
- Differentiate clinical manifestations of gastroenteritis
- Choose and interpret laboratory/diagnostic testing for gastroenteritis
- Describe appropriate treatment and referrals for gastroenteritis

Gastroenteritis is a common occurrence across all age groups, with young children and the elderly being particularly at risk. While it is most commonly caused by viruses, at times bacteria or parasites may be implicated.

Category	Microorganisms and significance
Bacteria	• *Campylobacter*: raw poultry, unpasteurized dairy products • *Clostridium difficile*: current or recent antibiotic use, current or recent hospitalization, older adults • *Escherichia coli*: O157:H7 or other Shiga toxin-producing *E. coli* may cause hemolytic uremic syndrome (*see Chapter 9, Lesson 1*) • *Salmonella*: food poisoning, contact with infected turtles and reptiles • *Shigella*: food poisoning • *Vibrio:* raw oysters
Virus	• Astrovirus: most common in winter; spread via contaminated food or water • Norovirus: more prevalent in cooler months; spread via contaminated food, water, or surfaces • Rotavirus: October–April, vaccine preventable, fecal/oral spread, and is found on hands, toys, hard surfaces • Rotavirus: October–April, vaccine preventable, found on toys and hard surfaces
Parasite	• *Giardia lamblia*: untreated well water, or lake/river water • *Cryptosporidium:* waterborne

Table 8.5.1 Causes of Gastroenteritis

Definitions
- **Rebound tenderness:** pain is felt when external abdominal applied pressure is released
- **Starvation stool:** continued watery stool occurring as a result of a prolonged liquid diet

Assessment

Subjective
Note risk factors such as travel on a cruise ship or to a foreign country, drinking well water, camping, recent antibiotic use, crowded living conditions, day care center attendance, or institutional living.

Symptoms
- Nausea, vomiting
- Diarrhea
- Abdominal pain or cramping
- Tenesmus
- Flatulence
- Possible fever (can be quite high with viral infections)

Review of Systems

- **Constitutional:** poor appetite, yet increased thirst, weakness, and malaise; for infants, irritability and disturbed sleep pattern; for children, decreased activity level
- **GU:** decreased urine output
- **MS:** myalgia
- **Neuro:** headache

> **Pro Tip**
> A child who urinated within the past few hours has a minimal degree of dehydration.

Objective

Objective findings may include diffuse abdominal tenderness, slight abdominal distention, hyperactive bowel sounds, anal skin irritation, sticky or dry mucous membranes, sunken eyes, poor skin turgor, and sunken fontanel (infant). Initial tachycardia and normal blood pressure progresses to bradycardia and decreased blood pressure with weak pulses and prolonged capillary refill as dehydration increases in severity.

> **Pro Tip**
> In the older adult, additional signs of dehydration include confusion, dizziness, muscle weakness, and fever.

Diagnosis

The diagnosis of gastroenteritis is based mainly upon the clinical presentation. Blood or pus in the stool is more representative of bacterial infection. Laboratory testing that may be useful in determining the cause of gastroenteritis includes:

- Leukocyte count in stool: elevated in bacterial infection; increased mononuclear cells is characteristic of *Salmonella* infection
- Real-time reverse transcriptase: polymerase chain reaction assay (RT-qPCR), detection of norovirus, rotavirus
- Stool culture: determines bacterial presence
- Stool for ova and parasites: to determine parasitic infection
- Stool guaiac: usually negative with viral infection; may be positive with bacterial

Plan

Treatment

Begin fluid and electrolyte replacement. In adults, use oral rehydration solutions such as Rehydralyte or sports drinks, add saltine crackers as tolerated. In children, use Pedialyte or Ricelyte, giving 5 mL orally every 5 minutes. Progress diet when diarrhea slows. If liquid diets are consumed for too long, starvation stools result.

> **Pro Tip**
> To make an oral rehydration solution at home, use 1 quart clean drinking water, 2 table-spoons sugar, and 1/2 teaspoon of salt. Mix well.

For dehydrated individuals who are unable to achieve rehydration orally, use intravenous (IV) isotonic fluids such as normal saline or Lactated Ringer solutions. Provide 20 mL/kg in an IV fluid bolus to dehydrated children. Dehydrated adults may require as much as 1–2 liters of isotonic fluid for volume restoration.

Resume diet slowly using small, frequent meals. Avoid milk in young children until diarrhea resolves. Continue breast-feeding in infants. The BRAT diet (banana, rice cereal, applesauce, and tea or toast) has not been demonstrated to change the course of the illness, is significantly nutrient-poor, and is not recommended.

In adults younger than 65 years of age, a two-day course of loperamide may be helpful. Avoid the use of antimotility and antidiarrheal agents in children and adults over 65 years of age. Antiemetics may control vomiting episodes, allowing for oral rehydration to be successful. Use only ondansetron in children.

For bacterial infection, prescribe trimethoprim-sulfamethoxazole. *Giardia* may be treated with metronidazole (Flagyl). Nitazoxanide (Nizonide) or paromomycin (Catenulin) should be used for *Cryptosporidium* infection (do not use paromomycin in patients under 1 year of age).

Education

Stress proper handwashing and food handling. Avoid drinking untreated water from wells or streams. While symptomatic, avoid spicy or greasy foods, caffeine, alcohol, and fruit juice and soda (increased sugar content may worsen diarrhea). Do not take non-steroidal anti-inflammatory drugs while symptomatic, as they may contribute to further gastrointestinal upset.

Referral

Refer to physician those patients with rebound tenderness, severe abdominal pain, neurological symptoms, immuno-compromise, or diarrhea lasting longer than 7 days. Refer patients with moderate dehydration not improving with rehydration efforts, patients with severe dehydration, and pregnant patients to the hospital. Infants and young children with paroxysmal abdominal pain and currant jelly stool should be referred to pediatric surgery to rule out intussusception.

Takeaways

- The vast majority of patients with gastroenteritis may be managed on an outpatient basis using appropriate oral rehydration measures.
- Antibiotics should only be prescribed for bacterial causes of diarrhea.
- Blood and pus in the stool may indicate bacterial infection.
- Occult blood is not usually present in the stool of those with viral gastroenteritis.

LESSON 6: GERD/PUD

Learning Objectives

■ Define the characteristics of gastroesophageal reflux disease (GERD) and peptic ulcer disease (PUD)

■ Identify diagnostic criteria of GERD and PUD

■ Select appropriate treatment options for GERD and PUD

Gastroesophageal reflux (GERD) occurs when the reflux of gastric contents into the esophagus causes symptoms or mucosal injury. Reflux by itself does not constitute GERD since non-pathological post-meal reflux is common after meals. Pathological reflux is symptomatic and can involve mucosal injury. A patient may report pyrosis (heartburn), regurgitation, and dysphagia. Pain may occur after large or fatty meals or during sleep.

Peptic ulcer disease occurs due to the action of pepsin and gastric acid and manifests as tears in the mucosal lining of the stomach or duodenum. Though peptic ulcers are most typically seen in the stomach (gastric ulcer) or duodenum (duodenal ulcer), they can occur in other areas such as the lower esophagus or the jejunum. Gnawing or burning abdominal pain is common and can intensify around meals. Those with duodenal ulcers may experience night pain.

ASSESSMENT

Risk Factors for GERD

- **Diabetes:** delays gastric emptying
- **Intra-abdominal pressure changes** caused by pregnancy, obesity, hiatal hernia, and asthmatic attacks may contribute to gastroesophageal reflux
- **Medications:** theophylline decreases lower esophageal sphincter contractility, and medications like iron, antibiotics (doxycycline), bisphosphonates (Fosamax), beta-adrenergic agonists (Albuterol), and NSAIDs can irritate or damage the gastric lining
- **Certain foods:** peppermint, chocolate, tomatoes, citrus fruits, fatty foods, onions, and caffeinated beverages
- **Cigarette smoking:** relaxes the lower esophageal sphincter permitting stomach acid to regurgitate; also believed to damage the gastric mucosa, impair esophageal muscle function, and reduce salivation

Risk Factors for PUD

- *Helicobacter pylori* (*H. pylori*)
- **NSAIDs:** inhibit prostaglandin synthesis causing mucosal damage and potential ulceration
- **Age:** peak incidence of PUD is ages 55–65. Older persons are more at risk for PUD as they are more likely to be long-term NSAID users and at high risk for *H. pylori* infection
- **Medications:** SSRIs, warfarin, and alendronate
- **Other:** alcohol abuse, smoking, Zollinger-Ellison syndrome (hypersecretory state that can damage the gastric lining), and radiation treatments

Subjective

Heartburn is common to patients with either GERD or PUD. Other symptoms differ:

- **GERD:** pain on swallowing, pharyngitis, globus sensation, and sour taste in mouth
- **PUD:** abdominal pain, loss of appetite, feeling bloated, early satiety, and fatigue and breathlessness (secondary to anemia)

Objective

Anemia is common to both GERD and PUD. Other signs differ:

- **GERD:** dysphagia, dysphonia, regurgitation, non-productive cough, peptic stricture, and esophagitis
- **PUD:** gastritis, eructation, blood in vomit or stool, syncope, unexplained weight loss, and postural hypotension

Gastric vs. Duodenal Ulcers

Gastric ulcers and duodenal ulcers have different clinical manifestations. Though these differences in symptoms should not lead to a final diagnosis, they can help focus attention on the suspected area of concern.

	Gastric ulcers	Duodenal ulcers
Pain	Dull, achy pain, directly after eating meal	Gnawing pain, 2–3 hours after a meal, or 1–2 hours in the morning
Eating	Does not tend to resolve pain	May relieve pain
H. pylori involvement	About 70%	About 90%

Table 8.6.1 Gastric vs. Duodenal Ulcers

Alarm Symptoms for GERD

Ongoing untreated GERD has serious consequences: esophagitis, peptic strictures (esophageal narrowing), and Barrett esophagus (where repeated acid damage causes esophageal cells to turn into cells similar to those in the intestine. This latter change is considered premalignant). Additional symptoms (below) should raise alarm:

- Pain or difficulty swallowing
- Anemia or other signs of bleeding
- Unexplained weight loss

> **Pro Tip**
> - Chest pain could also be a sign of angina or myocardial infarction. A myocardial infarction may feature additional symptoms such as diaphoresis, dyspnea, or pain radiating to the patient's arms, neck, or jaw
> - Pathology findings of Barrett's are indicative of GERD, but failing to find evidence of inflammation/erosion on pathological study does not exclude GERD

One out of four patients with PUD suffers a serious complication such as perforated ulcer, hemorrhage, or gastric outlet obstruction. Hemorrhage is the top cause of PUD-associated mortality and occurs in up to 20% of PUD patients.

Alarm Symptoms for PUD

- Family history of GI cancer

- Early satiety after meals

- Increasing difficulty swallowing food/pain on swallowing food

- Repeated vomiting

- Anemia or other signs of bleeding

- Unexplained weight loss

Pro Tip

- Not all patients who are infected with *H. pylori* will develop PUD; not all who have PUD are infected with *H. pylori*

- Nearly a third of older patients with PUD do not report pain

- The strict clinical definition of peptic "ulcer" requires the lesion to be 5 mm or greater in diameter and non-superficial. Without these traits, the lesion may be characterized as an erosion

---

Diagnosis

GERD is typically diagnosed clinically and confirmed empirically (by trialing the patient on anti-reflux medications). However, if complications from GERD develop, other studies may be needed. PUD diagnosis generally involves *H. pylori* testing and esophagogastroduodenoscopy (EGD) as applicable.

GERD	PUD
Diagnosis can be made clinically if the classic symptoms of heartburn and regurgitation are present without alarm symptoms	*H. pylori* testing: ELISA (serum enzyme-linked immunosorbent assay) can be used for initial testing, but the urea breath test tends to follow as a confirmatory test. All suspected PUD patients should undergo *H. pylori* testing, but it is especially appropriate as a first step for patients <55 years with no alarm symptoms
ECG, other cardiac studies if there is cause to suspect a cardiac etiology for chest pain or other adverse symptomology	Esophagogastroduodenoscopy (EGD) is appropriate for patients with evidence of unexplained weight loss, persistent nausea/vomiting, patient's refractory to medications, bleeding, any suspected PUD patient >55 years
Upper endoscopy if alarm symptoms or patient is high risk, i.e., family history of gastric cancer	Barium studies may be used in cases where the patient cannot tolerate EGD or if there is suspicion of underlying gastric outlet obstruction
Ambulatory esophageal reflux monitoring to confirm a hard-to-diagnose case of GERD, in patients who fail to respond to empiric therapy, and pre-surgically	

Table 8.6.2 GERD vs. PUD: Diagnostic Studies

Differential Diagnosis

Differential diagnoses for PUD: **gastroenteritis, GERD, gallstones/bile duct infection, inflammatory bowel disease, diverticulitis, viral hepatitis**

Differential diagnoses for GERD: **PUD, irritable bowel syndrome, achalasia, esophageal cancer**

Plan

Treatment

GERD

- Medical management with lifestyle changes is the gold standard treatment of GERD

    - Proton pump inhibitors (PPIs) such as omeprazole (Prilosec) are the gold standard treatments for GERD

    - Histamine-receptor antagonists (H2 blockers) such as famotidine (Pepcid) are second-line; they are not believed to be as effective as PPIs

    - Antacids such as calcium carbonate (Tums) may be suitable for mild forms of GERD

- Surgical options for refractory GERD include Nissen fundoplication and LINX reflux surgery

PUD

- PUD treatment depends on the cause

    - *H. pylori* eradication—a quadruple regimen (PPI, bismuth, tetracycline, and a nitroimidazole) is usually recommended; an alternate regimen—the triple regimen (PPI, clarithromycin, and amoxicillin or metronidazole)

    - NSAID cessation (unless ASA, an NSAID is used for cardiac prophylaxis)

- Medication management: PPIs, H2 blockers, sucralfate (Carafate)

- Surgical options for duodenal ulcer: vagotomy, partial gastrectomy; for gastric ulcer: partial gastrectomy with gastroduodenal or gastrojejunal anastomosis

> **Digital Resource**
>
> The American College of Gastroenterology maintains guidelines for treatment of both GERD and PUD at its website: **http://gi.org**.

Education

Lifestyle changes for GERD include avoiding heartburn food triggers (such as caffeine), avoiding meals 2–3 hours before bedtime, elevating the head of the bed, and weight loss, which can all help reduce heartburn episodes. For PUD—avoiding night shift work (since studies suggest sleep pattern instability contributes to ulcers), reducing stress, avoiding excessive alcohol. Although researchers now believe that factors such as caffeine and coffee do not *cause* ulcers, such factors can encourage susceptibility to ulcers.

If needed, use lowest dose of NSAIDs and always take with food. Educate patients to use enteric-coated medication.

Referral

A typical referral for GERD and PUD is gastroenterology. Other referrals may include:

- Oncology (if pre-malignant or malignant conditions associated with GERD or PUD develop)

- Other possible referrals include ENT, pulmonology, allergy depending on patient symptoms

Takeaways

- Some risk factors for GERD or PUD may not be avoidable (such as mandated NSAID use for cardiac prophylaxis), but many contributing factors to GERD/PUD (such as excessive ETOH use or smoking) can be avoided.
- Take careful patient histories to ascertain if lifestyle factors are contributing to the patient's GERD/PUD condition or thwarting management of it.

LESSON 7: HEMORRHOIDS/FISSURES

Learning Objectives

- ■ Differentiate between hemorrhoids and perianal/anal fissures
- ■ Identify diagnostic criteria of hemorrhoids and fissures
- ■ Select appropriate treatment options for hemorrhoids and fissures

Hemorrhoids and anal fissures are among two of the most common anorectal complaints.

Hemorrhoidal tissue is vascular tissue that helps buffer the anal canal. Hemorrhoids can develop from hard stools and straining. If the vasculature in the tissue becomes swollen and irritated, the tissue can become tender and is popularly described as hemorrhoids or piles. Internal hemorrhoids (Grade I) may be asymptomatic or may cause bleeding. External hemorrhoids can also bleed. Some prolapse out of the anal canal upon defecation; but reduce spontaneously (Grade II); some are only manually reducible (Grade III); some are irreducible and may even strangulate (Grade IV).

Perianal/anal fissures are linear tears in the skin lining of the anal canal. Perianal/anal fissures may result from increased anal pressure (sitting, pregnancy), trauma (hard stools), or an underlying condition (malignancy, Crohn's disease). Ninety percent of fissures are found in the posterior midline. Those found more laterally tend to be associated with STDs, Crohn's disease ulcerative colitis, tuberculosis, or HIV infection. One possible contributory condition—anal spasm—reduces blood flow to the fissure, making it more difficult to heal.

Assessment

Subjective

A patient may present perianal discomfort, pain, and pruritus; pain associated with anal fissures is typically more intense. Rectal bleeding is common to hemorrhoids and fissures.

Hemorrhoids commonly affect middle aged adults. Increased age, chronic constipation, pregnancy, prolonged sitting, poor hydration, low-fiber diet, anti-coagulation therapy, and portal hypertension are additional risk factors. Fissures most commonly affect infants and older adults. Risks include constipation, trauma, and childbirth.

Objective

Exam may reveal skin irritation, rectal bleeding, especially with defecation and fecal soiling.

> **Pro Tip**
>
> Blood from anal fissures and hemorrhoids tends to be bright red, as it is fresh from the lowest portion of the GI tract. Tarry black stools (melena) or dark red blood emanating from the rectum may be indicative of bleeding higher in the GI system. Occult blood testing, sigmoidoscopy, or colonoscopy may be warranted in case cancer or other conditions are at fault.
>
> Lateral anal fissures tend to be associated with disease conditions. A lateral anal fissure should prompt the provider to consider underlying conditions such as Crohn's disease/ulcerative colitis.
>
> Skin tags associated with Crohn's disease or ulcerative colitis can sometimes be confused with hemorrhoids.

Diagnosis

Diagnostic methods include:

- Digital/physical exam
- Visual exam
- Anoscopy
- Colonoscopy or sigmoidoscopy: typically for patients >50 years of age (unless occult bleeding or personal/family history of colon cancer warrants earlier testing)
- CBC with differential
- Serial fecal occult blood testing

Differential Diagnosis

Differential diagnoses for hemorrhoids: **rectal prolapse, fissure, polyps, skin tags, condyloma acuminatum, Crohn's disease, ulcerative colitis**

Differential diagnoses for anal fissures: **rectal cancer, polyps, Crohn's disease, ulcerative colitis, syphilis**

Plan

Treatment

Treatment options for hemorrhoids and anal fissures are similar. They include increased fiber and water intake, stool softeners or laxatives, analgesic creams (such as lidocaine), and anti-pruritic and anti-inflammatory creams. Topical nitroglycerin or nifedipine are sometimes used for thrombosed hemorrhoids and for anal fissures to promote relaxation of the anal sphincter. Warm sitz baths can reduce itchiness and irritation, and for the anal fissure, improve blood flow, promote healing, and relax the anal sphincter (helping to reduce spasms, which may impair healing).

Hemorrhoids	Perianal/anal fissures
Rubber band ligation	botulinum toxin injection (to promote relaxation of anal sphincter)
Cryosurgery, sclerotherapy	Lateral internal sphincterotomy
Strangulated hemorrhoids can become gangrenous and may need surgical removal (hemorrhoidectomy)	Anal fissures can usually be treated with medication, but if they become infected or even ulcerated they may require more invasive treatment, such as surgery

Table 8.7.1 Treatment Options for Hemorrhoids and Fissures

These conditions are not without complications:

- **Hemorrhoids**
  - Iron-deficiency anemia (from ongoing bleeding)
  - Thrombosis (leading to more pain)
  - Strangulation, gangrene (requiring surgery)
  - Post-surgical fecal impaction, bleeding, urinary retention, UTIs, surgical wound infection, and dehiscence
- **Perianal/anal fissures**
  - Hypertrophied papilla: accompanying internal (anal canal) tissue or sentinel piles/skin tags (external tissue)
  - Chronic fissure formation (can develop with repeated anal spasm or high anal pressure)
  - Post-surgical fecal incontinence

Education

Caution patients with hemorrhoids to avoid overuse of hydrocortisone creams, as these can cause skin atrophy. Remind patients taking fiber products to also increase water intake, as fiber alone can cause worsened constipation. Exercise can also help promote regular bowel movements.

Nitroglycerin ointment/cream is often applied to anal fissures. Educate patients that its vasodilatory effects can include headaches and hypotensive episodes (especially in patients who are already taking anti-hypertensive medication).

Referral

Strangulated hemorrhoids can become gangrenous and may need surgical removal. If conditions such as Crohn's disease are contributory, refer to gastroenterology.

Takeaways

- Hemorrhoids and anal fissures are generally mild conditions.
- Complications and underlying conditions require attention and follow-up.

LESSON 8: HEPATITIS

Learning Objectives

- Define the characteristics of the various types of hepatitis
- Identify the criteria for diagnosing hepatitis
- Select appropriate treatment options for hepatitis

Autoimmune Hepatitis

Autoimmune hepatitis (AIH) is a disease of unknown etiology in which the immune system attacks the body's own liver, often leading to chronic hepatitis, cirrhosis, and liver failure. The most common kind of autoimmune hepatitis (Type 1) can develop at any time throughout the life span, but typically affects teens and young adults. It tends to co-present with other autoimmune conditions, such as Sjögren syndrome, Grave disease, and ulcerative colitis. The second form of autoimmune hepatitis (Type 2) also features autoimmune destruction of liver cells. Type 2 tends to occur in children, be more severe, and co-present with other autoimmune conditions (like Type 1).

Diagnosis involves blood testing and liver biopsy. Symptoms for both forms of AIH can include hepatomegaly, jaundice, pruritic and/or rashy skin, spider angiomas, fatigue, dark urine, abdominal pain, joint pain, clay-colored stools, and appetite loss.

Caught early, both types of AIH can be treated with steroids and immunosuppressive medications. Some patients may progress to fulminant hepatic failure and may require a liver transplant.

Alcoholic Hepatitis

Alcoholic hepatitis (AH) is a form of chronic liver inflammation associated with a heavy intake of alcohol. Most AH patients consume at least 6–7 drinks daily, but AH can present in those who consume fewer drinks daily. African Americans and Hispanics with AH diagnoses tend to fare less well than Caucasians. Women fare worse than men, even with less consumption, due to their reduced body weight and higher proportion of body fat. AH tends to progress over time with continuing alcohol abuse. However, some patients suffer from sudden acute AH, which has a mortality rate of up to 50%.

Patients with mild forms of AH may be asymptomatic. As AH worsens, symptoms can include anemia, abdominal pain, hepatomegaly, jaundice, coagulation dysfunction, esophageal varices, ascites, and variceal hemorrhage. Those with advanced disease may progress to cirrhosis or even hepatocellular carcinoma.

Diagnosis involves taking a patient history (with the caveat that most alcoholics tend to underestimate their consumption), screening with tools such as the CAGE questionnaire (which screens for alcohol abuse), and lab testing. Liver enzymes and gamma-glutamyl transferase are typically elevated, with a ratio of AST/ALT greater than 2 (suspicious for AH).

Treatment is fairly simple: the patient needs to stop drinking. AH tends to resolve after months of alcohol abstinence, although those with more severe AH may end up with some cirrhosis. Detox programs may offer pharmacological aids in alcohol abstinence such as naltrexone (Vivitrol), acamprosate (Campral), or disulfiram (Antabuse). Of note, medications metabolized though the liver (see below) may overwhelm an already compromised liver.

> **Pro Tip**
> About 1 in 6 patients with chronic liver disease are found to be suffering from concurrent alcohol abuse and hepatitis C infection.
>
> It is estimated that anemia is present in over 90% of AH cases.

Drug-Induced Hepatitis

Many medications are metabolized through the liver and can cause medication-induced hepatic damage. Painkillers and acetaminophen are top culprits, but other offenders include NSAIDs, steroids, antibiotics like tetracycline and erythromycin, sulfa medications, statins, and methotrexate. Symptoms are similar to other kinds of hepatitis and include abdominal pain, dark urine, jaundice, and clay-colored stools.

Treatment can be straightforward: discontinue the offending medication. Most patients recover in weeks, but some unfortunate patients can develop liver failure.

Viral Hepatitis

Hepatitis A (HAV)

- **Transmission:** fecal-oral transmission; can also be contracted through food or beverages that have been contaminated by the blood and/or stool of an infected person
- **Prognosis:** symptoms usually show up 2–6 weeks after exposure, and most patients recover in 3–6 months; HAV does not cause chronic hepatitis; in those with weakened immune systems (the very young, the elderly, and those already suffering from liver compromise), adverse complications can develop, such as liver failure or fulminant hepatitis
- **Prevalence:** >180,000 HAV infections are seen in the U.S. yearly, with about one-third of these involving children under age 15
- **Immunization:** vaccines that protect against HAV infection are available; vaccine protects patients for 4 weeks after the first dose, and a booster shot is needed 6–12 months later for long-term protection; short-term protection is also available in the form of an immune globulin, which is about 85% effective in preventing HAV infection within 2 weeks; protection lasts about 3 months
- **Risk factors:**
  - Close and/or sexual contact
  - Travel to a country with a high incidence of hepatitis
  - Poor sanitation
  - Working in a healthcare setting, in sanitation, or in the food industry
  - Close contact with someone who has HAV
  - IV drug/illicit drug use

Hepatitis B (HBV)

- **Transmission:** through blood or body fluids; rarely through vertical transmission
- **Prognosis:** not all patients show symptoms, but for those that do, symptoms tend to appear 2–4 months after exposure; 30–50% of children over age 5 show symptoms, but infants, children under 5 years, and adults with immunosuppression may *not* show symptoms; most (95%) adult patients overcome infection and become immune; in contrast, 90% of infants and 30% of children under 5 who contract HBV will develop chronic infection (infection lasting more than 6 months)

- **Prevalence:** approximately 700,000 to 2.2 million persons in the U.S. have chronic HBV infection
- **Immunization:** universal vaccination of all infants is recommended starting at birth; adults at increased risk for infection (such as healthcare workers, adults with diabetes, and dialysis patients) should also be vaccinated; booster doses of the vaccination are recommended only in select population; additionally, people who succumb to chronic HBV infection who are not immune to hepatitis A should receive two doses of hepatitis A vaccine at least six months apart
- **Risk Factors:**
  - Newborn of infected mother (rare, transmitted during childbirth)
  - Infected person in household
  - Men who have sex with men
  - Injectable drugs
  - Piercings/tattoos
  - Blood transfusion/organ transplant
  - Travel to a country with a high rate of hepatitis B infection
  - Born in a country with a high rate of hepatitis B infection
  - Failed to be vaccinated in infancy
  - HIV positive

> **Pro Tip**
> Hepatitis B vaccination starts at birth. *See Chapter 3, Lesson 4, for the childhood immunization schedule.*

Hepatitis C (HCV)

- **Transmission:** exposure to blood or body fluid; in rare cases, HCV can be transmitted by sexual activity and vertical transmission (mother to baby during childbirth); note, it cannot be spread through breast milk, food, water, or casual contact
- **Prognosis:** six known genotypes of HCV have been identified; >95% of all U.S.-based infections are genotypes 1 (subtypes 1a and 1b), 2, or 3; acute HCV infection can lead to chronic infection, with acute symptoms appearing 1–3 months after virus exposure and lasting 2–3 months; about one-third of patients with HCV will develop cirrhosis, while 5–10% will develop liver cancer
- **Prevalence:** 3.2 million people in the U.S. are estimated to have HCV, with about 17,000 new cases identified yearly; the World Health Organization (WHO) estimates that 15–30% of chronic HCV cases progress to liver cirrhosis; on the bright side, timely treatment with antiviral medication can cure 95% of HCV cases
- **Immunization:** none
- **Risk Factors:**
  - User/past user of injectable drugs
  - Piercings/tattoos
  - Healthcare worker
  - Long-term recipient of hemodialysis treatment
  - Recipient of a blood transfusion/organ transplant before 1992

– Spent time in prison

– Born between 1945 and 1965

– Men who have sex with men (especially men who have HIV+)

Hepatitis D (HDV)

- **Transmission:** through blood or body fluids; rarely through vertical transmission (HDV transmission is the same as for HBV)

- **Prognosis:** HDV may worsen co-existing acute or chronic hepatitis B infection; it can even trigger symptoms in people who had sub-clinical hepatitis B; average incubation period for HBV/HDV co-infection is 90 days, with superinfection in approximately 2–8 weeks

- **Prevalence:** hepatitis D infects about 15 million people worldwide; as it only occurs in a small number of people who carry hepatitis B, HDV exists rarely in the U.S.

- **Immunization:** there is no specific immunization for HDV, but as HDV cannot be contracted unless one first contracts HBV, HBV immunization prevents HDV

- **Risk Factors:**

  – HBV infection

  – User of injectable drugs

  – Vertical transmission

  – Blood transfusions

  – Men who have sex with men

Hepatitis E (HEV)

- **Transmission:** fecal-oral transmission (usually due to drinking water with fecal contamination); much rarer causes include undercooked meat from infected animals or infected raw shellfish, vertical transmission, and transfusion with infected blood products

- **Prognosis:** HEV is self-limited; the incubation period after HEV exposure ranges from 2–10 weeks, with an average of 5–6 weeks; mortality is estimated to be 4%, with pregnant women and liver transplant recipients at higher risk (specifically, pregnant women who contract HEV in their second or third trimester can be at increased risk of acute liver failure, spontaneous abortion, and death); symptomatic infection is more likely to be seen in those 15–40 years, while children can experience asymptomatic infection or only mild symptoms

- **Prevalence:** there are believed to be about 3.3 million symptomatic cases of hepatitis E globally, but HEV is rare in the U.S.

- **Immunization:** there is a HEV immunization available in China, but not yet available globally

- **Risk Factors:**

  – Poor sanitation

  – Area with a high rate of HEV infection

Hepatitis G (HGV)

- **Transmission:** primarily parenteral (as through blood transfusion); rarely, vertical and sexual transmission; virus tends to show up in co-infection with other viruses such as HAV, HBV, or HIV

- **Prognosis:** can be acute but is self-limiting, but some patients have persistent years-long viremia; however, even long-term HGV infection does not appear to lead to liver damage or increased liver enzymes

- **Prevalence:** unknown, HGV is rare and self-limiting

- **Immunization:** none
- **Risk Factors:**
  - Injectable drug use
  - Previous infection with other viral hepatitis

Be aware, some researchers feel that HGV may not be a true hepatitis virus, as it does not appear to contribute to illness in humans. Also, as a point of interest, there is no hepatitis F.

Assessment

The symptoms of viral hepatitis tend to be similar, except in some cases, viral symptoms are self-limited.

Subjective

- Loss of appetite
- Fatigue
- Abdominal pain
- Joint pain

Objective

- Dark-colored urine
- Hepatomegaly
- Cirrhosis
- Elevated liver enzymes
- Hay or white colored stools
- Jaundice
- Low-grade fever
- Nausea/vomiting
- Splenomegaly (in cirrhosis)

Diagnosis

General Tests

- Elevated AST (SGOT) and ALT (SGPT)
- Reduced platelets (may sequester in the spleen)
- Low albumin (due to liver dysfunction)
- Anemia (can result from portal hypertension/splenomegaly)
- Prolonged prothrombin time (PT) may be present in those with severe hepatitis—more than three times normal may suggest fulminant hepatitis
- Ultrasound/CT scan: can show tumors, liver size
- Liver biopsy: evidence of inflammation and cirrhosis
- Elevated total bilirubin

Hepatitis A: immunoglobulin M (IgM) is typically elevated first, during acute illness; immunoglobulin G (IgG) then rises.

Hepatitis B: acute infection can be determined by the presence of HBsAg (surface antigen) and IgM antibodies (such as HBcAb, core antibody). HBsAb (surface antibody) may develop 4–5 months after exposure and is evidence of immunity. HBsAg (surface antigen) persisting past 6 months can indicate chronic infection.

Hepatitis C: a reactive HCV antibody test (anti-HCV) shows evidence of exposure/immune response to HCV but does not signify current infection. This antibody will typically become present 6 weeks to 3 months after infection. HCV RNA shows active virus and is usually detectable 1–3 weeks after infection.

Hepatitis D: HBsAg markers and HDV IgM

Hepatitis E: HEVAb IgM confirms acute HEV and may be detected 2–9 weeks after exposure.

Plan

Treatment
Hepatitis A: HAV is self-limiting and does not require any specific treatment besides supportive treatment, such as bed rest. Patients should avoid hepatotoxic medications such as acetaminophen.

Hepatitis B: for some patients, hepatitis B infection will resolve; they will become immune. Those who become chronically infected may be treated with peginterferon or antiviral medication.

Hepatitis C: the most recent standard treatments for chronic HCV were combination therapies with peginterferon (a drug that boosts the immune system), ribavirin (an antiviral), boceprevir or telaprevir (NS3A/4A protease inhibitors) OR peginterferon, ribavirin, and either sofosbuvir or simeprevir (nucleotide polymerase inhibitors). However, newer highly effective (but also very expensive) medications have now become the gold standard.

Patients with chronic HCV should receive genotype testing because medications regimens can be targeted according to genotype.

Hepatitis C treatment	Prognosis	Possible new medication regimen
Genotype 1	Accounts for up to 75% of U.S. HCV cases. With standard treatment, only 40% of these cases are resolved. With newer treatments, an estimated 95% of HCV patients resolve	Harvoni (ledipasvir/sofosbuvir) boasts a cure rate of up to 99%. Treatment duration can be as short as 8 weeks, but varies depending on factors such as whether the patient already has cirrhosis
Genotypes 2 and 3	Regimens as short as 24 weeks were estimated to eliminate the virus in about 80% of cases	Epclusa (sofosbuvir/velpatasvir) demonstrated 94–99% efficacy in a 12-week regimen

Table 8.8.1 HCV Genotype Treatments

> **Pro Tip**
> Interferon is well known to produce psychiatric side effects of anxiety and/or depression in up to 30% of the patients receiving it, creating a risk for suicide in some patients. It can also cause debilitating flu-like symptoms.

Hepatitis D: some patients may be prescribed alpha interferon for long-term HDV infection. If co-infection with HBV leads to acute liver failure, the patient may need a liver transplant.

Hepatitis E: there is no specific treatment regimen for HEV, as it is usually self-limiting. However, those in vulnerable populations such as pregnant women in their third trimester or patients evidencing fulminant hepatitis should be hospitalized. Rare cases of chronic HEV can occur in immunosuppressed patients: standard treatments for such patients include ribavirin as first-line and interferon as second-line therapy.

Hepatitis G: there is no specific treatment, just supportive care.

Education

Patient education for viral hepatitis may include making the patient aware about immunizations (and the immunoglobin) for HAV and immunization for HBV. For viral hepatitis transmitted by blood/body fluids, the patient should be made aware of the risks of dirty needles (such as for tattoos). For fecal-oral transmission, education about sanitary conditions is key, as is patient awareness of any travel-related risk, such as traveling to countries with endemic HAV.

Referral

- Gastroenterology
- Hepatology
- Oncology (in cases of carcinoma)

Takeaways

- Autoimmune hepatitis can be treated with steroids and immunosuppressive medications.
- Common symptoms of alcoholic hepatitis include anemia, abdominal pain, hepatomegaly, jaundice, esophageal varices, and ascites.
- Treatment for drug-induced hepatitis is to discontinue the offending medication.
- HAV and HEV are transmitted through the fecal-oral route.
- HBV, HCV, and HDV are transmitted through blood and body fluids.
- Immunizations are available for HBV.

LESSON 9: IRRITABLE BOWEL SYNDROME

Learning Objectives

- Accurately differentiate between IBS and IBD conditions
- Identify appropriate pharmacologic intervention corresponding to conditions and symptoms of condition
- Execute patient education on lifestyle behaviors to minimize acute exacerbation

Irritable bowel syndrome (IBS) is characterized by abdominal pain and discomfort accompanied by altered bowel habits. Traditionally, IBS has been defined as a functional bowel disorder lacking the structural or biochemical abnormalities typically noted in irritable bowel disorder (*discussed earlier in Lesson 2*). The psychosocial factors associated with the condition can induce and worsen it; managing these factors is an integral role of therapy.

IBS is typically a diagnosis of exclusion, and relies heavily upon the data collected during the history and physical examination. There are no structural or chemical markers for IBS, which limits the value of diagnostic studies. Its prevalence is estimated to be about 12% of Americans and the cause of 20–50% of referrals to gastroenterology specialists. Seventy percent of cases are women, and frequent comorbidities include fibromyalgia, chronic pelvic pain, chronic fatigue syndrome, migraine headaches, and mood disorders such as chronic depression and/or anxiety.

Assessment

Subjective

Common symptoms of IBS include:

- Change in the appearance or frequency of stools (patients may present with diarrhea, constipation, or both)
- Abdominal pain that is relieved with defecation
- Bloating
- Abdominal distention
- Mucus in the stool
- Fecal urgency
- Feeling of incomplete fecal evacuation

As a quick reminder, irritable bowel disease (IBD) typically manifests as ulcerative colitis or Crohn's disease. Onset of the disease generally occurs between ages 15–40 years. Substantial mucosal lining changes and dysfunction induced by autoimmune activity are the hallmarks of IBD.

Key elements of the medical history to be reviewed with patients when working toward a diagnosis of IBS include past history abdominal and bowel dysfunction during childhood, history of abdominal/pelvic trauma or surgery, or comorbidities noted above.

Objective

The physical exam should include a thorough exam of related systems to assist with the differential:

- **Eyes:** presence of episcleritis or exophthalmia could suggest IBD and/or hyperthyroidism
- **Lymph:** presence of adenopathy could suggest infection or malignancy
- **Skin:** presence of dermatitis herpetiformis can be seen among Celiac disease patients
- **GI:** assessment for scars, bowel sounds, tenderness, and masses are critical to differential
- **Rectal:** assessment for masses, rectal bleeding, ulcerations, stool impaction

Diagnosis

Diagnosis of IBS is driven by history and physical exam. CBC, erythrocyte sedimentation rate (ESR), TSH, and fecal occult blood stools may be helpful in early evaluation, but add little diagnostic value. Positive history findings consistent with either Manning or Rome III criteria, lacking alarm symptoms and a normal physical exam, yields a likelihood ratio of 3:5 favoring IBS.

Diagnostic Criteria for Irritable Bowel Syndrome
Manning criteria
• Onset of pain linked to more frequent bowel movements • Looser stools associated with onset of pain • Pain relieved with passage of stool • Noticeable abdominal bloating • Sensation of incomplete evacuation more than 25% of the time • Diarrhea with mucus more than 25% of the time
Rome III criteria
Symptoms of recurrent abdominal pain or discomfort and a marked change in bowel habits for a least six months, with symptoms experienced on at least three days per month for at least three months. Two or more of the following must apply: • Pain relieved by a bowel movement • Onset of pain is related to a change in frequency of stool • Onset of pain is related to a change in appearance of stool

Table 8.9.1

Differential Diagnosis

Differential diagnoses include: **IBS, Crohn's disease, gluten intolerance, lactose intolerance, endometriosis, malignancy, depression or anxiety**

> **DANGER SIGNS** Patients over the age of 50 and those exhibiting alarm features should be considered for colonoscopy. Alarming symptoms include:
>
> • Weight loss
> • Gastrointestinal bleeding
> • Anemia
> • Fever
> • Frequent nocturnal symptoms

Plan

Treatment

The treatment goal for IBS is aimed at symptom control and improved well-being. A stepwise approach is recommended to minimize need for multiple therapies and medication side effects.

Step 1: Gut Luminal and Mucosal Therapies

- **Dietary modification:** avoidance of food triggers
- **Osmotic laxatives:** polyethylene glycol, lactulose, magnesium products
- **Antidiarrheals:** loperamide, diphenoxylate/atropine
- **Antispasmodics (anticholinergics):** methscopolamine, hyoscyamine, dicyclomine
- **Probiotics**

Step 2: Gut-Directed Regulators

- **Guanylate cyclase C agents:** linaclotide
- **Chloride channel activators:** lubiprostone
- **Serotonin modulators:** alosetron
- **Antibiotics:** rifaximin, neomycin

Step 3: Centrally Acting Agents

- **Tricyclic antidepressants:** amitriptyline, nortriptyline
- **SNRI antidepressants:** venlafaxine, duloxetine
- **SSRI antidepressants:** citalopram, paroxetine, sertraline
- **Other centrally acting agents:** gabapentin, pregabalin, antiseizure agents

Step 4: Adjunctive and Complementary Therapy

- Psychotherapy
- Stress Reduction
- Acupuncture

Education

Patients with IBS benefit from education focused on diet and stress management. A review of diet triggers as well as education on a low FODMAP diet can aid in controlling symptoms. FODMAPs are short-chain carbohydrates that are known irritants of the GI tract. Foods included in FODMAP are high-fructose foods (juice, apples, cherries, pears), lactose (dairy), oligosaccharides (peaches, beans, rye, wheat), and sorbitol and mannitol (sugar-free products). Promoting regular exercise and good sleep hygiene can be helpful when counseling patients on stress management.

Referral

Refer all patients exhibiting alarm symptoms to gastroenterology. Patients who have been resistant to early IBS interventions such as diet modification and medication aimed at symptoms control should also be referred for GI specialty consultation. A consideration of referral to counseling is integral in all IBS patients, given its significant overlap with depression and anxiety.

Takeaways

- IBS is a diagnosis of exclusion; there are no structural or chemical markers for IBS.
- Extensive overlap exists among patients with IBS and mood disorders.
- Demonstration of alarm symptoms requires immediate referral to a gastroenterology specialist for consultation and consideration of a colonoscopy evaluation.

LESSON 10: PANCREATIC CANCER

Learning Objectives
- Identify risk factors for developing pancreatic cancer
- Discuss signs and symptoms of pancreatic cancer
- Choose the appropriate labs and diagnostic imaging for workup of pancreatic cancer

Pancreatic cancer is the fourth leading cause of cancer death in both sexes in the U.S. Most cases are diagnosed in adults over the age of 50, late in the course of the disease once it has spread and symptoms become more specific. Survival varies depending on tumor type and stage at time of diagnosis. In general, prognosis is poor, with less than 30% survival rate at 1 year and less than 10% at 10 years. Metastasis is common to the regional lymph nodes and liver, and less common to the lungs, abdomen, and skin.

Risk factors contributing to the development of pancreatic cancer include:

- Tobacco smoking
- Obesity
- Diet: low in fruits/vegetables, high in red meat
- Increased intake of alcohol, especially in the setting of chronic pancreatitis
- Family history of pancreatic cancer
- History of chronic pancreatitis
- History of diabetes mellitus, especially a recent diagnosis

Definition
- **Magnetic resonance cholangiopancreatography (MRCP):** a medical imaging technique used to visualize the biliary and pancreatic ducts in a noninvasive manner

Assessment

Subjective

The onset is subtle and asymptomatic. The most common presenting symptom is midepigastric abdominal pain that may radiate to the back. The pain may be described as severe, unrelenting, worse at night, postprandial, occurring when lying flat, and relieved when sitting forward.

Nonspecific symptoms such as anorexia, weight loss (may be significant), fatigue, and malaise are commonly reported. A recent diagnosis of diabetes mellitus or acute pancreatitis can be a diagnostic clue.

As the disease progresses, patients may experience diarrhea with greasy, malodorous stools. Severe pruritus and signs of obstructive jaundice, such as dark urine and light-colored stools, may also be present.

Objective

Physical symptoms are rarely found early in the course of the disease. Patients may appear thin and malnourished due to anorexia and significant weight loss. Migratory thrombophlebitis (Trousseau sign of malignancy) or venous thrombosis may be the first noticeable symptom. A palpable gallbladder (Courvoisier sign), ascites, palpable abdominal mass, and hepatosplenomegaly are indications of advanced disease.

Diagnosis

Pancreatic cancer is difficult to diagnose in its early stages. It should be suspected if a patient over the age of 50 presents with abdominal pain, weight loss, and acute pancreatitis.

Lab workup should include CBC, CMP, LFTs, GGT, amylase, lipase, CA 19-9, and CEA, though results are nonspecific.

National Comprehensive Cancer Network (NCCN) guidelines recommend a CT scan in conjunction with an endoscopic ultrasound (EUS) for diagnostic purposes.

Screening guidelines from the International Cancer of the Pancreas Screening (CAPS) Consortium recommend an EUS with either an MRI or MRCP if a patient:

- Has more than two relatives and at least one first-degree relative with pancreatic cancer
- Is a genetic mutation carrier of p16 (also referred to as CDKN2A), PALB2, or BRCA2, with a first-degree relative with pancreatic cancer
- Has Peutz-Jeghers syndrome
- Has Lynch syndrome and a first-degree relative with pancreatic cancer

A consensus has not been reached to determine the age to begin screening or how often one should be screened.

Differential Diagnosis

Differential diagnoses for pancreatic cancer: **AAA, intestinal ischemia, lymphoma, hepatocellular carcinoma, bile duct strictures or tumors, gastric cancer, peptic ulcer disease, pancreatitis (acute or chronic), cholecystitis**

Plan

Treatment

Surgical resection is the mainstay of treatment of pancreatic cancer if diagnosed at a resectable stage. Chemotherapy and radiation play important roles in treatment, as does palliative care for pain management.

Referral

Following diagnosis, depression and suicide rates are extremely high. Refer the patient for psychological services as appropriate. A multidisciplinary oncology team is essential in the treatment of pancreatic cancer. A referral to a dietician may also be necessary, due to malabsorption and malnutrition.

Takeaways

- The prognosis for pancreatic cancer is extremely poor, as most cases are diagnosed after metastasis.
- Primary risk factors include smoking, family history, and a personal history of DM and/or pancreatitis.
- The most common presenting symptoms are midepigastric abdominal pain, pruritus, anorexia, and significant weight loss.
- Diagnostic imaging includes CT scan in conjunction with EUS.

PRACTICE QUESTIONS

Select the ONE best answer.

Lesson 1: Acute Abdomen

1. A 22-year-old male complains of RLQ abdominal pain that started last night. The pain has progressively worsened throughout the night and he is now nauseated and vomiting. Vital signs: HR 110, BP 118/76, RR 16, SpO$_2$ 98%, and temp 101.8°F (38.8°C). Based on this information, which diagnosis is most likely?

   A. Viral gastroenteritis

   B. Acute diverticulitis

   C. Acute appendicitis

   D. Renal calculi

2. Which is the correct description of Rovsing sign?

   A. Palpate RLQ, holding pressure for 30 seconds with palm of hand and then release

   B. Palpate LLQ and patient complains of pain in RLQ

   C. Flex right hip and right knee and internally rotate right hip

   D. Palpate RUQ and monitor for inspiratory pause during palpation

3. Which test is frequently used to diagnose cholecystitis?

   A. Abdominal x-ray

   B. RUQ ultrasound

   C. Urinalysis

   D. MRI of abdomen

4. Which of the following patients is at risk of developing pancreatitis?

   A. 14-year-old female with history of iron deficiency, anemia, and strong family history of alcoholism

   B. 52-year-old female who smokes 1/2 pack per day, diagnosed with breast cancer 1 month ago

   C. 65-year-old male with serum triglyceride level of 1200 mg/dL

   D. 5-year-old with history of formula intolerance and esophageal reflux

5. Outpatient treatment for diverticulitis includes which antibiotic regimen?

   A. ciprofloxacin (Cipro) and doxycycline (Vibramycin) for 10 days

   B. amoxicillin-clavulanate (Augmentin) and ciprofloxacin (Cipro) for 10 days

   C. trimethoprim-sulfamethoxazole (Bactrim) and levofloxacin (Levaquin) for 10 days

   D. metronidazole (Flagyl) and ciprofloxacin (Cipro) for 10 days

6. Maiya is a 42-year-old female complaining of intermittent epigastric pain that she rates as 7/10. The pain started 2 days ago after eating a cheeseburger at a fast food restaurant. She has felt feverish but hasn't checked her temperature. She also complains of nausea and decreased appetite and denies diarrhea, change in bowels, dysuria, or vaginal complaints. Based on this information, you should begin a workup for which diagnosis?

   A. Acute cholecystitis

   B. Acute pancreatitis

   C. Acute diverticulitis

   D. Acute appendicitis

Lesson 2: Crohn's Disease

7. Crohn's disease typically:

    A. Is confined to the colon (beginning at the rectum)

    B. Involves noncontiguous inflammation of all tissue layers

    C. Affects only the mucosal layer of the colon lining

    D. Is noted for its hallmark feature of bloody diarrhea

8. All of the following are risks for IBD except for:

    A. Being of Caucasian or Ashkenazi Jewish descent

    B. The patient's age

    C. Having a first-degree relative with IBD

    D. Alcohol use

9. Bone loss from irritable bowel disease generally results from:

    A. Malabsorption from the inflamed GI tract

    B. Increased osteoblast activity related to insulin resistance

    C. Chronic antibiotic use

    D. NSAID use

10. On physical exam, a 53-year-old Caucasian female patient presents with an anterior perianal fistula, mouth ulcers, weight loss, fever, and crampy abdominal pain. The nurse practitioner will do more testing, but she suspects the patient has:

    A. Ulcerative colitis

    B. Crohn's disease

    C. Diverticulitis

    D. Irritable bowel syndrome

Lesson 3: Colorectal Cancer

11. Which of the following clinical symptoms is most commonly seen with the initial presentation of colorectal cancer?

    A. Iron deficiency anemia

    B. Nausea

    C. Flatulence

    D. Indigestion

12. A 68-year-old male presents to the clinic with complaints of a recent change in the shape and size of his bowel movements, along with lower abdominal pain. He is given a home stool collection kit and is instructed to collect at least two samples from three consecutive specimens. The results are positive for occult blood. What should be the nurse practitioner's next step?

    A. Order a CT scan

    B. Order a CEA, CBC, and abdominal x-ray series

    C. Order a colonoscopy

    D. Perform a DRE to confirm the gFOBT

13. Which of the following statements regarding colorectal cancer is false?

    A. Colon cancer is more common than cancers involving the rectum

    B. Early manifestations include colicky abdominal pain and constipation

    C. Most colorectal cancers are not found during physical examination

    D. Colorectal cancer is the third leading cause of cancer deaths for both sexes in the U.S.

14. All of the following are included in the treatment plan for early stage colorectal cancer except:

    A. Radiation and palliative care

    B. Surgery

    C. Smoking cessation

    D. Colostomy

15. Screening guidelines for colorectal cancer begin at age 50 and include a(n):

    A. Annual DRE and colonoscopy every 5 years

    B. Flexible sigmoidoscopy every 5–10 years

    C. Double-contrast barium enema every 10 years

    D. Annual gFOBT and a colonoscopy every 10 years

16. A nurse practitioner is obtaining a medical history from a patient. Which preexisting condition may lead the nurse practitioner to suspect that a patient has colorectal cancer?

    A. Polyps

    B. Duodenal ulcers

    C. Hemorrhoids

    D. Weight gain

Lesson 4: Constipation

17. Constipation is considered chronic if it lasts longer than _____ weeks.

    A. 8

    B. 10

    C. 12

    D. 14

18. Constipation is defined as hard, lumpy stool that occurs fewer than _____ times per week.

    A. two

    B. three

    C. four

    D. five

19. Based on the Rome III criteria, all of the following are considered diagnostic for constipation except:

    A. Hard, lumpy stool

    B. Straining

    C. Tenesmus

    D. Bright red rectal bleeding

20. A 68-year-old male presents to the clinic with complaints of abdominal pain and increased flatulence. He has only had 2 bowel movements in the past week. You diagnose him with constipation and recommend lifestyle changes for initial treatment. You recommend that he increase his water intake to at least 8 cups a day and ingest how many grams of fiber per day?

    A. 10–20 g/day

    B. 15–25 g/day

    C. 20–35 g/day

    D. 35–40 g/day

21. All of the following pharmacologic treatments have been approved for long-term use in the setting of constipation except:

    A. lubiprostone

    B. docusate

    C. polyethylene glycol

    D. psyllium

Lesson 5: Gastroenteritis

22. A stool culture reveals *Shigella*. What medication should the nurse practitioner prescribe?

    A. acyclovir (Zovirax)

    B. amoxicillin clavulanate (Augmentin)

    C. rimantadine (Zantac)

    D. trimethoprim-sulfamethoxazole (Bactrim DS)

23. Which of the following is true considering the use of antidiarrheal medication for the treatment of gastroenteritis?

    A. The drugs are curative for gastroenteritis

    B. Antidiarrheal medications are not recommended for use in children

    C. These medications help with hydration status

    D. Only bacterial causes require these drugs

24. What type of diet should the patient with gastroenteritis eat?

    A. Slow return to a regular diet

    B. Clear liquids until all diarrhea resolves

    C. Glucose-containing sports drinks

    D. Nothing by mouth until diarrhea resolves

25. A patient has a well at his home. Which of the following is the likely cause of his gastroenteritis?

    A. *Shigella*

    B. *Salmonella*

    C. *Rotavirus*

    D. *Giardia*

26. What should the nurse practitioner recommend to the parents of a 3-year-old with gastroenteritis?

    A. Provide sips of flat soda pop

    B. Allow sips of oral rehydration solution

    C. Nothing by mouth for 12 hours after a vomiting episode

    D. Any fluid she will drink is permissible

27. The nurse practitioner is ordering intravenous fluids for a child with severe dehydration secondary to gastroenteritis who weighs 10 kilograms. Which of the following is most appropriate?

    A. 5% dextrose in water at 35 mL/hour

    B. 3% normal saline at 40 mL/hour

    C. Lactated Ringer solution at 42 mL/hour

    D. Lactated Ringer solution 200 mL bolus

Lesson 6: GERD/PUD

28. A subtle sign of ongoing hemorrhage in silent peptic ulcer disease (PUD) is:

    A. Gnawing abdominal pain

    B. Repeated episodes of hematochezia

    C. Ongoing bouts of orthostasis

    D. Excessive salivation

29. A peak age group most likely to suffer from PUD is:

    A. 14–18, typically due to poor diet and junk food

    B. 20–30, typically due to ETOH use and stress

    C. 55–65, typically due to *H. pylori* infection and NSAID use

    D. 40–50, typically due to disruption of gut bacteria and food allergies

30. Duodenal ulcers often present with:

    A. Pain 1–3 hours after a meal that can typically be relieved by eating again

    B. Pain 1–3 hours after a meal that typically cannot be relieved by eating again

    C. Pain immediately after a meal that can be relieved by eating again

    D. Pain immediately after a meal that cannot be relieved by eating again

31. GERD food triggers include:

    A. Wintergreen

    B. Cheddar cheese

    C. Chocolate

    D. Saltine crackers

32. An undesirable late-onset complication of GERD is:

    A. Testicular torsion

    B. Gastroparesis

    C. Gastric structure

    D. Diverticulum formation

33. Which of the following symptoms is not common to GERD?

    A. Regurgitation

    B. Heartburn

    C. Diverticulitis

    D. Dysphagia

Lesson 7: Hemorrhoids/Fissures

34. Hemorrhoids and perianal/anal fissures have many characteristics in common, yet each condition has unique qualities. Which of the following statements is true regarding hemorrhoids?

    A. Hemorrhoids commonly affect infants and older adults

    B. Risks for hemorrhoids include constipation, trauma, and childbirth

    C. Blood from hemorrhoids tends to be tarry black

    D. Complications may include iron deficiency anemia

35. A patient reports to the nurse practitioner perianal discomfort and pain. The patient has a history of constipation. Which of the following traits has an increased risk for perianal fissures?

    A. Patients aged 45–65

    B. History of trauma and childbirth

    C. Intake of low-fiber diet and adequate hydration

    D. Presence of both internal and external hemorrhoids

36. Rectal bleeding associated with hemorrhoids is usually described as:

    A. Bloody clot with mucus

    B. Dark brown/black stool

    C. Tarry black stool

    D. Bright red streaks with normal appearing stool

37. Treatment for hemorrhoids includes:

    A. Adequate hydration and low fiber to bulk and soften the stool

    B. Cool sitz baths to reduce itchiness and irritation

    C. Analgesic creams for pain management

    D. Oral nitroglycerin to promote relaxation of the anal sphincter

Lesson 8: Hepatitis

38. The nurse practitioner knows the most likely patients to succumb to chronic viral hepatitis of the following are:

    A. Any patients with hepatitis A

    B. Adults with hepatitis B

    C. Adults with hepatitis C

    D. Any patients with hepatitis D

39. _____ is a medication that is not strongly associated with drug-induced hepatitis/hepatotoxicity.

    A. Metformin (Glucophage)

    B. Tetracycline (Sumycin)

    C. Morphine (Roxanol)

    D. Griseofulvin (Gris-PEG)

40. Type 2 auto-immune hepatitis (AIH) usually strikes _____.

    A. the elderly

    B. children and young women

    C. young adults, typically male

    D. middle-aged adults

41. Which is a true statement about viral hepatitis?

    A. 1 in 2 acute cases of hepatitis E will end with liver failure

    B. Concurrent hepatitis B and hepatitis D infection tends to result in a poorer prognosis than hepatitis B infection alone

    C. Hepatitis D can only be contracted by a patient who already has hepatitis A

    D. There is no immunization for hepatitis A

42. The first-line treatment for alcoholic hepatitis is:

    A. Paracentesis for the ascites

    B. Topical steroid ointment for the pruritic skin

    C. Opiates for the abdominal pain

    D. Cessation of alcohol intake

Lesson 9: Irritable Bowel Syndrome

43. Which of the following is more characteristic of irritable bowel syndrome than inflammatory bowel disease?

    A. Fecal urgency

    B. Bloody stools

    C. Weight loss

    D. Tenesmus

44. According to Rome III criteria, a patient diagnosed with irritable bowel syndrome must incur all of the following except:

    A. Weight changes of greater than 6 kg in the past 3 months

    B. A change in bowel habits for at least 6 months

    C. Recurrent abdominal pain or discomfort

    D. Symptoms on at least 3 days per month for 3 months

45. Which of the following is characteristic of irritable bowel syndrome?

    A. It is typically a diagnosis of exclusion

    B. It is induced by autoimmune activity

    C. Diagnosis relies heavily on data from labs and imaging

    D. Diagnosis is confirmed by colonoscopy and biopsy

46. A comorbidity frequently associated with irritable bowel syndrome is:

    A. Migraine headaches

    B. Diabetes mellitus

    C. Obstructive sleep apnea

    D. Cirrhosis

47. Irritable bowel syndrome is more prevalent in:

    A. Women

    B. Men

    C. Elderly

    D. Young children

48. Drug therapy for irritable bowel syndrome is dependent on whether the disorder manifests with diarrhea, constipation, or both. For IBS-D, which drug therapy would be most effective?

    A. eluxadoline (Viberzi)

    B. linaclotide (Linzess)

    C. lubiprostone (Amitiza)

    D. amoxicillin/clavulanate (Augmentin)

Lesson 10: Pancreatic Cancer

49. Metastasis of pancreatic cancer is common to the regional lymph nodes and the:

    A. Liver

    B. Brain

    C. Bones

    D. Kidneys

50. All of the following are risk factors for developing pancreatic cancer except:

    A. Obesity

    B. Family history

    C. History of Addison disease

    D. History of diabetes mellitus

51. The most common presenting symptom of pancreatic cancer is midepigastric pain that is characterized as being worse at all of the following times except:

    A. At night

    B. After eating

    C. When lying flat

    D. When sitting forward

52. A 72-year-old male presents to the clinic with a 2-month history of severe abdominal pain; greasy, malodorous stools; fatigue; and a 20-pound unintentional weight loss. He also complains of dry, itchy skin and was diagnosed with diabetes mellitus 3 months ago. You suspect pancreatic cancer as your leading differential based on which of the following diagnostic clues?

    A. Abdominal pain

    B. Recent diagnosis of diabetes mellitus

    C. Dry, itchy skin

    D. Greasy, malodorous stools

53. NCCN guidelines recommend which of the following to diagnose pancreatic cancer?

    A. CT scan and EUS

    B. MRI and EUS

    C. CT scan and MRCP

    D. Ultrasound and ERCP

54. Patients eventually diagnosed with pancreatic cancer may present with all of the following symptoms except:

    A. Rectal bleeding

    B. Dark-colored urine

    C. Jaundice

    D. Stomach bloating

ANSWERS AND EXPLANATIONS

Lesson 1: Acute Abdomen

1. C

Acute appendicitis **(C)** is characterized by RLQ pain, nausea and vomiting starting after the pain, and elevated temperature. Viral gastroenteritis (A) presents with generalized abdominal pain, and nausea and vomiting precede the abdominal pain. Acute diverticulitis (B) is characterized by LLQ pain and low-grade fever. Renal calculi (D) are characterized by colicky flank pain that often radiates to the groin. Fever can be present if coexisting UTI but not common.

2. B

Rovsing sign is a test for peritoneal irritation associated with appendicitis. The patient experiences pain in the RLQ when the LLQ is palpated **(B)**. If the patient experiences pain after relieving pressure (A), that is an example of rebound tenderness. The obturator sign is obtained by flexing the right hip and knee and internally rotating the right hip (C). If a patient experiences an inspiratory pause during palpation of the RUQ (D), then Murphy sign is positive.

3. B

RUQ ultrasound **(B)** will reveal gallstones, which commonly cause cholecystitis. Gallstones are not radiopaque and can not be visualized on an x-ray (A). Urinalysis (C) would be commonly done to rule out potential differentials, but it is not diagnostic for cholecystitis. An MRI of the abdomen (D) is costly and not always readily available, making it a poor choice.

4. C

The serum triglyceride level of 1200 mg/dl **(C)** is extremely elevated, and elevated triglyceride levels are a risk factor for developing pancreatitis. A personal history of alcoholism, not a family history (A), increases the risk of pancreatitis. In addition, pancreatitis is rare in children (A and D), and iron deficiency anemia does not increase.

5. D

Metronidazole and ciprofloxacin **(D)** are appropriate therapy for outpatient treatment of diverticulitis, and are given in combination. Ciprofloxacin (A) is given in combination with other medications, but not with doxycycline. Doxycycline is not an antibiotic of choice for treating diverticulitis. While both amoxicillin and ciprofloxacin (B) are appropriate therapy for diverticulitis, they are not given in combination. Amoxicillin-clavulanate is given as monotherapy. Trimethoprim-sulfamethoxazole (C) is appropriate therapy but is given in combination with metronidazole.

6. A

Acute cholecystitis **(A)** is characterized by right upper quadrant pain, anorexia, nausea, vomiting, and fever. The pain of acute pancreatitis (B) can be epigastric, but pain is constant and does not follow consumption of a high-fat meal. Acute diverticulitis pain (C) is located in the LLQ. The pain of acute appendicitis (D) is located in RLQ and is constant.

Lesson 2: Crohn's Disease

7. B

Crohn's disease typically involves noncontiguous inflammation of all intestinal tissue layers **(B)**. Ulcerative colitis typically is confined to the colon (A), affects only the mucosal layer of the colon lining (C), and is noted for bloody diarrhea (D).

8. D

Alcohol use **(D)** is not a risk for IBD. Risk factors for IBD include being of Caucasian or Ashkenazi Jewish descent (A), the patient's age (B), and having a first-degree relative with IBD (C).

9. A

Bone loss from irritable bowel disease generally results from malabsorption of calcium (primarily) from the inflamed GI tract **(A)**. Osteoblasts (B) build bone matrix, as opposed to reducing it. Bone loss is from chronic corticosteroid use, not chronic antibiotic use (C). NSAID use (D) does not pose a risk of bone loss.

10. B

The patient that presents with anterior perianal fistula, mouth ulcers, weight loss, fever, and crampy abdominal pain suggests Crohn's disease **(B)**. Ulcerative colitis (A) is typically confined to the colon; it does not affect the oral cavity. While diverticulitis (C) may present with fever, weight loss, and abdominal pain, it does not cause mouth sores or fistulas. Note that irritable bowel syndrome (D) is not the same as irritable bowel disease. While IBS does present with abdominal pain, it does not tend to cause the other symptoms listed. It typically presents with stool frequency changes, bloating, flatulence, and constipation and/or diarrhea.

Lesson 3: Colorectal Cancer

11. A

Upon initial presentation, vague abdominal complaints such as pain, constipation, diarrhea, change in bowel habits, and iron deficiency anemia **(A)** are normally seen. Nausea (B) and flatulence (C) aren't commonly seen in colorectal cancer. Indigestion (D) is more suggestive of GERD.

12. C

A colonoscopy **(C)** is the next step and the diagnostic method of choice. A CT scan (A) may show tumors but is not diagnostic for colorectal cancer. While a CEA, CBC, and abdominal x-ray (B) would be helpful, they are not diagnostic. There is no justification for repeating gFOBT (D) in response to a positive finding.

13. B

Early manifestations of colorectal cancer do not include colicky abdominal pain or constipation **(B)**. Choices (A), (C), and (D) are all true regarding colorectal cancer.

14. A

Radiation and palliative care **(A)** are used for late stage (III–IV) colorectal cancer. Treatment for colorectal cancer stages I–III includes surgery (B), smoking cessation (C), and, very likely, a colostomy (D).

15. D

Screening guidelines for colorectal cancer begin at age 50 for persons of average risk and include an annual gFOBT (or FIT) and a colonoscopy every 10 years **(D)**. A DRE (A) is not a recommended screening method. Alternative screening methods include an annual gFOBT (or FIT) plus one of the following every 5 years: a flexible sigmoidoscopy (B), a double-contrast barium enema (C), or a CT colonography.

16. A

Colorectal polyps **(A)** are common with colon cancer. Duodenal ulcers (B) and hemorrhoids (C) aren't preexisting conditions of colorectal cancer. Weight loss, not gain (D), is an indication of colorectal cancer.

Lesson 4: Constipation

17. C

Constipation is considered chronic if it lasts longer than 12 weeks **(C)**. Answers (A), (B), and (D) are incorrect.

18. B

Constipation is defined as fewer than three **(B)** bowel movements per week. Answers (A), (C), and (D) are incorrect.

19. D

Bright red blood per rectum **(D)** is not part of the diagnostic criteria for constipation. Hard, lumpy stool (A), straining (B), and tenesmus (C) are all included in the diagnostic criteria for constipation.

20. C

The recommended daily intake of fiber is 20–35g/day **(C)**. Answers (A), (B), and (D) are incorrect.

21. B

Docusate **(B)**, an emollient stool softener, has not been approved for long-term use for the treatment of constipation. Lubiprostone (A), polyethylene glycol (C), and psyllium (D) are all approved for long-term treatment of constipation.

Lesson 5: Gastroenteritis

22. D

Trimethoprim-sulfamethoxazole **(D)** is appropriate for the treatment of the bacteria *Shigella*. Acyclovir (A) is an antiviral drug often used in the treatment of herpes. Amoxicillin-clavulanate (B) is very likely to worsen the diarrhea. The antiviral drug rimantadine (C) is indicated for influenza infection.

23. B

Antidiarrheals are not routinely recommended for use in children **(B)** with gastroenteritis. The drugs do not cure gastroenteritis (A). They have no direct effect on hydration (C). It is not only bacterial (D) that require treatment with antidiarrheals, but viral and parasitic gastroenteritis as well.

24. A

Once vomiting has subsided, the patient with gastroenteritis should slowly return to his regular diet **(A)** as tolerated. Continuing clear liquids (B) may lead to starvation stools. The high glucose content in sports drinks (C) may worsen diarrhea. Nothing by mouth (D) would lead to dehydration.

25. D

Of the pathogens listed, *Giardia* **(D)** is the one most likely to contaminate the water supply. *Shigella* (A) and *Salmonella* (B) are common with typical food poisoning. *Rotavirus* (D) is very contagious and quite common in day care centers.

26. B

Sips of oral rehydration solution **(B)** allow young children to maintain their hydration status while suffering from diarrhea and vomiting. Soda pop (A) is not recommended, due to the sugar content contributing to further diarrhea. Nothing by mouth for 12 hours (C) places the child at significant risk for dehydration. Allowing all types of fluid intake (D) is not a correct choice, as fruit juice and milk can both contribute further to diarrhea.

27. D

Severe dehydration requires IV boluses of lactated Ringer solution or normal saline 20 mL/kg **(D)** until improvement is noted. It is inappropriate to use either a hypotonic solution (A) or a hypertonic solution (B). Lactated Ringer solution at 42 mL/hour (C) is appropriate for maintenance of hydration.

Lesson 6: GERD/PUD

28. C

Ongoing bouts of orthostasis **(C)** are a subtle sign of hemorrhage in PUD, in that persistent blood loss can lead to reduced circulating blood, predisposing a patient to postural hypotension. Gnawing abdominal pain (A) doesn't fit the definition of silent PUD, since pain is present. Repeated episodes of hematochezia (B) are a sign of bleeding, but are not subtle and would also not likely be silent since a patient would likely report it. Excessive salivation (D) is not a known sign of PUD, silent or otherwise.

29. C

Duodenal ulcers have been known to strike as early as 25, but overall PUD is considered a disease of older patients, peaking between ages 55–65 **(C)**. PUD rarely strikes under age 40 (A and B), and not for the reasons listed: poor diet, food allergies, etc. Disruption of gut bacteria and food allergies (D) are not common causes of PUD.

30. A

Duodenal ulcers often occur 1–3 hours after a meal and can be relieved by eating again **(A)**. With that, (B) is incorrect. Pain from a duodenal does not come immediately after a meal, making (C) and (D) incorrect.

31. C

Chocolate **(C)** is a known GERD trigger. Peppermint, not wintergreen (A), is a trigger. Neither cheddar cheese (B) nor saltine crackers (D) are triggers for GERD.

32. C

Gastric stricture (esophageal narrowing) **(C)** can result from repeated damage to the gastric lining. Testicular torsion (A) is not a condition associated with GERD, but is caused by twisting of the spermatic cord-cutting of blood flow to the scrotum. Gastroparesis (B) can contribute to heartburn episodes, but is not generally a result of them. Diverticulum formation (D) is associated with diverticulitis, not GERD.

33. C

Diverticulitis **(C)** is not a symptom of GERD. Regurgitation (A), heartburn (B), and dysphagia (D) are classic GERD symptoms.

Lesson 7: Hemorrhoids/Fissures

34. D

Complications from hemorrhoids may include iron deficiency anemia **(D)** from prolonged bleeding. Hemorrhoids commonly affect middle-aged adults; fissures are more often seen in infants and older adults (A). Risks for hemorrhoids include chronic constipation, pregnancy, prolonged sitting, poor hydration, and low-fiber diet; risk for anal lesions include constipation, trauma, and childbirth (B). Blood from hemorrhoids tends to be bright red; tarry black blood (C) tends to be indicative of bleeding higher in the GI system.

35. B

History of trauma and childbirth **(B)** increases one's risk of perianal/anal fissures. Patients aged 45–65 (A) are more at risk for hemorrhoids, not anal fissures. Intake of low fiber (C) puts one at risk for hemorrhoids; adequate hydration is a good thing, not a risk for hemorrhoids or fissures. Presence of both internal and external hemorrhoids (D) has no direct association with anal fissures.

36. D

Rectal bleeding associated with hemorrhoids is usually described as bright red streaks with normal appearing stool **(D)**. While a small amount of mucus in the stool may be normal, blood clots with mucus (A) are suggestive of Crohn's disease. Dark brown/black (B) and tarry black (C) stool may be suggestive of ulcerative colitis and possibly cancer.

37. C

Treatment for hemorrhoids includes analgesic cream **(C)**. Adequate hydration and a high-fiber diet will bulk and soften the stool, not a low-fiber diet (A). Warm (not cool) sitz baths (B) will reduce itchiness and irritation. Topical nitroglycerin (not oral nitroglycerin) (D) is sometimes used for thrombosed hemorrhoids.

Lesson 8: Hepatitis

38. C

Adults with hepatitis C **(C)** are likely to succumb to chronic viral hepatitis. Up to 30% of those who contract hepatitis C will progress to chronic infection. Hepatitis A (A) does not progress to chronic infection. Chronic hepatitis B (B) infection is primarily a disease of children, not adults. Only about 5% of adults who contract acute hepatitis B progress to *chronic* hepatitis B. Hepatitis D (D) is fairly uncommon in the U.S. and few patients are left with chronic disease.

39. A

Metformin **(A)** is not associated with drug-induced hepatitis/hepatotoxicity, as it is not metabolized in the liver—or in fact metabolized at all. It is excreted unchanged through the kidneys. Tetracycline (B) (especially high-dose tetracycline), morphine (C) (most opiates and painkillers), and griseofulvin (D) are all associated with hepatotoxicity and would be used with caution in patients with liver compromise.

40. B

Type 2 AIH is usually seen in children and young women **(B)**. The elderly (A), young adults (C), and middle-aged adults (D) are all incorrect. Type 1 AIH can affect patients through the life span (but often affects teens and young adults).

41. B

Concurrent hepatitis B and hepatitis D infection tends to lead to a poorer outcome **(B)**. Most cases of hepatitis E (A) are self-limited, although certain populations—pregnant women and liver transplant patients—may have worse outcomes. Hepatitis D infection (C) can only occur if hepatitis B infection preceded it. Hepatitis A has two vaccines, making (D) incorrect. Short-term protection can be conferred upon at-risk individuals with an immune globulin injection (such as patients allergic to some component of the hepatitis A immunization).

42. D

Cessation of alcohol intake **(D)** is the first-line treatment for alcoholic hepatitis. Stopping alcohol use will often reverse alcoholic hepatitis, although long-term heavy drinkers may suffer sequelae such as cirrhosis. Paracentesis for the ascites (A) can help with the abdominal discomfort and fluid buildup from ascites, but it will not stop the ongoing hepatic damage if the patient continues alcohol use. Topical steroids (B) can help in reducing pruritis associated with liver dysfunction, but their use will not address the ongoing hepatic damage. Opiates (C) could potentially help with pain, but would probably not be advised for a patient with alcohol hepatitis, as (1) both opiates and alcohol depress the nervous system, potentially leading to respiratory depression, and (2) opiates are used with caution in patients with hepatic dysfunction as they can prove hepatotoxic.

Lesson 9: Irritable Bowel Syndrome

43. A

Fecal urgency **(A)** is typically present in IBS. Bloody stools (B), weight loss (C), and tenesmus (D) could be indicative of IBD and would require further evaluation by a gastroenterology specialist.

44. A

Weight change **(A)** is not a defining characteristic of IBS. A change in bowel habits (B), recurrent abdominal pain or discomfort (C), and symptoms on at least 3 days per month for 3 months (D) are all elements of Rome III criteria defining a patient's condition as IBS.

45. A

IBS is typically a diagnosis of exclusion **(A)**. IBD, rather than IBS, is characterized by biochemical and mucosal lining abnormalities often induced by autoimmune activity (B), which is measured by abnormal lab and stool tests (C). Diagnosis of IBS is driven by history and physical exam; IBD is confirmed by colonoscopy and biopsy (D).

46. A

Frequent comorbidities of IBS include chronic pelvic pain, chronic fatigue syndrome, depression, anxiety, fibromyalgia, and migraine headaches **(A)**. There is no evidence of correlation between IBS and diabetes (B), obstructive sleep apnea (C), or cirrhosis (D).

47. A

IBS is more prevalent in women **(A)**. About twice as many women as men (B) have the condition. There are theories to support the idea that changing hormones in the menstrual cycle may provoke the disorder. IBS can affect people of all ages, but it's more likely for people in their teens through their 40s, rather than the elderly (C) and young children (D).

48. A

Eluxadoline **(A)** is a mu opioid receptor agonist. It also is a delta opioid receptor antagonist and a kappa opioid receptor agonist. The multiple opioid activity is designed to treat the symptoms of IBS-D while reducing the incidence of constipation that can occur with unopposed mu opioid receptor agonists. Linaclotide (B) and lubiprostone (C) are drugs used to treat irritable bowel syndrome with constipation. Amoxicillin/clavulanate (D) is an antibiotic used to treat bacterial overgrowth.

Lesson 10: Pancreatic Cancer

49. A

Metastasis of pancreatic cancer is common to the liver **(A)** and less common to the lungs, abdomen, and skin. Metastasis of pancreatic cancer do not often travel to the brain (B), bones (C), or kidneys (D).

50. C

A history of Addison disease **(C)** is not a risk factor for developing pancreatic cancer. Obesity (A), family history of pancreatic cancer (B), and a personal history of diabetes mellitus (D) are all risk factors for developing pancreatic cancer.

51. D

The pain associated with pancreatic cancer is usually relieved when sitting forward **(D)**. It is often described as being worse at night (A), postprandial (B), and when lying flat (C).

52. B

A recent diagnosis of diabetes mellitus **(B)**, in the setting of the patient's other symptoms, serves as a diagnostic clue for pancreatic cancer. Abdominal pain (A); dry, itchy skin (C); and greasy, malodorous stools (D) are concerning, but not diagnostic.

53. A

NCCN guidelines recommend a CT scan in conjunction with an EUS **(A)** for diagnosing pancreatic cancer. An MRI (B), MRCP (C), and ultrasound and ERCP (D) are not recommended for diagnosis.

54. A

It is not likely that the patient eventually diagnosed with pancreatic cancer will present with rectal bleeding **(A)**. While symptoms of pancreatic cancer are often nonspecific, patients may present with dark-colored urine (B), jaundice (C) (as bilirubin levels in the blood increase), and stomach bloating (D) (as the tumor grows).

CHAPTER 9

GU/Reproductive

LESSON 1: RENAL

Learning Objectives

- Differentiate clinical manifestations of various renal and urinary tract disorders
- Choose and interpret laboratory/diagnostic testing for renal and urinary tract disorders
- Describe appropriate treatment and referrals for renal and urinary tract disorders

A number of disorders may occur within the urinary tract. Disorders primarily affecting the lower urinary tract include cystitis, urinary incontinence, and bladder cancer. Disorders primarily affecting the upper urinary tract are acute pyelonephritis, nephrolithiasis, acute kidney injury, renal insufficiency, and chronic kidney disease (also termed failure).

Cystitis occurs when the bladder epithelium becomes invaded by bacteria, most frequently *Escherichia coli*. **Pyelonephritis** results when the bacteria ascend into the upper urinary tract. **Urinary incontinence** may occur due to weakness of the pelvic floor muscles in women or following prostate surgery in men. It can also result from lack of awareness or inability to reach the toilet in a timely fashion or be transient in nature (related to other illness, medications, etc.). Urinary incontinence may affect quality of life, resulting in social isolation and/or depression and anxiety. **Bladder cancer** usually occurs over the age of 65 years and more frequently in men.

Renal stones (nephrolithiasis) develop secondary to an accumulation of crystals in the urine (the most common being calcium oxalate) and may obstruct urinary flow. **Acute kidney injury** results from either blockage in the urinary tract, decreased blood flow to the kidneys, or direct injury to the kidneys. Decreased renal blood flow may occur with hypotension, shock, myocardial infarction, heart or liver failure, or overuse of NSAIDs. Direct damage to the kidneys may occur with sepsis, nephrotoxic medication use, radiographic contrast administration, vasculitis, acute glomerulonephritis, or hemolytic uremic syndrome. **Chronic kidney disease** is caused by diabetes, chronic hypertension, urinary tract abnormalities, nephrosis (nephrotic syndrome or associated with lupus), or glomerulonephritis.

Definitions

- **Acute kidney injury (AKI):** sudden onset of elevated blood urea nitrogen (BUN) and creatinine
- **Anuria:** absence of urine output
- **Azotemia:** elevation of BUN with or without increased creatinine levels
- **Chronic kidney disease (CKD):** glomerular filtration rate (GFR) is <60 mL/minute for at least 3 months
- **Oliguria:** urine output <400 mL/day in the adult, <0.5 mL/kg/hr in children, <1 mL/kg/hr in infants
- **Renal failure:** kidney functioning is <10% (end-stage renal disease)
- **Uremia:** the accumulation of urea and other nitrogenous wastes in the blood as a result of kidney failure

Assessment

Risk Factors for Urinary Tract Disorders

Urinary Tract Infection (Cystitis)

- PMH of prior urinary infections, constipation, DM
- Urogenital anomalies and disease
- Females—due to anatomy/additional risk with:
  - Pregnancy
  - Spermicide use, anal intercourse
  - Vaginal atrophy
- Males with uncircumcised penis
- Others: catheterization, poor hygiene, age (elderly)

Urinary Incontinence

- Females—h/o vaginal delivery, increased parity; vaginal atrophy
- Obesity
- Older age
- Caucasian
- Caffeine intake and tobacco use

Bladder Cancer

- Cigarette smoking (most significant)
- FH of bladder cancer or arsenic exposure
- Males/advanced age
- Industrial chemical use/exposure; history of cyclophosphamide treatment

Pyelonephritis

- Previous UTI
- Chronic constipation (children)
- PMH: sickle cell disease, DM, HIV
- Incomplete bladder emptying, urinary obstruction, vesicoureteral reflux, neurogenic bladder
- Urinary catheterization
- Pregnancy

Nephrolithiasis

- Males
- Chronic underhydration
- Hypercalciuria, hyperparathyroidism, gout, renal tubular acidosis, cystinuria, cystic kidney disease
- High protein, sodium, sugar diet
- Personal or FH of renal calculi

Acute Glomerulonephritis
- Antecedent skin or upper respiratory infection (post-streptococcal)
- Other: bacterial endocarditis, autoimmune disorders, HTN, DM, viral infections (HIV, hepatitis)

Hemolytic Uremic Syndrome
- Exposure to undercooked meat, unpasteurized dairy
- Recent petting zoo or water park visit
- Prior streptococcal infection

Component	Result
Color	Yellow
Clarity	Clear or cloudy
pH	4.5–8
Specific gravity	1.010–1.030
Glucose	≤130 mg/d
Ketones	None
Nitrites	Negative
Leukocyte esterase	Negative
Bilirubin	Negative
Urobilinogen	Small amount (0.2–1) mg/dL
Blood	≤3 RBCs
Protein	≤150 mg/d
WBCs	≤15–20 WBCs/hpf
Squamous epithelial cells	≤15–20 cells/hpf
Casts	0–5 hyaline casts/hpf
Crystals	Occasionally
Bacteria	None
Yeast	None

Table 9.1.1 Normal Urinalysis Results

Item	Adult value	Pediatric value
Blood urea nitrogen (BUN)	Females: 6–21 mg/dL Males: 8–24 mg/dL	*1–17 years: 7–20 mg/dL
Creatinine (serum)	Females 16 years or older: 0.6–1.1 mg/dL Males 16 years or older: 0.7–1.3 mg/dL	Females *1–15 years: 0.1–0.7 (varies by age) Males *1–15 years: 0.1–0.9 (varies by age)
Creatinine clearance	#Females • 18–29 years: 78–161 mL/min/BSA • 30–39 years: 72–154 mL/min/BSA • 40–49 years: 67–146 mL/min/BSA • 50–59 years: 62–139 mL/min/BSA • 60–72 years: 56–131 mL/min/BSA #Males 19–75 years: 77–160 mL/min/BSA	Reference values have not been established for females <17 years and males <18 years
Glomerular filtration rate	≥60 mL/min	≥75 mL/min

Table 9.1.2 Renal Function Test Results

*Reference values have not been established for children less than 12 months of age.
#Reference values have not been established for females 73 years and older, and males 76 years and older.

App Alert

For more info on GRF/eGFR including eGFR calculator app for iPhone/iPad, go to **www.kidney.org/professionals/KDOQI/gfr**.

Pro Tip
For current hemodialysis patients, assess the arteriovenous fistula or graft for presence of a bruit and a thrill. Do not take blood pressures on the side with the graft to avoid clotting it.

Diagnosis

Symptoms	Objective findings	Laboratory and diagnostic results
Urinary tract infection (cystitis) • Dysuria, urgency, frequency, fever (particularly in infants and children) • May report strong/foul smelling urine	Suprapubic tenderness, cloudy urine	• UA (usually dipstick in clinic setting): positive nitrites, leukocyte esterase, blood, and protein • Urine culture: if recurrent UTI
Bladder cancer Painless/bloody urine (most frequent), urinary frequency, or dysuria (occasionally)	Gross hematuria, abdominal mass if advanced disease	UA: positive blood
Urinary incontinence • Functional incontinence: inability to reach toilet on time/unaware of need to void • Stress incontinence: leaking urine with cough, sneeze, exercise (increases in intra-abdominal pressure) • Urge incontinence: overactive bladder, strong sensation of a need to urinate/ may or may not leak urine • Urethral obstruction: overflow incontinence dribbling post void	• Functional incontinence: limited mobility and/or altered cognition • Stress, urge incontinence, and urethral obstruction: no particular findings	• Ensure negative urinalysis and urine culture • Pelvic exam may demonstrate vaginal atrophy (urge incontinence) • Urodynamic study may assist in diagnosis

Table 9.1.3 Clinical Manifestations of Lower Urinary Tract Disorders

Pro Tip
Elevated BUN with a normal creatinine level may occur with significant dehydration or with a diet very high in protein.

Symptoms	Objective findings	Laboratory and diagnostic results
Glomerulonephritis Swelling of hands or feet, fatigue, decreased urine output, bloody urine, lethargy, anorexia, nausea, abdominal pain	Hypertension, pink/cola/tea-colored urine, periorbital edema, dyspnea, cough, pallor	Proteinuria, hematuria, elevated BUN and creatinine; renal ultrasound may ascertain amount of renal damage; kidney biopsy confirms diagnosis
Hemolytic uremic syndrome Decreased urine output, bloody diarrhea, fever, irritability, fatigue	Hypertension, bruising, edema, pallor	Proteinuria, hematuria, elevated BUN and creatinine, anemia (may be significant), thrombocytopenia

Table 9.1.4 Clinical Manifestations of Upper Urinary Tract Disorders

Symptoms	Objective findings	Laboratory and diagnostic results
Nephrolithiasis (renal calculi) Flank pain (moderate to severe—may radiate to groin), dysuria, frequency, urgency, nausea, vomiting Note: patient may be asymptomatic when stone is in the renal pelvis	CVA tenderness, blood-tinged urine	• Renal ultrasound or CT may verify presence of stones • UA—acidic pH with calcium oxalate stones, alkalotic pH with struvite and calcium phosphate stones • 24-hour urine—calcium citrate, oxalate, other sediment
Nephrotic syndrome Decreased urine output, facial puffiness, weight gain	Widespread edema, foamy urine	Significant proteinuria, hypoalbuminemia, elevated BUN and creatinine, anemia, hyperlipidemia, vitamin D deficiency
Pyelonephritis • Adults: Fever, chills, flank or groin pain, urinary urgency or frequency; nausea or vomiting; may report visible pus in urine • Children: Fever may be only symptom; also nausea, vomiting, diarrhea, poor feeding, irritability	CVA tenderness, guarding	• UA—positive leukocyte esterase; proteinuria • CBC with diff—leukocytosis, neutrophilia, bandemia • Serum procalcitonin level >0.5 ng/mL

Table 9.1.4 Clinical Manifestations of Upper Urinary Tract Disorders (Continued)

Patients with mild to moderate acute kidney injury may be asymptomatic, diagnosed solely by laboratory results (elevated BUN and creatinine, worsening glomerular filtration rate).

Disorder	Symptoms	Objective findings	Laboratory and diagnostic results
Mild to moderate AKI	Asymptomatic		Elevated BUN, elevated creatinine, worsening glomerular filtration rate
Severe AKI and chronic kidney disease	Oliguria, anuria, fatigue, anorexia, nausea, vomiting, weight gain	Edema (may be widespread); bleeding (with hemolytic uremic syndrome)	Anemia, electrolyte/acid-base imbalance, elevated BUN, elevated creatinine, worsening glomerular filtration rate

Table 9.1.5 Clinical Manifestations of Acute Kidney Injury and Chronic Kidney Disease

> **DANGER SIGN** Patients with acute kidney injury or chronic kidney disease may present with uremic encephalopathy noted by neurological symptoms such as a decline in mental status, flapping hand tremors, seizures, or coma. Refer immediately for dialysis in order to decrease the uremia and reverse the neurological symptoms.

Plan

Causes of proteinuria	Next steps
Orthostasis (increased protein secretion when upright—most common in older children and adolescents), fever, increased exercise, stress	Repeat urine protein check on first void upon arising, when afebrile, or compare pre- and post-vigorous exercise urine samples
Diabetes, hypertension, systemic lupus erythematosus, congestive heart failure, vasculitis	Consider referral if kidney damage is progressing
Preeclampsia	If protein >1+, assess for edema, headache, visual changes, hypertension—consult with MFM specialist; monitor urine protein and BP at each visit
Group A beta-hemolytic *Streptococcus*, HIV infection, hepatitis B and C, malaria, viral infections, syphilis	Determine infection presence, treat appropriately
Medication use: ACE inhibitors, allopurinol, amphotericin B, aminoglycosides, antiretroviral drugs, cimetidine, cisplatin, NSAIDs, penicillamine, quinolones, sulfonamides	Monitor protein in urine while on the medication
Substance abuse (heroin)	Refer for substance abuse treatment
Heavy metal exposure	Refer for chelation as needed, and/or to nephrologist if kidney failure present

Table 9.1.6 Approaches to Proteinuria

> **DANGER SIGN** When hematuria accompanies proteinuria, renal compromise is nearly always present. Refer to nephrology.

Causes of hematuria	Next steps*
Pigmentation (medications such as phenazopyridine, quinine sulfate, rifampin, or food such as blueberries or beets), recent circumcision, vaginal bleeding	This is false hematuria; repeat specimen when issue resolved
Collagen vascular disease, hemophilia, idiopathic thrombocytopenia purpura, sickle cell disease, Wilms tumor	Determine known history; further investigate for these diseases if not known by history
Anticoagulant drugs	Refer to urology or nephrology
BPH, cystitis, epididymitis, prostatitis, renal calculi, ureteritis, urethritis	Explore history and physical exam to diagnose causes
Fever, strenuous exercise such as a marathon	Recheck when resolved
Trauma	Abdominal/pelvic CT for further evaluation

Table 9.1.7 Approach to Hematuria

*Patients 35 years of age and younger, with a normal physical examination may need only electrolytes and a CBC, whereas those over 35 years of age should have a more detailed investigation.

Treatment	Patient education	Referral
Urinary tract infection Adult: • Acute, uncomplicated: 3-day course of trimethoprim-sulfamethoxazole; if sulfa-allergic, 5–7 day course of nitrofurantoin (Macrobid); fosfomycin in TMP-SMX resistance • Pyridium for bladder spasm (can cause orange-red color in urine, sweat, tears) • UTI prophylaxis for recurrent infections (≥3 per year); after acute treatment, maintain on PO once daily: trimethoprim 100 mg, cephalexin 250 mg, or ciprofloxacin 125 mg; may also use single-dose antibiotic after intercourse Children: • Uncomplicated cystitis: >2 years old, 3–5 days of antibiotics; 2–24 months, 7–14 days of antibiotics • In a first febrile UTI in infants and children, when urine sterile for 6 weeks, order renal and bladder ultrasound; if abnormal, order a voiding cystourethrogram	• Increase PO fluid intake • Do not stop antibiotic once the symptoms resolve/complete the prescription • Proper hygiene in females and uncircumcised males • Void after intercourse • Cranberry products are not proven to be effective	To urologist if persistent bacteriuria, recurrent UTI, or to rule out bacterial prostatitis in men
Bladder cancer		If suspected, refer to urologist for biopsy and diagnosis
Urinary incontinence • Anticholinergics: tolterodine (Detrol), oxybutynin (Ditropan), darifenacin (Enablex), solifenacin (Vesicare) • Pelvic floor support (i.e., pessary, etc.) • Kegels • Surgery—such as InterStim device placement	• Pelvic floor muscle training • Avoid bladder irritants such as caffeine and alcohol • Decrease fluid intake before bed • Importance of good glycemic control if diabetic • Weight loss if obese	• Urogynecology consult • Biofeedback training

Table 9.1.8 Treatment and Referral Plan for Lower Urinary Tract Disorders

Treatment	Patient education	Referral
Glomerulonephritis • Treat/manage underlying pathophysiology • Address HTN and DM if applicable • Antibiotics, corticosteroids, immunosuppressants may be utilized • Dialysis with renal failure	Sodium, protein, potassium restriction dependent upon lab results	• Refer to nephrologist; kidney biopsy will confirm diagnosis • Dialysis
Hemolytic uremic syndrome Antihypertensives	Sodium, protein, potassium restriction dependent upon lab results	Consult with nephrology and hematology; will likely require dialysis

Table 9.1.9 Treatment and Referral Plan for Upper Urinary Tract Disorders

Treatment	Patient education	Referral
Nephrolithiasis • Analgesics for pain • Alpha-blocker to relax ureter muscle for quicker passage of stone; intravenous hydration if patient unable to hydrate adequately orally • allopurinol (gout)	• Strain/screen urine for stones • Aggressively increase PO fluids, preferably with water and citrus fluids • For calcium oxalate/phosphate stones, decrease oxalate rich foods (rhubarb, spinach, okra, chocolate, etc.); decrease animal protein and sodium intake • For uric acid stones, decrease animal protein intake	• As needed for lithotripsy, ureteroscopy, or percutaneous nephrolithotomy • ER admission for patients with fever/chills, severe pain, acute renal failure
Nephrotic syndrome Sodium restriction during active disease • Diuretics • ACE inhibitors or ARBs • Anticoagulant therapy if needed • Monitor kidney function/electrolytes	• Weigh daily • Signs/symptoms of thrombus & DVT	Refer to nephrologist, possibly hematology
Pyelonephritis • Adults: ciprofloxacin 500 mg twice daily for 7 days, or levofloxacin 750 mg once daily for 5–7 days, or trimethoprim-sulfamethoxazole (TMP-SMX) 160 mg and 800 mg twice daily for 7–10 days; do not use nitrofurantoin • Children >3–6 months who are well hydrated, not vomiting, and without abdominal pain: oral cefixime, cefdinir, or ceftibuten for 7–14 days or once daily IM gentamicin or ceftriaxone until afebrile 24 hours, then switch to oral antibiotic For outpatient management, short term surveillance in 12–24 hrs	Encourage hydration • Return to office if fever persists >48 hrs after antibiotic initiated • Increase PO fluids	• Uncomplicated cases may be treated as outpatient; otherwise, inpatient evaluation/treatment is needed • Appropriately refer for pregnant women, children, elderly patients
Acute kidney injury and chronic kidney disease • Treatment will be based on Stage (1–5) • Discontinue any nephrotoxic meds • Antihypertensive therapy, erythropoietin if Hgb <20 g/dL • Address fluid/electrolyte imbalances	• Low sodium, low potassium, low protein diet as prescribed • Avoids NSAIDs and imaging contrast dye/agents • Importance of managing HTN and/or DM if applicable	Nephrology consult; referral—dialysis if GFR 15–29 mL/min

Table 9.1.9 Treatment and Referral Plan for Upper Urinary Tract Disorders (Continued)

DANGER SIGN Worsening kidney injury results in further decreases in urine output, blood in the urine, and increased edema, fatigue, nausea, and vomiting. Instruct patient to report these changes.

Takeaways

- Uncomplicated cases of urinary tract infection in children and adults may be treated with a short course of antibiotics.

- In general, UTIs are not expected in male patients—look for other pathology/underlying etiology.

- In addition to the use of anticholinergic medication, urge incontinence may be managed with pelvic floor strengthening, avoidance of caffeine and alcohol ingestion, and glycemic control in diabetes.

- When hematuria accompanies proteinuria, renal damage is nearly always present. Refer to nephrology.

LESSON 2: MEN'S HEALTH

Learning Objectives

- ■ Identify pertinent questions to include in a review of systems of the male patient
- ■ Diagnose and treat the most common anogenital, breast, scrotal, sexual, and urinary complaints of male patients
- ■ Define common presentation of testicular torsion
- ■ Order the appropriate screening tests based on age and risk factors

Adult male health focuses on conditions that specifically relate to and affect the male reproductive organs. The NP must be able to safely and accurately diagnose and treat these concerns, as some may lead to serious complications such as infertility and even death. Understanding the most common male complaints is the first step toward providing patients with best care.

Definitions

- **Anorchia:** absence of both testicles
- **Asthenozoospermia:** decreased sperm motility
- **Azoospermia:** absent sperm
- **Cryptorchidism:** failure of one or both testicles to descend into the scrotum
- **Cremasteric reflex:** contraction of the scrotum in response to stroking the inner thigh
- **Epididymitis:** inflammation of the epididymis
- **Epispadias:** urethral development above its typical placement
- **Hypospadias:** urethral development below its typical placement
- **Infertility:** inability to conceive after 1 year of timed or frequent unprotected intercourse
- **Oligospermia:** low sperm count
- **Orchitis:** inflammation of the testicles; may involve either one or both
- **Paraphimosis:** occurs with excessive inflammation of the glans penis that pushes the foreskin down and keeps it beneath the glans, causing further pain and inflammation

Assessment

Subjective

Health History

A complete adult male health history should include, but not be limited to, the following:

- **Allergies** to medications
- **PMH:** cancer of the prostate or testicles, congenital anomalies of the urethra (hypospadias, epispadias) or testicles (anorchia, cryptorchidism, undescended testes), depression, diabetes, heart disease, infertility, STIs, urinary retention, urinary tract infection(s)
- **PSH:** surgeries involving the penis, prostate, testicles, or contiguous structures
- **FH:** cancer of the breast, colon, prostate, or testicles; diabetes, heart disease (include ages of diagnosis when known)
- **SH:** alcohol, drug and tobacco use, sexual partner and gender preference, intimate partner violence screen, exercise habits
- **Current medications**, including compliance and satisfaction with those medications

Review of Systems

An adult male health-focused ROS should include, but not be limited to, the following:

- Recent fever, chills, body aches, swollen lymph nodes
- Fatigue, loss of libido, or lack of interest in intimacy
- New onset back or abdominal pain
- Change in urinary frequency, urgency or pressure, difficulty either initiating a urine stream or emptying the bladder, hematuria, abnormal penile discharge
- Difficulty generating or maintaining an erection
- Painful intercourse
- Anogenital lesions
- Penile or testicular malformations

Objective

The physical exam should be focused on the patient's chief complaint (CC). Assessments should include evaluation of the body systems above and below the area of concern. An example of a focused exam for a CC of scrotal pain is as follows:

- **VS:** BP, height, weight, BMI
- **General:** well appearing and in no acute distress
- **MS:** no CVAT
- **GI:** soft, non-tender × 4 quadrants
- **GU:** penis with no noted anomalies, varicosities are seen on the distal side of the left side of the scrotum; pain was reproduced with standing and resolved in the sitting position; bilateral testicles palpable, smooth, round, mobile and non-tender; vas deferens without abnormality; prostate normal size, non-tender

Diagnosis

Anogenital Lesions and Dermatoses

	Subjective	Objective	Diagnostic test
Chancroid	Sore(s) on the genital area	• Ulcerating lesion(s) on the genitals • Common on foreskin and the tip of the penis	Bacterial culture for *H. ducreyi*
Balanitis	Penile itching, irritation, or pain	• Redness of the glans penis • May see evidence of yeast or bacterial infection, depending on cause	• Physical exam • Testing for yeast and STIs to rule out causative pathogens
Herpes Simplex Virus 1/2	• Penile or anal itching, burning, or pain • "Bump(s)" on penis • Painful urination	Ulcerating lesion(s), may be in varying stages of healing, painful to touch	Viral culture for HSV 1/2
Human Papilloma Virus (genital warts)	Growth on penis, perineum, or near the anus	Flesh-colored growth(s) of varying presentations	• Physical exam • Skin biopsy may be useful in some cases
Primary syphilis	Painless "sore" or "bump" anywhere in anogenital region	• Single lesion, also known as a "chancre" • Swollen lymph nodes proximal to chancre common	Serum nontreponemal (screening) test with reflex treponemal (diagnostic) test

Table 9.2.1 Common Anogenital Lesions and Dermatoses

Breast Complaints

- **Gynecomastia:** complaints of thickened breast tissue or breast swelling (can be unilateral or bilateral); order a diagnostic mammogram and breast ultrasound to rule out pathology
- **Male breast cancer:** complaints of non-painful, hard mass; noted palpable mass, often underneath the areola; tissue biopsy to confirm diagnosis
- **Prolactinoma:** complaints of nipple discharge, enlarged breasts, and sexual dysfunction; noted reproducible leaking of fluid from the nipples; diagnosed with serum prolactin level >20 ng/dL, MRI for detection of pituitary tumor

Refer to Chapter 9, Lesson 3, for more information related to breast assessment, imaging, diagnosis, and management.

Scrotal Complaints

- **Acute epididymitis:** complaints of diffuse scrotal pain and urinary urgency, frequency, and pressure; on exam, painful, tender, and swollen scrotum (epididymo-orchitis); diagnosed by history (recent trauma, history of aggravating factors that may cause reflux of urine into the epididymis), bacterial cultures for *C. trachomatis* and *N. gonorrhea*, and urinalysis with culture
- **Testicular cancer:** complaints of painless, swollen, or enlarged testicle; on exam, palpable, non-tender mass; diagnosed with ultrasound or MRI
- **Varicocele:** complaints of scrotal pain, worse with standing, better at rest; history of infertility; on exam, appearance of varicose veins in the scrotum; diagnosed with physical exam and scrotal ultrasound

> **DANGER SIGN**
>
> **Testicular torsion:** sudden onset of severe pain and/or swelling of the testes. Left uncorrected, it can cause irreversible ischemia, leading to the loss of the affected testicle. Pain may be intermittent (due to twisting and un-twisting of testes) or constant (due to a full twist and the associated ischemia).
>
> Other symptoms include: fever, abdominal pain, and dysuria. Diagnosed by scrotal ultrasound. Surgery may be required for treatment.
>
> **Priapism:** painful, persisting erection (>4 hours); may be related to a side effect of ED medication; however, may not be associated with sexual activity and can be caused by other medical condition; represents a medical emergency.

Sexual Dysfunction

Condition	Subjective	Objective	Diagnostic tests
Ejaculatory disorders premature retrograde	• Ejaculating quickly (≤1 minute) • Anxiety related to the above symptoms; retrograde ejaculation typically occurs after surgery for BPH	Normal exam	• Patient's description of events • Thorough history (1 in 3 men with PE also have ED) • Urine culture and serum testosterone to rule out pathology
Erectile dysfunction (ED)	• Inability to produce or maintain an erection • Inability to ejaculate	• Vascular ED: auscultation of bruit in bilateral femoral arteries • Hypogonadism: testes and hair are smaller/lighter than expected for the patient's age; gynecomastia may be present; peripheral vision may be compromised in patients with a pituitary tumor • Impaired cremasteric reflex may be present in patients with compromised thoracolumbar erection center	• Physical exam findings guide the need for further testing • Blood work may be necessary to identify underlying cause (examples: diabetes, hypertension, hypogonadism)
Peyronie disease	• Curved penis • Painful erection • May be unable to have intercourse or unable to maintain erection	• Degree of bend & direction can vary • May shorten penile length	• History & exam findings • Ultrasound
Low testosterone	• Fatigue • Loss of/lowered libido	Typically, no physical impairments noted	Serum total testosterone <300
Sperm malfunction *Asthenospermia* *Azoospermia* *Oligospermia*	Infertility	Typically, no physical impairments noted	Semen analysis

Table 9.2.2 Sexual Dysfunction

Urinary Symptoms
Acute and chronic prostatitis

- Complaints of urinary urgency, frequency, pressure, difficulty emptying, dysuria, turbid urine, hematuria; penile/testicular/perineal pain; abdominal/pelvic/groin pain; painful ejaculation; fever, chills, body aches
- On exam: swollen, firm, warm, and extremely tender prostate
- Diagnosed by urinalysis with culture

Benign prostatic hyperplasia (BPH)

- Complaints of urinary frequency with incomplete emptying; urinary urgency, frequency; hematuria or hematospermia
- On exam: enlarged prostate on exam, may have a rubber-like texture
- Diagnosed by digital rectal exam

Prostate cancer

- Often asymptomatic
- On exam, enlarged prostate
- Diagnosed by digital rectal exam; biopsy is most specific; serum prostate-specific antigen (PSA) is controversial, as it is highly sensitive

Urethral stricture

- Complaints of multiple UTIs, difficulty emptying bladder despite feeling of urgency (which may lead to urinary frequency), decreased urine stream, spraying of urine, slower speed of ejaculation
- Exam may be normal
- Diagnosed by uroflowmetry, post-void bladder ultrasound

Urethritis *Gonococcal/Nongonococcal*

- Complaints of abnormal urethral discharge, dysuria, postcoital penile itching or burning; acute epididymitis or lymphogranuloma venereum often present with *C. trachomatis*
- On exam, urethral meatus may be red or swollen; clear or mucopurulent discharge may be visible (may be produced with gentle pressure toward the glans)
- Diagnosed by urinalysis with culture; urethral cultures for *N. gonorrhea, C. trachomatis,* and *trichomonads*

Plan

Routine Screening Tests and Treatment

Only a few screening tests specifically relate to the male reproductive system: testing for prostate and testicular cancers as well as sexually transmitted infections.

Treatment of the most common male concerns is multifaceted, as the complaint may not be reflective of the ultimate diagnosis. Some of the diagnoses relate to body systems that have been covered in other chapters, and when appropriate will be identified as such.

Age	Test	Frequency of testing
Male breast cancer	• Self breast exam • BRCA gene testing	• Men with elevated breast cancer risk (strong family history, obesity, alcoholism and liver disease, age >65, Klinefelter syndrome) should consider monthly breast self-exams • Men with a family history of BRCA gene mutation should consider speaking with a genetic counselor about their individual risk and the pros and cons of BRCA gene testing (American Cancer Society [ACS])
Prostate cancer	• PSA • Digital rectal exam	• Individuals with elevated risk (African American men and men with a family history of prostate CA) should start discussing pros and cons of testing at age 45 • The general population should start this conversation at age 50 (ACS)
		• Age <40 or >70: Screening not typically recommended • Age 40–55: Screen based on individual risk only • Age 55–69: Men should discuss risks and benefits of testing with their providers before deciding whether to proceed (American Urologic Association [AUA])
		Do not use PSA to screen for prostate cancer, as it is associated with over-diagnosis. Also, at this time, the risks associated with treatment by radiotherapy and/or surgery outweigh the risks of having undiagnosed prostate cancer (U.S. Preventive Services Task Force [USPSTF])
Testicular cancer	• Self testicular exam • Clinical testicular exam	Men with higher risk (history of cryptorchidism without pre-pubertal surgical correction, previous personal history, or strong family history of testicular cancer) may benefit from monthly self-testicular exams (ACS)
		Men with a history of cryptorchidism: monthly self testicular exams (AUA)
		Asymptomatic men should not be screened (USPSTF, American Academy of Family Physicians, American Academy of Pediatrics)

Table 9.2.3 Adult Male Health Cancer Screening Guidelines

Refer to Chapter 6, Lesson 4, for lung cancer screening guidelines and Chapter 8, Lesson 3, for colon cancer screening guidelines.

Benign Prostatic Hyperplasia (BPH)

Treatment of BPH should be considered for individuals who are experiencing a significant alteration in quality of life due to their condition.

Behavioral modifications	Medications
• Avoidance of food and beverages that have a diuretic effect and bladder irritants, such as caffeine and alcohol • Avoidance of medications with anticholinergic properties such as antihistamines, tricyclic antidepressants, and opioids, that may cause urinary retention • Urinating twice in a row so that the bladder may be emptied completely • Decreasing oral intake of fluids before departing any location and prior to sleeping	• Alpha 1 adrenergic antagonists: terazosin, doxazosin, alfuzosin, tamsulosin, silodosin • 5-alpha-reductase inhibitors: finasteride, dutasteride; may also be used in conjunction with tamsulosin • Anticholinergic agents: (*refer to Chapter 9, Lesson 1*) • Phosphodiesterase-5 inhibitor*: tadalafil; may be used in combination with finasteride** • Herbal remedies: not recommended despite popular use

Table 9.2.4 Behavioral and Medication Management of BPH

*Do not prescribe for men with a creatinine clearance of <30 mL/min.
**When tadalafil and finasteride are used together, treatment should be ≤26 weeks.

Sexual Dysfunction

Treatment of sexual dysfunction aims to improve a man's ability to achieve and maintain an erection, improve sexual desire, and prevent premature ejaculation.

Condition	Treatment
Ejaculatory disorders Premature ejaculation	• Selective serotonin reuptake inhibitors (SSRIs) (first-line): paroxetine, sertraline, fluoxetine, citalopram • Serotonergic tricyclic antidepressant (only if patient is intolerant of SSRIs): clomipramine • Analgesic: tramadol 1–2 hours prior to intercourse • Other: topical anesthetics or creams may help diminish sensation • Therapy in combination with medication appears to be most effective treatment
Erectile dysfunction	Phosphodiesterase-5 (PDE) inhibitors: sildenafil, vardenafil, tadalafil, avanafil (30 minutes to 1 hour before intimacy)
Decreased libido	• Psychotherapy • Testosterone replacement therapy • If safe to do so, stop use of medications with this side effect (SSRIs, opioids)
Low testosterone	Testosterone replacement therapy

Table 9.2.5 Management of Sexual Dysfunction

Uro-Genital Infections
Non-Sexually Transmitted Infections

Balanitis may result from poor hygiene (treatment: wash with saline solution twice per day) or *Candida* (treatment: clotrimazole or miconazole); balanitis typically occurs in uncircumcised men; severe cases may lead to paraphimosis. Treatment for acute and chronic epididymitis includes ice, elevation, NSAIDs, and antibiotics (with consideration for the individual at risk for STIs and those engaging in anal sex).

Sexually Transmitted Infections

Men should be tested for STIs based on risk factors. The frequency of testing is also influenced by number of partners and whether or not he is using condoms. STI blood work should be considered in addition to cultures for men who have sex with men.

Treatment of the following STIs is the same for both men and women (*refer to Chapter 9, Lesson 4*).

Urinary Tract Infections

Treatment of urinary tract infections is covered in Chapter 4, Lesson 2.

Male Fertility Control Methods

Method	First year failure rate	Considerations
Condoms	• Perfect use: 3% • Typical: 14%	• Convenient • May dull sexual pleasure
Vasectomy	• Perfect use: 0.10% • Typical use: 0.15%	• Outpatient procedure • Performed by specialist • Some degree of pain following the procedure (may be treated with ice and NSAIDs) • 3-month gap between the procedure and complete sterilization • Permanent

Table 9.2.6 Male Fertility Methods

Education
- Proper genital hygiene: should be reviewed with at-risk individuals
- Sexual health: yearly discussion of condom use, STI prevention, relationship safety

Referral
- Malformations or strictures associated with the urinary tract, cancer, male factor infertility, paraphimosis: urologist
- Palpable breast mass: breast surgeon
- Pituitary tumor: ophthalmologist, endocrinologist, neurosurgeon

Takeaways
- Healthcare that is specific to the adult male involves evaluation and treatment of the reproductive organs and surrounding structures.
- Patients may present with symptoms that only reflect a small portion of a larger problem.
- Follow-up is often necessary to evaluate efficacy of treatment.

LESSON 3: BREAST

> ### Learning Objectives
> - Create a treatment plan for a patient with a breast problem
> - Determine and order appropriate breast imaging
> - Identify when referral for further evaluation is needed

Given that breast cancer is the most common cancer in women, the nurse practitioner must be diligent in evaluating, treating, and/or referring patients with abnormal breast findings. In addition, patients (both male and female) do present with episodic complaints dealing with specific breast issues/problems.

Assessment

Subjective
- Pertinent information to elicit: PMH or FH of breast cancer; any prior breast biopsy or surgery; past exposure to chest wall irradiation (such as part of treatment for Hodgkin lymphoma); if the patient is pregnant or lactating

> **Digital Resource**
>
> Calculate your patient's lifetime risk of a sporadic breast cancer using these free resources:
>
> - Gail score: **www.cancer.gov/bcrisktool**
> - Tyrer-Cuzick: **www.ems-trials.org/riskevaluator**
> - Multiple models including Gail, BRCAPRO, Claus and Tyrer-Cuzick: **www.hughesriskapps.com**
>
> Identify patients who should consider genetic testing due to a PMH and/or FH of certain cancers:
>
> - National Comprehensive Cancer Network: **www.nccn.org/professionals/physician_gls/f_guidelines.asp#detection** (this site is also free but requires the user to create a username and password)

Breast Pain

- Location: specific area of a breast vs. global pain; unilateral vs. bilateral pain
- Timing: pain related to menses/cyclical; new initiation of hormone replacement therapy or hormone-based contraception
- Frequency/intensity/duration
- Associated aggravating or alleviating factors

Nipple Discharge

- Note if the discharge is spontaneous or elicited with compression
- Update the patient's medication history—certain medications can contribute to nipple discharge

> **Pro Tip**
> Bilateral, multicolored nipple discharge as well as discharge only elicited with compression are usually benign variants.

Breast Mass and/or Skin Change

- Determine how long the patient has appreciated the finding on self-exam
- Have the patient describe size/shape/texture
- Note if the finding has increased, decreased, or remained stable in size

Infection

Mastitis is commonly associated with breastfeeding. However, breastfeeding is not a requirement for a breast infection, and mastitis can occur in male and female patients. Examples include an infected breast cyst, subareolar abscess (common in smokers), infected nipple piercing(s), etc. In addition to the subjective information regarding pain, discharge, mass, and skin change (noted above), you also need to determine the following:

- Is the patient pregnant or breastfeeding?
- Are systemic symptoms such as fever, nausea, or diarrhea present?

> **DANGER SIGN** Inflammatory Breast Cancer (IBC) is always a differential diagnosis if your patient presents with an erythematous, edematous breast.

Objective

Inspection

- Symmetry: mild asymmetry is a normal variation; a breast should not appear distended with edematous skin and/or erythema
- Peau d'orange is a suspicious finding; although this can be seen with mastitis, it raises a red flag for breast cancer
- Retraction of the nipple or retraction/dimpling of a focal area of the breast is an abnormal finding
- Nipple discharge: elicited from a central duct vs. multiple ducts; discharge can vary in color from clear to white, from yellow to green, from rust-colored to bright red/overt blood
- Crusted skin/lesions could represent eczema or contact dermatitis, but Paget's disease would be a differential diagnosis
- Sebaceous cysts, epidermal inclusion cysts, folliculitis and hidradenitis suppurativa can involve the skin of the breast

- An ulcerated lesion is not an expected finding; this could represent skin involvement from an invasive breast cancer
- Document location/size/shape of any skin lesion or skin color change

> **Pro Tip**
> An advantage of EMR is the ease of downloading digital photos into the patient's chart. Photograph your patient's breast finding(s) to have as a comparative baseline.

Palpation

- Palpate all 4 quadrants and the retroareolar aspect; breast tissue can vary from firm to dense; areas of nodular tissue/nodularity are a normal variation
- If a mass is present, document location/size/shape as well as noting if the mass is either mobile or fixed; tender or non-tender
- In addition, palpate the axilla as well as the supraclavicular fossa to assess for adenopathy
- If the breast is erythematous, palpate to assess for warmth as well as tenderness

Diagnosis

The clinical findings and pertinent imaging studies (see "Plan" below) will assist you in making a diagnosis.

Differential Diagnosis

Mastodynia, gynecomastia, breast mass, breast cyst, diffuse cystic mastopathy (fibrocystic change), skin/nipple change, nipple discharge, mastitis, abscess, localized/regional adenopathy, breast cancer

Plan

Mastodynia

- The etiology of breast pain is usually benign/physiologic, such as fibrocystic breast change
- Order age-appropriate/risk-appropriate imaging studies (see below)
- Comfort measures: decrease caffeine intake, daily primrose oil supplementation and/or vitamin E, essential oils (such as lavender or peppermint), OTC anti-inflammatory PRN, good bra support
- If imaging studies are negative for correlation, have the patient RTC in 2–3 months to assess for regression/resolution of symptoms; if pain persists or worsens rather than improves, refer to a breast specialist

Nipple Discharge

- Perform a hemoccult of the nipple discharge to rule out occult blood
- Assess prolactin and TSH levels—especially if the discharge is bilateral and milky
- Order age-appropriate/risk-appropriate imaging studies (see below)
- If the above points are negative, advise the patient to avoid compressing/checking for the nipple discharge and have the patient RTC for short-term clinical surveillance in 2–3 months; if symptoms persist or progress, refer to a breast specialist

> **DANGER SIGN** Unilateral, spontaneous, clear to bloody discharge requires further imaging evaluation and referral to a breast specialist.

Breast Mass

- Order age-appropriate/risk-appropriate imaging studies (see below)
- Refer the patient to a breast specialist for further evaluation, even if the imaging study is negative as breast cancer is always a differential diagnosis

Mastitis

- Order age-appropriate/risk-appropriate imaging studies (see below); for the breastfeeding woman, do not order mammography—rather, begin with breast ultrasound
- Appropriate course of antibiotic therapy, such as: dicloxacillin, trimethoprim/sulfamethoxazole (Bactrim), or clindamycin (Cleocin); Bactrim should not be used in women who are breastfeeding infants <2 months of age
- OTC anti-inflammatory for discomfort PRN
- For the breastfeeding woman, consider referral to a lactation specialist; measures/teaching to consider include:
  - Massage or apply warm compresses prior to nursing/pumping to assist with let-down
  - Advise that the breast needs to feel softened after nursing/pumping
  - Use cabbage leaves to address swelling/engorgement
  - Take lecithin if she is experiencing recurrent plugged ducts
  - For the mother taking antibiotic therapy, the baby may develop GI symptoms or thrush/diaper dermatitis (unless the patient is pumping/dumping)
- Reassess the patient for resolution of symptoms in 1–2 weeks; if there has not been complete regression in all symptoms, you must refer the patient to a breast specialist
- If the clinical picture is consistent with mastitis but a mass is present as well, abscess is the differential diagnosis; can be confirmed with ultrasound; refer patient to a breast specialist as ultrasound guided aspiration or I & D may be required

Gynecomastia

- Can be unilateral or bilateral; often tender/painful
- Order a diagnostic mammogram and breast ultrasound to rule out a solid mass
- Review the patient's medication list; certain meds contribute to the development of gynecomastia, including, but not limited to: antihypertensives, H2 blockers, anabolic steroids and androgens, and recreational drugs
- If symptomatic, consider treating the patient with endocrine therapy such as tamoxifen or an aromatase inhibitor
- If significant asymmetry or significant bilateral breast enlargement is present, refer the patient to a plastic surgeon for consultation

Imaging Studies

Screening for Breast Cancer

Guideline recommendations apply to women with "average risk" for developing breast cancer.

- **The Guide to Clinical Preventative Services Task Force:** at least biennial mammography is recommended for woman ages 50–74. For women ages 40–49, mammography may also be beneficial, especially for women above average risk. For women >75 years of age, a recommendation was not made for or against screening. The decision should be individualized according to the patient and her individual risk
- **The American Cancer Society:** annual mammogram screening by age 45, changing to biennial mammography by age 55. The ACS does advise that a woman should have the option to begin annual screening at age 40

- If the patient has an estimated lifetime risk for a sporadic breast cancer at 20% or higher, supplemental breast MRI should be considered. Tools for calculating risk include the Gail score, Claus, BRCAPRO, and Tyrer-Cuzick. Other factors that significantly elevate a woman's risk include gene mutations such as BRCA 1 and 2 and prior exposure to chest wall irradiation

- The American College of Radiologists created the reporting system Breast Imaging Reporting and Data Systems (BI-RADS), which includes categories, assessments, and recommendations

Category	Assessment	Recommendation
0	Incomplete	Additional imaging or comparison with prior studies needed
1	Negative	Screening protocol
2	Benign finding	Screening protocol
3	Probable benign finding	Imaging surveillance in 3, 6, or 12 months
4	Suspicious	Appropriate biopsy
5	Highly suspicious	Appropriate biopsy
6	Known biopsy proven malignancy	Appropriate clinical management

Table 9.3.1 Breast Imaging Report and Data Systems
www.acr.org/~/media/ACR/Documents/PDF/QualitySafety/Resources/BIRADS/Posters/BIRADS-Reference-Card_web_F.pdf?la=en

Diagnostic Imaging Workup

- For a breast complaint, diagnostic mammogram and/or ultrasound should be pursued for further evaluation

- For women under the age of 40, begin with a breast ultrasound as mammography will likely be of limited utility

- If the imaging is abnormal (such as BI-RADS 4 or 5), then refer the patient for biopsy. If the imaging is negative for correlate (BI-RADS 1 or 2) OR if a benign imaging finding has been seen (BI-RADS 3), the patient needs to be re-evaluated in a short-term interval, such as 3 months. A referral to the breast surgeon should be considered, even if the imaging is negative for correlate

Takeaways

- With mastitis, if the symptoms do not resolve with a course of antibiotic therapy, immediate referral is needed to rule out inflammatory breast cancer.

- Even in the presence of normal breast imaging, always consider referral to a breast specialist for any focal breast finding or persisting patient complaint.

- Known risk factors for breast cancer:

  - FH of breast cancer including a male relative, female relative under age 50, 2 or more female relatives diagnosed with breast cancer

  - FH or PMH of ovarian cancer

  - Hormonal influences—early menarche or late menopause; nulliparous; postmenopausal weight gain/obesity (increased peripheral conversion of estrogen)

  - Prior breast biopsy with pathology findings of atypical ductal hyperplasia, atypical lobular hyperplasia, or LCIS

  - Prior chest wall irradiation

  - Gene mutation carrier such as BRCA 1 or BRCA 2

LESSON 4: WOMEN'S HEALTH—GYN

Learning Objectives

- Identify the components of a routine well-woman exam, as well as GYN-specific components of the patient's health history
- Order the appropriate screening tests based on the age and risk factors
- Demonstrate knowledge of fertility control methods and peri-menopausal therapies
- Diagnose and treat the most common gynecological complaints

The annual well-woman exam is often the only time a woman will see a primary care provider each year. Therefore, this visit functions as a critical opportunity to perform a thorough H & P, as well as to screen for genetic risk factors, endocrine disorders, GYN-cancers, STIs, and other social concerns. It is important to have a concrete understanding of reproductive illness and disease so that when a woman presents with a GYN problem, you may accurately diagnose and treat each patient.

Definitions

- **Bacterial vaginosis (BV):** an imbalance of the vaginal pH caused by a loss of lactobacillus that leads to an overgrowth of certain bacteria and the development of unpleasant symptoms
- **Clue cells:** epithelial cells with fuzzy borders
- **Puberty:** the period during which adolescents reach sexual maturity and become capable of reproduction
  - **Menarche:** age of first period
  - **Thelarche:** development of breast tissue; average age 9–17
  - **Adrenarche:** hair growth, specifically pubic and axillary; starts after thelarche begins
  - **Menstrual cycle:** average cycle is 28 +/− 2 days; cycle length is measured by counting the days from the first day of bleeding in one month to the first day of bleeding the next consecutive month; each period of bleeding is 4–6 +/− 2 days; volume is approximately 40 cc
- **Menorrhagia:** heavy and/or long bleeding during periods
- **Metrorrhagia:** abnormal uterine bleeding
- **Primary amenorrhea:** absence of initial menses by age 16
- **Secondary amenorrhea:** absence of menses in a woman who previously experienced regular cycles
- **Oligomenorrhea:** periods less frequent than every 35 days but more often than every 6 months
- **Infertility:** inability to conceive after 1 year of actively trying
- **Perimenopause:** begins 2–8 years before menopause and lasts on average 4 years; characterized by significant hormone shifts and their corresponding physical signs and symptoms
  - Hormone shifts include declining estrogens and androgens, which cause a reflexive rise in LH/FSH
  - Symptoms: irregular menses, hot flashes, sleep disturbance, vaginal dryness, atrophic vaginitis, dyspareunia, dysuria, stress incontinence related to weakened urethral muscles and diminished perception of need to void, decreased genital sensation, longer time to orgasm

- Physical signs associated with changes to the reproductive system: vaginal atrophy (pale appearance, smooth rugae), increased vaginal pH ($\geq$5.0), smaller cervix/stenosis of the cervical os, decreased size of the ovaries and uterus, thinning pubic hair, smaller breast/ptosis with less fibroglandular tissue
  - Lab findings: FSH >40 mIU/mL, LH 20–100 mIU/mL, Estradiol <20 pg/mL
- **Menopause:** diagnosed after 1 full year without periods; average age 51.3 years
- **Postmenopause:** after menopausal symptoms are complete
- **Reproductive years:** from menarche to menopause

Assessment

Subjective

Health History

The health history should include, but not be limited to, the following:

1. **Allergies** to medications
2. **PMH:** abnormal PAP results, anxiety/depression, asthma, blood clots or blood disorders, cancer, dense breast tissue on mammography, diabetes or prediabetes, heart disease/HTN, headaches or migraines (specifically with or without aura), obesity
3. **PSH:** abdominal surgery, breast surgery (including tissue biopsy), cervical cone biopsy, cryotherapy, laser treatment or LEEP procedure, uterine surgery or surgery on contiguous structures (including endometrial biopsy, myomectomy, tubal ligation, oophorectomy)
4. **FH:** breast/ovarian/endometrial cancer, blood clots or blood disorders, diabetes, heart disease, multiple miscarriages, polycystic ovarian syndrome (PCOS), thyroid disorders
5. **SH:** sexual habits and partner preference, intimate partner violence, substance use
6. **Obstetrical history:** gravida, parity, term, preterm, abortions, living children (GTPAL)
7. **Current medications** and compliance and satisfaction with those medications

Review of Systems

A GYN-focused ROS should include, but not be limited to, the following:

- New pelvic/back pain, persistent abdominal bloating/fullness/pressure/decreased appetite
- Urinary urgency/frequency/pressure/pain
- Vaginal itching/irritation/abnormal discharge/odor
- Abnormal uterine bleeding, LMP, frequency/length/quality of periods
- Peri/postmenopausal: hot flashes/night sweats, vaginal dryness, painful intercourse, vaginal bleeding of any kind

Objective

The exam should be tailored to the type of chief complaint (CC) given. During an annual well-woman exam, this typically includes 10 body systems. When a woman presents for a GYN "problem visit," her examination should be focused on not only the body system of concern, but also those above and below. For example, a woman presenting with pelvic pain may have the following exam documented (normal findings listed):

- BP, height, weight, BMI, LMP, breastfeeding status
- **Gen:** well appearing and in no acute distress

- **MS:** no CVAT
- **GI:** soft, non-tender × 4 quadrants, no masses palpated, no supra-pubic tenderness
- **GU:** normal appearance, no lesions or other skin abnormalities noted
- **Cervix:** normal appearance, vaginal discharge is thin, white, non-odorous
- **Bimanual:** cervix without cervical motion tenderness (CMT); uterus small, mobile, non-tender, smooth contours; adnexa non-tender, no masses palpated

Diagnosis

Condition	Chief complaint	Exam findings	Diagnostic tests
Abnormal Uterine Bleeding			
Pregnancy	• Missed period • Abdominal pain • Persistent bloating • N/V • Breast tenderness • Inter-cycle bleeding	• Positive urine pregnancy test • Enlarged uterus • Adnexal mass/tenderness (concern for ectopic)	• Ultrasound showing pregnancy • Fetal cardiac activity by doppler • Fetal movement noted on palpation of abdomen
Unscheduled or postcoital bleeding due to cervicitis or STI	• Postcoital bleeding • Inter-cycle bleeding	• Cervical inflammation/redness • Cervical friability • Vaginal discharge may be thick, frothy, malodorous, or normal	• Positive cultures for GC/CT/*Trichomonas* • Findings associated with BV/yeast
Unscheduled or absent bleeding due to birth control	• Irregular menses • Breakthrough bleeding • Secondary amenorrhea	Typically no anomalies noted	The patient reports the following chief complaint and is taking one of the corresponding medications: • Absent bleeding: continuous COCs, LNG IUDs (after 12 months of use), Depo-Provera (after 12 months of use) • Unscheduled/excessive bleeding: Depo-Provera (first 6 months), implants (first 6–12 months), copper IUD • Unscheduled bleeding/intermittent spotting: POPs, Depo, implants, IUDs
Endometrial carcinoma	• Painless, unscheduled bleeding in women >35 years old (median age is 63; only 5% of cases occur in women <40) • Lower abdominal pain (10%) • Infertility	• Vaginal bleeding may be present • Uterus may be enlarged/soft	Gold standard: • Fractional dilation and curettage Also useful: • Transvaginal ultrasound • Sonohysterogram • Endometrial biopsy

Table 9.4.1 Most Common GYN Complaints

Condition	Chief complaint	Exam findings	Diagnostic tests
Polycystic ovarian syndrome (PCOS)	• Irregular menses • Oligomenorrhea • Amenorrhea • Infertility	• Hirsutism • Thinning head hair • Acne • Deep voice • Obesity (40%) • Acanthosis nigricans	Two out of three of the following must be met: • Oligo/amenorrhea • Physical or laboratory findings consistent with hyperandrogenism • Polycystic ovaries on ultrasound Other causes must also be excluded: • Thyroid disorders • Obesity • Hyperprolactinemia • Androgen-secreting tumors • Cushing disease • Pregnancy
Vaginitis			
Bacterial vaginosis (BV)	• Abnormal vaginal odor • Vaginal irritation • Increased vaginal discharge • Dyspareunia	• Moderate white-gray discharge • Amine or "fishy" odor on exam	Three of the following criteria must be met: • Visualization of moderate white-gray discharge coating the vaginal walls • Vaginal pH $\geq$4.5 • Positive whiff test (amine odor produced by applying 10% KOH to the discharge) • Clue cells seen on wet mount
Trichomoniasis	• Sudden increase in vaginal discharge • Vaginal itching/irritation • Postcoital bleeding • Dyspareunia • Many patients are asymptomatic	• Yellow-green or gray vaginal discharge that may also be frothy in appearance • Strawberry cervix (30%) • Friable cervix • Vaginal pH $\geq$5	• Positive DNA culture • WBCs and motile trichomonads on wet mount (60–70% sensitive)
Vulvovaginal candidiasis (VVC)	• Mild to severe external or internal vaginal itching • Thick, clumpy, white vaginal discharge • Labial swelling • Burning on urination • Dyspareunia	• Redness/swelling of the labia minora or majora • External abrasions secondary to the patient scratching • Scant to copious thick white clumping vaginal discharge, often adhering to the walls • Discharge may be tinted yellow or green	• Wet mount plus 10% KOH shows mycelia, spores, and pseudohyphae • Positive fungal culture

Table 9.4.1 Most Common GYN Complaints (Continued)

Condition	Chief complaint	Exam findings	Diagnostic tests
Vulvar Lesions and Dermatoses			
Chancroid or HSV lesion(s)	• "Bump on vagina" • Burning on urination • Painful lump in groin	Chancroid: • Deep ulcerating lesion with irregular borders • Swollen inguinal lymph nodes (30–60%) HSV: • Single or multiple painful, blistering, or ulcerating lesions • Lesions may be in various stages of healing Both conditions may be found on the labia, in the vagina, on the cervix, and/or in the peri-anal area	Culture of lesion(s) should show *H. ducreyi* for chancroid and HSV-1 or 2 for herpes
Condyloma and molluscum	Non-painful bump(s) in anogenital area	Genital warts: • Single or multiple wart-like lesions with rough texture • May be cone shaped, pedunculated, or have a cauliflower appearance • May be macular or with a cobblestone appearance Molluscum: • Multiple round papules with an umbilicated center • Waxy/smooth/firm to palpation • May be yellow or reddish in color	• Physical exam • Tissue biopsy
Lichen sclerosus	• Vaginal and/or anal itching • Vulvar pain • Dysuria • Dyspareunia	• Diffuse white papules or plaques on the vulva, possibly extending down the perineum and around the anus • Excoriation may be visible from where the patient was scratching	Physical exam plus tissue biopsy
Syphilis	Painless ulcer (chancre) on the genitals, anus, or mouth	Exam findings, staging, and diagnostic criteria are discussed in Table 9.4.7	
Pelvic Pain			
Endometriosis	• Dysmenorrhea with back pain • Dyspareunia • Infertility	• Tenderness on bimanual exam • Adnexal mass • Fixed, retroverted uterus • May have normal exam if disease is mild	Laparoscopic visualization of extra-uterine endometrial stroma and glands

Table 9.4.1 Most Common GYN Complaints (Continued)

Condition	Chief complaint	Exam findings	Diagnostic tests
Leiomyomata uteri (fibroid myoma)	• Menorrhagia • Dysmenorrhea • Dyspareunia • General persistent feeling of fullness or bloating Severe cases: • Signs of intestinal or urethral obstruction	Enlarged, bulky, firm, irregular uterus	• Transvaginal ultrasound • Sonohysterogram • CT or MRI may be helpful with larger fibroids
Ovarian cyst	Unilateral or bilateral pelvic pain • Pain may worsen with intercourse or certain position changes • Pain may be sharp, dull, or aching • Pain may be severe if cyst ruptures or ovarian torsion occurs	• Unilateral tenderness on palpation of adnexa • Adnexal mass on palpation	Transvaginal ultrasound
Ovarian carcinoma	• Most women in early stages are asymptomatic • Irregular, mild abdominal discomfort or persistent feeling of fullness or bloating • Increased sensation of bladder/rectal pressure *Late stage:* • More constant, persistent, and painful symptoms • Decreased appetite • Chronic heartburn	Ovarian/adnexal mass on palpation; typically fixed, firm, non-tender and bilateral Late stage: • Ascites Very late stage: • Pleural effusion • Lymphadenopathy • Wasting syndrome (cachexia)	• Transvaginal ultrasound, CT, or MRI will identify the presence of a tumor • Laparotomy will confirm diagnosis of cancer
Pelvic inflammatory disease	• Diffuse abdominal and/or pelvic pain • Back pain • Dyspareunia • Abnormal vaginal discharge and/or odor • Irregular vaginal bleeding/spotting (30%) • Fever • Dysuria • Nausea, vomiting	One or more of the following findings is considered to be the minimum criteria for treatment: • Lower abdominal tenderness • Cervical motion tenderness • Uterine/adnexal tenderness Findings that further support diagnosis include: • Temp >101°F (38°C) • Mucopurulent cervical discharge • Friable cervix • WBCs on wet mount • Elevated erythrocyte sedimentation rate • Elevated C-reactive protein • GC/CT positive by culture	

Table 9.4.1 Most Common GYN Complaints (Continued)

> **Pro Tip**
> Patients will often present to the office with multiple concerns. When appropriate, triage the problems by most to least urgent, address the top issues, and bring the patient back for a follow-up visit to discuss the rest.

Plan

Screening Tests and Treatment

The annual well-woman exam is in fact a primary care visit, and therefore includes screening for GYN-related illness and disease. As a nurse practitioner, you will assess each patient based on her age and risk factors to determine which tests to order.

Treatment plans in gynecology are often "rolling," which means you will send the patient home with one plan and then make a new one once test results are complete. It is also common to request follow up anywhere from a few days to a month later to determine whether symptoms have improved. If the patient is not better, more tests may be ordered or referrals may be given.

GYN-Specific Screening Tests by Age Group

Age (years)	Screening test and frequency of testing	Management of abnormal testing
20	Clinical breast exam—yearly	*See Chapter 9, Lesson 3*
21	Pelvic exam—yearly	Transvaginal ultrasound should be considered for women with a palpable pelvic mass, enlarged/irregularly shaped uterus, and/or adnexal tenderness
21–29	Pap smear—if normal, cytology screening every 3 years	*See Table 9.4.3*
30–65	Pap smear—if normal, either cytology screening every 3 years or cytology and HPV screening every 5 years (preferred)	*See Table 9.4.3*
≤24—sexually active teens and women **≥25—sexually active women with more than 1 partner, or a partner who has been diagnosed with an STI**	*N. gonorrhoeae, C. trachomatis*—yearly	*See Table 9.4.7*

Table 9.4.2 Routine GYN Screening Tests

Age (years)	Screening test and frequency of testing	Management of abnormal testing
Any age—women with a history of vaginal lesions of unknown type, or women who have had a partner with HSV-2	HSV IgG (HSV 1, HSV 2)	Serum herpes 1 or 2 IgG positive: • HSV 1 or 2 IgG positive with no personal history of a lesion: counsel the patient that while she has been exposed to the virus, it does not mean she will ever have an outbreak • HSV 1 or 2 positive in the context of oral or vulvar lesions: if vulvar HSV 1 or oral HSV 2, recurrence is uncommon and may typically be treated episodically Plan: • HSV 1 primary outbreak: acyclovir **or** famciclovir **or** valacyclovir (all regimens are for 7–10 days) • HSV 1 recurrent outbreak: acyclovir (5 days) **or** famciclovir (1-day dosing) **or** valacyclovir (1-day dosing) *For treatment of HSV 2, refer to Table 9.4.7 in this chapter.*
Please see Chapter 3, Lesson 3, for a complete discussion on screening tests.		

Table 9.4.2 Routine GYN Screening Tests (Continued)

Cervical Cancer Prevention

Gardasil 9 is the only cervical cancer vaccine available in the U.S. at the time of this publication. Gardasil and Cervarix are two other HPV vaccinations that may be available in other countries. The main difference between these injections is the number of HPV strains covered: Cervarix is bivalent (HPV 16, 18), Gardasil is quadrivalent (HPV 6, 11, 16, 18), and Gardasil 9 is 9-valent (HPV 6, 11, 16, 18, 31, 33, 45, 52, 58). Vaccination is recommended starting at 11–12 years of age for both girls and boys (UPDATE: as of 10/2018, the FDA approved the HPV vaccine for adult patients between the ages of 27 and 45). Young women and men who have yet to be vaccinated are generally recommended to receive the injection series by age 26. Injections are given either two or three to a series and the vaccination schedules are as follows:

- Patients <15 years of age: first dose at any time, second dose 6 to 12 months later
- Patients >15 years of age, or immunocompromised patients at any age: first dose any time, second dose 1–2 months after the first, and third dose 6 months after the first

Management of Abnormal Cytology Results

Management of abnormal cytology results for women who have had no prior abnormal cervical cancer screening tests is noted in the table below. Follow-up for women who have had prior abnormal results is different and is beyond the scope of an entry-level FNP.

Result	ASCCP management guidelines			
	Ages 21–24	**Ages 25–29**	**Ages 30 and older (HPV negative)**	**Ages 30 and older (HPV positive)**
Normal Pap test results	Routine screening: Pap test every 3 years	Routine screening: Pap test every 3 years	Routine screening: Preferred: co-testing (combined Pap test and HPV test) every 5 years Acceptable: Pap test alone every 3 years	• Co-testing in 12 months OR • HPV typing
ASC-US	Preferred: repeat Pap test in 12 months Acceptable: reflex HPV test	Preferred: reflex HPV test Acceptable: repeat Pap test in 12 months	Repeat co-testing in 3 years	Colposcopy
LSIL	Repeat Pap test in 12 months	Colposcopy	Preferred: repeat Pap test in 12 months Acceptable: Colposcopy	Colposcopy
ASC-H	Colposcopy	Colposcopy	Colposcopy	Colposcopy
HSIL	Colposcopy	Immediate excisional treatment or colposcopy	Immediate excisional treatment or colposcopy	Immediate excisional treatment or colposcopy
AGC	AGC has several subcategories. The type of follow-up tests depends on the AGC subcategory. Tests performed include colposcopy, endocervical sampling, and endometrial sampling			

- **HPV:** Human Papilloma Virus
- **ASC-US:** Atypical Squamous Cells of Undetermined Significance on Cytology—changes in the cervical cells are present. Changes are most often a sign of HPV infection. This is the most common abnormal Pap test result
- **LSIL:** Low-grade Squamous Intraepithelial Lesions—cervical cells show changes that are mildly abnormal. LSIL is often caused by HPV infection and that often resolves on its own
- **ASC-H:** Atypical Squamous Cells: Cannot exclude high-grade LSIL—changes in the cervical cells suggestive of the presence of HSIL
- **AGC:** Atypical Glandular Cells

Table 9.4.3 Management of Abnormal Cytology Results

American College of Obstetricians and Gynecologists (2016)
www.acog.org/Patients/FAQs/Abnormal-Cervical-Cancer-Screening-Test-Results

Fertility Control Methods

Method	Considerations
Abstinence Avoidance of penile-vaginal or penile-rectal intercourse	None
Barrier methods Cervical cap Diaphragm Female condom Male condom	• Latex allergy • Interference with spontaneity • Decreased sexual experience of the male partner • First year failure rate with perfect condom use: female 5%, male 3%; typical use: female 21%, male 14%
Combined oral contraceptive pill (COC) Estrogen-progesterone Monophasic Triphasic Extended cycle	• Compliance with taking a daily medication *For a complete list of contraindications to estrogen-containing medications as well as directions for use, refer to Chapter 4, Lesson 9*
Progesterone-only pill (POP) (Micronor, "mini pill", Camila)	• Compliance with taking a daily medication • Requires patient to take her pill at the exact same time every day • Increased likelihood of breakthrough bleeding • Acceptable for breastfeeding women
Vaginal insert Combined estrogen-progesterone (NuvaRing)	• Patient must be comfortable placing the ring inside her vagina • Same contraindications as combined oral contraceptives
Contraceptive patch Combined estrogen-progesterone (Ortho-Evra)	• Patch sites can become irritated and/or itchy • Same contraindications as combined oral contraceptives
Progesterone-only injection (Depo-Provera)	• Needle phobia • Patient must present to the office every 3 months for injection • Potentially delayed return to fertility after cessation • Acceptable for breastfeeding women
Progesterone-only implant (Implanon, Nexplanon)	• Needle phobia • Significant unscheduled bleeding • Potentially delayed return to fertility after cessation/removal • Acceptable for breastfeeding women
Intrauterine devices (IUD) Progesterone-only (LNG IUS) (Skyla, Kyleena, Liletta, Mirena) Copper (ParaGard)	• Abnormal uterine bleeding (with LNG IUS this is predictably limited to the first 6 months) • Insertion/removal must be performed by a trained provider • Insertion is typically more painful for nulliparous women • Women must feel comfortable checking for strings • Acceptable for breastfeeding women
Female sterilization Transabdominal approach (Surgical ligation, electrocauterization, tube resection, occlusion) Transcervical approach (Essure)	• Permanent method • Patient must be 100% certain she does not want to conceive in the future • Outpatient surgical procedure • Essure may be done in the office, but can be painful • There is also a 3-month period between the procedure and effectiveness

Table 9.4.4 Fertility Control Methods

Method	Considerations
Male sterilization Vasectomy	3-month period between procedure and effectiveness
Emergency contraception POP, Plan B COC Copper IUD	• Plan B or COC must be started within 3 days, or IUD must be inserted within 5 days after intercourse • Pills may cause heavy bleeding • Pills decrease chance of pregnancy to ~25% • IUD decreases chance of pregnancy to ≤1%
Abortion First trimester: Misoprostol Dilation & curettage (D&C) Second trimester: Dilation & evacuation (D&E)	• Medication can cause heavy bleeding and moderate to severe cramping • Surgical management involves analgesia or anesthesia • Pills are 95% effective when administered ≤7 weeks and 80% effective at 9 weeks • Surgery is 100% effective

Table 9.4.4 Fertility Control Methods (Continued)

Pharmacological and Non-Pharmacological Relief Measures for Peri- and Postmenopausal Symptoms

Symptom	Relief measure (Dosing ordered from most to least effective)
Vasomotor Hot flashes, night sweats	Medication (estrogen): • Oral conjugated estrogen* • Oral 17-estradiol • Transdermal 17-estradiol Medication (Selective Estrogen Receptor Modulator, or SERM): • Bazedoxifene (SERM) plus conjugated estrogen (Duavee) Medication (non-hormonal methods): • venlafaxine (Effexor), sertraline (Zoloft), or paroxetine (Paxil)** • Phytoestrogens, botanicals, and natural therapies Lifestyle changes: • Avoid or limit spicy foods, chocolate, caffeine, and alcohol • Avoid overeating/large meals • Avoid or limit time spent in hot/humid environments, including hot baths/showers, jacuzzis, and saunas • Avoid wearing restrictive clothing • Wear clothing in breathable fibers; dress in layers that can be easily removed • Initiate smoking cessation plan • Regularly engage in moderate exercise • Participate in activities that promote relaxation and decrease stress

Table 9.4.5 Relief Measures for Peri- and Postmenopausal Symptoms

Symptom	Relief measure (Dosing ordered from most to least effective)
Urological and vulvovaginal Vaginal itching, irritation, dryness; dyspareunia; urinary urgency, frequency, pain	Medication (hormonal methods): • Oral estrogen/progesterone • Ospemifene (*Osphena*) • Vaginal estrogen creams • Estrogen vaginal ring (Estring, Femring*) • Topical sprays Medications (non-hormonal methods): • OTC Replens, or other vaginal moisturizers Lifestyle changes: • Regular intimacy and sexual activity; use water-soluble lubricants
*If uterus is intact, requires additional progestin in order to prevent endometrial hyperplasia. **Paroxetine, fluoxetine, and bupropion are specifically contraindicated in women taking tamoxifen; escitalopram, duloxetine, and sertraline should be used with caution; venlafaxine is the safest option.	

Table 9.4.5 Relief Measures for Peri- and Postmenopausal Symptoms (Continued)

Management of Select GYN Complaints

Diagnosis	Treatment
Endometriosis	Hormonal contraception is first-line; progesterone will decrease the effect of the endometrial lining, which should in turn limit the proliferation of tissue
Lichen sclerosis	• Topical corticosteroids • Injected corticosteroids for thicker areas
Polycystic ovarian syndrome (PCOS)	Infertility • metformin (especially helpful for regulating periods in women who also have insulin resistance) • Weight loss for women who are overweight • clomiphene citrate or letrozole (off-label) for ovulation induction; clomiphene preferred for women with BMI <30, and letrozole for women BMI >30 • Reproductive endocrinology referral for women who either do not respond to ovulation induction and/or are candidates for intrauterine insemination (IUI) or in-vitro fertilization (IVF) Endometrial protection • Combined oral contraceptives (may also help with acne) • Progesterone-only methods for women who are not candidates for oral estrogen Hyperandrogenism • COCs • Antiandrogens: spironolactone, finasteride • Gonadotropin Releasing Hormone Agonists (GnRH; less common) • Waxing or laser treatments for hirsutism • Dermatology referral for acne or alopecia

Table 9.4.6 Management of Select GYN Complaints

Management of Genitourinary Infections in Non-Pregnant Adult Patients

Condition/pathogen	Recommended treatment*
Bacterial vaginosis (BV) Caused by an imbalance of normal vaginal flora, allowing for certain bacteria to overgrow Common pathogens: *G. vaginalis* and *M. hominis*	• metronidazole (Flagyl) 500 mg PO BID × 7 days, **or** • metronidazole (MetroGel) gel 0.75%, one full applicator (5 g) PV daily × 5, **or** • clindamycin cream 2% (Cleocin), one applicator (5 g) PV nightly × 7
Vulvovaginal candidiasis (VVC) Common pathogens: *C. albicans, C. glabrata, c. tropicalis*	Over-the-counter: • clotrimazole, miconazole, tioconazole, butoconazole creams and vaginal suppositories; dosing is 3–14 days, depending on medication and strength Prescription: • diflucan 150 mg PO × 1 (may repeat in 3 days prn) • Lotrisone topical cream prn itching
Chancroid *H. ducreyi*, gram-negative anaerobe, STI	• azithromycin 1 g PO × 1, **or** • ceftriaxone 250 mg IM × 1, **or** • ciprofloxacin 500 mg PO BID × 3 days, **or** • erythromycin base 500 mg PO TID × 7 days
C. trachomatis Intracellular organism, STI	Adolescents and adults: • azithromycin 1 g PO × 1, **or** • doxycycline 100 mg PO BID × 7 days
Condyloma acuminata (genital warts) Human papillomavirus (HPV), STI	Patient-applied: • imiquimod 3.75% or 5% cream,** **or** • podofilox 0.5% solution or gel, **or** • sinecatechins 15% ointment** Provider-administered: • Cryotherapy with liquid nitrogen or cryoprobe, **or** • Surgical removal, **or** • trichloroacetic acid (TCA) or bichloroacetic acid (BCA) 80–90% solution
Genital herpes Herpes simplex virus (HSV) type 2, STI	First episode: • acyclovir 400 mg PO TID × 7–10 days, **or** • valacyclovir 1 g PO BID × 7–10 days Recurrent episode: • acyclovir 400 mg PO TID × 5 days, **or** • valacyclovir 500 mg PO BID × 3 days, **or** • valacyclovir 1 g PO daily × 5 days Daily suppression: • acyclovir 400 mg PO BID, **or** • valacyclovir 500 mg, or 1 g PO daily
HIV	Treatment of HIV is complicated and multifaceted. Women diagnosed with this disease should be referred to a specialist for management of care.
N. gonorrhea Gram-negative bacteria, STI	• ceftriaxone 250 mg IM × 1, **plus** • azithromycin 1 g PO × 1

Table 9.4.7 Management of Genitourinary Infections in Non-Pregnant Adult Patients

Condition/pathogen	Recommended treatment*
Pelvic inflammatory disease (PID) *C. Trachomatis, N. gonorrhea, E. coli, G. vaginalis, H. influenzae, Mycoplasma,* and *Ureaplasma* species Can be caused by sexually transmitted organisms, vaginal douching, or sex during menstruation	Outpatient regimens: • ceftriaxone 250 mg IM × 1, **plus** • doxycycline 100 mg PO BID × 14 days, **with or without** • metronidazole 500 mg PO BID × 14 days for coverage of anaerobes
Syphilis	*Please see Table 9.4.8*
Trichomoniasis Anaerobic flagellated protozoan parasite, STI	• metronidazole 2 g PO × 1, **or** • tinidazole 2 g PO × 1
*Alternative and inpatient regimens may be found by visiting **www.cdc.gov**. **May weaken condoms and diaphragms	

Table 9.4.7 Management of Genitourinary Infections in Non-Pregnant Adult Patients (Continued)

Diagnosis and Management of Syphilis in Non-Pregnant Adult Patients

Stage and diagnosis	Signs and symptoms	Treatment
Primary Positive RPR/VDRL confirmed by an FTA-ABS or TP-PA	Localized infection: Chancre within 10–90 days of exposure, painless lymphadenopathy, or asymptomatic; may last 1–6 weeks	benzathine PCN G 2.4 million units IM × 1
Secondary Seropositive	Systemic infection: Starts after chancre disappears; maculopapular rash on palms/soles, swollen lymph nodes, fever, fatigue, joint pain, headaches; may last 1–8 weeks	benzathine PCN G 2.4 million units IM × 1
Latent Seropositive	Asymptomatic	Early latent: • benzathine PCN G 2.4 million units IM × 1 Late latent or latent syphilis of unknown duration: • benzathine PCN G 7.2 million units total, administered as 2.4 million units IM weekly × 3 doses
Tertiary syphilis Dark field microscopy of fluid from lesions will show T. pallidum; CSF exam is negative	Diffuse nodular lesions that eventually necrose (gummas), cardiac symptoms	benzathine PCN G 7.2 million units total, administered as 2.4 million units IM weekly × 3 doses
Neurosyphilis and ocular syphilis CSF exam is positive for T. pallidum	Tabes dorsalis, general paralysis, mental status changes, ocular inflammation, Argyll Robertson pupil, seizures, leukoplakia	• aqueous crystalline PCN G 18–24 million units per day, administered as 3–4 million units IV every 4 hrs, or continuous infusion for 10–14 days **or** • procaine PCN G 2.4 million units IM daily × 10–14 days, **plus** Probenecid 500 mg po 4 × day × 10–14 days

Table 9.4.8 Diagnosis and Management of Syphilis in Non-Pregnant Adult Patients

> **App Alert**
>
> The Center for Disease Control has numerous mobile apps for healthcare providers, two of which focus on the safe prescribing of birth control methods and treatment of STIs. You can find more information here: **www.cdc.gov/reproductivehealth/contraception/ mmwr/mec/summary.html**.

Education

Annual Visit

- **Ages 13–20:** normal body changes, the menstrual cycle, HPV vaccination, underaged substance use, healthy relationships, pregnancy, STI and hepatitis B prevention, introduction to the speculum and pelvic exams, domestic violence assessment
- **Ages 21–40:** Pap guidelines, substance use risk reduction, basic pre-conceptive counseling, fertility control, STI and hepatitis B risk reduction, domestic violence assessment
- **Ages 40–50:** perimenopausal symptoms, breast/colon cancer screening
- **All ages:** STI prevention, intimate partner violence, diet/exercise

Proper administration of birth control pills

1. Combined oral contraceptive pills

- **Initiation of treatment:** Patients may use the "quick start" method, "Sunday start" method, or initiate treatment on the first day of her cycle. "Quick start" means she begins her pill pack at any time (sometimes even in the office with the provider), but she must use a back-up method for at least seven days, and she must be educated that her period will likely be irregular for up to three months after beginning the pills. "Sunday start" is a popular method because it is easy to remember, but women should be counseled to use a back-up method or abstain for seven days. Many COC manufacturers recommend initiating treatment on the very first day of a woman's period because this will help the placebo week to align with the woman's regular cycle and decrease the chance of breakthrough bleeding. How you choose to counsel your patient will depend on whether she is at high risk for pregnancy or not
- **How to take:** COCs must be taken in a specific order, starting with those containing hormones and ending with the placebo or iron pills. With triphasic or extended cycle methods, extra teaching must be given so that the pills are taken in the correct order. Patients should also be warned that many generic pill packs will only have three weeks of hormone tablets included, and no placebo pills will be provided for the last week. Each pill should be taken at the same time of day
- **Missed pills:** If one pill is missed, the patient should take that pill as soon as she remembers and then continue the rest of her pack as usual. If two pills are missed, she should take two pills daily for the next two days, which will get her back on track. She should also use condoms as a back-up method for seven days. If any pills are missed specifically during the third week, the placebo week should be skipped and she should instead start a new pack immediately following the third week

2. Progesterone-only pills

- **Initiation of treatment:** Similar to COCs, patients may use the "quick start" or "Sunday start" methods with a seven-day back-up, or begin on the first day of her period
- **How to take:** Each pill must be taken at exactly the same time per day; if a pill is taken even three hours late, the patient should use a back-up method or abstain from intercourse for two days
- **Missed pills:** If one pill is missed, the patient should use condoms or abstain for at least two days. If two or more pills are missed, she should take both pills as soon as she remembers and also use a back-up method for two days

> **DANGER SIGN** Women taking medication containing estrogen should seek emergency care immediately if experiencing the following symptoms: *Severe **A**bdominal pain, **C**hest pain/shortness of breath, severe unilateral **H**eadache/sudden onset dizziness, **E**ye problems/vision changes, **S**evere pain and/or swelling in calf or thigh (**ACHES**).*

Referral

As a nurse practitioner providing women's health services, you will be a member of a diverse network of medical providers who will often refer patients to each other. Some examples of necessary referrals include:

- Enlarged thyroid with abnormal thyroid blood work results: endocrinologist
- Persistently palpable breast mass at any age: breast surgeon
- Abnormal Pap results requiring colposcopy: gynecologist or gynecologist-oncologist
- Enlarged, painful external hemorrhoids not responding to traditional treatment: rectal surgeon
- Persistent UTI symptoms with negative cultures: urologist
- Urinary incontinence due to vaginal muscle weakness: physical therapist who specializes in pelvic floor strengthening
- Pre-conceptive counseling for a patient with a complicated health history: maternal fetal medicine
- PCOS with a desire for pregnancy: reproductive endocrinologist
- Undesired pregnancy: GYN provider who performs family planning procedures

Takeaways

- Women's health is a division of healthcare that often overlaps with other areas of study, and often includes the evaluation of multiple body systems.
- The annual GYN exam is an opportunity to review and perform a complete health history and physical exam. Social habits and risk for intimate partner violence should be evaluated. Medication compliance and side effects should be addressed.
- GYN problem visits are rarely straightforward, and often require examination of multiple body systems in an effort to narrow down differential diagnoses. Sometimes a definitive diagnosis is not able to be made at the visit, and follow-up is required once test results are received.

LESSON 5: WOMEN'S HEALTH—OB

Learning Objectives
- Identify the components of a routine healthy pregnant woman exam
- Order the appropriate screening tests based on the woman's gestational age and risk factors
- Demonstrate knowledge of the most common discomforts of pregnancy and their treatment options
- Confidently diagnose complications of pregnancy

Pregnancy is a normal part of human life; however, for many women, it can feel very abnormal and foreign. As a nurse practitioner, promoting education and safety are your primary goals with each visit. You must not only ensure that the woman and fetus are healthy, but also that, during the weeks in-between her appointments, she knows what symptoms may warrant further exploration. In terms of pregnancy complications, you must have the knowledge to identify dangerous symptoms and initiate the care required to diagnose high-risk illness. Even though you will be collaboratively managing or transferring care of high-risk women, you must be able to recognize when the health and safety of your patients may be compromised.

Definitions

- **First trimester:** conception through 13 weeks, 6 days (13w6d)
- **Second trimester:** 14w0d through 27w6d
- **Third trimester:** 28w0d through delivery
- **Preterm:** 24w0d (viability) through 36w6d
- **Periviable:** 20w0d through 25w6d
- **Early term:** 37w0d through 38w6d
- **Term:** 39w0d through 40w6d
- **Late term:** 41w0d through 41w6d
- **Post-term:** >42 weeks gestational age
- **Nulliparous:** used to describe a woman who has either never been pregnant or who has not carried a pregnancy past 20-weeks gestation
- **Primiparous/primigravida:** used to describe a woman who has been pregnant once or is in her first pregnancy
- **Multiparous:** used to describe a woman who has delivered a baby after 20-weeks gestation
- **GTPAL:** used to communicate a woman's obstetrical history (gravida, term, preterm, abortions, living children)
- **Oligohydramnios:** decreased amniotic fluid volume of either a maximum vertical pocket (MVP) <2cm, or an amniotic fluid index (AFI) <5 cm
- **Polyhydramnios:** elevated amniotic fluid volume of either an MVP >8cm, or an AFI >25 cm
- **Quickening:** pregnant woman's first perception of fetal movement
- **Chadwick's sign:** bluish discoloration of the vagina and cervix
- **Goodell's sign:** softening of the vaginal portion of cervix
- **Hegar's sign:** softening and compressibility of the isthmus of uterus
- **Uterine fundus:** the top of the uterus, the location of which is measured during antepartum visits to assess fetal growth; fundal height is also assessed postpartum to evaluate potential for maternal bleeding

Assessment

Signs of pregnancy are categorized as presumptive, probable, and positive.

Presumptive	Probable	Positive
Signs and symptoms that may resemble pregnancy signs and symptoms, but may be caused by something else: • Amenorrhea • Breast tenderness • Fatigue • Frequent urination • Nausea, vomiting • Quickening	Signs that indicate pregnancy the majority of the time, with the chance they can be false or caused by something else: • Positive pregnancy test • Chadwick sign • Goodell sign • Hegar sign • Uterine enlargement	Signs that cannot be mistaken for other conditions; evidence that pregnancy has occurred: • Fetal heart tones • Fetal outline noted on palpation • Ultrasound of fetal outline

Table 9.5.1 Signs of Pregnancy

Subjective

The first prenatal visit is essentially a complete well-woman exam with a focus on history that may impact the current pregnancy. Similar to the GYN health history, the pertinent positives are listed below along with their significance to pregnancy.

- **Medication allergy:** you now have two patients who may be affected by the management and complications of an allergic reaction
- **PMH:**
  - **Anxiety/depression:** symptoms may worsen during or after pregnancy
  - **Asthma:** pregnant women have diminished lung capacity in the third trimester, which can predispose them to respiratory infections, asthma exacerbations, and complications during delivery
  - **Blood clots:** pregnancy is a hypercoagulable state; if a woman has a history of a DVT or PE, she may need to be on anticoagulant therapy during pregnancy
  - **Diabetes, heart disease, thyroid disorder, HTN:** women must have excellent control of these conditions during pregnancy to prevent both maternal and fetal complications
- **PSH:**
  - **Uterine surgery:** may require a cesarean delivery
  - **LEEP procedure:** increases the risk of premature shortening of the cervix
  - **Oophorectomy:** increases the risk of ectopic pregnancy
- **FH:** first-degree relative with history of spontaneous blood clot and/or diagnosis with a clotting disorder may warrant a maternal-fetal medicine (MFM) consultation/referral
- **SH:**
  - **Sexual habits:** will influence STI screening
  - **Partner preference:** always ask who is in the room, never assume
  - **Intimate partner violence:** studies have shown that domestic violence worsens during pregnancy
  - **Substance abuse:** women who are taking illicit substances during pregnancy should be strongly encouraged to stop, and resources given to assist in their sobriety; this may include referral to a detox and/or long-term drug maintenance program like a methadone clinic

- **Obstetrical history:** GTPAL
- **Medications:** a thorough medication history will alert you to any potential risks to the baby

How to Calculate GTPAL

Term	Significance
Gravida	Total number of pregnancies
Term	Total number of pregnancies delivered at 37w0d or later (multiple gestations are only counted *once*)
Preterm	Total number of pregnancies delivered between 20w0d and 36w6d (multiple gestations are only counted *once*)
Abortion	Total number of pregnancies that ended before 20w0d, including: • Miscarriages • Ectopic pregnancies • Second-trimester losses • Terminations
Living	Total number of children born who are living today (this number will be higher than the "G" if twins/triplets are born, and lower than the "G" if any losses or deaths have occurred)
Example: A woman has been pregnant 5 times. Her first child was born at 41w3d. She then had 2 miscarriages. Her fourth pregnancy was twins delivered at 35w6d. All 3 of her children are still living. Based on this information, she is a G5 T1 P1 A2 L3. Often, the abbreviation is shortened to just G (number of pregnancies) & P (number of deliveries); so for this woman, the notation would be shortened to G5P2.	

Table 9.5.2 Calculating GTPAL

Naegele's rule is a standard way of calculating the due date for a pregnancy. The rule estimates the expected date of delivery (EDD) by adding one year, subtracting three months, and adding seven days to the first day of a woman's last menstrual period (LMP).

Review of Systems

The pregnant woman's ROS evolves throughout the pregnancy based on her gestational age and the risks associated with that age.

First and Second Trimesters

- Vaginal bleeding
- Moderate to severe abdominal cramping
- Moderate to severe nausea, which may affect hydration/nutrition status

Third Trimester

- Vaginal bleeding or leaking of fluid
- Uterine contractions, especially when accompanied by back pain
- Headaches, scotoma, epigastric or RUQ pain
- Fetal movement (categorized as present, absent, or decreased)
- Swelling of extremities or face

Objective

Every woman has a minimum of five pieces of information collected at every prenatal visit: blood pressure, weight, urine protein and glucose, fundal height, and fetal heart rate. Fetal movement, fetal presentation, and maternal cervical exam are added when appropriate. The earliest a fetal heartbeat can be heard by external Doppler is 9 weeks. Measuring fundal height with a measuring tape is a valuable assessment; however, it may lose accuracy close to term. Many pregnancies are tracked using a chart to show progress over time. Using this type of chart, the NP can clearly see the frequency of visits, which typically begins as every 4 weeks during the first and second trimesters, then increases to every 2 weeks from 28–36 weeks, and then weekly from there on.

Blood Pressure Evaluation

Maternal blood pressure $\geq 140/90$ is considered to be elevated in pregnancy and requires follow-up.

Maternal Weight Gain

The Institute of Medicine (IOM) has set weight gain goals for pregnancy, which are based on pre-pregnancy BMI:

Singleton Pregnancy

- <18.5: 28–40 lb
- 18.5–24.9: 25–35 lb
- 25–29.9: 15–25 lb
- ≥ 30: 11–20 lb

Twin Pregnancy

- <18.5: Not enough research has been completed to make a recommendation
- 18.5–24.9: 37–54 lb
- 25–29.9: 31–50 lb
- ≥ 30: 25–42 lb

Urine Evaluation

Proteinuria may be significant, especially in the context of an elevated blood pressure or diabetes mellitus, but it is especially concerning for poorly controlled diabetes or undiagnosed gestational diabetes. Ketones may be associated with dehydration or overexertion.

Assessing Fundal Height

Fundal height is evaluated by hand from 12–24 weeks gestation. After 26 weeks, a measuring tape with centimeters is used and the number of centimeters from the top of the woman's pubic bone to the top of her fundus should equal her weeks of gestation. Measurements may be $+/-$ 2 weeks and still considered to be normal. Hand measurements are as follows:

- 12 weeks: just above the pubic symphysis
- 16 weeks: four finger breadths below the umbilicus
- 20 weeks: at the umbilicus
- 24 weeks: four finger breadths above the umbilicus
- Using the measuring tape: 30 cm = 30 weeks gestation

Assessing Fetal Position Using Leopold Maneuvers

The fetal position is determined using Leopold maneuvers, a series of hand assessments that will help you to discern between the fetal head and buttocks, as well as recognize the location of limbs.

STEP 1

Find the uterine fundus, palpate for a large, firm, non-movable part consistent with the fetal buttocks.

If you feel a round, ballotable part it may be the fetal head.

STEP 2

Slowly work your hands down either side of the uterus, careful to notice any bony prominence(s) that would clue you in to where a foot or hand may be.

If you don't feel any limbs, you can always ask the mother where she typically feels kicking movements.

STEP 3

On the opposite side of the abdomen from the bony prominence, a smooth, firm fetal back may be felt.

This is where you are going to listen for the fetal heartbeat (*see Table 9.5.3 for specific location*).

STEP 4

Just above the pubic symphysis, a round, ballotable part consistent with the fetal head should be felt.

If presenting part is unclear, consider ordering an ultrasound to confirm.

Assessing Fetal Heart Rate

The normal range for the fetal heart rate is 110–160. However, very early in pregnancy, rates up to 170 may be considered normal. Up until 30 weeks, fetal position is difficult to assess by hand; therefore, you may choose to start listening for the heartbeat in the middle of the abdomen and work your way out from there. Once the fetus is large enough to palpate position, it is easiest to hear the heartbeat through the baby's back.

Fetal position	Where to listen
Left occiput anterior (LOA) and left occiput posterior (LOP)	Maternal LLQ
Right occiput anterior (ROA) and right occiput posterior (ROP)	Maternal RLQ
Left sacral anterior (LSA)	Maternal LUQ
Right sacral anterior (RSA)	Maternal RUQ

Table 9.5.3 Where to Listen for Fetal Heart Rate Based on the Fetal Position

Diagnosis

Human chorionic gonadotropin (HCG) is a hormone made during pregnancy. It can be detected in the blood 10–11 days after ovulation. In general, the HCG level doubles every 2–3 days in early pregnancy. The level peaks around 8–10 weeks of pregnancy and then declines.

Pregnancy is an experience that affects every single body system during the 10 months of gestation. For you to identify when complications arise, you must first understand what the normal physical changes are and why they happen.

Normal Physiologic Changes of Pregnancy: The Basics

Body system	Changes with pregnancy
Cardiovascular	Maternal blood volume increases by 1.5 times by 20 weeks gestation
Gastrointestinal	• High levels of progesterone slow GI motility, leading to constipation and contributing to the presence of hemorrhoids • In the third trimester, the uterus presses up against the stomach, leading to heartburn
Genitourinary	• The weight of the uterus presses on the bladder, increasing urinary urgency • The size of the uterus limits the ability for the bladder to expand, increasing urinary frequency
Integumentary	• Stretch marks are common, as the skin is forced to rapidly accommodate the growing uterus and body weight changes • Hair growth continues normally; however, the shedding cycle halts, which may make some women feel that their hair is fuller
Musculoskeletal	• Increased levels of the hormone relaxin contributes to pubic symphysis separation • Kyphosis of the spine in the third trimester can contribute to poor posture; use of muscles that are not typically used and therefore weaker can lead to lower back pain • Carpal tunnel occurs due to fluid retention in the connective tissue
Respiratory	As the uterus grows, it expands upwards and presses on the diaphragm, which can limit lung expansion

Table 9.5.4 Normal Physiologic Changes of Pregnancy

Complications of Pregnancy

Complication	Signs and symptoms	Diagnostic tests
Anemia of pregnancy	• Fatigue • Palpitations and/or shortness of breath if severe	Hemoglobin and hematocrit
Deep vein thrombosis (DVT)	Unilateral swollen, painful extremity that is hot to the touch	Venous doppler/ultrasound
Ectopic pregnancy	• Unilateral pelvic pain (severe pain if ruptured) • Spotting • Missed period and/or positive pregnancy test	Ultrasound
SAB threatened, inevitable, complete, incomplete	• Vaginal bleeding • Uterine cramping/pain	Clinical Findings • Cervical os closed (threatened) • Cervix dilated, cannot stop contractions (inevitable) • Products of conception; fetus/placenta expelled (complete) • Retained products of conception/placenta (incomplete)
Gestational diabetes	• Rapid weight gain • Uterine size > gestational age • Glucose on urine dip • Polyhydramnios	• Screening: 50 g glucose challenge test (GCT) • Diagnosis: 100 g glucose tolerance test (GTT)

Table 9.5.5 Complications of Pregnancy

Complication	Signs and symptoms	Diagnostic tests
Gestational hypertension	• Elevated blood pressure • Often asymptomatic	Either a systolic BP of ≥140 or a diastolic BP of ≥90 on 2 separate occasions greater than 4 hours apart and in the absence of proteinuria
Gestational thrombocytopenia	Asymptomatic	Persistent platelets <140
Intrahepatic cholestasis of pregnancy (ICP)	• Generalized itching, which includes the palms and soles, and is worse at night • Absence of a rash	• Screening: liver function tests • Diagnostic: elevated serum bile acids Order labs together; bile acid results may take up to a week to be processed. Elevated LFTs may help guide early treatment
Preeclampsia	• Headache unrelieved by acetaminophen • Scotoma • Epigastric or RUQ pain • Sudden onset significant lower extremity swelling • Facial swelling	Clinical findings • BP ≥140/90, and proteinuria • BP ≥160/100 Laboratory findings • Urine protein-creatinine ratio >0.3 or urine protein DIP >+3 • Elevated LFTs (worrisome for HELLP syndrome) • Platelets trending downwards (worrisome for HELLP syndrome) Eclampsia is a severe complication of preeclampsia and is diagnosed by the presence of seizures
Premature rupture of membranes (PROM)	Leaking of fluid from the vagina	Sterile speculum exam • Pooling of fluid • Nitrazine paper with pH of 7 • Ferning pattern on slide preparation
Preterm labor	• Abdominal and back pain that comes and goes • Pink-tinged discharge	• 24–32 weeks: transvaginal ultrasound for cervical length • 32w1d–term: digital cervical exam
Pruritic urticarial papules and plaques of pregnancy (PUPPP)	Red, raised, itchy rash that starts around the umbilicus and moves outwards; typically found in the striae	Physical examination

Table 9.5.5 Complications of Pregnancy (Continued)

Plan

Treatment

Common complaints or discomforts	Relief measures	Medication management
Bloating	• Small frequent meals • Avoid legumes and cruciferous vegetables • Avoid caffeine	simethicone
Braxton Hicks contractions	• Hydration • Rest • Empty bladder	diphenhydramine or doxylamine to promote rest
Carpal tunnel	• Soft wrist brace • Ice packs • Increase hydration	acetaminophen 650 mg PO q 6 hours prn pain
Constipation	• Increase dietary fiber • Increase hydration	docusate sodium 50 mg PO daily; can increase to TID
Edema	• Increase hydration • Elevate legs when able • Supportive shoes • Compression socks or stockings	No medication available
Fatigue	Nap as often as able	220 units of caffeine per day is acceptable
Heartburn	• Avoid spicy or fatty foods • Avoid eating within 2 hours of bedtime • Remain upright for 1 hour after eating • Space out consumption of beverages and food	• calcium carbonate • ranitidine • famotidine
Insomnia	• Develop a bedtime routine • Avoid use of electronics within 30 minutes of bedtime • Keep room dark and quiet • Try a white-noise maker to drown out distracting sounds	• doxylamine • diphenhydramine
Lower back pain	• Heating pad • Massage	acetaminophen
Melasma (aka: "mask of pregnancy")	Wear sunscreen before going outside to prevent darkening of the area	N/A
Nausea and vomiting	• Ginger-containing products • Coca-Cola • Eating crackers before getting out of bed in the morning • Taking a walk	• doxylamine/pyridoxine (Diclegis) 10mg/10 mg, 2 tablets at night; may add 1 tablet in the AM and 1 in the afternoon if needed • ondansetron 4–8 mg PO q 8 hours for moderate to severe nausea and vomiting • compazine
Round ligament pain	Pregnancy belt or belly band	acetaminophen
Sciatic pain	• Hamstring stretch • Massaging area with a tennis ball • Heating pad on affected area	acetaminophen

Table 9.5.6 Common Discomforts of Pregnancy and Relief Measures

Treatment of Select Complications of Pregnancy

Condition	Treatment
Anemia	Slow-release or extended-release iron • 140 to 160 mg (45 mg) PO daily or BID depending on severity
Intrahepatic cholestasis of pregnancy (ICP)	ursodeoxycholic acid (UCDA) • 300 mg po TID or 15 mg/kg PO daily diphenhydramine • 25 mg PO TID prn itching
Gestational diabetes	• Diet modification is sufficient for most women • If insulin is necessary, it should be managed by a specialist
Gestational hypertension	Beta-blockers are first-line treatment
Preeclampsia	• Delivery of the baby and placenta is the only "cure" for preeclampsia • Women who are preterm with mild preeclampsia may be managed outpatient with beta-blockers to control their blood pressure • Women who are early term or later should be delivered
PUPPS	• Sarna lotion • Oatmeal-based lotions • diphenhydramine

Table 9.5.7 Treatment of Select Complications of Pregnancy

For information related to HIV and the pregnant woman, refer to Chapter 15, Lesson 2.

> **DANGER SIGN** In addition to the conditions in Table 9.5.7 above, pregnancy can be complicated by:
>
> • **Placenta previa**: painless vaginal bleeding in the third trimester
> • **Placenta abruptio**: vaginal bleeding and painful contractions in the third trimester
> • **HELLP syndrome:** occurs in women with preeclampsia; hemolysis, elevated liver enzymes, low platelets
> • **Rh incompatibility/ABO incompatibility**: potential complications are hydrops fetalis and erythroblastosis fetalis

The nurse practitioner may treat high-risk pregnancies with the collaboration of an obstetrician or MFM. Specific treatment regimens are not discussed in this text, as they are out of the scope of practice for the independent family nurse practitioner.

Patient Education and Screening Tests Organized by Gestational Age

Gestational age	Education and testing
0–14 weeks	**Prenatal vitamins:** • All will have a minimum of 400 mcg folic acid; some women need more than this based on their medical history • Some women may need iron or a stool softener **Medications/substances:** • Discuss all medications prior to use (both prescribed and over-the-counter) • Do not drink alcohol or use drugs • Discuss smoking cessation, if applicable **Dietary avoidances:** • Raw or undercooked meats/fish (use a meat thermometer to assess "done-ness") • Large fish, such as swordfish or mackerel, which have high levels of mercury • Cold cuts • Unpasteurized dairy products • Raw honey • Loose-leaf teas **Exercise:** • Pregnant women should not be sedentary; however, they will likely need to modify their exercise routines • Avoid strenuous activity or any activity which includes bearing down • Drink 8–10 glasses of water per day, increase with activity **Environmental concerns:** • Cats who go outdoors may carry toxoplasmosis which can be transmitted to humans through their stool • Old homes may have lead paint; walls can easily be tested by anyone, but removal must be done by a professional service • Dye hair and paint nails in a well-ventilated space • Patient's occupation should also be considered and screened for risk factors **Genetic testing:** • First trimester screen: recommended for women ≤35 years old at the time of delivery; consists of a blood test and an ultrasound to measure the fetal nuchal translucency; goal is to determine risk of the fetus having trisomy 18 or 21 • Cell-free DNA testing: recommended for women >35 years old at the time of delivery; consists of a blood test only; typically tests for trisomy 13 (Patau syndrome), 18 (Edwards syndrome), 21 (Down syndrome); can be expanded to include microdeletions, monosomies, and sex-linked disorders • Chorionic villus sampling: can be performed from 10–12 weeks (cervical or transabdominal approach) **New OB labs (may be limited to or expanded upon the following based on the patient's individual risk factors and geographic location):** • CBC with differential and RBC, ABO/Rh, HIV, hepatitis B surface antigen, syphilis, CG, chlamydia, GBS, rubella titer, varicella, urinalysis, and culture **Other education:** • Recommend the flu vaccine per CDC guidelines • If rubella negative, will need an MMR postpartum • If Rh negative, will need a RhoGAM injection at 28 weeks and postpartum • Discuss common early pregnancy symptoms and relief measures

Table 9.5.8 Patient Education and Screening Tests Organized by Gestational Age

Gestational age	Education and testing
14–20 weeks	Alpha-fetal protein (AFP) test for neural tube defects • Optimal time to test is 15–18 weeks Quad screen (AFP, hCG, estriol, inhibin-A) • Also completed between 15–18 weeks • Tests for trisomy 18–21, as well as AFP Fetal anatomy scan • Completed between 17–20 weeks Amniocentesis • Can be performed 15–18 weeks Education: • Quickening occurs around 18 weeks
20–28 weeks	Second-trimester labs • Completed between 26–28 weeks • Include a CBC and a glucose challenge test (GCT) • Screening for HIV and RPR a second time may be recommended based on patient population
28–34 weeks	Education: • Fetal movement counts (FMCs) • Signs and symptoms of preterm labor: painful, regular contractions, especially with lower back pain; leaking of amniotic fluid; vaginal bleeding • Common discomforts of pregnancy • Childbirth, breastfeeding, newborn, and sibling education classes • Choosing a pediatrician • Tdap vaccine is due between 28–34 weeks
34–42 weeks	Education: • Labor and delivery process and pain relief options • Induction of labor • Newborn care • Breastfeeding • Circumcision Testing: • Group B *Streptococcus* vaginal/rectal culture at 36 weeks (if positive, treated with antibiotic (PO PCN or clindamycin); woman must receive an IV antibiotic during labor)

Table 9.5.8 Patient Education and Screening Tests Organized by Gestational Age (Continued)

Labor

It is important to teach the woman about signs of impending labor. Lightening usually occurs a few weeks before labor. Passage of the mucus plug happens a few days prior to delivery. Teach the woman to time her contractions; with true labor, the contractions occur at regular intervals and, as time goes on, get closer together (lasting about 30–70 seconds). With false labor, contractions will stop with activity/walking; however, in true labor, the contractions will persist. The pain originates in the woman's back and moves toward her abdomen. On exam, there will be cervical effacement ($\geq$50%) and cervical dilation ($\geq$2 cm).

Postpartum

Breastfeeding	*Refer to the online bonus content "Developmental Considerations in Childhood: Lesson 1: Development of the Newborn & Infant."*
Mastitis	*Refer to Chapter 9, Lesson 3, "Mastitis."*
Depression	*Refer to Chapter 12, Lesson 3, "Postpartum Depression."*
Follow-up care	A postpartum checkup should be scheduled within the first 3 weeks. ACOG's latest recommendations regarding postpartum care are available here: **https://www.acog.org/Clinical-Guidance-and-Publications/Committee-Opinions/Committee-on-Obstetric-Practice/Optimizing-Postpartum-Care**.

Table 9.5.9 Postpartum Care

Referrals

Referral to a specialist or to a higher level of care is not uncommon during pregnancy. Pregnant women are systematically screened for illness that could put them or their fetuses at risk. Therefore, when a concern is discovered it is critical that the woman be swiftly transferred or, at minimum, co-managed by the appropriate team of providers. Some conditions, such as diet-controlled gestational diabetes, can be easily managed by a nurse practitioner after consultation with an endocrinologist. Other conditions, such as gestational hypertension requiring medication management, should be monitored and treated with the collaboration of an obstetrician.

Takeaways

- Pregnancy is a normal part of the human experience, although it may make women feel like their bodies are not their own.
- Pregnant women are a protected population, which means that the safety of many products and medications is unknown.
- For information regarding prescription medications related to pregnancy, *see Chapter 4, Lesson 9.*
- Be aware of conditions for which consultation/referral is needed.

PRACTICE QUESTIONS

Select the ONE best answer.

Lesson 1: Renal

1. An adult male has been diagnosed with nephrolithiasis. Which of the following is the correct patient education?

    A. Take cranberry supplements on a daily basis

    B. Once the stone passes, recurrence is unlikely

    C. Increase daily amounts of fluid intake

    D. Avoid eating bananas, potatoes, and oranges

2. An 8-year-old has been diagnosed with acute poststreptococcal glomerulonephritis. Which finding does the nurse practitioner anticipate?

    A. Blood pressure 128/88

    B. Blood pressure 105/73

    C. Heart rate 80

    D. Urine output 2 mL/kg/hr

3. The nurse practitioner is assessing the results of a urine dipstick for a patient with a suspected renal disorder. The urine is 3+ for blood. This finding rules out which disorder?

    A. Glomerulonephritis

    B. Nephrolithiasis

    C. Nephrotic syndrome

    D. Urinary tract infection

4. An adult patient is being scheduled for an intravenous pyelogram (IVP). What is an important pre-procedure assessment the nurse practitioner should make?

    A. Ability to urinate independently

    B. Mobility status

    C. Oral fluid intake

    D. Current medication list

5. The nurse practitioner is reviewing the results of a urinalysis. Which set of results is most indicative of urinary tract infection?

    A. Protein 2+, blood 2+, nitrites negative

    B. Protein negative, nitrites 2+, leukocyte esterase 2+

    C. Bacteria 1+, nitrites negative, leukocyte esterase negative

    D. Protein negative, blood negative, WBC 4

6. The nurse practitioner has diagnosed a young adult with acute uncomplicated pyelonephritis. Which is the appropriate first-line treatment?

    A. amoxicillin-clavulanate (Amoxil)

    B. trimethoprim-sulfamethoxazole (Bactrim DS)

    C. nitrofurantoin (Macrobid)

    D. ciprofloxacin (Cipro)

Lesson 2: Men's Health

7. A 56-year-old male presents to the office with complaints of painful, frequent, and urgent urination. He also states that sometimes when he tries to void he has difficulty emptying. This is the third time he has been seen with these same symptoms in the last 8 months, and each time his urine culture showed *E. coli*. Based on his symptoms, you know that your patient is most likely suffering from which of the following conditions?

    A. Asymptomatic bacteriuria

    B. Interstitial cystitis

    C. Chronic prostatitis

    D. Varicocele

8. A 22-year-old male calls the answering service at 2 AM with a report that he was awakened from sleep with severe, debilitating testicular pain that lasted 10 minutes and then spontaneously resolved. He denies pain at this time but is afraid it will happen again. Which of the following is the nurse practitioner's best response?

   A. Go to the emergency room now for further evaluation

   B. Take acetaminophen 650 mg PO × 1 in case the pain comes back, and make an appointment to be seen as soon as the office opens

   C. Explain that this can be a normal symptom that is more common with younger men and it is nothing to worry about

   D. Prescribe azithromycin (Zithromax) 1 gram PO × 1, as this is a symptom of chlamydia

9. A 60-year-old male presents to the office with complaints of sexual dysfunction. He reports that over the past 6 months he has had difficulty maintaining an erection. He denies any UTI symptoms and denies any recent trauma or psychological component, but does feel anxious about his situation. After examining the patient, you find no physical abnormalities and decide to start him on which of the following medications?

   A. sertraline (Zoloft)

   B. sildenafil (Viagra)

   C. ciprofloxacin (Cipro)

   D. testosterone (AndroGel)

10. A 36-year-old man presents to the office with complaint of a lump in his chest. On exam, you note a 1 cm × 1 cm hard, non-tender mass beneath the right areola at 3 o'clock. Based on these findings, you make which of the following plans?

    A. Schedule the patient for a right-breast ultrasound

    B. Refer to a breast surgeon for removal

    C. Continue to monitor for one month, and return for care if still present

    D. Schedule the patient for a diagnostic mammogram and breast ultrasound

11. A 30-year-old man presents to the office for an annual visit. His best friend was recently diagnosed with testicular cancer and is asking whether he should get himself tested. He states he has completed a thorough testicular self exam and has not felt any masses, but he is still worried. Based on the current cancer screening guidelines, you give him what advice?

    A. Asymptomatic men such as himself are low-risk and should not undergo testing

    B. Even though he is low-risk, it doesn't hurt to send him for a baseline testicular ultrasound just in case

    C. As long as he did not have cryptorchidism as a child, he will not get testicular cancer

    D. The average age of diagnosis is 50–69, which makes his friend an exception, so he shouldn't worry about it

12. A diagnosis of benign prostatic hyperplasia includes all of the following except:

    A. Urinary urgency and frequency

    B. Slow urination, occasional spraying of urine

    C. Painful urination

    D. Enlarged prostate on digital rectal exam

Lesson 3: Breast

13. A 35-year-old female presents to the clinic for evaluation of recent onset of right-nipple discharge. This discharge is elicited with manipulation and is green to yellow in color. Her paternal grandmother was diagnosed with breast cancer at the age of 65. Which of the following is best for the nurse practitioner to include in the treatment plan?

    A. Schedule the patient for a diagnostic mammogram

    B. Perform a hemoccult of the nipple discharge

    C. Reassure the patient that her nipple discharge is benign

    D. Refer the patient to a breast specialist

14. The nurse practitioner ordered a diagnostic mammogram and breast ultrasound to further evaluate a palpable area of concern for a 55-year-old female patient. The patient reported feeling a mass during her recent self-breast exam. The nurse practitioner appreciated thickening on exam but no obvious mass. The imaging report notes that there is no visible correlate for the palpable finding with a BIRADS category 2 and recommendation for a screening mammogram in one year. What will the nurse practitioner do next?

    A. Reassure the patient, as her imaging was normal and she has no family history of breast cancer

    B. Schedule the patient for return appointment with a screening mammogram in one year

    C. Schedule a short-term follow up appointment in 6 months

    D. Schedule a consult with a breast surgeon

15. The patient states "I am really fearful of breast cancer. I have so much cancer in my family." How should the nurse practitioner respond?

    A. Perform a three-generation family pedigree

    B. Refer the patient to a breast surgeon

    C. Prescribe tamoxifen (Nolvadex) for risk reduction

    D. Include breast MRI as part of the patient's annual imaging surveillance

16. A 30-year-old breastfeeding patient was diagnosed with mastitis and treated with dicloxacillin (Dynapen) for 7 days. She presents for reassessment. The patient reports, "I think things are getting better." The affected breast remains erythematous throughout. Which of the following is best for the nurse practitioner to do?

    A. Discontinue the dicloxacillin and prescribe trimethoprim/sulfamethoxazole (Bactrim)

    B. Advise the patient to use cabbage leaves for her engorgement

    C. Refer the patient to a breast surgeon

    D. Schedule the patient for a mammogram

17. Mammograms do not always identify cancer in dense breast tissue. All of the following are more effective at detecting breast cancers in women with dense breasts except:

    A. Ultrasound

    B. MRI

    C. CT scan with contrast

    D. 3-D mammogram

18. Which is the safest contraceptive method for a woman with active breast cancer?

    A. Copper IUD (Paragard)

    B. Depo-Provera

    C. Combined oral contraceptives

    D. Mirena IUD

Lesson 4: Women's Health—GYN

19. A 19-year-old female presents to the office for a well-woman exam. She has been sexually active with her first partner for 6 months. She denies any complaints and states, "I'm just here for my birth control refill." Her exam should include which of the following?

    A. Pap smear, gonorrhea test, and chlamydia test

    B. Full physical exam including clinical breast exam and pelvic exam

    C. Complete health history and vital signs only; no physical exam is necessary

    D. Gonorrhea test and chlamydia test

20. A 53-year-old female presents to the office with complaints of vaginal discomfort and burning on urination. Her last period was two years ago. Your exam findings are as follows: pregnancy test is negative, external vagina with normal appearance, internal vagina is pale light pink, cervix with mild stenosis, scant clear vaginal discharge, bimanual exam without tenderness, vaginal pH is 5, whiff test is negative, wet mount shows no buds/clue cells/trichomonads, urine DIP is negative. Which of the following prescriptions do you recommend for this patient?

    A. hydrocortisone 1% topical cream (Cortef)

    B. metronidazole gel 0.75% (MetroGel)

    C. estradiol 0.01% cream (Estace)

    D. clotrimazole 1% cream (Cleocin)

21. A 36-year-old G3P2 female presents to the office with pelvic and back pain, as well as painful intercourse and burning on urination. Your exam reveals tenderness in the LLQ and RLQ of the abdomen, cervical motion tenderness, and exquisite pain on palpation of the uterus and right adnexa. Her urine dipstick is positive for leukocytes and ketones and negative for blood and nitrites. Based on these findings, you diagnose and treat her with which of the following?

    A. Urinary tract infection: nitrofurantoin (Macrobid) 100 mg PO BID × 5 days

    B. Pelvic inflammatory disease: ceftriaxone (Rocephin) 250 mg IM × 1 and doxycycline (Vibramycin) 100 mg PO BID × 14 days

    C. Trichomoniasis: tinidazole (Tindamax) 2 g PO × 1

    D. Endometriosis: continuous combined oral contraceptives

22. A 23-year-old female presents to the office with a desire for birth control. She is generally healthy and has no drug allergies but is lactose intolerant. She denies any PMH/PSH and denies smoking cigarettes. She takes a multivitamin "most of the time," though she often forgets. She reports her period is regular and she likes having it because it reassures her she's not pregnant. Based on this information, the nurse practitioner recommends which of the following birth control methods?

    A. Combined oral contraceptive pills

    B. DMPA (Depo-Provera) injections

    C. Vaginal ring (NuvaRing)

    D. LNG-IUD (Skyla)

23. A 60-year-old female presents to the office for follow-up after being seen two weeks ago for a painless labial lesion and associated swollen, though non-painful, inguinal lymph nodes. She had a VDRL drawn, which resulted positive, so reflex testing was performed. Today you will tell her that her FTA-ABS was also positive and give her which of the following diagnoses?

    A. Primary syphilis

    B. Hepatitis B virus

    C. Human immunodeficiency virus

    D. Herpes zoster virus

24. A 22-year-old nulliparous female presents to the office with complaints of burning on urination and vaginal itching. She broke up with her boyfriend three months ago and recently became sexually active with someone new. Her symptoms began three days ago and she has already tried OTC miconazole, which made the burning worse. She denies any urinary frequency, urgency, pressure, vaginal odor, or postcoital bleeding. On exam, you note multiple blistering lesions with red, swollen bases, in varying stages of healing. You culture the lesions, but tell her you are most confident she has which diagnosis?

    A. Molluscum

    B. Secondary syphilis

    C. Primary HSV infection

    D. Condyloma acuminatum caused by HPV

25. A 41-year-old female calls the answering service to report a possible anxiety attack. She is feeling short of breath and has palpitations and mild chest pain. The symptoms began this evening when she got home from the airport after traveling on a business trip. A thorough review of her chart reveals she is a healthy nonsmoker and that her only medication is combined oral contraceptives. Based on this information, you give her which advice?

    A. Make an appointment in the office as soon as it opens tomorrow

    B. Practice slow deep breaths, take a warm shower, and try to rest

    C. Call in a prescription for alprazolam to the pharmacy

    D. Do not take any more COCs and go immediately to the nearest emergency department

26. A 30-year-old female was recently seen for her annual well-woman exam. As is recommended by the ASCCP, she had a Pap smear with HPV co-testing completed. Her results are ASCUS and HPV negative. You take which of the following actions?

    A. Refer the patient for a colposcopy

    B. Repeat Pap with co-testing in three years

    C. Return for cytology only in six months

    D. Repeat Pap with co-testing in one year

Lesson 5: Women's Health—OB

27. Select the appropriate GTPAL score for the woman with the following obstetrical history: vaginal births at 39w3d and 40w0d, cesarean delivery for twins at 35w4d, miscarriage at 11 weeks, termination at 6 weeks, all children born are still alive.

    A. G5T2P1A2L4

    B. G6T2P1A2L4

    C. G5P4

    D. G6P2

28. Every prenatal visit includes the following information except:

    A. Fundal height

    B. Fetal heart rate

    C. Temperature

    D. Blood pressure

29. After performing the Leopold maneuvers, you determine that the fetus is in the LOA position. Based on this information, you listen for fetal heart tones in which abdominal quadrant?

    A. RLQ

    B. LLQ

    C. LUQ

    D. RUQ

30. A 32-year-old G1P0 presents to the office with complaints of daily heartburn. She is already taking calcium carbonate several times a day and is asking if there is anything else she can do. You write which of the following prescriptions as your first-line treatment?

    A. pantoprazole (Protonix) 40 mg PO daily

    B. doxylamine (Unisom) 10 mg qhs

    C. diphenhydramine (Benadryl) 25 mg PO TID

    D. ranitidine (Zantac) 75 mg PO qhs

31. The diagnosis of preeclampsia can be made with which of the following findings?

    A. BP 150/92 and UPCR 0.4

    B. BP 140/90 and +2 protein on dipstick

    C. BP 142/96 and +3 bilateral pitting edema

    D. BP 150/78 and trace urine protein on dipstick

32. A 28-year-old G3P2 at 16w5d presents to the office for a prenatal visit. You are sure to offer which test appropriate for her gestational age before she leaves?

    A. Group B strep swab

    B. Cell-free DNA

    C. Alpha-fetoprotein

    D. Ultrasound anatomy scan

33. The Tdap vaccine should be encouraged at which time?

    A. Anytime, as long as it is during the pregnancy

    B. 28–34 weeks

    C. Immediately postpartum

    D. During the first trimester

ANSWERS AND EXPLANATIONS

Lesson 1: Renal

1. C

Adequate fluid intake **(C)** decreases the risk of further stone formation and maintains good hydration. Cranberry supplements (A) and cranberry juice have not been shown to have an effect on stones. The recurrence rate for kidney stones may be as high as 50% (B). Bananas, potatoes, and oranges (D) are high in potassium, which is an issue in renal insufficiency, not nephrolithiasis.

2. A

Hypertension is a likely finding with glomerulonephritis; blood pressure 128/88 **(A)** is high for an 8-year-old. Blood pressure 105/73 (B) is within the higher range of normal limits for an 8-year-old. Heart rate 80 (C) is within normal range for an 8-year-old. Glomerulonephritis may result in renal failure: urine output of 2 mL/kg/hr (D) is normal in children.

3. C

Nephrotic syndrome **(C)** is not associated with occult or frank hematuria. Hematuria may occur with glomerulonephritis (A), nephrolithiasis (B), and urinary tract infection (D).

4. D

Review the patient's current medication list **(D)** for nephrotoxic drugs, as IV contrast also carries the potential for nephrotoxicity. While adequate urine output is necessary for elimination of IV contrast, the ability to urinate independently (A) is not necessary. Mobility status (B) has no effect on the IVP. Adequate fluid intake (C) post-procedure is important for appropriate elimination of the contrast material.

5. B

The presence of nitrites and leukocyte esterase **(B)** on the urinalysis is most indicative of a urinary tract infection, as nitrites indicate the presence of bacteria that reduce nitrates, and leukocyte esterase is indicative of inflammation. Proteinuria and hematuria (A) are consistent with glomerulonephritis. The presence of bacteria (C) in the urinalysis as the only positive finding does not necessarily indicate infection, as a small amount of bacteria can be a common finding upon urinalysis, especially with a clean-catch specimen. WBC <5 (D) is a normal finding.

6. D

Ciprofloxacin **(D)** is effective against gram-negative organisms and should be prescribed for 5–7 days. Amoxicillin-clavulanate (A) is not an appropriate choice for gram-negative infection. Trimethoprim-sulfamethoxazole (B) is considered the first-line treatment for acute uncomplicated urinary tract infection, while nitrofurantoin (C) may be prescribed for those with sulfa allergy.

Lesson 2: Men's Health

7. C

Recurrent UTI symptoms and difficulty emptying are two common symptoms of chronic prostatitis **(C)**. Urine cultures also often result with the same offending bacteria. Asymptomatic bacteriuria (A) is diagnosed after three urine cultures are positive for bacteria, despite the patient denying any symptoms. Interstitial cystitis (B) is an inflammatory disease characterized by recurrent UTI symptoms in the absence of positive urine cultures. Varicocele (D) occurs when vein distention is present in the scrotum.

8. A

Sudden onset of scrotal pain may be a sign of testicular torsion **(A)**, a medical emergency that must be evaluated immediately, as it may lead to permanent ischemia and loss of the affected testes. Telling the patient to be seen tomorrow (B) ignores the fact that this may be a medical emergency. Severe testicular pain warrants investigation, it is not a "normal" symptom (C). Untreated chlamydia (D) may cause pelvic pain, urethral inflammation, and abnormal discharge. The patient should be evaluated prior to treatment.

9. B

The patient is reporting symptoms of erectile dysfunction, a condition for which the first-line treatment is phosphodiesterase-5 inhibitors, including sildenafil **(B)**. Sertraline (A) is an SSRI is used to treat ejaculatory disorders. Ciprofloxacin (C) may be ordered for a complicated UTI. Testosterone (D) is used to treat hypoandrogenism.

10. D

When suspicious for male breast cancer, a diagnostic mammogram and ultrasound **(D)** should be ordered to more clearly visualize the tissue, although a biopsy will ultimately be needed to confirm the diagnosis. An ultrasound (A) is not the most appropriate "standalone" diagnostic tool. Referral to a breast surgeon is an excellent use of community resources; however, planning for removal (B) is presumptive. (C) Waiting another month before further examination may delay diagnosis of a breast cancer, as the mass described is worrisome for a malignancy.

11. A

Current guidelines according to the ACS, AUA, and USP-STF state that asymptomatic men should not be tested for testicular cancer **(A)** because screening, including ultrasound (B), has not been proven to improve cure rates. While cryptorchidism (C) is a major risk factor for testicular cancer, it is not the only one. Age (nearly 50% of cases occur in men 20–34 years old, not 50–69 years [D]), race (African American men are at greatest risk), and family and personal history are also considered risk factors.

12. C

BPH does not cause painful urination **(C)**, although alterations to voiding patterns may cause a urinary tract infection, which may present with dysuria. BPH is diagnosed by taking a thorough history of symptoms related to urine storage (A) and patterns of urination, as well as difficulty controlling urine (B). Some patients may be asymptomatic, but all patients with BPH will have an enlarged prostate (D) on exam.

Lesson 3: Breast

13. B

The nipple discharge described is likely benign, and performing a hemoccult **(B)** will rule out occult blood, supporting the diagnosis. Since the patient is under age 40, mammogram (A) is not useful for imaging evaluation of nipple discharge; rather, a retroareolar breast ultrasound would be ordered. Although the patient's discharge is likely benign, further evaluation is warranted to support the diagnosis; reassurance is not enough (C). Further evaluation is needed prior to referral (D). If the hemoccult is positive or breast ultrasound is abnormal, then referral would be appropriate.

14. D

Refer the patient to a breast specialist with an area of palpable concern **(D)**, even if the imaging study is negative. Normal imaging and no FH of breast cancer are indeed "reassuring"; however, the patient has reported a mass and the NP palpated thickening on exam—choice (A) is not the next best step. If the patient had a normal breast exam, a screening mammogram in one year (B) would be appropriate. With an area of concern on the patient's SBE and focal thickening on exam, clinical surveillance in 6 months (C) is not appropriate.

15. A

Assessing a detailed FH **(A)** will allow the NP to determine if further intervention, such as referral to a genetic counselor and/or enhanced imaging surveillance (with breast MR for example), is warranted. If there is a significant FH and genetic testing is needed, the best referral would be to a genetic counselor, not a surgeon (B). Tamoxifen (C) is appropriate if the woman has elevated risk; the NP would need to calculate a Gail score, Tyrer-Cuzick, or something similar to determine this OR if the woman had a genetic predisposition identified by genetic testing. The patient's lifetime risk would need to be determined first; risk of 20% or greater indicates consideration for MRI surveillance (D).

16. C

An erythematous breast that does not respond to antibiotic therapy may not reflect mastitis; rather, this could be inflammatory breast cancer; you must refer the patient to a breast surgeon **(C)**. Changing antibiotic therapy (A) is not sufficient given the findings on exam. The clinical findings are not suggestive of engorgement (B). Mammograms (D) are often not helpful in ruling in/ruling out inflammatory breast cancer, nor are they a useful tool in diagnosing mastitis.

17. C

CT **(C)** is not an ideal imaging modality for the breast. It can be utilized as part of staging studies in a woman diagnosed with breast cancer. Ultrasound (A), MRI (B), and 3-D mammogram (D) (also referred to as "tomosynthesis") are better options for imaging the woman with dense breast tissue. The ASTOUND study, published online on March 9, 2016, by the *Journal of Clinical Oncology* found that adding 3-D mammography or breast ultrasound to regular screening mammograms can detect more cancers in dense breasts. Ultrasound was slightly better at detecting cancers in dense breasts than 3-D mammography, and both screening methods had similar false-positive rates. Breast MRI is another alternative; given the rate of false positives, recommendation for inclusion of MRI is for the woman with a lifetime risk of breast cancer of 20% or greater.

18. A

The Copper IUD **(A)** is the safest contraceptive method for a woman with active breast cancer. According to the WHO Medical Eligibility Criteria for Contraceptive Use, neither combined oral contraceptives (C) nor Depo-Provera (B) should be initiated or continued in a woman with active breast cancer. Mirena IUD (D) is not approved for use in women with a history of breast cancer.

Lesson 4: Women's Health—GYN

19. D

All sexually active teens and young women 24 years of age and younger should be screened for GC/CT at every visit **(D)**. Pap smears (A) do not start until age 21. A pelvic exam (B) is not necessary for women <20 years of age, unless they are reporting specific complaints. A consultation visit (health history and vital signs without CBE or pelvic exam) (C) is appropriate for healthy women <20 years of age.

20. C

The patient is exhibiting symptoms of atrophic vaginitis due to menopause; therefore, a topical estrogen cream **(C)** is an appropriate intervention. Hydrocortisone cream (A) may be recommended for hemorrhoids. Metronidazole gel (B) is used for bacterial vaginosis, and clotrimazole (D) treats yeast.

21. B

The minimum criteria for PID **(B)** are lower abdominal tenderness, cervical motion tenderness, and uterine or adnexal tenderness. A UTI (A) is not likely given the absence of bacteria and nitrites. Trichomoniasis (C) may be causing the PID; however, when a presumptive diagnosis of PID is made, the patient should be treated with antibiotics that cover anaerobic bacteria. Endometriosis (D) may present with pelvic and back pain; however, cervical motion tenderness and uterine or adnexal tenderness are not seen. All of the medications listed are appropriate for their corresponding diagnoses.

22. C

The patient would be most successful on a continuous birth control method that would also keep her periods regular, such as NuvaRing **(C)**. CCOs (A) require daily administration, and therefore would not be the best option for her since she often forgets her vitamin. Both DMPA (B) and LNG-IUD (D) have the common side effects of irregular bleeding and possible cessation of menses. The DMPA also carries a risk of bone demineralization; therefore, a patient who ingests limited dietary calcium should consider this method with caution.

23. A

A chancre is a classic sign of primary syphilis **(A)**, and diagnosis is confirmed by performing a nontreponemal screening test (VDRL), which then reflexes to a treponemal test (FTA-ABS) if positive. The tests used to diagnose hepatitis B (B) are HBsAg/IgM anti-HBc. Testing for HIV (C) involves an enzyme immunoassay screening test and Western blot diagnostic test. Herpes zoster virus (D) can cause both varicella (chicken pox) and shingles; diagnosis is typically made by physical exam.

24. C

The question stem describes the classic presentation of a primary HSV outbreak **(C)**. Molluscum (A) are waxy, painless lesions. Secondary syphilis (B) is not associated with genital lesions, but rather a full-body rash as well as other systemic symptoms. Condyloma acuminatum (genital warts) (D) have a clustered or cauliflower presentation with a grainy appearance.

25. D

Your patient should immediately present to the nearest emergency department **(D)** due to the fact that she is experiencing symptoms of a possible pulmonary embolism (PE). Other clues include recent airplane travel and taking estrogen-containing medication. Making an appointment tomorrow (A) ignores the fact that the patient is in a potentially life-threatening situation. Practicing yoga breaths (B) and prescribing alprazolam (Xanax) (C) assume that the patient is experiencing anxiety; however, a PE needs to be ruled out first because it poses the largest threat.

26. B

The recommended follow-up for a cytology result of ASCUS combined with a negative HPV test is to repeat both cytology and HPV testing in three years **(B)**. A colposcopy (A) would only be necessary if the HPV test was positive. Returning for cytology in six months (C) is not part of the current ASCCP guidelines for these results. Had the patient not been tested for HPV and you only had ASCUS as a result, you could have chosen to repeat cytology in one year. Since the patient's HPV status was determined to be negative, repeating co-testing in one year (D) is unnecessary.

Lesson 5: Women's Health—OB

27. A

GTPAL stands for Gravida, Term, Preterm, Abortion, and Living. This woman was pregnant 5 times total (twin pregnancies are only counted once), she had two term births, one preterm birth, two abortions (miscarriages are included here), and all four of her children are still living. This makes her a G5T2P1A2L4 **(A)**. If using just GP to score her OB history, this woman would be G5P2, making (C) and (D) incorrect.

28. C

Maternal temperature **(C)** is not a standard component of the prenatal visit. Fundal height (A), fetal heart rate (B), blood pressure (D), weight, and urine should be assessed each appointment.

29. B

Since the fetal heartbeat is easiest to hear through the fetal back, when in the left occiput anterior (LOA) position, the heartbeat is best heard in the LLQ **(B)**. Heart tones are best heard in RLQ (A) if the fetus is in the ROA position and in LUQ (C) and RUQ (D) if the fetus is breach.

30. D

Although the H2 receptor antagonists are chemically similar to each other, and it is probable that they will affect a baby in the womb in the same way, we cannot be 100% certain of this. Ranitidine **(D)** is the H2 receptor antagonist that has been best studied in pregnant women and has not been shown to harm a developing baby in the womb. Ranitidine is therefore generally preferred over other H2 receptor antagonists for use in pregnancy when lifestyle changes (such as avoiding spicy foods and raising the head of the bed) and antacid or alginate medicines have not helped. It is recommended only to use Pantoprazole (A), a PPI, during pregnancy as needed, when no other options are available. Doxylamine (B) is used as an antihistamine and sleeping aid, and diphenhydramine (C) is an antihistamine.

31. A

Preeclampsia is diagnosed as an elevated BP $\geq$140/90 with either +3 protein on dipstick or $\geq$0.3 random urine protein-creatinine ratio (UPCR) **(A)**. The amount of proteinuria (B and D) is not diagnostic for preeclampsia. Edema with preeclampsia is central (facial) as well as peripheral, making (C) incorrect.

32. C

The alpha-fetoprotein blood test **(C)** for neural tube defects like spina bifida should ideally be drawn between 15–18 weeks. It is an optional test that should be offered to all women. The GBS swab (A) is collected universally at 36 weeks. Cell-free DNA (B) is a blood test for chromosomal anomalies, sex-linked disorders, and microdeletions, and should be offered in the first trimester. The anatomy scan (D) is typically done between 18–20 weeks.

33. B

The Tdap vaccine should be administered between 28–34 weeks **(B)** in order to allow for maternal antibodies to build and subsequently cross through the placenta to the baby prior to delivery. The timings in (A), (C), and (D) are inappropriate.

CHAPTER 10

Musculoskeletal

LESSON 1: ARTHRITIS OVERVIEW

Learning Objectives

- Distinguish the differences between non-inflammatory, inflammatory, and crystal-induced arthritic conditions
- Discuss assessment, diagnosis, and treatment of arthritic conditions

Arthritis can be broken down into three categories: non-inflammatory, inflammatory, and crystal-induced. This lesson will focus on osteoarthritis (non-inflammatory), rheumatoid arthritis (inflammatory), and gouty arthritis (crystal-induced). Understanding the differences can assist in assessment, diagnosis, and treatment.

Assessment

Pay particular attention to the joints during the physical assessment. Objective findings will be obtained from visual inspection and palpation.

Pro Tip: Assessment Hot Spots

- Gait pattern, use of assistive devices such as cane, crutches, and wheelchair
- Active range of motion
- Passive range of motion
- Joints for erythema, swelling, crepitus, synovitis, warmth, and tenderness

Osteoarthritis can be primary or secondary. Primary osteoarthritis is degenerative and occurs from wear and tear of the joints. Secondary osteoarthritis typically occurs from trauma to the joint.

Rheumatoid arthritis is an autoimmune disorder leading to symmetric inflammation.

Gouty arthritis is a metabolic disorder occurring when the body does not properly manage uric acid. This is manifested as decreased uric acid excretion, which allows uric acid to accumulate in the joints, subcutaneous tissues, and bones.

Characteristic	Osteoarthritis	Rheumatoid arthritis	Gouty arthritis
Onset	• >50 years • Onset is slow	• 20–40 years • Onset rapid: weeks to months • May occur at any time in life	• 30–50 years • Onset sudden: frequently occurs at night • More common in men and postmenopausal women
Systemic symptoms	None	Fatigue, low-grade fevers, muscle aching, anemia, and rheumatoid nodules	None
Joint symptoms	• Joint pain • Joint swelling less common • Asymmetric joint involvement	• Joint pain, swelling, and stiffness • Joints are tender, red, warm, and swollen • Symmetrical joint involvement	Joint pain, inflammation, redness, tenderness, decreased range of motion, and possible development of tophi
Joints involved	Neck, back, shoulders, PIP/DIP/CMC joints of the hands, hips, knees, and MTP joints of the great toes	Jaw, neck, shoulders, elbows, wrists, MCP/PIP joints of the hands, hips, knees, ankles, tarsal joints, and MTP joints of the feet (primarily small joints)	Commonly the great toe, but also occurs in ankle, heel, knee, wrist, fingers, and elbows
Morning stiffness	<30 minutes	>1 hour	None
Movement	Increases pain	Decreases pain	Increases pain

Table 10.1.1 Differentiation of Arthritis Types

Diagnosis

Osteoarthritis: radiographic evaluation reveals loss of articular cartilage, joint space narrowing, and/or osteophytes in painful joint(s). Laboratory testing is needed for diagnosis, but certain tests may be used to rule out other causes of joint pain, such as rheumatoid arthritis (see below).

Rheumatoid arthritis: combination of subjective and objective findings (as noted above). Supporting findings such as elevation of the ESR and CRP, along with positive RF and anti-CCP antibodies, and radiographic findings such as periarticular osteopenia and erosions.

Gouty arthritis: needle-aspiration to identify monosodium urate crystals in synovial fluid (obtained either from the joint or gouty tophi). X-rays are initially negative, but as the disease progresses, erosions or "rat-bite lesions" are noted.

American College of Rheumatology Criteria for the Diagnosis of Rheumatoid Arthritis
1. Morning stiffness lasting for >1 hour 2. Swelling of 3 or more joints (observed by provider) 3. Symmetric distribution 4. Involvement of hand joints and wrists, including MCP joints, PIP joints, and sparing of the DIP joints 5. Positive RF 6. Rheumatoid nodules (found on extensor tendon surfaces, specifically the olecranon) 7. Radiographic changes (periarticular osteopenia and erosions) For diagnosis, patient must meet 4 of the 7 criteria. Criteria 1–4 must be present for at least 6 weeks.

Table 10.1.2

Plan

Treatment

Osteoarthritis

- Goal: pain management
- acetaminophen for mild/moderate osteoarthritic pain without apparent inflammation. If the clinical response to acetaminophen is inadequate or if the presentation is inflammatory, a nonsteroidal anti-inflammatory drug (NSAID) is the better alternative; topicals such as menthol, lidocaine, or capsaicin; local cortisone injections
- Supportive braces
- Heat
- Weight management and low-impact exercise

Rheumatoid Arthritis

- Goal: pain management, decrease joint damage/deformity, control inflammation
- NSAIDs and disease modifying medications (DMARDs)
- Oral corticosteroids are used as an adjunct treatment
- Weight management and low-impact exercise

Gouty Arthritis

- Goal: treat flares, lower uric acid levels
- Rule out septic arthritis prior to treatment
- NSAIDs, corticosteroids, or colchicine to treat gouty flares
- Allopurinol, febuxostat, or probenecid to prevent flares by lowering uric acid production
- Dietary: avoid foods high in purines

Pro Tip: Disease Modifying Medication (DMARD)

- Chemical (methotrexate—first-line treatment)
- Biologic (anti-TNF agents [adalimumab], non-TNF agents [abatacept, rituximab], and oral JAK inhibitors [tofacitinib])

Prior to starting therapy: (1) obtain baseline chest x-ray and baseline CBC, liver, and kidney function tests, screening for hepatitis B and C, (2) update immunizations prior to initiation of chemical DMARD therapy, (3) obtain tuberculin PPD test or a QuantiFERON TB blood test.

Routine lab monitoring should occur for all patients on DMARD therapy.

Referral

- Osteoarthritis: refer to orthopedics when pain is not controlled with acetaminophen, NSAIDs, activity modification, exercise, heat, or bracing; referral may also be necessary for a patient with decreased range of motion or decreased function
- Rheumatoid arthritis: refer to rheumatology for further evaluation and management
- Gouty arthritis: refer to rheumatology if symptoms are frequent and not controlled or if the patient has gouty tophi

Takeaways

- A thorough history and review of systems can assist in differentiation of arthritis types.
- Osteoarthritis is degenerative. Rheumatoid arthritis is systemic, autoimmune, and inflammatory. Gouty arthritis is crystal induced.
- Low-impact exercise, weight management, and a healthy diet can be beneficial for all types of arthritis.

LESSON 2: MISCELLANEOUS MUSCULOSKELETAL DISORDERS

Learning Objectives
- Understand various disorders that present with musculoskeletal (MS) complaints
- Differentiate among MS disorders based on symptoms and exam findings
- Recognize treatment options for MS disorders

There are a variety of disorders that are directly or indirectly related to the MS system. These disorders are indirectly related to the MS system, yet present with MS complaints. In this chapter, the following conditions will be discussed: systemic lupus erythematosus (SLE), fibromyalgia, reactive arthritis, and septic arthritis.

Definitions

- **Malar rash:** erythema to the cheeks and across the bridge of the nose, spares nasolabial folds; often called "butterfly rash" because it resembles a butterfly on the face
- **Discoid rash:** raised erythematous disc-shaped patches
- **Keratoderma blennorrhagica:** rash that may be present with reactive arthritis that initially appears as papules and vesicles with a waxy texture on palms and soles; can progress to scaling and crusted patches and nodules, and extend to other parts of the body
- **Serositis:** inflammation of a serous membrane (tissue lining the lungs, heart, abdominal organs)
- **Enthesitis:** inflammation of insertion sites of ligaments and tendons
- **Dactylitis:** inflammation of a digit ("sausage" shaped)
- **Vasculitis:** inflammation of blood vessels

Assessment

Subjective

In the case of SLE and fibromyalgia, common complaints include muscle/joint pain and fatigue. Reactive and septic arthritis complaints include joint pain; however, septic arthritis is typically monoarticular. The cause of these disorders is often multifactorial.

Symptoms

	SLE	Fibromyalgia	Reactive arthritis	Septic arthritis
Cause	Unknown; autoimmune but there is a genetic component and possible hormonal component. In addition, it is theorized that certain medications and viruses can cause the illness	Unknown	Recent genitourinary (*Chlamydia trachomatis*) or gastrointestinal infection (*Shigella, Salmonella, Yersinia, Campylobacter*)	Various bacterial agents; most commonly gram-positive bacteria
Age at onset/ gender prevalence	More common in women, reproductive years	More common in women, age 20–50	More common in young adults	Age varies, no gender prevalence
Fever/weight loss	Common/common	Absent/absent	Common/common	Common/absent
Fatigue	Common	Common	Common	Absent
Joint pain	Polyarticular	Polyarticular	Polyarticular—often lower extremity joints	Monoarticular (most often)
Muscle pain	Common	Common	Absent	Absent
Muscle weakness	Rare	Rare	Absent	Absent
Rash	Common (malar rash, discoid rash, or photosensitive rash)	Absent	Keratoderma blennorrhagica may be present	Absent; affected joint may be erythematous, warm and edematous
Other body systems affected	MS, dermatologic (both commonly affected); can also effect cardiovascular, renal, hematologic, neurologic systems; serositis, vasculitis	Neurologic: headache, cognitive disturbances, paresthesia; psychologic: depression/anxiety	Enthesitis, dactylitis, back pain, and conjunctivitis may be present	None

Table 10.2.1 Comparison of MS Symptomatology

Review of Symptoms

- **PMH:** recent illness (gastrointestinal or genitourinary); history of recurring muscle or joint pain; depression; medications that can induce SLE (procainamide, hydralazine, minocycline); recent hospitalization or frequent urinary tract infections (guides choice of treatment for septic arthritis); diabetes, rheumatoid or osteoarthritis (increases risk of septic arthritis); seizures (SLE)

- **PSH:** previous or recent musculoskeletal surgery; joint surgery (septic arthritis); recent abdominal surgery (guides choice of treatment for septic arthritis)

- **FH:** autoimmune disease, arthritis

- **SH:** smoking (to prevent complications if disease exists); IV drug use (septic arthritis); high-risk sexual behavior (reactive arthritis)

Objective

- **Constitutional:** fever, weight loss
- **EENT:** nystagmus, visual field defects (SLE), conjunctivitis (reactive arthritis); painless oral or nasal ulcers (SLE)
- **CV:** presence of murmurs, tachycardia, arrhythmia (SLE), HTN (SLE nephritis), pericardial friction rub (pericarditis-SLE), lower extremity edema (SLE nephritis), Raynaud phenomenon (SLE)
- **Resp:** decreased breath sounds, pleural friction rub (SLE serositis)
- **GI:** pain on palpation (SLE serositis)
- **Urinary:** proteinuria, hematuria (SLE nephritis)
- **MS:** examine affected joints (erythema, edema, warmth, ROM, weakness), palpation for tender points (fibromyalgia)
- **Neuro:** cranial nerve deficits (SLE)
- **Lymphatic:** generalized lymphadenopathy (SLE) or localized lymphadenopathy (septic arthritis)
- **Skin/hair:** rash (SLE or reactive arthritis), thinning hair, alopecia (SLE)
- **Psychiatric:** depression or anxiety (fibromyalgia, SLE), psychosis (SLE)

Diagnosis

Lab results must be interpreted in light of the clinical scenario. Many of the lab tests used for MS conditions are nonspecific for a particular disease and can be positive in some patients without clinical illness.

SLE: laboratory tests include antinuclear antibody (ANA), anti-dsDNA, anti-Smith antibodies, CBC/diff (anemia, thrombocytopenia, leukopenia), creatinine, U/A (proteinuria), ESR, CRP; testing for complications associated with SLE: echocardiogram, ECG, CXR, renal ultrasound, x-ray (swollen and painful joints).

The American College of Rheumatology (ACR) has criteria to establish a diagnosis of SLE, and 4 of the 11 criteria must be present to establish a diagnosis:

ACR SLE Criteria
Malar rash
Discoid rash
Photosensitivity
Oral ulcers
Arthritis that is nonerosive ($\geq$2 peripheral joints)
Serositis (pleuritis or pericarditis)
Renal disorder characterized by persistent proteinuria (>0.5 gm/day or 3+) or presence of urinary casts
Neurologic disorder characterized by seizures or psychosis unattributed to any other cause
Hematologic disorder characterized by hemolytic anemia, leukopenia, lymphocytopenia, or thrombocytopenia
Immunologic disorder characterized by positive anti-DNA, anti-SM, or phospholipid antibodies
Positive ANA

Table 10.2.2

www.rheumatology.org/Portals/0/Files/1982%20SLE%20Classification_Excerpt.pdf

> **Pro Tip**
> SLE can co-exist with other autoimmune conditions such as rheumatoid arthritis and Sjogren syndrome.

Fibromyalgia: the ACR established criteria in 1990 to diagnose fibromyalgia; there is a new preliminary set of criteria the ACR established in 2010, but this criteria needs further validation. Criteria from 1990 include complaint of widespread MS pain that affects both sides, upper and lower portions of the body; pain is present in 11 of 18 tender points (*see Figure 10.2.1*: pressure should be placed on the tender points to whiten the nail bed of the examiner). Pain should be present for three months or longer; other differentials must be ruled out prior to making the diagnosis of fibromyalgia. There is no single test in making the diagnosis.

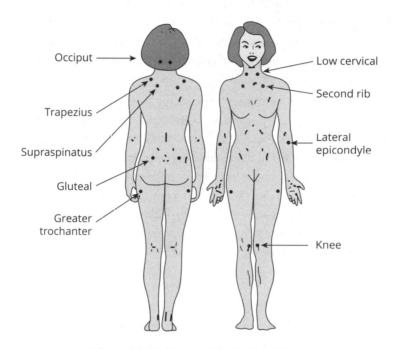

Figure 10.2.1 Fibromyalgia Tender Points

Reactive arthritis: consider if multiple arthralgias in a patient with recent GI or GU infection; testing includes CBC/diff, ESR, CRP, HLA-B27, and other testing to rule out differentials (rheumatoid factor, anti-SM, anti-DNA); if gastrointestinal symptoms present, stool cultures for *Shigella*, *Campylobacter*, *Yersinia*, and *Salmonella*; genitourinary testing for *Chlamydia*; x-rays of affected joints; if joint effusion present, schedule for arthrocentesis (check for WBC, crystals, bacteria; infectious agents are not present in joints with reactive arthritis)

Septic arthritis: joint aspiration for gram stain, culture and sensitivity, and WBC count; CBC/diff, blood cultures, ESR, CRP; x-ray of affected joint

Plan

Treatment

- **SLE:** course of SLE is often variable among patients with remissions and exacerbations; treatment is based on severity and involvement of other organ systems; NSAIDs (if no HTN or renal disease) for joint and muscle pain; prevent and treat complications (smoking cessation, exercise, heart-healthy diet); antihypertensives if HTN present; treat anemia; minor exacerbations can be treated with hydroxychloroquine and/or low dose prednisone; more severe exacerbations treated with high-dose glucocorticoid (prednisone, methylprednisolone), immuno-suppressants (methotrexate, cyclophosphamide), or belimumab (a biologic); update immunizations prior to treatment with an immunosuppressant or biologic agent

- **Fibromyalgia:** initial treatment involves improving sleep with good sleep hygiene and exercise; if initial measures are ineffective, medications can be used; medications that are the most effective are tricyclic antidepressant (amitriptyline [Elavil]), cyclobenzaprine (Flexeril), SNRIs (duloxetine [Cymbalta], milnacipran [Savella]) and gabapentinoids (pregabalin [Lyrica], gabapentin [Neurontin]); many patients benefit from a combination of medications, and often treatment is decided based on additional symptoms; tricyclics improve pain and sleep, SNRIs are good with depression and fatigue, and gabapentinoids are good choices for sleep difficulty; NSAIDs and tramadol can be used for widespread pain; extreme caution must be exercised when prescribing opioids

- **Reactive arthritis:** if chlamydia present, treat infection; treatment of GI tract infections generally not indicated; treat pain (NSAIDs: naproxen, diclofenac, indomethacin); pain that does not respond to NSAIDs can be treated with intra-articular glucocorticoid (triamcinolone) or systemic glucocorticoid (prednisone); for chronic or unresponsive arthritis, DMARDs (such as sulfasalazine, methotrexate) or anti-tumor necrosis factor medications (etanercept, infliximab) to prevent joint destruction

- **Septic arthritis:** treatment with IV antibiotics depending on suspected organism; use antibiotic therapy guided by culture and sensitivity results; gram-positive organism (streptococci or staphylococci): vancomycin, clindamycin, or third-generation cephalosporin are appropriate empiric choices until culture results are available; suspect MRSA infection (in nursing home residents, recent inpatient hospitalizations, or presence of leg ulcer or urinary catheter), where empiric treatment is vancomycin or clindamycin; suspect gram-negative organisms (in older, frail patients and patients with recurrent UTIs or recent abdominal surgery); empiric treatment for gram-negative organism includes third-generation cephalosporin or ciprofloxacin; IV antibiotics are used for approximately 2 weeks, then followed by PO antibiotics for approximately 2–4 weeks; suspect *Pseudomonas aeruginosa* in IV drug users, treat with ceftazidime and gentamicin

Education

- **SLE:** encourage healthy sleep habits to combat fatigue and use of sunscreen/protective clothing to prevent photosensitive rash; advise of risk of infection with immunosuppressive or biologic agent; encourage good handwashing, avoiding those with acute illness and keeping immunizations up to date

- **Fibromyalgia:** encourage patients to perform gentle exercise (water aerobics, yoga, stretching); educate regarding sleep hygiene; focus on stress-reduction measures

- **Reactive arthritis:** symptoms occur one to four weeks after infection; symptoms resolve in less than six months in half of all patients; rest affected joints during initial illness

- **Septic arthritis:** high risk for joint destruction and joint disability; must take full course of antibiotics

Referral

- **SLE:** rheumatology for complex cases and multi-organ involvement

- **Fibromyalgia:** refer to rheumatologist for poor response to treatment or multiple comorbidities; physical therapist for tailored exercise program; psychiatrist or psychologist for cognitive behavioral therapy, biofeedback, or treatment of comorbid depression and/or anxiety; pain management and sleep specialist

- **Reactive arthritis:** rheumatology

- **Septic arthritis:** orthopedic surgeon for joint aspiration; infectious disease consultation for IV drug users, penicillin or cephalosporin allergy, and ICU patients

Takeaways

- Avoid sulfa-based medications with SLE because of risk of exacerbation of disease.
- Reactive arthritis is rare. If symptoms last more than six months, it is considered chronic.
- Fibromyalgia is a diagnosis of exclusion.
- Diagnosis and definitive treatment of these conditions is best done in consultation with a specialist.

LESSON 3: CONDITIONS SPECIFIC TO THE NECK & SPINE

Learning Objectives
- ■ Know the components to assess for a patient reporting a musculoskeletal (MS) neck and spine complaint
- ■ Understand common MS conditions affecting the neck and spine
- ■ Prescribe proper treatment for MS conditions of the neck and spine

Musculoskeletal complaints related to the neck and spine are commonly seen in practice. These complaints can range from mild muscle strains to more serious conditions involving the spinal cord. Neck pain is less prevalent than back pain, and most episodes of back pain will heal with time.

A thorough understanding of the anatomy of the neck and spine is needed to appropriately diagnose these conditions. Common causes/differential diagnoses of neck and back pain include: **disc herniation, bulging disc, degenerative disc disease, spondylolisthesis, facet joint arthropathy, ankylosing spondylitis, osteoarthritis, osteoporosis, synovial cyst, fracture,** and **spinal mass**.

Definitions

- **Dermatome:** sensory group(s) and their corresponding spinal nerves; alteration in sensation in the associated sensory area can indicate spinal nerve involvement (*see Figure 10.3.1*)
- **Kyphosis:** outward curve (thoracic spine normally exhibits slight kyphosis)
- **Lordosis:** inward curve (cervical and lumbar spine normally exhibit slight lordosis)
- **Myotome:** motor group(s) and their corresponding spinal nerve(s); alteration in strength/reflex of the associated muscle group can indicate spinal nerve involvement (*see Table 10.3.1*)
- **Patrick sign or FABER test** (for Flexion, **AB**duction, and External **R**otation): assesses for hip joint or the sacroiliac pathology; flex the leg and abduct and externally rotate the thigh; pain elicited on the ipsilateral side anteriorly suggests a hip joint disorder, and pain elicited on the contralateral side posteriorly around the sacroiliac joint suggests SI joint dysfunction
- **Radiculopathy:** radiating extremity pain secondary to compression or inflammation of a spinal nerve, which may also be accompanied by numbness and tingling, muscle weakness, and loss of specific reflexes
- **Sciatica:** pain often originating in the low back that radiates down the leg(s)
- **Scoliosis:** side curvature of the spine, always abnormal
- **Spondylolisthesis:** a condition where a vertebra slips forward on the vertebrae below it
- **Spondylosis:** age-related degenerative changes that occur in the spine

- **Spurling test:** test for cervical radiculopathy; with neck neutral, push down on top of patient's head; if symptoms reproduced, test is positive; can also have patient turn head to affected side with neck hyperextended while pushing down if initial test is negative
- **Straight leg raise:** assess for discogenic cause of back pain; if the patient experiences leg pain when the straight leg is at an angle of between 30–70 degrees, then the test is positive and a herniated disc is a possible cause of the pain

Assessment

Subjective

Risk/contributing factors for neck and back pain include:

- **PMH:** weight loss, previous or current malignancy, current trauma or injury, previous neck or back injury, recent illness, osteopenia, osteoporosis
- **PSH:** neck or spine surgery
- **FH:** arthritis, rheumatologic diseases
- **SH:** smoking, sports involvement (football, weight lifting, gymnastics)
- **Age:** wear and tear over time (disc degeneration, stenosis, osteoarthritis)
- **Genetics:** degenerative disc disease
- **Occupational hazard:** jobs consisting of repetitive bending and lifting (e.g., construction worker, nurse), or that require long hours of standing without a break (e.g., security guard, barber), or sitting in a chair
- **Sedentary lifestyle:** linked to obesity; increases risks for occurrence and likely severity of the pain
- **Excess weight:** increases stress on the lower back, as well as other joints (e.g., knees)
- **Poor posture**
- **Pregnancy**

Symptoms

Patients with neck or back pain can present in a variety of ways:

- **Onset:** when the pain began, initial episode, repeat episode
- **Location:** spine, extremities, unilateral/bilateral
- **Quality:** dull, aching, sharp, burning, stabbing, sharp, pins/needles, tingling, electrical, cramping
- **Timing/setting:** length of pain episodes, intermittent, constant, time of day, related to temperature changes, exertional, at rest, positional, during sleep, daytime, nighttime
- **Severity:** intensity on scale of 0–10 or visual analogue scale
- **Radiation:** to extremities, chest
- **Aggravating factors:** activity, sitting, standing, walking, lying down, bending, twisting
- **Alleviating factors:** rest, stretching, sitting, lying down, medications (NSAIDs, ASA, acetaminophen, topical creams), ice, heat
- **Associated symptoms:** headache, dizziness, visual changes, dyspnea, shortness of breath, falls, bowel or bladder changes (retention, incontinence), changes in handwriting, dropping objects frequently

> **DANGER SIGNS** The following may indicate a serious medical condition requiring immediate medical care:
>
> - Acute, severe, continuous abdominal and low back pain (dissecting abdominal aneurysm)
> - Difficulty passing urine or having a bowel movement and/or incontinence
> - Progressive weakness in the arms or legs, frequent falls, or foot drop
> - Other unexplained symptoms accompanying the pain, including fever, night sweats, history of cancer, recent unexplained weight loss, pain that awakens them at night, or pain after a trauma
>
> Cauda equina syndrome (CES): a medical emergency that calls for urgent surgical intervention. The cauda equina can become damaged due to lumbar disc herniation, lumbar spinal stenosis, tumors, trauma, and infection. Onset of symptoms can be acute or gradual and may include:
>
> - Severe pain
> - Weakness, tingling, or numbness in the legs and/or feet (unilateral or bilateral)
> - Loss of bowel or bladder function
> - Saddle anesthesia (numbness of the groin, buttocks, and genitals, and/or the upper inner thighs)
>
> Early recognition and treatment are crucial for making as full of a recovery as possible. If left untreated, it can lead to paralysis, impaired bladder and/or bowel control, difficulty walking, and/or other neurological and physical problems.

Objective

- **VS:** no specific changes anticipated unless physiological responses to pain: increased heart rate, blood pressure, and respiratory rate
- **Head:** signs of trauma, bruising, bleeding, abrasions, occipital tenderness
- **Neck:** bruising, erythema, deformity, cervical spine tenderness, altered lordosis, paravertebral muscle tenderness, palpable muscle spasm, facet columnar tenderness, trapezius tenderness, range of motion (flexion, extension, side bending, and rotation), Spurling test; if concern over infection, check for nuchal rigidity, Kernig sign, and Brudzinski sign (*see Chapter 11, Lesson 6*)
- **Back:** bruising, erythema, deformity, thoracic, lumbar or sacral spine tenderness, paravertebral muscle tenderness, palpable muscle spasm, facet columnar tenderness, presence of spinal abnormalities (kyphosis), range of motion (flexion, extension, rotation, and side bending), ability to walk on heels and toes, straight leg raise, strength of legs, reflexes (patellar, Achilles)
- **GI/GU:** bowel or bladder changes (i.e., retention, incontinence, perianal numbness)
- **Neuro:** check sensation along affected dermatomes (sharp, dull, cold, warm stimuli), motor function and strength of upper and lower extremities, reflexes (biceps, brachioradialis, triceps, patellar, and Achilles), and muscle atrophy of the extremities

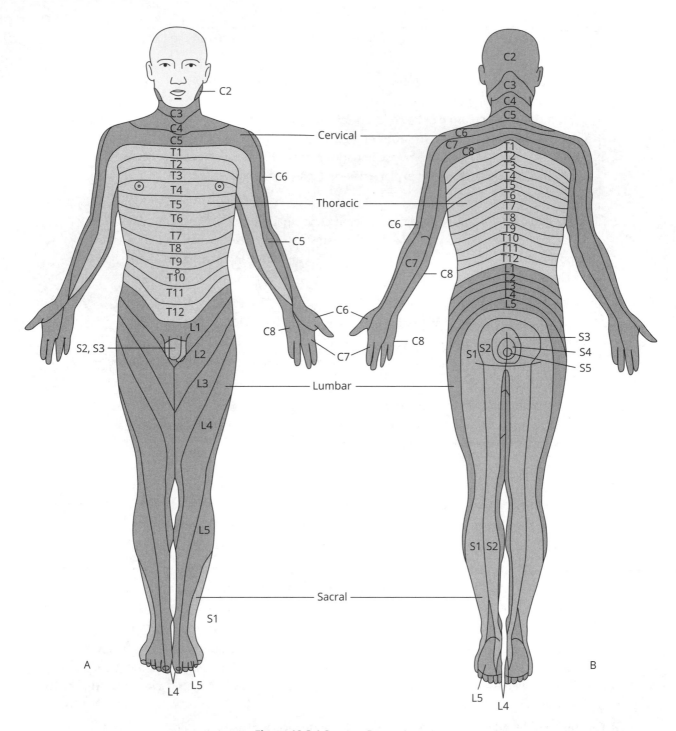

Figure 10.3.1 Sensory Dermatomes

Level	Function	Reflex
C5/C6	Deltoid/biceps: shoulder shrug/elbow flexion	Biceps (C5)/Brachioradialis (C6)
C7/C8	Triceps: elbow extension	Triceps (C7)
C8/T1	Finger flexion, extension; thumb opposition, abduction	
T1–T12	Intercostal and abdominal muscles	
L2/L3	Hip flexion	
L2/L3/L4	Hip adduction/quadriceps	
L4/L5	Ankle dorsiflexion (heel walking), great toe dorsiflexion	Patellar (L4)
S1/S2	Ankle plantar flexion (toe walking)	Achilles (S1)
S2/S3/S4	Rectal tone	

Table 10.3.1 Myotomes of Spinal Nerves

Diagnosis

The clinical diagnosis is usually arrived at through a combination of the patient's history (including a description of the pain) and a physical exam. Labs are not typically indicated upon initial presentation. Imaging studies are indicated for symptoms persisting longer than 6 weeks, neurologic deficits, recent trauma, and/or suspected malignancy or infection. Helpful diagnostic tests include:

- X-ray (AP, lateral, flexion, extension)
- MRI
- CT scan
- CT myelogram
- Discography

With regard to lumbar radicular symptoms, it's important to rule out other causes of leg/foot pain including peripheral vascular disease, diabetes, and DVT.

Plan

Treatment

Initially, a course of conservative treatment is usually recommended for 6–8 weeks. These include:

- Physical therapy
- Acupuncture
- Manipulation
- Electrical stimulation
- Massage
- Ultrasound therapy
- Ice/heat

Medications include:

- NSAIDs (ibuprofen, naproxen)
- Acetaminophen
- Muscle relaxants (cyclobenzaprine, tizanidine, baclofen)
- Opioids (oxycodone, hydrocodone, codeine)—use with caution due to risk of abuse/dependence
- Steroids (prednisone)
- Topical creams (capsaicin, lidocaine)
- Antidepressants (SSRIs)

More invasive interventions include MUA (manipulation under anesthesia), selective spinal injects (epidural/facet block/nerve block), and percutaneous decompression.

Patients that are exhibiting any danger signs should be referred to the emergency department or for immediate consultation with a specialist (orthopedist, neurosurgeon). In addition, those that are not responding to conservative measures may warrant a referral to a spine specialist.

Education

Inform patients that bed rest is not recommended. Activities (bending, twisting, climbing, crawling, overhead reaching, heavy lifting) may need to be restricted for 3–6 weeks. They should understand when to seek follow-up care, including worsening of their condition and any of the "danger signs."

General preventative measures include:

- Weight loss
- Maintaining physical fitness
- Smoking cessation
- Stress reduction
- Improved ergonomics and posture
- Activity modification, as appropriate
- Avoidance of aggravating tasks (e.g., heavy lifting, bending, twisting)

Referral

- Neurologist
- Physiatrist/physical therapist
- Pain management
- Spine specialist (orthopedic surgeon, neurosurgeon)
- Oncologist (if applicable)

Takeaways

- Put the puzzle together when considering spinal complaints. Do radicular symptoms and weakness correspond to appropriate dermatomes and myotomes?
- Weakness in great toe dorsiflexion may be only sign of L4–L5 disc bulge.
- Be on the lookout for "danger signs," as they require immediate medical care.

LESSON 4: CONDITIONS SPECIFIC TO THE UPPER EXTREMITY JOINTS

Learning Objectives

■ Differentiate clinical manifestations of conditions commonly associated with joints of the upper extremity

■ Choose and interpret diagnostic testing for common upper extremity joint conditions

■ Describe appropriate treatment, referral, and patient education for common upper extremity joint conditions

The upper extremity joints include the shoulder, elbow, wrist, and hand. Common upper extremity joint disorders often result in pain, decreased range of motion, and subsequent decreased use of the joint. Many times, these disorders are related to overuse or injury.

Fractures often occur as a result of a fall or direct blow. The bone may bow (especially in younger children), make a clean break, or result in a fragmented bone (compound fracture). In the case of a hand or wrist fracture, the injury may include crushing or twisting of the region. A sprain often results from trauma: the associated joint's ligaments are over-stretched. Inflammatory conditions such as tendonitis, bursitis, and epicondylitis frequently result from overuse of the associated joint. Nerve impingement may also occur particularly in the wrist/hand or elbow regions. Carpal tunnel syndrome occurs when the median nerve is compressed, while cubital tunnel syndrome results from ulnar nerve compression. Young children may present with radial head subluxation (nursemaid's elbow) resulting from pulling on the forearm via a variety of mechanisms.

Definitions

- **AC joint injury** (acromioclavicular joint separation or injury): the clavicle separates from the scapula; common with athletes/physically active; associated with falls

- **Adhesive capsulitis:** commonly called frozen shoulder; adherence of the capsule to the humeral head with subsequent diminished ROM and pain

- **Avascular necrosis:** also called osteonecrosis; injury or fracture impairs blood supply to the bone, leading to tissue death; common in the hip

- **Boutonnière deformity:** deformed position of finger(s) or toe(s); pathologic flexion at the proximal interphalangeal joint and hyperextension at the distal interphalangeal joint

- **Colles fracture:** fracture of the radius near the wrist with upward deviation of the fractured bone; associated with a fall onto an outstretched hand

- **Dupuytren contracture:** abnormal, gradual thickening of the tissues in the palm of the hand, leading to a permanent flexion of the finger(s)

- **Ganglion cyst:** cysts that develop on the joints/tendons of the hand or wrist

- **Mallet finger:** deformity results from injury to the extensor tendon of the finger; common athletic injury

- **Swan neck deformity:** deformity created by hyperextension of the proximal interphalangeal joint and flexion of the distal interphalangeal; commonly associated with rheumatoid arthritis

- **Paresthesia:** numbness, tingling

- **Trigger finger:** (stenosing tenosynovitis) pain and stiffness with "locking" or "catching" of the finger with flexion/extension

Assessment

Subjective

Pain over the injury or area of concern is common among upper extremity conditions, as is swelling and possible bruising. When an injury precedes the onset of the condition, it is important to explore the history for the mechanism of injury, as it may be helpful in guiding the diagnostic process.

Risk Factors

- Falls
- Awkward posture
- Repetitive exertion of prolonged duration
- Stress or force to the extremity
- Other vascular, metabolic, inflammatory, or anatomical factors (nerve impingements)

Objective

Test	Condition	How to perform	Positive result
Finkelstein test	De Quervain tenosynovitis	Have the patient make a fist enclosing the thumb and then ulnar flex the wrist	Significant increased pain with test
Median compression test	Carpal tunnel syndrome	Examiner holds pressure with thumbs over the patient's carpal tunnel for 30 seconds	Pain, paresthesia in the median nerve distribution
Phalen test	Carpal tunnel syndrome	Passively bring the patient's wrist to maximum flexion, while maintaining the shoulder in neutral and elbow in extension; keep this position for ≥60 seconds	Numbness or tingling in the median nerve distribution
Tinel sign	Carpal tunnel syndrome, cubital tunnel syndrome	Tap over the median nerve in the wrist or the ulnar nerve	Numbness or tingling in the median nerve distribution (carpal tunnel) or the fourth and fifth fingers (cubital tunnel)
Pressure provocative test	Cubital tunnel syndrome	Apply sustained manual pressure to the ulnar groove	Pain and paresthesia of the fourth and fifth fingers
Painful arc	Rotator cuff impingement	Have patient abduct arms above head	Pain at 60–120° arc in shoulder
Hawkins-Kennedy	Rotator cuff impingement	Position arm at 90° in the scapular plane, bend the elbow 90°, and passively take into internal rotation	Pain is produced
Neer	Rotator cuff impingement	Lift the arm in the scapular plane with the arm internally rotated	Pain during the test
Drop arm	Rotator cuff tear	Instruct patient to slowly lower arm to side from abduction	Cannot bring down in a slow arc (arm falls down)

Table 10.4.1 Orthopedic Testing of Upper Extremity Joints

Test	Condition	How to perform	Positive result
Anterior apprehension test	Anterior shoulder instability or torn labrum	Abduct arm to 90° and externally rotate humerus; apply forward pressure to humeral head	Patient apprehension with test and resistance of further external rotation
Posterior apprehension test	Posterior humerus instability or dislocation	Elevate the patient's shoulder in the plane of the scapula to 90° while stabilizing the scapula; apply force posterior on the patient's elbow while horizontally adducting and internally rotating the arm	Patient apprehension with test

Table 10.4.1 Orthopedic Testing of Upper Extremity Joints (Continued)

Diagnosis

Disorder	Symptoms	Objective findings	Diagnostic test results
Sprain	Pain, swelling, decreased use of joint	Edema, ecchymosis, decreased range of motion	• X-ray is negative for fracture • Rotator cuff injury: positive drop arm test, positive MRI
Fracture	Pain, possible swelling, decreased use of affected area, or deformity	Edema, ecchymosis, decreased range of motion, possible tenting of skin over fracture or deformity	• X-ray demonstrates fracture • With radial head neck fractures, a positive "fat pad" sign may be diagnostic • CT or MRI may be necessary for diagnosis of shoulder and wrist region fractures
Tendonitis, bursitis, epicondylitis	Pain, decreased use	Decreased range of motion • Lateral epicondylitis: exquisite tenderness to palpation • De Quervain tenosynovitis: tenderness with palpation of the radial styloid region	• Rotator cuff: positive Neer and Hawkins test • Lateral epicondylitis: Increased pain with resisted flexion and extension of the wrist • De Quervain tenosynovitis: positive Finkelstein test
Nerve impingements	Numbness, tingling, pain	• Carpal tunnel: thumb, second, third, and fourth fingers • Cubital tunnel: elbow, fourth, and fifth fingers	• Carpal tunnel: positive median compression test, Phalen test, and Tinel sign • Cubital tunnel: positive Tinel sign (ulnar area), positive pressure provocative test • EMG is diagnostic for both
Radial head subluxation	Little distress but does not use affected arm	Observed to hold affected arm close to body; pain with mild passive supination of the forearm; absence of bony tenderness, deformity, edema	X-ray is negative

Table 10.4.2 Diagnosis of Upper Extremity Joint Conditions

DANGER SIGN When neurovascular compromise is noted, refer to orthopedic surgeon immediately.

Plan

Pain management for upper extremity joint disorders may be achieved with the use of acetaminophen, NSAIDs, or opioid analgesics.

Disorder	Treatment	Patient education
Fractures	• Shoulder: swathe and sling • Elbow or wrist: splint • Fingers: immobilize above and below the injury	• Keep affected area elevated for period instructed • Do not place any item inside splint
Sprains	Rest, ice, compression, elevation; buddy tape fingers; physical therapy is needed in some cases	• Instruct to return slowly to full use and range of motion
Tendonitis, bursitis, epicondylitis	Physical therapy; brace lateral epicondylar area; thumb spica splint for De Quervain	• Avoid aggravating factors • Forearm muscle strengthening exercises (epicondylitis)
Nerve impingement	Night splints, physical therapy	Avoid aggravating factors

Table 10.4.3 Treatment of Upper Extremity Joint Conditions

Pro Tip

Following splinting, ensure neurovascular status is intact.

Referrals

Refer patients with a suspected labral tear for a magnetic resonance arthrogram (MRA). Refer patients with the following conditions to orthopedics:

- Fractures
- Sprains that do not resolve within a couple of weeks
- Tendonitis, bursitis, epicondylitis, or nerve impingement that does not improve with conservative treatment
- Suspected infection

Takeaways

- Most upper extremity disorders benefit from pain management and rest.
- Use the particular physical diagnostic tests to distinguish various upper extremity disorders.
- Splint fractures and refer to orthopedics.
- Physical therapy is helpful for tendonitis, bursitis, epicondylitis, and nerve impingements.

LESSON 5: CONDITIONS SPECIFIC TO THE LOWER EXTREMITY JOINTS

Learning Objectives
- Differentiate clinical manifestations of conditions commonly associated with the lower extremities
- Choose and interpret diagnostic testing for common lower extremity conditions
- Describe appropriate treatment, referral, and patient education for common lower extremity conditions

The lower extremity joints include the hip, knee, ankle, and foot joints. Pain in a lower extremity joint is common and often occurs from an injury, as do the decreased range of motion and subsequent decreased use of the joint. Osteoarthritis is a common cause of hip and knee pain in middle-aged and older adults (*see Chapter 10, Lesson 1*).

Fracture in the hip joint is most common in the older population. Knee pain from osteoarthritis, sprains, and other injuries is one of the most common concerns in primary care. Plantar fasciitis is caused by inflammation of the plantar fascia and is one of the most common causes of foot pain (particularly in the middle-aged adult).

Definitions
- **Achilles tendinopathy:** pain and swelling and stiffness of the Achilles tendon; thought to be caused by repeated injury
- **Baker cyst:** fluid-filled cyst behind the knee
- **Compartment syndrome:** increased pressure within a compartment that results in decreased blood supply to the tissue
- **Hip impingement:** also known as femoroacetabular impingement (FAI); abnormal contact between the ball and socket of the hip joint resulting in increased friction and wearing that may damage the joint
- **Intertrochanteric fracture:** one of three common types of hip fractures; a fracture involving the femoral head, femoral neck, and trochanteric region
- **Legg-Calvé-Perthes:** avascular necrosis of the femoral head resulting from interrupted blood supply
- **Morton neuroma:** thickening of the tissue around a nerve leading to the toes
- **Osgood-Schlatter:** inflammation of the patellar ligament at the tibial tuberosity
- **Patellar dislocation:** kneecap slips out of its normal position, resulting in pain and swelling
- **Pes anserinus:** also known as goose foot; conjoined tendons of three muscles that insert onto the anteromedial surface of the proximal extremity of the tibia
- **Pes cavus:** foot type in which a high arch of the foot does not flatten with weight-bearing
- **Pes planus:** flat foot, no arch to the foot
- **Shin splints:** also known as medial tibial stress syndrome (MTSS); pain along the inner edge of the shinbone (tibia)

Assessment

Subjective
Pain, bruising, and swelling over the injury or area of concern is common with lower extremity joint conditions.

Risk Factors

Explore the patient's health history for the following risk factors:

- Older age: hip fracture

- Osteoporosis: fractures

- Athlete or sports enthusiast: sprains, fractures

- Fall, other trauma: sprains, fractures

- Overuse: tendonitis, bursitis, sprains, fractures

- Reduced ankle dorsiflexion, prolonged standing or jumping, flat feet, or obesity (plantar fasciitis)

Objective

With knee pain, the following tests assist with pinpointing anatomical locations of knee issues.

Test/anatomy	How to perform	Positive result
Anterior drawer/anterior cruciate ligament (ACL)	With patient supine and knees flexed to 90°, sit on patient's foot to stabilize tibia, grasp posterior proximal tibia, and pull forward like a drawer	Greater anterior movement or translation of the tibia compared to the opposite side
Lachman/ACL	With patient supine and knee flexed to 30°, use one hand to stabilize distal femur while using other hand to pull proximal tibia anteriorly	Greater anterior movement compared to opposite knee
McMurray/meniscus	With knee maximally flexed and internally rotated as leg is passively extended, simultaneously externally rotate leg while palpating tibial joint line; repeat with leg externally rotated, internally rotating while extending	Palpable click or tibial joint line pain
Moving patellar apprehension/ patellar subluxation	With patient's knee in full extension, push the patella laterally while the knee is flexed to 90° and then return to full extension; repeat and push the patella medially	Apprehension or resistance with lateral movement, but not medial movement
Posterior drawer/posterior cruciate ligament (PCL)	With patient supine and knees flexed to 90°, sit on patient's foot to stabilize tibia, grasp posterior proximal tibia, and push posteriorly	Greater posterior movement of the tibia compared to opposite knee
Valgus stress/medial collateral ligament (MCL)	With knee in 20–30° of flexion, stabilize leg with one hand while applying direct lateral pressure to the joint; repeat in full extension	Elicits pain at MCL
Varus stress/lateral collateral ligament (LCL)	As with valgus stress, but stress at joint is directed from medial to lateral	Elicits pain at LCL

Table 10.5.1 Orthopedic Tests for Knee Injury/Pain

App Alert

Does this ankle need an x-ray? There's an app for that!

The Ottawa Rules app can be downloaded from the:

- Apple App Store **https://itunes.apple.com/ca/app/the-ottawa-rules/ id1104004722?mt=8**

Diagnosis

Disorder	Symptoms	Objective findings	Diagnostic tests
Sprain	Pain, swelling, decreased use of joint	Edema, ecchymosis, decreased range of motion	X-ray is negative for fracture
Fracture	Pain, possible swelling, decreased use of affected area, or deformity	Edema, ecchymosis, decreased range of motion, possible deformity or tenting of skin over fracture	X-ray demonstrates fracture
Tendonitis/bursitis	Pain, decreased use	Altered gait, decreased range of motion	X-ray is negative for fracture
Plantar fasciitis	Heel pain typically worse after a period of inactivity or with first steps in the morning; pain lessens throughout the day, worsening again with prolonged weight-bearing	With toes dorsiflexed, tenderness upon palpation of the affected heel and forefoot; palpate using thumb and forefinger	Radiographic and laboratory tests not indicated
Patellar dislocation/ subluxation	• Dislocation: severe pain following giving way, reported audible pop or tear • Subluxation: pain, popping, catching, stiffness, swelling	• Dislocation: observe knee held at 20–30° flexion; palpate patella laterally • Subluxation: high-riding or laterally displaced patella, effusion, abnormal patellar tracking	• Dislocation: x-ray not needed • Subluxation: positive moving patellar apprehension test

Table 10.5.2 Diagnosis of Lower Extremity Joint Conditions

Pro Tip

High impact injuries should raise suspicion for other injuries: neurovascular, soft tissue damage, etc.

Plan

Pain management for lower extremity joint disorders may be achieved with the use of acetaminophen, NSAIDs, or opioid analgesics. Further specific treatment is noted below.

Disorder	Treatment	Patient education
Fractures	Immobilization, cold therapy initially, buddy tape fractured toe	• Keep affected area elevated for period instructed • Do not place any item inside splint
Sprains	Rest, ice, compression, elevation, buddy tape toe	• Return slowly to full range of motion and use affected extremity as symptoms improve
Tendonitis/bursitis	Heat therapy	• Perform stretching exercises
Plantar fasciitis	Short course of NSAIDs; rest and cold therapy initially	• Perform calf and plantar fascia stretching exercises • Avoid walking barefoot or wearing flat shoes • Use prefabricated heel cups or arch supports inside shoes • Decrease aggravating or causative activities
Patellar dislocation/subluxation	• Dislocation: patellar reduction • Subluxation: refer to orthopedics	• Perform strengthening exercises • Wear knee brace • May return to sports in 6 weeks if improved

Table 10.5.3 Treatment of Lower Extremity Joint Conditions

Referral

If the patient with a knee sprain is not improving, refer for magnetic resonance imaging (MRI) to rule out torn ligament or meniscus. When tendonitis or bursitis is not improving with conservative treatment, refer for physical therapy. Refer patients with the following conditions to orthopedics:

- Fractures
- Sprains that do not resolve within a couple of weeks
- Suspected ligament, tendon, or meniscus tear, or Achilles tendon rupture
- Tendonitis or bursitis that does not improve (possible cortisone injections)
- Patellar subluxation and non-reducible dislocation

Takeaways

- Sprains and strains are treated with rest, ice, therapy, and elevation (RICE).
- Refer all patients with fractures to orthopedics.
- Stretching and/or strengthening exercises are useful in tendonitis, bursitis, plantar fasciitis, and patellar dislocation/subluxation.
- Utilize the orthopedic knee tests to potentially rule out ligament, tendon, or meniscal tear in patients with apparent sprains.
- After application of splints, immobilization, or reduction, assess neurovascular status distal to the affected area.

PRACTICE QUESTIONS

Select the ONE best answer.

Lesson 1: Arthritis Overview

1. A 52-year-old woman presents to the clinic with a three-month history of pain in the MCP joints of both hands with synovitis. She has associated fatigue and morning stiffness lasting for one hour. Which tests would be most beneficial to assist in diagnosis?

   A. Rheumatoid factor, anti-CCP antibodies, x-rays of the hands

   B. Rheumatoid factor, x-rays of the hands

   C. CBC, rheumatoid factor

   D. CBC, ESR, CRP

2. A 70-year-old man presents to the office with a three-year history of bilateral knee pain, exacerbated by walking for long periods of time. He denies any new injuries, but he did play football in high school. He has no joint swelling, but reports some stiffness in the mornings for approximately 30 minutes and every time he rises from a sitting position. Based on the history, what diagnosis is suspected and what testing would be most beneficial?

   A. Osteoarthritis; x-rays of the knees

   B. Osteoarthritis; x-rays of the knees, CBC, ESR, RF, anti-CCP

   C. Rheumatoid arthritis; x-rays of the knees, CBC, ESR, RF, anti-CCP

   D. Gouty arthritis; aspiration of the knee joints

3. A 47-year-old obese man presents to the clinic with nocturnal acute onset pain and swelling to the right foot. He denies previous incidence of symptoms and denies known injury. The patient is on high blood pressure medication, is a borderline diabetic, and consumes alcohol regularly. What diagnostic test is essential for diagnosis of this patient's condition?

   A. CBC

   B. Uric acid

   C. X-ray of the foot

   D. Aspiration of the joint

4. A 54-year-old woman with known rheumatoid arthritis is in the office for a routine visit. She has swelling in her 2nd and 3rd MCP joints bilaterally and reports morning stiffness lasting for more than 1 hour. She has been taking naproxen twice daily for the past several years, but she no longer feels this medication is helping with her arthritis. Which DMARD medication would you consider using for treatment of this patient?

   A. leflunomide (Arava)

   B. etanercept (Enbrel)

   C. methotrexate (Rheumatrex)

   D. adalimumab (Humira)

Lesson 2: Miscellaneous Musculoskeletal Disorders

5. B.W. is a 34-year-male who complains that his left knee has been painful for three days and is getting progressively worse. He describes the pain as throbbing and rates the pain as a 7/10. ROS is positive for fever. He denies fatigue, weight loss, and rash. PMH is unremarkable. He denies past gastrointestinal or genitourinary infection. Surgical history includes previous arthroscopic surgery to left knee two years ago. Social history includes smoking 2 packs per day. On exam, the left knee is erythematous, warm, and edematous. Which diagnosis is most probable?

   A. Septic arthritis

   B. Fibromyalgia

   C. Reactive arthritis

   D. SLE

6. Which is not included in the ACR criteria to diagnose SLE?

   A. Proteinuria

   B. Leukopenia

   C. Elevated potassium

   D. Malar rash

7. Which type of bacteria is a common cause of reactive arthritis?

    A. *Pseudomonas aeruginosa*

    B. *Mycobacterium tuberculosis*

    C. Beta-hemolytic *Streptococcus*

    D. *Chlamydia trachomatis*

8. Kallie is a 35-year-old female who complains of widespread musculoskeletal pain and fatigue for the last year. After ruling out other possible diagnosis, she is diagnosed with fibromyalgia. You are educating her on her diagnosis. Which information is correct teaching for fibromyalgia?

    A. Adequate sleep and exercise are often first-line treatment

    B. Opioid medications are first-line treatment for pain control

    C. She should avoid sulfa antibiotics going forward to prevent exacerbations

    D. She will need to have her ANA level checked every three months to predict exacerbations

Lesson 3: Conditions Specific to the Neck & Spine

9. A 45-year-old female complains of neck pain after lifting boxes while moving into a new apartment. Sharp pain radiates down the left arm, 8/10, aggravated by flexion and rotation. She has a history of a cervical fusion at C5–C6 three years ago. On exam, how you would anticipate C4–C7 radiculopathy to present?

    A. Tingling that starts at the neck and radiates down the shoulder, to the back of the left arm, to the tips of fingers 1–3

    B. Left biceps reflex 2+

    C. Positive Patrick sign

    D. Decreased sensation to left ear

10. Which of the following is not a danger sign for neck or back pain?

    A. Patient with neck pain who was involved in an MVA two days ago

    B. Patient with low back pain who is currently taking chemotherapy for stage III colon cancer

    C. Patient with neck pain and a history of smoking two packs per day for 30 years

    D. Patient with neck pain that is worsening and radiates to the left jaw

11. A 45-year-old male presents with low back pain that radiates down the posterior right buttock and the thigh to his knee. He noticed the pain when lifting heavy boxes while helping a friend move late yesterday afternoon. He reports urinary incontinence since the onset of pain and now notices decreased sensation in the perianal region. On exam, straight-leg raises cause an increase in pain in the leg and posterior thigh. These symptoms suggest:

    A. Spondylolisthesis

    B. Lordosis

    C. Sciatica

    D. Cauda equina syndrome

12. A 74-year-old female complains of low back pain. She reports a history of osteopenia, steroid use for her chronic rheumatoid arthritis, and a fall yesterday down the back two steps. What is the likely cause of her low back pain?

    A. Kyphosis

    B. Spinal fracture

    C. Poor posture

    D. Cauda equina syndrome

Lesson 4: Conditions Specific to the Upper Extremity Joints

13. To perform the Phalen test, the nurse practitioner maintains the patient's shoulder in neutral and the elbow in flexion. The NP then passively brings the patient's wrist to maximum flexion for what length of time?

    A. 3 minutes

    B. 5 minutes

    C. 30 seconds

    D. 60 seconds

14. Which of the following signs is highly suspicious for radial head subluxation?

    A. Numbness and tingling in the affected hand

    B. Noticeable deformity of the affected arm

    C. Fixed, straight position of the affected arm by the side

    D. Significant edema of the affected arm

15. The nurse practitioner has just splinted a patient's wrist. What should the NP assess next?

    A. Finger sensation and color

    B. Ability to lift the arm

    C. Pain relief

    D. Sensation of the elbow

16. Which nerve's compression is responsible for the pain and tingling associated with carpal tunnel syndrome?

    A. Axillary nerve

    B. Median nerve

    C. Radial nerve

    D. Ulnar nerve

Lesson 5: Conditions Specific to the Lower Extremity Joints

17. Which test is used to rule out a meniscal tear?

    A. Lachman

    B. McMurray

    C. Moving patellar apprehension

    D. Valgus stress

18. The nurse practitioner is evaluating a patient who has presented with knee pain. The Lachman test is positive. Which of the following structures is likely involved?

    A. Medial collateral ligament

    B. Lateral collateral ligament

    C. Posterior cruciate ligament

    D. Anterior cruciate ligament

19. All of the following are risk factors for plantar fasciitis except:

    A. Flat feet

    B. Obesity

    C. Osteoporosis

    D. Prolonged standing

20. For which of the following would the nurse practitioner not recommend stretching exercises as a part of the initial treatment plan?

    A. Tendonitis

    B. Sprain

    C. Plantar fasciitis

    D. Bursitis

ANSWERS AND EXPLANATIONS

Lesson 1: Arthritis Overview

1. A

MCP joint pain with synovitis, the systemic finding of fatigue, morning stiffness lasting greater than one hour, and positive RF, anti-CCP, and x-ray findings **(A)**, assist in the diagnosis of rheumatoid arthritis. Rheumatoid factor and x-rays of the hands (B) are lacking anti-CCP antibodies (90% specific for rheumatoid arthritis), making it a less precise answer choice. While the CBC (C), ESR, and CRP (D) are beneficial to assist in the diagnosis of RA, the RF, anti-CCP, and x-rays are the most beneficial.

2. A

Based on the history, this patient most likely has osteoarthritis, and x-rays of the knees **(A)** would be the best diagnostic test for this patient. ESR, RF, and anti-CCP (B) and (C) support the diagnosis of rheumatoid arthritis. And, while aspiration of the joint is appropriate for gouty arthritis (D), this history is specific to osteoarthritis.

3. D

Aspiration of the joint **(D)** is essential for the diagnosis of gout. The aspirate will reveal intracellular monosodium uric acid crystals. A CBC (A) may show an elevation of the white blood cell count, but does not help in establishing the diagnosis. Uric acid levels (B) may not be elevated during an acute gout attack. An x-ray of the foot (C) may be beneficial in determining chronic gout changes, osteoarthritis, or rheumatoid arthritis, but is not considered essential.

4. C

Methotrexate **(C)** is considered the gold standard DMARD treatment for rheumatoid arthritis. Leflunomide (A), Enbrel (B), and Humira (D) are DMARDs and are also effective for treatment of rheumatoid arthritis, but methotrexate is considered the gold standard and should be utilized as a first-line DMARD treatment.

Lesson 2: Miscellaneous Musculoskeletal Disorders

5. A

The complaint of left knee pain (monoarticular) of short duration (three days), fever, erythema, warmth, and edema of affected extremity make the diagnosis of septic arthritis **(A)** most probable. Fibromyalgia (B) is characterized by widespread pain of 3 months or more. Reactive arthritis (C) is caused by recent genitourinary or gastrointestinal infection. SLE (D) is characterized by polyarticular pain and fatigue.

6. C

Elevated potassium **(C)** is not listed in the ACR criteria to diagnose SLE. Proteinuria (A), leukopenia (B), and malar rash (D) are all listed as criteria.

7. D

Chlamydia trachomatis **(D)** is a common cause of reactive arthritis. *Pseudomonas aeruginosa* (A) can be a cause of reactive arthritis but it is not a common cause. It is only suspected in IV drug users. *Mycobacterium tuberculosis* (B) and beta-hemolytic *Streptococcus* (C) are not common causes of reactive arthritis.

8. A

Adequate sleep and exercise **(A)** are used as first-line treatments prior to medication therapy. Opioid medications (B) are not used as first-line treatments for pain. NSAIDs are often used for pain relief prior to opioids. It is not necessary to avoid sulfa antibiotics (C). There is no correlation between sulfa antibiotic use and exacerbations of fibromyalgia. ANA levels (D) do not need to be checked to predict exacerbations with fibromyalgia. There is no single blood test to detect fibromyalgia, and blood tests are often normal.

Lesson 3: Conditions Specific to the Neck & Spine

9. A

Tingling that starts at the neck and radiates down the left arm to the tips of fingers 1–3 **(A)** follows predicted patterns of sensory dermatomes and/or myotomes. The C4–C7 dermatomes include sensation of the neck, shoulders, arms, and fingers. A biceps reflex of 2+ (B) is a normal finding and doesn't exclude radiculopathy. However, a normal finding does not support radiculopathy. Patrick sign (C) is a test for sacroiliac joint dysfunction. It gives no information regarding cervical radiculopathy. Sensation of the left ear (D) is innervated by the C2 dermatome.

10. C

Smoking two packs per day **(C)** is not a danger sign with neck or back pain. However, a recent trauma or injury such as an MVA two days ago (A), a current cancer diagnosis like stage III colon cancer (B), or worsening pain (D) are all danger signs. In addition, the patient in choice (D) could have a cardiac cause for their pain.

11. D

Low back pain that radiates down the posterior leg, accompanied by urinary incontinence and numbness in the perianal region is suggestive of cauda equina syndrome **(D)**. Onset of symptoms can be gradual or acute. Spondylolisthesis (A) is a condition where a vertebra slips forward on the vertebrae below it. Lordosis (B) is an inward curve; cervical and lumbar spine normally exhibit slight lordosis. Sciatica (C) that radiates along the path of the sciatic nerve may involve low back pain and radiating pain, but would not result in urinary incontinence or saddle anesthesia.

12. B

Given the osteopenia, steroid use, and recent fall, it is likely the patient has an underlying spinal fracture **(B)**. Kyphosis (A), an outward curve of thoracic spine, is common and does not generally result in pain. Poor posture (C) may result in low back pain, but does not address the patient's past medical history. Cauda equina syndrome (D) generally presents as severe pain; weakness, tingling, or numbness of the legs or feet; loss of bowel and bladder function; and even saddle anesthesia.

Lesson 4: Conditions Specific to the Upper Extremity Joints

13. D

The NP maintains the patient's wrist in maximum flexion for 60 seconds **(D)**. The remaining answer choices are not the correct amount of time for the Phalen test.

14. C

With radial head subluxation, a child will hold the affected arm in a fixed, straight position by their side **(C)**. Numbness and tingling (A), deformity (B), and swelling (D) are not typically found in radial head subluxation.

15. A

Immediately after splinting, neurovascular status should be assessed. Finger sensation and color **(A)** are neurovascular assessments. The patient's ability to lift the arm (B) would not be affected by a wrist splint. Pain relief (C), while important, should not be assessed prior to ensuring that neurovascular status of the distal hand is intact. While sensation of the elbow (D) would be a neurovascular check, it is not an appropriate check for a wrist splint. Neurovascular assessment is done distal to a splint.

16. B

The median nerve **(B)** innervates the flexors in the forearm responsible for the wrist; thumb; and second, third, and fourth digit movement. The axillary nerve (A) is responsible for the deltoid and teres minor muscles. The radial nerve (C) innervates the back of the arm (triceps). The ulnar nerve (D) is responsible for the medial elbow and the fourth and fifth digits.

Lesson 5: Conditions Specific to the Lower Extremity Joints

17. B

The McMurray test **(B)** is used for determining involvement of the meniscus in knee pain. Use Lachman test (A) for evaluation of the anterior cruciate ligament, the moving patellar apprehension test (C) to determine patellar subluxation, and the valgus stress test (D) to evaluate the medical collateral ligament.

18. D

A Lachman test is for the anterior cruciate ligament **(D)**. The medical collateral ligament (A) is tested with valgus stress and the lateral collateral ligament (B) with varus stress. To evaluate the posterior cruciate ligament (C), use the posterior drawer test.

19. C

Osteoporosis **(C)** is a risk factor for fracture, not plantar fasciitis. Flat feet (A), obesity (B), prolonged standing (D) or jumping, and reduced ankle dorsiflexion are risk factors for the development of plantar fasciitis.

20. B

Sprains **(B)** are initially treated with rest, ice, compression, and elevation. Tendonitis (A), plantar fasciitis (C), and bursitis (D) may all benefit from the use of stretching exercises.

CHAPTER 11

Neurologic

LESSON 1: CRANIAL NERVE OVERVIEW

Learning Objectives
- Identify the function of each of the 12 cranial nerves
- Define the proper means to test each of the 12 cranial nerves
- Recognize the diagnostic characteristics of Bell palsy

The cranial nerves (CNs) are made up of 12 pairs of nerves, numbered using Roman numerals (I–XII). CNs are classified as sensory, motor (connected to glands or organs), or both. A commonly used mnemonic for the cranial nerves is **On Old Olympus's Towering Top, A Finn And German Viewed Some Hops**. The first letter stands for the name of the cranial nerve. The word order corresponds to the sequential numbering of the cranial nerves.

- **Olfactory nerve (CN I):** located in the nose, CN I controls the sense of smell (sensory); the nerve is not usually tested unless the patient complains of loss or change in smell or appetite

- **Optic nerve (CN II):** located in and behind the eyes, CN II controls central and peripheral vision (visual acuity and visual fields; motor/sensory)

- **Oculomotor nerve (CN III):** located in and behind the eyes, CN III controls pupil reaction, extraocular eye movements, eyelid elevation, and lens adjustment (motor)

- **Trochlear nerve (CN IV):** controls movement of the eye inward and downward (motor)

- **Trigeminal nerve (CN V):** covers most of the face (ophthalmic, maxillary, and mandibular nerves) and controls motor strength of temporalis and masseter muscles and sensation (temperature, pain, and tactile)

- **Abducens nerve (CN VI):** controls the lateral movement of the eyes (motor)

- **Facial nerve (CN VII):** controls the corneal reflex, facial movements and expression (motor), secretion of tears and saliva, and taste on the anterior two-thirds of the tongue and salivary glands (sensory)

- **Acoustic nerve (CN VIII)** (also known as vestibulocochlear or auditory nerve): located in the ears, CN VIII controls hearing and also balance/equilibrium (sensory)

- **Glossopharyngeal nerve (CN IX):** located in the tongue (glosso) and throat (pharynx); its function affects the soft palate and uvula movement, gag reflex, swallow (motor), and taste on the posterior one-third of the tongue (sensory)

- **Vagus nerve (CN X):** from the Latin term for "wandering," CN X wanders from the base of the brain linking the neck, heart, lungs, and abdomen to the brain; provides visceral sensation to the laryngopharynx, heart, lungs, and abdomen (sensory), and provides taste sensation behind the tongue (special sensory); its function is critical to swallowing and speech phonation (motor) and is responsible for respiration, heart rate, and digestive tract function (parasympathetic)

- **Spinal accessory nerve (CN XI):** controls neck and shoulder movement (motor)
- **Hypoglossal nerve (CN XII):** innervates the tongue, speech, and swallow (motor)

CN	Assessment	Normal finding
I	Test each nostril with a strong smell such as coffee, vanilla, peppermint	Identifies the difference in smells with each nostril
II	Test each eye separately with Snellen eye chart/card using eye cover (visual acuity/central vision); examine visual fields (peripheral vision) by confrontation Have the patient cover one eye and look directly at your nose. Move your fingers from outside the vision field into the patient's line of sight. Test the nasal, temporal, superior, inferior, and oblique angles one at a time. Ask the patient to note any movement in the peripheral vision fields	Visualizes examiner's fingers entering the visual fields symmetrically and from all directions
III IV VI	Pupil reaction: shine light in from the side to gauge pupil's light reaction. Assess both direct and consensual responses Cardinal fields of gaze: have the patient follow your fingers through the six cardinal fields of gaze Test convergence by moving finger toward the patient's nose Test accommodation by having the patient look into the distance and then to about 5 inches from the nose midline	Pupils equal and constrict to direct and consensual light, constrict when looking at near object, and dilate when looking at distant object Smooth and symmetrical eye movement through all fields and converge at the nose
V	Corneal reflex: patient looks up and away. Touch wisp of cotton wool to cornea. Repeat other side Motor: observe during normal conversation—smiles, frowns, raises eyebrows, wrinkles forehead, shows teeth, and puffs out cheeks With patient closing eyes tightly, try to open them by pulling up on the eyebrow and down on the cheeks Sensory: place sterile sharp item on forehead, cheek, jaw. Repeat with dull object. Ask the patient to report sharp or dull. If abnormal, then use temperature (heated/water-cooled tuning fork) and light touch (cotton) Sensory: test tip of tongue for sweet and salty taste, borders at the tip for sour, and back of tongue and soft palate for bitter	Blinks both eyes Symmetrical movements and strength Equal strength Intact and equal sensation bilaterally or sharp, dull, and light touch stimuli Taste sensation intact bilaterally
VII	Corneal reflex is tested with CN V Check sensation of each area (ophthalmic, maxillary, and mandibular) with light touch, superficial pain, and temperature Assess facial expression (open/close eyes, smile/frown) Ask the patient to clench the teeth and move the jaw side to side against the resistance of your hands	Blinks both eyes Intact and equal sensation Symmetrical movements Symmetrical jaw strength

Table 11.1.1 Cranial Nerve Assessment

CN	Assessment	Normal finding
VIII	Test gross hearing by rubbing your fingers together by each ear Perform Weber test (holding tuning fork on top of patient's head at midline) Perform Rinne test (stem of tuning fork at mastoid process until sound stops, then tines in front of auditory meatus; air conduction should be heard twice as long as bone conduction) Perform Romberg test (with eyes closed, have patient stand with feet together and arms extended to the front, palms up)	Hears fingers rub 3–4 inches from ear bilaterally Hears tone centrally Air conduction (ear) longer than bone conduction (mastoid) Maintains balance
IX	Ask the patient to open his mouth and say "AHHHHHH" Assess gag reflex by *lightly stimulating* the back of the throat on each side Observe the patient's ability to swallow Assess the sense of taste on the back of the tongue	Uvula midline, and the palate rises symmetrically Reflexes present or symmetrically diminished
X	(Same as IX)	
XI	Ask the patient to raise shoulders against your hands to assess the trapezius muscle and to turn head against your hand (resistance) to assess the sternocleidomastoid muscle	Symmetrical movements and strength
XII	Listen to articulation. Note lateral movement and protrusion of the tongue With tongue in mouth, ask the patient to press it against the cheek on each side and have the patient touch the roof of the mouth with the tongue	Symmetrical movements and strength

Table 11.1.1 Cranial Nerve Assessment (Continued)

Bell Palsy

Bell palsy is a diagnosis of exclusion. When a patient presents with facial weakness, differentiate between an upper and lower motor neuron lesion of the facial nerve (CN VII). An upper motor neuron lesion is indicative of a cerebrovascular accident, whereas a lower motor neuron lesion occurs with Bell palsy.

Assessment

Bell palsy is characterized by an abrupt onset of symptoms, which often peak in less than 48 hours. The patient commonly presents with an acute onset of **unilateral** upper and lower facial weakness or paralysis. Other symptoms include posterior auricular pain, taste disorders, sagging eyelid, dryness or excessive tearing of one eye, inability to fully close the eye and raise the corner of the mouth, and loss of taste.

The patient may have experienced a recent viral infection or received an immunization. PMH may also include heredity, autoimmune, or vascular ischemia. A history of tick bite, arthritis, or facial swelling may raise suspicion of Lyme disease. Other risk factors include diabetes mellitus and pregnancy.

Objective
See CN VII assessment above.

Diagnosis
A lower motor neuron lesion causes weakness of the frontalis muscle and muscles used in facial expression.

Differential Diagnosis

1. Concurrent limb weakness, hyperreflexia, upgoing plantar, and ataxia, with facial weakness suggests an *upper motor neuron lesion.*

2. Recurrent ipsilateral facial paralysis or hearing loss may suggest *tumor of the facial nerve or parotid gland.*

3. Severe pain and associated hyperacusis and presence of rash may indicate *herpes zoster.*

Plan

Treatment

Two-thirds of patients with Bell palsy recover spontaneously. Most patients have some improvement within three weeks; the rest demonstrate improvement in three to six months. Because of this, treatment is controversial.

- Any patient with an inability to completely close their eye should have eye care: lubricating ocular drops a minimum of three times a day, ointment at night, and padding the eye shut at night

- Evidence is strong for the use of corticosteroids for patients who present within 3 days of symptom onset; prednisolone: 1 mg/kg/day (to a maximum of 80 mg per day) PO daily for 10 days

- There is no compelling evidence to support antiviral therapy

- Non-pharmacological treatment may include physical therapy (facial exercises, neuromuscular retraining) or acupuncture

- Patients with incomplete recovery of the facial nerve damage should be referred to an ophthalmologist

Takeaways

- Cranial nerves are listed by number (not by name) on the test; knowing the correct chronological order is important.

- A commonly used mnemonic for the cranial nerves is: "On Old Olympus's Towering Top, A Finn And German Viewed Some Hops."

- The actual name of each CN lends a clue as to its function.

- Bell palsy is a form of temporary (usually unilateral) facial paralysis resulting from damage or trauma to the facial nerves.

LESSON 2: CVA & TIA

Learning Objectives
- Recognize the symptoms of stroke and respond appropriately
- Define measures to minimize the risk of a secondary cerebrovascular event or myocardial infarction

A transient ischemic attack (TIA) is a temporary blockage of blood flow to the brain, without acute infarction as seen in stroke. Symptoms, including motor, sensory, speech/language, vision, or cerebellar disturbances, often resolve within minutes. Even with the resolution of symptoms, an infarct may have occurred. A relatively brief ischemia can lead to permanent damage. As such, no longer is TIA defined as an episode lasting less than 24 hours.

A stroke results in permanent neurologic damage caused by obstruction of blood flow to an area of the brain. The majority of strokes are ischemic (blockage within the blood vessel) or due to hemorrhage of a weakened blood vessel. Rarely (about 5% of cases), carotid artery dissection in a young adult leads to stroke.

The initial investigations for emergent TIA and a suspected acute stroke are the same. The following table defines the range of risk factors; uncontrolled hypertension is the most common cause.

Non-modifiable	Modifiable
• Age (60+ years) • Atrial fibrillation • Ethnicity (Asian, Hispanic, African American) • Gender (men) • Family history • Previous stroke or TIA	• Alcohol consumption • Atherosclerosis • Bleeding abnormalities • Cardiac disease • Carotid stenosis • Cigarette smoking • Diabetes • Hypertension • Hyperlipidemia • Illicit drug use • Medication use—estrogen replacement, combined OCPs • Obesity • Sedentary lifestyle • Stress

Table 11.2.1 Risk Factors: TIA and Stroke

Assessment

The patient may present with new onset of focal abnormalities. Depending on severity of the TIA, the signs and symptoms can be subtle to severe:

- Numbness/weakness of one side of the body or face
- Flaccidity
- Visual changes
- Severe headache, nausea, vomiting
- Ataxia
- Dysarthria
- Confusion
- Altered level of consciousness

Objective

The acronym FAST can identify neurological changes:

- **F**ace drooping
- **A**rm weakness/pronator drift
- **S**peech difficulty (slurred or strange)
- **T**ime to call 911

Diagnosis

Further testing is used to rule out conditions that can mimic TIA/stroke, such as complex migraine, seizures, hypoglycemia, and to identify underlying etiology.

Test category	Test
Laboratory tests	• CBC • Electrolytes: sodium, potassium • Creatinine and eGFR • Coagulation: INR, aPTT • Troponin • Lipids—full profile • Fasting blood glucose OR hemoglobin A1c
ECG	• Echocardiogram: considered when a cardiac source of embolism is suspected (e.g., dysrhythmia, heart failure, left ventricular dysfunction, post myocardial infarction state) • Holter monitor: considered when cardioembolic mechanism or paroxysmal atrial fibrillation is suspected
Neuroimaging	• Noncontrast computed tomography (NCCT) is the standard test to diagnose stroke; the NCCT has high sensitivity for hemorrhage initially; its sensitivity for ischemia increases after 24 hours • Diffusion MRI, though more complicated and time-consuming, shows a clearer image of the brain and is more useful to diagnosis ischemic strokes in the first 12 hours

Table 11.2.2 Diagnostic Tests: TIA/Stroke

Plan

Treatment

As a stroke represents a medical emergency, refer/transport the patient to the nearest ER if clinical findings are suggestive of a stroke. For TIA, prompt imaging workup is needed within 24 hours of symptom onset.

Once diagnosed, determine the patient's eligibility for tissue plasminogen activator (tPA) therapy. Benefits of tPA are time critical. TPA is most effective if used within 4.5 hours of clearly defined symptom onset. If tPA is not available, consult a stroke neurologist.

- Manage hypertension, dyslipidemia, and diabetes (to control atherosclerosis)
- Antiplatelet therapy with aspirin or aspirin with extended release dipyridamole OR clopidogrel (Plavix) for the patient with peripheral arterial or multivessel atherosclerotic disease
- Warfarin (Coumadin) with a goal INR of 2.0–3.0; newer oral anticoagulants: dabigatran (Pradaxa), rivaroxaban (Xarelto), and apixaban (Eliquis) may be used

Takeaways

- TIA/CVA have sudden onset of focal neurological deficits associated with a specific cerebral vascular territory.
- tPA is best when used within 4.5 hours of onset of symptoms.
- Lifestyle changes must accompany pharmacological interventions.

LESSON 3: DEMENTIA/DELIRIUM

Learning Objectives

■ Determine clinical manifestations representative of dementias, including Alzheimer's disease

■ Identify appropriate treatment options

■ Differentiate between dementia and delirium

Dementia is not a specific disease, but rather an umbrella term describing a pathological process defined as a decline in mental ability severe enough to interfere with daily life. Dementia affects 15% of older Americans.

There are many types of dementia. The table below defines their characteristics.

Dementia	Characteristics
Vascular (15–20%)	• Can be gradual or abrupt • Caused by cerebral infarcts secondary to atherosclerosis • Risk factors include being male, history of hypertension, arrhythmias, MI, peripheral vascular disease, hyperlipidemia, diabetes mellitus, and smoking • Often occurs in conjunction with Alzheimer's dementia (mixed dementia)
Lewy body (10%)	• Usual onset between 55–70 • Presence of Lewy bodies causing a loss of dopamine-producing neurons
Frontotemporal	• Usual onset between 45–60 with positive family history found in up to 40% of cases • Heterogeneous disorder characterized by focal degeneration of the frontal and/or temporal lobes
Creutzfeldt-Jakob disease	• Rare and rapidly progressive • Caused by infection by a prion, leading to rapid destruction of neurons and formation of plaques and vacuoles in the neurons
Alzheimer's disease	• Progressive disease, symptoms gradually worsen over a number of years

Table 11.3.1 Types of Dementia

Dementia results from cell damage in particular regions of the brain. The hippocampus, the brain's center of learning and memory, is often the first damaged. Most changes in the brain are permanent and worsen over time. However, thinking and memory problems caused by the following conditions may improve when the condition is treated or addressed:

- Depression
- Disorders/conditions that may affect the brain: AIDS, syphilis, hydrocephalus, head injury, lupus, intracerebral vasculitis, intracranial masses
- Medication side effects
- Excess use of alcohol
- Hypothyroidism
- Vitamin B deficiency
- Lyme disease

Definitions

- **Aphasia:** an inability to comprehend and formulate language because of damage to specific brain regions
- **Apraxia:** an impaired ability to perform motor activities
- **Agnosia:** inability to interpret sensations and recognize objects

Assessment

Symptoms of dementia can vary greatly depending on the type.

Alzheimer's disease is a progressive disease, where symptoms gradually worsen over a number of years. In its early stages, memory loss is mild. As the disease progresses, individuals lose the ability to carry on a conversation and respond to their environment. Alzheimer's disease typically progresses slowly in three stages. Symptoms worsen over time, but the rate of progression varies between individuals.

Mild	Moderate	Severe
• May function independently • Forgetfulness • Problems with word finding • Difficulty remembering names • Increasing trouble with planning or organizing • Difficulty with complex tasks • Apathy • Poor attention • Losing or misplacing a valuable	• Forgetfulness of events or about one's own personal history • Disorientation to person, place, and time • Difficulty performing ADL/IADL • Changes in sleep patterns • Wandering • Speech difficulty • Restlessness • Personality and behavior changes (e.g., withdrawn, compulsive, suspiciousness, delusions, repetitive behavior)	• Agnosia • Apraxia • Aggression • Increasing difficulty communicating • Changes in physical abilities, including the ability to walk, sit, and, eventually, swallow • May need round-the-clock assistance with daily activities and personal care • Significant personality changes

Table 11.3.2 Stages of Alzheimer's Disease

For any patient thought to have dementia, ask about:

- **PMH:** HTN, CAD, hyperlipidemia, DM, stroke, head trauma, hypothyroidism, hydrocephalus, syphilis, Lyme disease
- **PSH:** CABG, angiography, PCI
- **FH:** dementia
- **SH:** diet high in saturated fats or trans fat, high intake of refined carbohydrates, sedentary lifestyle, smoking, alcohol use, illicit drug use, stress

Objective

The physical exam should include a thorough exam of related systems.

- **Vital signs:** hypotension, orthostatic changes, hypoxemia
- **Neuro:** disorientation, confusion, restlessness

Diagnosis

Diagnosis of dementia requires significant impairment in two or more areas:

- Memory
- Communication and language
- Ability to focus and pay attention
- Reasoning and judgment
- Visual perception

Diagnostic tests may help to determine a physiological etiology for the patient's change in cognition.

Category of test	Specific test
Blood test	• CBC • CMP • Urinalysis • Thyroid function • Syphilis • B12 • HIV • Lyme
Tests	• Mini Mental Status Exam (MMSE) • Mini-Cog • Geriatric Depressions Scale (GDS) • Neuropsychologic testing • EEG
Imaging studies	• Head CT • MRI

Table 11.3.3 Diagnostic Tests

Plan

Treatment

Currently, there is no cure for Alzheimer's nor dementia, but there are pharmacological and non-pharmacological treatments that may help with both cognitive and behavioral symptoms.

Behavior and Supportive Therapies

Typically, the patient responds to pain, discomfort, frustration, change in environment, temperature extremes, or anxiety with a change in behavior. Behaviors can be unpredictable and difficult for the caregiver to control. Identifying what has triggered a behavior can often help in selecting the best interventions. Examples include:

- Evaluation for contributing factors (e.g., medication side effects, discomfort from infection, urinary retention or constipation, hearing or visual problems)
- Creating a calm environment
- Avoiding being confrontational
- Remaining flexible, patient, and supportive by responding to the emotion, not the behavior
- Not taking behavior personally

Medications for Alzheimer's Disease

Current medications cannot cure Alzheimer's disease or stop it from progressing, but may help lessen symptoms. The FDA has approved two types of medications (cholinesterase inhibitors and memantine) to treat cognitive symptoms of Alzheimer disease (memory, thinking, language, judgment, thought process).

Three **cholinesterase inhibitors** are commonly prescribed: donepezil (Aricept) is approved for all stages of Alzheimer's disease and rivastigmine (Exelon) and galantamine (Razadyne) are approved to treat mild to moderate Alzheimer's disease.

Memantine (Namenda) may be prescribed. It can be used alone or with other Alzheimer's disease treatments.

Medications commonly used to treat behavioral and psychiatric symptoms of Alzheimer's disease include:

- Antidepressants
- Anxiolytics
- Antipsychotics

Education

Educate the patient's caregiver about identifying and addressing needs that the patient may have difficulty expressing as the disease progresses. Talk to the caregiver about the following:

- Recognizing the behavior is not just "acting out," but a result of further symptoms of the disease
- Changing the environment to resolve challenges and obstacles to comfort and security
- Avoiding being confrontational
- Looking for reasons behind behavior and exploring various solutions
- Redirecting the patient's attention
- Creating a calm environment with little noise, glare, and too much background distraction
- Allowing for adequate rest

Referral

- Neurologist
- Psychiatrist
- Psychologist

Delirium

Delirium and dementia are unique disorders, but often difficult to distinguish. Both affect cognition, yet delirium is characterized primarily by inattention (difficulty focusing or maintaining attention). The following table may help to differentiate the disorders.

Feature	Delirium	Dementia
Onset	Sudden, defined beginning	Insidious
Cause	Underlying cause (infection, dehydration, drugs—anticholinergics, psychotropics, opioids, hospitalization, sleep deprivation, emotional stress)	Various, usually chronic brain disorder
Duration	Minutes to hours to days	Weeks to months to years (usually permanent)
Course	Usually reversible	Slowly progressive
Attention and awareness	Difficulty focusing; reduced orientation	Unimpaired until late stage
Memory	Varies	Greatly impaired, especially recent memory
Perception	Disturbed (hallucinations, paranoia, false beliefs)	Unimpaired until late stage
Psychomotor	Hyperkinetic, hypoactive, mixed, no change (rare)	No changes

Table 11.3.4 Delirium vs. Dementia

Consider delirium in patients (particularly older adults) who present with impaired memory or attention. Diagnosis is made through history and physical exam, mental status exam, diagnostic criteria, and tests (CT, MRI, drug screen, CBC, blood cultures, ABG, etc.) to determine underlying cause.

Treatment involves correcting the cause (hydration, antibiotics, nutritional deficits) and removing aggravating factors (drugs). Low-dose haloperidol, atypical antipsychotics, and benzodiazepines are the drugs of choice for delirium. Reorientation cues (clocks, calendars) may be helpful.

Takeaways

- The onset of Alzheimer's disease or dementia cannot be stopped or reversed.
- An early diagnosis allows patients with dementia and their families a better chance of benefiting from treatment, including care and support services, making it easier for them and their family to manage the disease.
- Behavioral changes are unpredictable; identifying what has triggered a behavior can often help in selecting the best approach to deal with it.
- Thoroughly assess the patient with delirium to determine etiology: infection, dehydration, drugs, and neurological trigger.

LESSON 4: NEUROLOGIC EXAM

Learning Objectives

■ Outline a systematic approach to neurological assessment

■ Differentiate normal from abnormal findings associated with a neurological examination

The neurological exam is generally integrated with a complete examination. It may not be necessary to complete a full neurological exam, but for the patient with a deficit or neurological complaint or finding, an expanded exam is needed.

The minimal screening exam should include an assessment of mental status and cerebellar functioning; the latter includes coordination, motor function, reflexes, and sensation. Testing the cranial nerves is part of a full neurological examination (*see Chapter 11, Lesson 1*).

Assessment

Mental Status

A mental status examination includes detailed (but simple) questions designed to assess cognitive ability.

- Awareness, response to the environment
- Appearance, hygiene, general behavior
- Mood, content of thought, and orientation to person, place, and time
- Speech, ability to follow commands and respond appropriately
- Rapport, facial expression, eye contact

A mini mental exam should be performed if the patient is not oriented to person, place, and time. Test recall and memory (have patient recall three random words immediately and then again in five minutes), concentration/attention (have patient count backwards from 100 in multiples of 7), and abstraction skills ("What do people mean when they say…").

Cerebellar Function

Balance

Normal: smooth, coordinated gait, with equal steps and swing of the arm

- **Romberg test:** with eyes closed, stand with feet together and arms extended to the front, palms up
- **Heel to toe:** walk heel to toe in a straight line, forwards and backwards; then, walk on heels and then on toes

Coordination

Normal: each of these tests completed without missing the mark

- **Rapid alternating movements (RAM):** place the palm of the hands on the lap and turn the hands onto the dorsal surface; repeat the process
- **Heel to shin test:** assess coordination of the lower extremities; place the right heel on the left knee and slide it down the left shin; repeat for the right side
- **Finger to nose test:** with eyes closed, touch the tip of the nose with the index finger of each hand

Motor System

Normal: muscle strength, size, and tone equal bilaterally; tics and tremors are abnormal findings

- Strength in upper and lower extremities: test against resistance using a 0–5 scale, with 0 being no movement and 5 being strong muscle strength
- Observe and palpate muscle size (noting atrophy or hypertrophy) and tone (noting flaccidity, spasticity, and rigidity)

Reflexes

Normal: equal reflexes bilaterally; alterations in reflexes are an early sign of neurological dysfunction

The major deep tendon reflexes are the Achilles (S1), patellar (L4), biceps (C5, C6), and triceps (C7) reflexes. The limb should be relaxed. Briskly strike the selected tendon with a reflex hammer and observe muscle contraction. Grade the response on a scale from 0–5.

- 0 = no contraction (absent reflex)
- 1+ = diminished, but present
- 2+ = normal
- 3+ = brisk
- 4+ = hyperactive with clonus (a repetitive vibratory contraction)
- 5+ = sustained clonus

Compare each side—they should be equal. Asymmetric reflexes or a large difference between limbs can indicate neurologic (or muscular) dysfunction in the pathway that produces the affected reflex. Ratings of 0, 4+, and 5+ are abnormal. Reflexes can be influenced by age, thyroid dysfunction, electrolyte imbalance, or anxiety level of the patient.

Babinski reflex: hold the patient's foot with one hand and stroke the lateral aspect of the sole from heel to the ball of the foot with a pointed object. Expected finding is plantar flexion of the toes. A positive test is characterized by dorsiflexion of the great toe with fanning of the other toes. This indicates an upper motor neuron lesion.

Sensation

Complete sensory testing of the dermatome is often unnecessary.

- **Light touch, sharp touch, and temperature:** test affected and adjacent dermatomes bilaterally
- **Stereognosis:** with eyes closed, have the patient identify a familiar object, such as a key placed in the patient's hand
- **Graphesthesia:** with eyes closed, have the patient "read" a number "written" in the palm
- **Vibration sense:** place a tuning fork on patient's great toe; if no vibration is noted, move the tuning fork back to the bony malleolus of the ankle, the tibial shaft, and anterior iliac crest
- **Proprioception:** (joint position sense) with eyes closed, have patient note if the toe is up or down when the examiner moves the toe in the corresponding direction

Takeaways

- A basic neurological exam is generally integrated with a complete examination.
- For the patient with a neurological deficit, a comprehensive exam is needed.
- A minimal screening exam should include an assessment of mental status and cerebellar functioning.

LESSON 5: HEADACHES

> **Learning Objectives**
> - Accurately characterize headache as acute vs. chronic and primary vs. secondary type
> - Differentiate the characteristics and exam findings among the various types of primary headaches
> - Identify the red flags of headaches
> - Categorize therapies as abortive or prophylactic for each primary headache type

The headache diagnosis is primarily influenced by the patient history. Differentiating between an acute and chronic headache and assessing for signs and symptoms of a dangerous headache are the critical first steps. Once characterized as dangerous or low-risk, the evaluation proceeds to distinguish presentation as representative of a primary vs. secondary headache.

Definitions

- **Acute headache:** abrupt onset of pain anywhere in head region with no known previous headache diagnosis
- **Chronic daily headache:** headache present for 15 days or more per month for at least three months
- **Primary headache:** headache with no apparent underlying organic disease process (migraine, tension, and cluster headache)
- **Secondary headache:** headache caused by an underlying organic disease process (subarachnoid hemorrhage, temporal arteritis, etc.)
- **Short duration:** headaches lasting less than four hours
- **Long duration:** headaches lasting longer than four hours

Assessment

Subjective

At the time of presentation, a thorough headache history is vital to diagnosis and includes detailed information regarding headache pain, past medical history, social history, and previously tried self-treatment strategies and their efficacy. Pain details should include information about its onset, location, characteristics, severity, duration, and frequency. PMH elements to address include head trauma, head/facial surgeries, prior CVA/TIA, prior headache diagnosis, comorbid conditions, and NSAIDs and anticoagulant use. While obtaining a social history, be sure to inquire about occupational and travel exposures.

Review of Systems

Inquire about the following to help determine if the headache could be related to another pathology outside of the neurosystem:

- **Constitutional:** fever, chills, fatigue, weight loss, anorexia
- **Skin:** rash
- **HEENT:** vision changes, ptosis, ear pain, tinnitus, lacrimation, sinus pain, rhinorrhea, facial swelling, throat pain, dysphagia
- **CV:** palpitations, chest pain, discolored/cold extremities
- **Resp:** dyspnea, orthopnea, cough
- **GI:** nausea, vomiting

- **MS:** weakness, myalgias, arthralgias, nuchal rigidity
- **Neuro:** disorientation, memory changes, speech changes, balance disturbances, gait changes, sensory changes, dizziness, paresthesia, numbness, loss of consciousness

Objective

- **Vitals:** with specific attention to temperature, BP, and weight
- **HEENT:** specifically noting facial symmetry, TM characteristics, optic disc characteristics, vision field, facial/scalp contusions or laceration, sinus or temporal tenderness, TMJ function, nuchal musculature
- **CV:** specifically noting heart rate and regularity, cardiac murmurs, carotid bruits
- **Resp:** specifically breathing effort, adventitious sounds
- **Neuro:** specifically cranial nerves, cerebellar function, motor and sensory function, memory, cognition, speech, mood, orientation, extremity strength, and symmetry

Red Flags among Headache Signs and Symptoms

- First and/or worst headache of patient's life
- Presence of focal or lateralizing neurologic signs
- Headache triggered by Valsalva maneuver
- Neck stiffness
- New onset of headache during pregnancy or postpartum
- Abrupt onset of headache in patient >50 years of age
- Papilledema
- Headache with systemic illness (fever, rash, weight loss)
- Tenderness over temporal artery
- Headache with change in personality, mental status, or level of consciousness
- New headache in a patient with:
  - Cancer
  - Human immunodeficiency virus infection
  - Lyme disease

Table 11.5.1

Source: Hainer, B.L. & Matheson, E. M. (2014). Approach to Acute Headache in Adults. *American Family Physician, 87*(10), 682–7.

Diagnosis

As previously mentioned, headache diagnosis is most determined by patient history. In the setting of primary headaches, imaging is of little diagnostic value. However, in those patients presenting with signs or symptoms of dangerous headache, neuroimaging is warranted. The most useful test is an MRI. Contrast should be included if there is concern for a mass. In the setting of intracranial bleeding, CT is the preferred imaging modality. Lumbar puncture should be considered for those patients whose laboratory or image testing has revealed changes suggestive of infection, bleeding, or CNS malignancy.

Classification of headaches as primary vs. secondary relies upon the suspicion of an underlying organic disease (i.e., infection or vascular).

Criteria exists to aid in identifying low-risk headache:

- Younger than 30 years old
- Features typical of primary headaches (*see Table 11.5.3*)
- History of similar headache
- No abnormal neurologic findings on physical exam
- No abnormal changes in usual headache pattern
- No high-risk comorbid conditions

Type	Danger sign or symptom	Example
Infectious	Neck stiffness, meningism	Meningitis
Altered intracranial pressure	Visual disturbance, confusion, altered speech pattern, recent lumbar puncture/epidural intervention	Increased or decreased intracranial pressure
Medication related	First or worst headache of patient's life	Intracranial hemorrhage secondary to anticoagulation
Metabolic	Tachycardia, increased BP, profound fatigue, anergy	Hypoxia, obstructive sleep apnea
Posttraumatic	Head injury/laceration/hematoma	Traumatic brain injury
Structural/vascular	• Headache with change in personality, mental status, level of consciousness • Headache triggered by cough or exertion, or during intercourse	• CNS infection, intracerebral bleed, mass/lesion • Subarachnoid hemorrhage, mass/lesion

Table 11.5.2 Types of Secondary Headaches

Source: Hainer, B.L. & Matheson, E. M. (2014). Approach to Acute Headache in Adults. *American Family Physician, 87*(10), 682–7.

In the setting of acute headache with concerns for potential secondary causes, the American College of Radiology recommends neuroimaging for the following: immunocompromised patients, patients older than 60 years with suspected temporal arteritis, those with suspected meningitis, pregnant and postpartum women, and those experiencing the worst headache of their life.

In patients with localized headaches, the American College of Rheumatology says a temporal arteritis diagnosis is imminent when three of the following five criteria are met:

1. Age of onset 50 years
2. New onset of localized headache
3. Temporal artery tenderness or decreased pulsation
4. ESR >50 mm/hour
5. Abnormal artery biopsy

Diagnosis	Headache characteristics	Associated symptoms	Patient profile
Cluster headache	Sudden onset, unilateral severe headache, duration 15–180 minutes, typically reoccurs around same time daily	Ipsilateral autonomic symptoms (e.g., watering eye)	Onset typically age 20–40; more common in men
Migraine headache	Sudden onset, unilateral, throbbing headache	Nausea, vomiting, photo- or phonophobia; 20% have visual aura	Onset typically in adolescence or young adult; more common in women
Tension headache	Gradual onset, constant bilateral ache or band-like squeezing	Pericranial and neck muscle tenderness	Slightly more common in women
Trigeminal neuralgia	Sudden onset, paroxysmal, stabbing pain in trigeminal nerve distribution	Pattern is inconsistent and irregular	Onset typically after age 50; slightly more common in women

Table 11.5.3 Differential Diagnosis of Primary Headaches

Source: Weaver-Agostoni, J. (2013). Cluster Headache. *American Family Physician, 88*(2), 122–8.

Plan

Treatment

When formulating a treatment plan for headache pain, there are two distinct approaches. Abortive therapy is aimed at alleviating the headache symptoms acutely, whereas prophylaxis treatment is aimed at minimizing headache occurrence. Patients whose abortive therapy use is equal to or greater than twice per week should be considered for prophylaxis treatment. With triptan medications, be aware that there is a max daily dose for each preparation.

Headache type	Abortive therapy	Prophylaxis treatment

Cluster headache	• Oxygen: 100% via non-rebreather face mask at 12–15 L/min for 15–20 min
	• sumatriptan:
	  – SQ; may repeat once at 1 hour later
	  – Nasal spray
	• zolmitriptan
	  – Nasal spray; may repeat once in 2 hours
	  – PO
	• lidocaine
	  – 1 mL 10% solution intranasally, bilaterally applied with swab for 5 minutes
		• verapamil daily in single or divided doses
		• valproic acid daily
		• topiramate daily

Migraine headache	• Combination analgesic: acetaminophen/aspirin/caffeine (Excedrin Migraine)
	• NSAIDs:
	  – ibuprofen
	  – naproxen
	• Triptans:
	  – almotriptan
	  – eletriptan
	  – frovatriptan
	  – naratriptan
	  – rizatriptan
	  – sumatriptan
	  – zolmitriptan
		• amitriptyline daily
		• propranolol divided doses
		• timolol BID
		• topiramate BID
		• valproic acid BID

Tension headache	• ibuprofen • acetaminophen • Adjunctive therapy includes promethazine, diphenhydramine, caffeine, or aspirin	• amitriptyline @ HS • paroxetine • venlafaxine • fluoxetine

Table 11.5.4 Pharmacologic Management of Common Primary Headaches

Education

Educating patients on "rebound" headache phenomena associated with excessive analgesic use is a critical teaching point. Patients can reduce its occurrence by limiting analgesic use to two times per week. Smoking cessation is also vital, since tobacco use is strongly correlated with headache index score and frequency of headaches. Other non-medication therapies practitioners should counsel patient on include identification and avoidance of triggers, relaxation training, cognitive therapy, acupuncture, and chiropractics. Educating patient on proper posture, home exercise/stretches, and good work ergonomics can also reduce headache occurrence.

Referral

All headache patients presenting with red flag symptoms should be referred for emergency imaging and evaluation. Consideration of neurology consultation should occur with diagnostic uncertainty, refractory to abortive and/or prophylaxis outpatient therapy, and progressing symptoms or neurologic change.

Takeaways

- Be familiar with the red flag signs and symptoms of acute headaches warranting emergency imaging and evaluation.
- In assessing patients with headaches, it is critical to discern between acute and chronic onset, and if symptoms are representative of primary or secondary headache.
- For many patients, headache management may include abortive therapy aimed at relieving symptoms upon onset and prophylaxis therapy aimed at minimizing headache events.

LESSON 6: MENINGITIS

Learning Objectives
- Identify clinical manifestations of meningitis
- Choose and interpret laboratory/diagnostic testing for meningitis
- Differentiate appropriate treatment and referrals for meningitis

Meningitis is an inflammation of the meninges resulting from bacterial or viral invasion, or as a result of other causes such as drug-related aseptic meningitis. Generally, aseptic meningitis (viral or other nonbacterial causes) is self-limiting, whereas bacterial meningitis is an emergency. Early treatment is needed to prevent serious complications from bacterial meningitis.

Definitions
- **Meningism:** signs of meningeal irritation such as headache, neck ache, stiff neck
- **Nuchal rigidity:** stiff neck
- **Opisthotonos:** backward arching of spine, neck, and head due to muscle spasm
- **Photophobia:** profound sensitivity to light

Assessment

Subjective

The health history may include known exposure to an infectious agent. Determine immunization status, particularly for *Haemophilus influenzae* type B, *Streptococcus pneumoniae,* and *Neisseria meningitidis.* In the newborn, history may include maternal infection or fever at delivery. Obtain mother's group B *Streptococcus* status. Evaluate for the presence of risk factors:

- Children <5 years of age and adolescents/young adults
- Communal living such as college dormitories or in the military
- Day care, school, or camp attendance
- Antecedent bacterial otitis media, rhinosinusitis, dental infection, or varicella infection

- Sickle cell disease, asplenia
- Immunosuppression or immunodeficiency
- Penetrating wound, head trauma, lumbar puncture, ventriculoperitoneal shunt

Symptoms
- Fever
- Headache
- Nuchal rigidity

Review of Systems
- **Constitutional:** fever, chills, anorexia, lethargy, poor feeding (infant)
- **EENT:** photophobia, ear pain, difficulty swallowing
- **GI:** vomiting
- **MS:** neck ache, backache
- **Neuro:** irritability; with the infant, inconsolability (especially while lying down)
- **Skin:** rash

Objective
- **Resp:** respiratory distress in the infant
- **MS:** infant: hypotonia or opisthotonos
- **Neuro:** altered mental status or decreased level of consciousness, confusion, positive Kernig and/or Brudzinski sign (see chart), seizure; infant: high-pitched cry, bulging fontanel
- **Skin:** petechiae; purpura; or macular, maculopapular, or vesicular rash

Kernig	Brudzinski
• With the patient lying supine, keep one leg straight while flexing the other knee and hip to a 90° angle, then slowly extend the lower leg • A positive response is pain and spasm in the hamstring muscle. The patient may also resist the extension	• With patient lying supine, flex the head upward • A positive response is flexion of hips/knees/ankles

Table 11.6.1 Meningeal Irritation Tests

Diagnosis

Bacterial meningitis may quickly result in complications such as need for mechanical ventilation, seizures, coma, septic shock, and hearing or brain damage. In bacterial meningitis, the onset of fever, headache, and nuchal rigidity is usually abrupt, as compared to viral meningitis.

A lumbar puncture is performed, with opening pressure obtained (usually elevated) and cerebrospinal fluid (CSF) sampled. The following chart provides a comparison of laboratory testing results for bacterial and aseptic meningitis.

Laboratory test	Bacterial meningitis	Aseptic meningitis
White blood cell count	Elevated (polymorphonuclear leukocytosis with a left shift)	May be elevated
CSF opening pressure	Elevated	Usually normal
CSF gram stain	Positive for bacteria	Negative
CSF glucose	Low	Normal
CSF protein	High	Normal
CSF WBC count	Greatly elevated (neutrophilic pleocytosis)	May be elevated (lymphocytic pleocytosis)
CSF culture	Positive for bacteria	No bacteria identified

Table 11.6.2 Laboratory Results for Bacterial and Aseptic Meningitis

Lumbar puncture and initiation of antibiotics in the case of suspected bacterial meningitis should not be delayed for neuroimaging studies to be obtained. Magnetic resonance imaging (MRI) demonstrates meningeal enhancement more clearly than does computed tomography (CT) and is useful for determining complications related to bacterial meningitis.

Plan

Treatment

Empiric broad-spectrum intravenous antibiotics are administered until CSF culture and sensitivities are returned. For culture-documented bacterial meningitis, change to sensitive antibiotic (usually narrower spectrum) when the results are obtained. Early dexamethasone may decrease the incidence of neurologic sequelae in pneumococcal meningitis. For bacterial culture-negative meningitis (aseptic, usually viral), discontinue antibiotics. Herpes simplex viral meningitis is treated with acyclovir; other viruses do not require antiviral medication, and the patient should receive supportive care.

Education

Advise patients with *Haemophilus influenzae* type B or meningococcal meningitis to have close contacts of the patient receive antibiotic prophylaxis or the meningococcal polysaccharide vaccine (depending upon the strain of meningococcus).

Prevent meningitis caused by *Haemophilus influenzae* type B, *Streptococcus pneumoniae,* and *Neisseria meningitidis* by receiving recommended immunizations (*see Chapter 3, Lesson 4, for further information*).

Referral

For an infant less than 3 months old, meningitis can represent an urgent situation—refer to the nearest emergency room for further evaluation. Consult with the physician for an infant over 3 months of age or a child.

Takeaways

- Bacterial meningitis is a serious illness requiring prompt treatment in order to minimize complications.
- The onset of symptoms with bacterial meningitis is usually much more rapid than with aseptic meningitis.
- Treatment for viral meningitis is usually only supportive care.

LESSON 7: MULTIPLE SCLEROSIS

Learning Objectives
- Understand the neurological basis of multiple sclerosis
- Recognize risk factors for multiple sclerosis and expected disease progression
- Identify and implement appropriate treatment options depending on the stage of multiple sclerosis

Multiple sclerosis (MS) is believed to be an autoimmune disease in which the body's own immune system attacks the myelin sheath protecting nerve fibers (a neurodegenerative disease).

Assessment

No single etiologic factor has been implicated in MS. Several risk factors have been identified, including demographics (age, gender, ethnicity), geography, genetics, viral infections, and certain autoimmune diseases (diabetes, thyroid disorders). Smoking and vitamin D deficiency are also noted risk factors.

Subjective

Symptoms differ from person to person and depend on the location of the affected nerve fibers and the progression of the disease.

- Fatigue
- Tingling, numbness, weakness, or pain in one or more extremities
- Changes in vision (partial or complete loss, double vision)
- "Clumsiness" (with possible frequent falls)
- Dizziness
- Bowel and bladder problems
- Heat sensitivity

Objective

Classic signs of multiple sclerosis include: (1) transverse myelitis (inflammation of the spinal cord) with subsequent replacement by scar tissue and (2) optic neuritis, which is one of the earliest signs of MS. Other hallmark signs include ataxia (the loss of control of body movements) and spasticity (continuous contraction of specific muscles), irregular eye movements (e.g., nystagmus), and imbalance/uncoordinated movement.

Diagnosis

A comprehensive history, physical, and neurological exam may provide enough evidence to meet the diagnostic criteria of MS. No definitive blood test will confirm MS, but blood tests may rule out other conditions.

According to the National Multiple Sclerosis Society, to arrive at a diagnosis of MS the provider should first consider and rule out other differential diagnoses, discover nerve deterioration in at least two areas of the CNS, and find evidence that the damage (i.e., two lesions) developed at least one month apart.

> **Pro Tip**
>
> For more specific guidelines on MS diagnosis and treatment, providers often consult the McDonald Criteria as outlined by the International Panel on the Diagnosis of Multiple Sclerosis. Most recent guidelines were published at the end of 2017.

Test	Expected outcome
MRI (spinal cord)	Can show demyelination
MRI (brain)	Can show hyperintense areas in the periventricular white matter of the brain (that is, lesions next to ventricles of brain)
CBC	Normal (not expecting underlying hematologic disorder)
CSF	Normal protein, glucose, and cell counts expected; about 80% of MS cases show evidence of elevated CSF IgG and IgG synthesis
Vitamin B12	Normal (not expecting evidence of alcoholic neuropathy)
TSH	Normal (not expecting evidence of thyroid issues)
CMP	Normal (not expecting metabolic disturbance)
Evoked potentials	Measures the electrical activity of sensory nerve pathways; slowed electrical impulses may point to damaged nerves

Table 11.7.1 Diagnostic Tests for Multiple Sclerosis

Multiple sclerosis has different types. Relapsing-remitting MS has the most inflammatory activity and is characterized by periods of remission and exacerbations. Secondary progressive MS is inflammatory; symptoms worsen and increase over time with few remissions. Primary progressive MS is degenerative (and rare); the patient worsens over time without remission.

Differential Diagnosis

- **Fibromyalgia:** features widespread musculoskeletal pain and nonspecific white matter changes
- **Cervical spondylosis:** features compressed spinal cord
- **Sjögren syndrome:** autoimmune disorder affecting moisture-producing glands and featuring increased levels of autoantibodies (anti-Ro/SSA and anti-La/SSB)
- **Ischemic stroke:** sudden loss of blood circulation to a brain area due to embolus or thrombus
- **Guillain-Barré syndrome:** autoimmune disorder resulting in damage to the peripheral nervous system, featuring ascending paraplegia and potentially fatal respiratory muscle weakness
- **Acute disseminated encephalomyelitis (ADEM):** a demyelinating autoimmune disorder with damage typically seen in white matter of the brain and spinal cord; seen predominately in children/teens
- **Amyotrophic lateral sclerosis (ALS):** both upper and lower motor neurons affected, leading to hyperreflexia, atrophy, and fasciculations
- **Neuromyelitis optica (Devic disease):** autoimmune disorder with myelin damage typically to optic nerves and spinal cord; median age of onset around 30–40 years

Plan

Treatment

Medications are used to modify the disease course, treat relapses, and manage symptoms.

Immunomodulatory therapy is aimed at reducing the number of relapses and exacerbations and may be effective in slowing progression of the disease. Relapse is often caused by inflammation of the CNS. The most common treatment for relapse is corticosteroids. Symptom management addresses pain, spasticity, tremor, gait and motor dysfunction, fatigue, and mood disorders.

For nerve pain, medications such as gabapentin can be considered. Stretching, and medications such as baclofen, can address increased muscle tone/muscle spasms. Primidone, propranolol, and clonazepam can be used for tremor. For gait and motor dysfunction, physical therapy and dalfampridine may be helpful. Adjunct medications such as amantadine, modafinil, or armodafinil can be considered for fatigue.

Education

- On average, a patient with MS has only a slight decrease in life expectancy (5–7 years), but the typically progressive nature of the disease can have implications for mobility (about one-third of MS patients lose the ability to walk), employment, and even cognition
- Research suggests MS patients have a higher prevalence of depression than the general population, though there is an overlap between signs of MS and signs of depression (such as fatigue)
- Not all MS patients experience remissions
- MS patients are often at risk for falls; physical therapy/conditioning can be helpful in improving motor function

Referrals

Neurology and physical therapy consultations are typical. Psychiatry consultation can also be sought as needed.

Takeaways

- Classic signs of multiple sclerosis include inflammation of the spinal cord (transverse myelitis) and optic neuritis.
- Immunomodulatory therapy and immunosuppressive therapy are aimed at reducing exacerbations and remissions and slowing the progression of the disease, not curing it.
- Adjunctive pharmacological therapy may include anti-epileptic medications, muscle relaxants, anticonvulsants, sedatives, beta-blockers, muscle strengtheners, dopamine promoters, and stimulants.
- The nurse practitioner can help MS patients and their families develop realistic expectations about the progression and management of MS.

LESSON 8: PARKINSON DISEASE

Learning Objectives
- Understand the neurological basis of Parkinson disease
- Recognize risk factors for Parkinson disease and expected disease progression
- Identify and implement appropriate treatment options depending of the stage of Parkinson disease

Parkinson disease (PD) has been described as a neurodegenerative disease with loss of dopaminergic neurons in the substantia nigra causing hallmark symptoms of rigidity, slowed movements (bradykinesia), resting tremor ("pill rolling" is common), and postural/gait impairment. The most common neurodegenerative disorder after Alzheimer disease, it is thought to have a mean onset in the early to mid 60s and is estimated to affect 1% of adults over 60 years old. Its etiology is unknown, but it is thought to result from a combination of environmental and genetic factors. It is progressive and currently cannot be cured. Treatment is symptomatic.

Subjective

Symptoms are vague. Patients may present with fatigue and depression.

Risk factors include gender (being male), ethnicity (being Hispanic), age (60 years of age and older), exposure to N-methyl-4-phenyl-1, 2, 3, 6-tetrahydropyridine (MPTP) (a street drug), and having mutations in the gene encoding glucocerebrosidase (GBA mutations).

Objective

The following signs are common in Parkinson disease:

- Resting tremor
- Slowed movements (bradykinesia)
- Rigidity (and freezing)
- Postural impairment (stooped posture)
- Reduced facial expression (masked facies)
- Low volume speaking voice (hypophonia)
- Small cramped writing (micrographia)
- Gait impairment (shuffling/short steps)
- Asymmetric onset: for example, resting tremor in one hand

Diagnosis

A diagnosis for Parkinson disease is achieved clinically. Laboratory tests are not used to confirm the diagnosis, but are used in the differential.

A patient may be trialed on a dopaminergic medication such as levodopa. Since Parkinson disease is a condition of dopamine depletion, it stands to reason that the patient will improve if dopamine replacement is instituted. A scratch-and-sniff ancillary smell test may be used to identify a change in olfactory function. Over 80% of Parkinson sufferers report reduced ability or complete loss of ability to detect odors. Loss of smell is not specific to the disease, so it must be considered in the broader context.

Differential Diagnosis

Parkinsonism is the appearance of Parkinson disease type signs/symptoms with an underlying cause that is not true Parkinson disease. Drug-induced parkinsonism motor difficulties may be caused by a medication that affects dopamine levels. This disorder, for example, is generally reversible if the medication is withheld.

Parkinson-plus syndromes can be differentiated from Parkinson disease by symptoms such as short or complete lack of response to levodopa and early deterioration into dementia.

- **Dementia with Lewy bodies (DLB):** an adult-onset, progressive, multisystem fatal disorder of unknown etiology featuring Parkinson-like symptomology and corticospinal, cerebellar, and autonomic dysfunction
- **Corticobasal ganglionic degeneration (CBD):** progressive condition featuring both motor movement and cognitive dysfunction
- **Progressive supranuclear palsy (PSP):** condition with parkinsonian gait and motor issues, but with unique differences such as supranuclear ophthalmoplegia (the "hallmark" gaze palsy associated with this condition) and axial rigidity
- **Vascular parkinsonism:** Parkinson-type symptoms caused by multiple small strokes
- **Multiple system atrophy (MSA):** progressive neurodegenerative disorder affecting both the autonomic nervous system and motor function

Some conditions, signs, and symptoms point to a diagnosis other than Parkinson disease. For example:

- **Encephalitis** presents as confusion, slow movements, hallucinations (but also fever, irritability, photosensitivity)
- **History of repeated head injuries** can cause dementia-like symptoms
- **Oculogyric crisis** is an acute dystonia of the ocular muscles resulting in involuntary intermittent or sustained deviation of the eyes. One cause is neuroleptic drug treatment
- **Babinski sign** is abnormal for patients >2 years of age and could indicate upper motor neuron disease
- **History of multiple strokes** could cause neurological and cognitive deficits, but does not originate from dopamine deficiency
- **Poor response to levodopa** may indicate a Parkinson-plus syndrome

Plan

Treatment

Treatment for Parkinson disease depends on the stage.

Medications for Early Parkinson Disease	
Monoamine oxidase-B (MAO-B) inhibitor	rasagiline (Azilect), safinamide (Xadago)
Dopamine agonists	pramipexole (Mirapex), ropinirole (Requip)
Anticholinergic medications	benztropine mesylate (Cogentin)

Table 11.8.1

Anticholinergic agents are adjunctive and generally appropriate only for younger patients with mild tremor. They can increase fall risk and cause adverse anticholinergic effects in older patients.

> **Pro Tip: Side Effects of Anticholinergic Agents**
> - Blind as a bat: mydriasis, blurred vision
> - Mad as a hatter: delirium, psychosis, memory loss
> - Red as a beet: flushing
> - Hot as a hare: fever
> - Dry as a bone: dry mouth, dry eyes, decreased sweat

Medications for Moderate Parkinson Disease	
Dopamine replacement	carbidopa/levodopa (Sinemet)
Catechol-o-methyltransferase (COMT) inhibitors	entacapone (Comtan); tolcapone (Tasmar)
Anticholinergic medications	benztropine mesylate (Cogentin)

Table 11.8.2

Providers generally wait until it is absolutely necessary to prescribe levodopa, as it tends to "wear out" in effectiveness in under 10 years. Levodopa will eventually cause dyskinesias. COMT inhibitors prevent the breakdown of levodopa and are to be taken concurrently with the drug.

Medications for Late Parkinson Disease	
Dopamine replacement	carbidopa/levodopa (Sinemet)

Table 11.8.3

All treatment for Parkinson disease is symptomatic. No known medications reverse the condition. Even after taking medications, the patient may experience severe motor difficulties. The injectable form of dopamine, apomorphine, can be used in late Parkinson disease for patients who are "freezing" (having difficulty starting movement) or suffering from dysphagia. Similarly, dissolvable carbidopa/levodopa (Sinemet) and/or selegiline (Eldepryl) can also be used with patients who are having difficulty swallowing.

Non-pharmacological/surgical treatments include the following:

- **Deep brain stimulation (DBS)** delivers electrical pulses to brain cells and can offer improvement in Parkinson symptoms; evidence that DBS alters disease progression is lacking
- **Pallidotomy** is a surgery to the globus pallidus, which can reduce rigidity
- **Thalamotomy** is rarely performed; it destroys part of the thalamus to block signals to the muscles causing tremors

Education
- Many antiemetics, such as metoclopramide (Reglan), are antidopaminergic medications and contraindicated in Parkinson disease
- Anticholinergic medications can help Parkinson symptoms, but are generally not recommended in older patients due to the potential for fall risk and causing adverse anticholinergic symptomology
- Drooling can be another concern with Parkinson disease; tricyclic antidepressants such as Elavil (with a side effect of dry mouth) can be useful, as the provider can treat both drooling and depression; tricyclics can come with the side effect of orthostatic hypotension, causing an increased falling risk in the already at-risk Parkinson patient

- Parkinson patients can become socially isolated because others may interpret their slowed movement as evidence of slowed thinking and their stony expressions as evidence of a lack of social engagement, which is unfortunate; it is estimated only about 20% of Parkinson sufferers develop severe dementia

Referrals

Parkinson patients may benefit from evaluation by neurology, especially in patients with polypharmacy concerns or comorbid psychiatric concerns.

Physical therapy referral may also be helpful, as treadmill training and physiotherapy can help with gait and balance in early and moderate Parkinson disease.

Takeaways

- Treatment for Parkinson disease is symptomatic. Medications do not reverse the condition.
- Diagnosis is clinical. No definitive diagnostic tests or laboratory results confirm this condition.
- Part of the NP's role is to educate Parkinson patients and their families to not only manage motor deficits and avoid falls, but also to help the Parkinson patient avoid social isolation.

LESSON 9: MYASTHENIA GRAVIS

Learning Objectives
- Recognize risk factors for myasthenia gravis and expected disease progression
- Differentiate between the clinical manifestations of myasthenia gravis and other neurological disorders
- Differentiate between myasthenic and cholinergic crisis
- Identify appropriate diagnostic tests and disease management

Myasthenia gravis (MG) is a chronic autoimmune neuromuscular disease that causes weakness in the voluntary skeletal muscles. With MG, antibodies destroy or block the receptor sites for acetylcholine at the neuromuscular junction, which prevents the muscle from contracting. It is characterized by fluctuating skeletal muscle weakness of the extraocular, pharyngeal, facial, and respiratory muscles. Myasthenia gravis occurs in all races, both genders, and at any age. Risk factors include:

- Age: women >40, men >60
- Family history
- Other autoimmune disease

Assessment

Subjective

History
- **PMH:** autoimmune thyroid disorder, thymoma, lupus, Sjögren syndrome, recent vaccination
- **FH:** myasthenia gravis, rheumatoid arthritis, scleroderma, lupus

ROS

- **HEENT:** photophobia, frequent changes in eyeglasses
- **Neuro:** painless, severe, generalized muscle weakness (as opposed to fatigue); progressive weakness of muscles with repeated use that improves with rest

Symptoms

Although MG may affect any skeletal muscle, those typically involved include the extraocular muscles, facial muscles, and muscles utilized for swallowing. Onset may be sudden; symptoms are rarely immediately recognized as MG. In most cases, the first noticeable symptom is ptosis or double/blurry vision. Painless/specific muscle weakness, difficulty swallowing, and slurred speech are also common. Weakness can fluctuate throughout the day, worsen with prolonged activity, and improve with rest. Patients may have asymptomatic periods. Additional symptoms may include:

- Difficulty chewing
- Facial weakness
- Extremity weakness
- Chronic muscle fatigue
- Difficulty breathing

Exposure to bright sunlight, surgery, immunization, emotional stress, menstruation, and increased temperature might trigger or worsen exacerbations.

Objective

With mild presentations of MG, there may be only subtle findings. Findings may not be apparent unless muscle weakness is triggered by repetitive use of the involved muscles and strength is recovered after a period of rest. Variability in weakness can be significant and findings may be absent during examination, often leading to misdiagnosis.

- **VS:** bradypnea, cyanosis, hypoxemia
- **HEENT:** mask-like face with ptosis, nystagmus, impaired EOM, nasal twang to the voice, hypophonia, slurred speech, hanging jaw sign, snarling expression, difficulty holding head upright
- **Resp:** dyspnea, decreased respiratory effort
- **Neuro:** weakness, poor muscle tone

> **DANGER SIGN** Myasthenic crisis is a medical emergency. Muscle weakness produces respiratory insufficiency that can lead to respiratory failure. May be triggered by infection, stress, surgery, or an adverse reaction to medication. Signs and symptoms include:
>
> - Dyspnea
> - Difficulty speaking
> - Daytime fatigue
> - Morning headaches
> - Increased respiratory secretions
> - Use of accessory muscles
> - Increasing difficulty chewing or swallowing
> - Weight loss

Diagnosis

Signs and symptoms may mimic other neurological disorders; therefore, certain patterns can help the NP to differentiate MG from other disorders:

- Ptosis
- Facial weakness
- Fluctuating extremity weakness

Helpful diagnostic tests include:

- Tensilon (edrophonium) test
- Nerve conduction velocity (NCV) test
- Acetylcholine receptor antibody test
- Anti-MuSK antibody test
- Ice pack test
- Lumbar puncture
- EMG
- Chest CT/MRI (may identify the presence of a thymoma)
- Pulmonary function testing
- ABG

Plan

Treatment

There is no known cure for MG, but there are treatments that lessen the severity of the illness. Treatment goals are individualized. Initial stabilization may require hospitalization/ICU admission. Treatment includes:

- Anticholinesterase medications
- Thymectomy
- Immunosuppressive drugs: steroids, azathioprine, mycophenolate mofetil, tacrolimus, and rituximab
- Plasmapheresis
- High-dose immunoglobulin therapy
- Mechanical ventilation in those with respiratory compromise (tracheostomy for prolonged intubation)
- PT/OT

> **DANGER SIGN** Cholinergic crisis: overstimulation at a neuromuscular junction due to an excess of acetylcholine, typically as a consequence of overmedication. As a result, the muscles stop responding to the bombardment of acetylcholine, leading to flaccid paralysis and respiratory failure. Other signs and symptoms include:
>
> - Diaphoresis
> - Miosis
> - Increased salivation
> - Lacrimation
> - Diarrhea
> - Urination
> - Abdominal cramping
> - Emesis
> - Muscle spasm
> - Increased respiratory secretions
> - Respiratory failure

Education

Discuss with the patient that with treatment, most individuals with muscle weakness from MG can lead full lives. Some cases of MG may go into remission and muscle weakness may disappear completely. Teaching should include:

- Stay active, but don't overexert
- Alternate activities with periods of rest
- Take fall precautions, as patients are prone to falls or injury
- Use caution with eating and drinking, as coughing or choking while doing so can occur and lead to aspiration
- Report increasing difficulty with chewing or swallowing
- Report signs and symptoms of myasthenic crisis
- Report signs and symptoms of cholinergic crisis

Referral

- Neurologist
- Ophthalmologist
- Pulmonologist
- PT/OT

Takeaways

- Be on the lookout for myasthenic and cholinergic crisis. Difficulty breathing necessitates urgent or emergent evaluation and treatment. Patients may require mechanical ventilation support until the crisis resolves.
- Edrophonium can help discriminate between a myasthenic and a cholinergic crisis. When edrophonium exacerbates paralysis, it indicates that a true cholinergic crisis is present. Muscle strength improvement after administration of edrophonium suggests myasthenic crisis.

LESSON 10: GUILLAIN-BARRÉ SYNDROME

Learning Objectives

■ Identify risk factors associated with Guillain-Barré syndrome

■ Differentiate between the clinical manifestations of Guillain-Barré syndrome and other neurological disorders

Guillain-Barré syndrome (GBS) is a disorder in which the body's immune system attacks the myelin of the peripheral nervous system. It is a rare syndrome that can affect people at any age, and both sexes are equally prone to the disorder. GBS typically occurs a few days or weeks after the patient has had symptoms of a respiratory or gastrointestinal viral infection. In rare cases, surgery or vaccinations may trigger the syndrome.

Assessment

Subjective

Initial symptoms include varying degrees of lower extremity weakness or tingling sensations. Subsequent symptoms can progress over the course of hours, days, or weeks. In many instances, the symmetrical weakness and abnormal sensations ascend to the upper body and upper extremities. Symptoms can become life-threatening, potentially interfering with breathing and hemodynamic status, including blood pressure or heart rate.

History

- **PMH:** recent upper respiratory or gastrointestinal infection, Epstein-Barr virus and cytomegalovirus, infection with the bacterium *Campylobacter jejuni*, recent vaccination
- **PSH:** recent surgery

Symptoms

- Ascending muscle weakness
- Dysesthesias
- Paresthesia
- Pain (back, legs)
- Dysphagia
- Shortness of breath
- Dysarthria

Objective

- **VS:** labile BP, orthostatic hypotension, cardiac arrhythmias
- **Neuromuscular:** acute symmetric ascending weakness of limbs, hyporeflexia, areflexia, decreased vibratory sense, gait abnormality, pain

Diagnosis

Since signs and symptoms can vary and mimic other neurological disorders, it may be difficult to diagnose GBS in its earliest stages. Certain patterns can help differentiate GBS from other disorders. These include:

- Bilateral symptoms
- Ascending muscle weakness
- Quickness with which the symptoms appear

Helpful diagnostic tests include:

- Nerve conduction velocity (NCV) test: slowed or blocked relay of nerve impulses indicate a positive test
- Lumbar puncture: elevation in CSF protein (>0.55 g/L) without an elevation in white blood cells indicates a positive test
- EMG
- EPS

Plan

Treatment

There is no known cure for GBS, but there are treatments that lessen the severity of the illness and accelerate the recovery in most patients. Most individuals have a good prognosis, even the most severe cases, though some continue to have a certain degree of weakness.

Initial stabilization may require ICU admission. Treatment includes:

- Plasmapheresis
- High-dose immunoglobulin therapy
- Steroids
- Mechanical ventilation in those with respiratory compromise (tracheostomy for prolonged intubation)
- Management of hypo/hypertension
- Arrhythmia management (bradycardia, tachycardia)
- Pain management
- Catheterization for urinary retention
- Prevention of complications of immobility: atelectasis/pneumonia, pressure injury, thromboembolism, atrophy, ileus/constipation
- PT/OT

Education

Explain to the patient that GBS is a temporary illness, with most people returning to normal and having no further problems. Others may have some permanent nerve damage. Encourage the patient to:

- Stay active, but don't overexert themselves
- Alternate activities with periods of rest
- Be patient, as recovery from nerve damage is a slow process
- Be careful if they are still experiencing numbness and weakness, as they are prone to falls or injury

Referral

- Neurologist
- Physical therapist
- Occupational therapist

Takeaways

- GBS signs and symptoms may mimic other neurological disorders; therefore, a thorough history and physical is vital.
- Look out for signs of autonomic dysfunction including blood pressure lability and arrhythmias.

LESSON 11: SEIZURE DISORDERS

Learning Objectives

■ Recognize signs and symptoms to help diagnose seizures/epilepsy
■ Identify risk factors associated with epilepsy
■ Know common anti-epilepsy medications
■ Be able to educate patient/family on seizure safety

Seizures and epilepsy are not synonymous. Seizures are described as isolated events featuring abnormal electrical brain activity. In contrast, epilepsy is described as at least two unprovoked seizures 24 hours apart. Thus, a single unprovoked seizure would not garner a patient a diagnosis of epilepsy.

One way of categorizing seizures is to establish which are generalized (caused by entire brain electrical instability), as opposed to local or partial (those caused by localized instability). A third category includes "unclassified" seizures (seizures that do not fit the previous categories).

Types of seizures	Description
Generalized seizures	
Myoclonic	• Brief twitching of a muscle or muscle group, usually on both sides of body at the same time • May last only a few seconds • Patient typically awake and able to return to normal activity right away
Tonic	• Muscle stiffening • Generalized: the entire body stiffens • Focal: the seizure may affect only one area of the body • Typically short, <20 seconds • Patient typically does not lose consciousness/awareness
Clonic	• Jerking movement (muscle stiffening and relaxing) • Rarely alone, usually part of tonic-clonic seizure • Generalized: patient is not awake • Focal: patient is often awake
Tonic-clonic (grand mal)	• Muscle stiffening (tonic movements) and jerking movements (clonic movements) • Can last up to 3 minutes • A tonic-clonic seizure >5 minutes is a medical emergency (status epilepticus) • Loss of consciousness; may lose bladder control and be confused after the seizure

Table 11.11.1 Seizures

Types of seizures	Description
Absence (petit mal)	• Generalized onset • Typically last only a few seconds • Involves a loss of awareness, sometimes with staring, with patient appearing to possibly daydream • More common in children
Atonic (drop attack)	• Can be focal or generalized; if generalized, patient tends not to be aware during seizure, may be confused afterward • Usually last <15 seconds • Muscles suddenly become limp
Focal seizures	
Focal onset aware seizure	• Originates in one area of the brain (focal) • Typically short; <2 minutes • Patient stays alert and able to interact
Focal onset impaired awareness seizures	• Originates in one area of the brain (focal) • Typically short; 1–2 minutes • Patient can experience decreased awareness or complete unawareness of surroundings • Can involve an aura, such as a visual disturbance • Can involve automatisms—purposeless movements (such as lip repetitive tapping, fumbling, or lip smacking)
Focal to bilateral tonic-clonic seizures	• When a focal seizure spreads to both sides of the brain
Unclassified seizures	• When there is not enough information to categorize the seizure as above

Table 11.11.1 Seizures (Continued)

Assessment

Subjective

Patients may report **prodromal** signs like irritability, aura, lightheadedness, or difficulty concentrating. **Ictal** symptoms include changes in thinking or awareness, difficulty breathing, or muscle weakness, and **postictal** (post-seizure) symptoms include confusion, memory loss, or anxiety and/or depression.

Some patients report having seizures after exposure to certain stimuli or triggers:

- Failing to take anti-seizure medication
- Stress
- Alcohol use
- Caffeine
- Nicotine
- Visual stimuli
- Recreational "street" drugs
- Lack of sleep
- Hypoglycemia

Objective

Objective findings may include abnormal EEG readings, brain scans (MRI/CT), and motor activity (tonic, clonic). In addition, there may be loss of consciousness or decreased awareness, loss of muscle tone (with accompanying signs such as loss of bladder control or falling), and postictal signs of neurological deficit (such as continuing motor dysfunction or memory loss).

Common causes of seizures by age group are listed below.

Newborns	Infants and children	Adults
• Traumatic brain injury during birth • Abnormalities in brain structure • Metabolic disorder (such as hypoglycemia) • Hypoxia	• Fever (febrile seizures) are the top reasons for seizures in infants and children • Infection • Medication • Brain tumor/brain scarring • Head trauma • Genetic disorder	• Head trauma • Brain tumor/brain scarring • Stroke • Abnormalities in brain structure

Table 11.11.2 Common Cause of Seizure by Age Group

> **Pro Tip**
>
> Seniors experience the highest incidence of epilepsy. Past age 60, the risk of seizure increases; tumors and strokes are more likely with this population.

Diagnosis

To make a diagnosis of epilepsy, the nurse practitioner must take into account clinical signs such as confusion, diagnostic tests such as the EEG, and underlying issues that may contribute to epileptogenesis, such as previous stroke. Additionally, the nurse practitioner should exclude alternative diagnoses such as syncope or even malingering.

Diagnostic and lab tests may include: electroencephalogram (EEG), MRI/CT, BUN/creatinine, blood glucose, CBC with differential, alcohol and drug levels, electrolytes, liver function tests (LFTs).

Differential Diagnosis

Differential diagnoses for seizure: **syncope, hyperventilation, alcoholism, illicit drug use, TIA/stroke, brain tumor, metabolic disturbance, motor disorder, trauma**

> **Pro Tip**
>
> Status epilepticus is defined as 5 minutes or more of either continuous seizure activity or repetitive seizures without regaining consciousness. This constitutes a medical emergency. Besides the danger of physical injury from ongoing convulsions, the patient is at risk for hypoxia from ineffective respiratory effort, with resulting brain damage.

Plan

Treatment

Medication selection for seizures depends on various factors. For example, the nurse practitioner will consider the type of seizure, whether the medication is a maintenance medication or being administered in an emergency setting, and other medications the patient may be already taking, along with other factors.

Examples of pharmacological treatment include:

- carbamazepine (Tegretol): multiple drug interactions; helpful to manage mood
- lamotrigine (Lamictal): useful for severe seizures; use caution in prescribing; taper up slowly to avoid skin rash
- levetiracetam (Keppra): few medication interactions; no need to check drug levels
- lorazepam (Ativan): often administered in an emergency setting—for example, to halt an intractable seizure
- phenytoin (Dilantin): careful blood monitoring, as this medication has a narrow therapeutic window; several drug interactions
- topiramate (Topamax): can concurrently treat migraines and seizures; does not require blood level monitoring
- valproic acid (Depakote): requires monitoring of blood levels; can concurrently treat migraines; can cause significant weight gain

Some of the drugs are narrow therapeutic index drugs: blood levels must be monitored. Be aware of drug:drug and food:drug interactions.

Non-pharmacological treatment is not usually intended as standalone treatment, but is considered adjunctive. Biofeedback and relaxation techniques can reduce stress. A ketogenic diet (a special low-protein, low-carbohydrate, high-fat diet) is thought to help control seizure activity.

Education

- Family should be made aware of the latest recommendations on seizures: move nearby dangerous objects out of reach; assist the patient (as needed) to lie down and loosen restrictive clothing; do not restrain the patient; do not put tongue blades, other objects, or fingers in the patient's mouth; protect the head from injury with a soft object, like a pillow; turn the patient's head to the side to help with breathing, especially to avoid aspiration from saliva
- Hypoxia, post seizure, poses a risk for subsequent seizures
- Patients/family should be made aware to note the start time of any witnessed seizures; ongoing seizure activity (>5 minutes) represents status epilepticus and is a medical emergency

Referrals

If a patient's seizures/epileptic episodes have underlying causes, referral may be needed. For example, seizures triggered by hypoglycemic episodes may require referral to endocrinology.

Takeaways

- Seizures and epilepsy are not synonymous: seizures are isolated events; epilepsy is two or more unprovoked seizures.
- While some seizure activity is idiopathic (of unknown cause), in many cases seizures have identifiable underlying etiology (including but not limited to stress, stimulants, sleep disturbance, fever, infection, and head trauma). Treatment and management depend on addressing the underlying condition.
- Patient safety during the seizure should be addressed.

LESSON 12: BRAIN TUMORS

Learning Objectives
- Differentiate between primary and secondary central nervous system (CNS)/brain tumors
- Recognize signs/symptoms of brain tumors
- Identify treatment options for CNS/brain tumor patients

The incidence of brain tumors is approximately 29 per 100,000 people. The most common type of brain tumor is a secondary tumor and originates from another site in the body (lung, breast, and melanoma are most common). Primary brain tumors (originating in the CNS or brain) are less common in older adults, but more common in adolescents and young adults. Historically CNS/brain tumors were categorized primarily on histological similarities. The latest World Health Organization (WHO) classifications take into account genetic features as well. The greatest risk of developing a brain tumor is exposure to ionizing radiation. Hereditary causes account for only about 5–10% of brain tumors. Congenital causes are possible, but rarer.

Assessment

Signs and symptoms depend on the location of the tumor, and the patient may be asymptomatic.

Subjective
- Headache or change in previous headache pattern
- Nausea
- Muscle weakness
- Insomnia
- Fatigue
- Personality and cognitive changes

Objective
- Seizures—most common
- Cognitive difficulties (memory loss, altered mental status)
- Vomiting
- Abnormal gait/weakness on one side of body
- Vision changes (such as double vision)
- Speech difficulties (such as aphasia)
- Hearing difficulties
- Difficulty swallowing (associated with brain stem tumor)
- Increased intracranial pressure (ICP)—papilledema may be seen on ophthalmoscopic exam
- Abnormal neurological exam/cranial nerve exam depending on location of tumor and size
- Loss of consciousness related to increased ICP after position change

Patients may present with symptoms reflective of the area of the brain affected by the tumor.

Area of brain	Presentation
Frontal lobe	Changes in personality, communication, higher order thinking
Temporal lobe	Changes in hearing, understanding language
Parietal lobe	Loss of sensation and perception
Occipital lobe	Changes in vision and color perception
Cerebellum	Loss of balance and coordination
Brainstem	Alterations in breathing, heart rate, and temperature regulation

Table 11.12.1 Presentation Related to Affected Area of Brain

Diagnosis

The WHO (2016) brain tumor classifications signaled a new approach to brain tumor classification with implications for diagnosis, where both histological and genetic features of tumors are taken into consideration.

Diagnostic Testing

- **MRI** with contrast (gadolinium): imaging modality of choice; creates detailed imagery and measures tumor size
- **CT** scan with contrast: done if MRI contraindicated; creates three-dimensional image to locate and size tumors; CT of pelvis, abdomen, and chest to find primary tumor if brain tumor is suspected to be secondary
- **Biopsy:** can be done as open biopsy or stereotactic biopsy; determines histopathology and molecular structure of the tumor; if tumor is suspected to be a secondary tumor, assess for primary tumor first, as a biopsy is not needed if the brain tumor is secondary
- **Other testing:** cerebral arteriogram (evaluates arteries in brain), lumbar puncture (evaluates cerebral spinal fluid for tumor markers), electroencephalography (evaluates brain waves/monitors for seizure activity)

After diagnosis, the tumor is graded and a treatment plan is established.

Brain Tumor Grading	
Grade I	Least malignant; associated with long-term survival
Grade II	Slow-growing, but can invade nearby tissue
Grade III	Technically malignant, though Grade II and Grade III tumors are similar
Grade IV	Malignant; reproduces rapidly; creates its own blood vessels to aid growth; features areas of necrosis

Table 11.12.2

Differential Diagnosis

Differential diagnoses for brain tumor: **migraine headache, meningitis, encephalitis, pseudotumor cerebri, neuro-sarcoidosis, CVA, brain aneurysm, sinusitis, abscess**

Plan

Treatment

Treatment (and prognosis) for brain tumors depends on many factors, including type of tumor, size, grade, location (tumors may be close to delicate structures, such as the optic nerve, speech center), patient's age, and metastasis.

Treatment Options
High-dose glucocorticoids can decrease cerebral edema and subsequently decrease neurological deficits and headaches (contraindicated if lymphoma or infection is suspected)
Antiseizure medication
Surgical resection/removal
Chemotherapy
MRI-guided laser ablation
Radiation therapy
Tumor-treating fields, also known as alternating electric field therapy (uses electrical fields to disrupt cancer cells ability to multiply)
Debulking can reduce the size of a tumor without the intent of complete removal; provides for improved quality of life and length of life; generally done when tumors are incurable
Palliative care

Table 11.12.3

Following a craniotomy, monitor patient for adverse outcomes including DVT, PE, intracranial bleed, systemic infection, and worsening neurological status.

Education

- Patients with neurological deficits may require supportive therapies such as physical therapy, occupational therapy, speech therapy, or cognitive rehabilitation
- Patients who have survived brain tumors can expect regular follow-up (several months and sometimes years) after the initial diagnosis. Follow-up tests may include MRIs, eye/ear exams (sudden hearing or vision changes could represent brain compromise from new cancer activity), and regular follow-up with neurologist/neurosurgeon
- Brain tumor treatment is constantly evolving and improving; not all CNS tumor prognoses are grim

Referrals

- Oncology
- Neurology/neurosurgery
- Psychiatry
- Support groups
- Physical/speech/occupational or other supportive therapies

Takeaways

- The World Health Organization considers both histological and genetic features of tumors when classifying them.
- Brain tumors are rare. However, improved diagnostic and treatment options mean affected patients may enjoy higher recovery rates and better treatment outcomes.
- Presenting signs and symptoms may give clues as to which area of the brain has been affected by the tumor.

PRACTICE QUESTIONS

Select the ONE best answer.

Lesson 1: Cranial Nerve Overview

1. Audrey, a 53-year-old woman, reports a rapid onset of right-sided facial weakness. She is unable to turn a smile on the right side and unable to close her right eye fully. This presentation is likely paralysis of which cranial nerve?

   A. CN V

   B. CN VII

   C. CN IX

   D. CN X

2. In prescribing prednisone for the patient with Bell palsy, the nurse practitioner considers that:

   A. Early implementation of treatment is correlated with better recovery of nerve function

   B. Treatment for Bell palsy is controversial, and little data exists that suggests the drug will be effective

   C. A low dose steroid over four weeks is recommended

   D. Medication will strengthen the nerve to help eliminate facial and eye drooping

3. Which cranial nerves are associated with extraocular movements?

   A. CN II, III, IV

   B. CN II, IV, V

   C. CN III, IV, V

   D. CN III, IV, VI

4. The nurse practitioner asks the patient to "open up and say AHH." This assesses which cranial nerves?

   A. CN IX and XI

   B. CN IX and X

   C. CN X and XI

   D. CN XI and XII

Lesson 2: CVA & TIA

5. A 72-year-old patient presents with unilateral facial drooping, slurred speech, and vision changes. The first step in management is:

   A. Aspirin

   B. Echocardiogram

   C. Referral to the emergency department

   D. CBC, CMP, and troponin levels

6. When considering the diagnosis of acute stroke, which of the following are likely to be a part of the presentation?

   A. Ataxia, unilateral facial numbness, headache

   B. Slurred speech, coordinated gait, orientation × 3

   C. Severe headache, confusion, bilateral facial weakness

   D. Myopia, altered level of consciousness, severe headache

7. An 82-year-old patient presents with a history of TIA and confusion. Which test is the most sensitive for stroke?

   A. Ataxic gait

   B. Troponin, elevated

   C. Arm weakness/pronator drift

   D. Facial drooping, bilateral

8. George, age 65, has had several transient ischemic attacks. After a complete physiological exam and workup, the nurse practitioner would prescribe which medication?

   A. atenolol (Tenormin)

   B. warfarin (Coumadin)

   C. clopidogrel (Plavix)

   D. nitroglycerine (Nitrostat)

Lesson 3: Dementia/Delirium

9. The NP is aware that in order to make a diagnosis of dementia as per DSM-5 criteria, a decline in memory and a decline in at least one of the following must be present except the ability to:

   A. Generate coherent speech and understand spoken or written language

   B. Recognize or identify objects

   C. Execute motor activities

   D. Think objectively without prejudice

10. A medication like donepezil can be useful to treat mild and moderate dementia because it:

    A. Blocks cholinesterase, resulting in a reverse of cognitive symptoms

    B. Stimulates the release of cholinesterase, stopping the progression of cognitive decline

    C. Blocks cholinesterase, resulting in stabilization of cognitive decline

    D. Stimulates the release of cholinesterase, improving cognitive function

11. A 72-year-old male is brought in by his daughter who reports that her father seems to have had some changes in his memory. He recently lost his car downtown and had to take a cab home. She asks if her father has Alzheimer's dementia. What response by the NP is best?

    A. "Don't worry. This is a normal part of aging."

    B. "As long as he can still perform activities of daily living, this is not dementia."

    C. "We will need further testing."

    D. "Probably not, since women are more likely to develop dementia."

12. The NP is providing care for a patient diagnosed with Alzheimer's dementia. The patient's son states that his mom often wanders. The NP discusses with the son ways to ensure that his mom remains safe. Which response requires immediate follow-up by the NP?

    A. "I heard that using motion detectors on doors within the home can be helpful."

    B. "I usually leave the house keys and car keys on a rack by the door because I often misplace them."

    C. "I keep emergency phone numbers posted on the refrigerator."

    D. "I was able to get a home health aide to stay with my mom during the day when I am not home."

13. The NP is aware that which of the following are appropriate techniques for communicating with patients with dementia?

    A. Ask open-ended questions

    B. Maintain good eye contact and use a relaxed and unhurried approach

    C. Rephrase a statement if the patient does not seem to understand

    D. Finish the patient's statements

14. Which of the following is most indicative of delirium (as opposed to dementia)?

    A. Memory impairment

    B. Sleep disturbance

    C. Permanence

    D. Inattention

Lesson 4: Neurologic Exam

15. The nurse practitioner asks the patient to perform a rapid alternating movement (RAM) test to evaluate:

    A. Cerebral functioning

    B. Deep tendon reflexes

    C. Cerebellar functioning

    D. Frontal lobe functioning

16. Which documentation reflects a positive Romberg test?

    A. Unable to walk heel to toe in a straight line

    B. Unable to maintain balance with one foot outstretched

    C. Unable to maintain upper arms outstretched (i.e., one arm drops suddenly) with eyes closed

    D. Unable to maintain balance when standing with feet together with arms extended and eyes closed

17. When assessing the patient's deep tendon reflexes, the nurse practitioner notes the reflexes are normal. The nurse practitioner documents them as

    A. 0

    B. 1

    C. 2

    D. 3

18. During the neurological exam, the nurse practitioner asks the patient to walk heel to toe. This test assesses which function of the cerebellar system?

    A. Mental status

    B. Coordination

    C. Motor strength

    D. Reflex system

Lesson 5: Headaches

19. A headache induced by uncontrolled hypertension would be described as a:

    A. Primary headache

    B. Secondary headache

    C. Tertiary headache

    D. Chronic headache

20. A 27-year-old female presents to the clinic with a chief complaint of unilateral, frontal headaches. She reports the headaches occur 3–4 times per month and have not responded well to OTC ibuprofen therapy. Which of the following is a critical data element of her history of present illness?

    A. Pregnancy status

    B. Diet changes

    C. Sensitivity to high-pitched sound

    D. Immunization status

21. Which of the following would not meet the criteria identifying low-risk headache?

    A. History of similar headache

    B. A 27-year-old patient with new onset headache

    C. A pericranial headache associated with neck muscle tenderness

    D. Headaches triggered by the Valsalva maneuver

22. In a patient using zolmitriptan 2.5 mg tablets more than twice per week, the nurse practitioner knows to start which of the following medications?

    A. Amlodipine (Norvasc) 10 mg daily

    B. Trazodone (Desyrl) 150 mg daily

    C. Propranolol (Inderal) 80 mg per day

    D. Tramadol (Ultram) 50 mg twice daily

Lesson 6: Meningitis

23. Which of the following tests may be positive in the patient with meningitis?

    A. Kernig and Barlow

    B. Galeazzi and Brudzinski

    C. Galeazzi and Trendelenburg

    D. Kernig and Brudzinski

24. When considering the possibility of bacterial meningitis, which is the most likely presentation?

    A. Intermittent fever, neck pain

    B. Rapid onset of fever, headache, and nuchal rigidity

    C. Severe headache with low-grade fever

    D. Gradual onset of fever, headache, and nuchal rigidity

25. Of the following cerebrospinal fluid (CSF) results, which is most consistent with bacterial meningitis?

    A. Low opening pressure

    B. Lymphocytosis

    C. Low glucose, high protein

    D. Normal protein, normal glucose

26. Of the following bacterial causes of meningitis, which is not vaccine-preventable?

    A. *Neisseria meningitidis*

    B. Group B *Streptococcus*

    C. *Haemophilus influenzae* type B

    D. *Streptococcus pneumoniae*

Lesson 7: Multiple Sclerosis

27. Multiple sclerosis can be described as a(n):

    A. Autoimmune disorder typically featuring upper and lower motor neuron dysfunction, hyperreflexia, atrophy, and fasciculations

    B. Demyelinating autoimmune disorder with damage typically seen in the white matter of the brain and spinal cord; seen predominately in children/teens

    C. Autoimmune disorder typically featuring inflammation of the spinal cord, an inflamed optic nerve, and ataxia

    D. Autoimmune disorder typically featuring ascending paraplegia and potentially fatal respiratory muscle weakness

28. A 40-year-old Caucasian male with hypertension who presents with fatigue, tingling, numbness in the left lower extremity, and changes in vision asks the nurse practitioner if he has multiple sclerosis. Which of the following additional risk factors below are also symptoms that are suggestive of the disorder?

    A. Age, ethnicity

    B. Ethnicity, gender

    C. Gender, medical condition

    D. Medical condition, age

29. Which is most accurate about the progression of multiple sclerosis?

    A. All MS patients experience occasional remissions

    B. Most MS patients completely lose the ability to walk

    C. About one-half of MS patients eventually experience cognitive deficits

    D. MS patients' life expectancy is the same as the general population

30. Primary progressive multiple sclerosis (PPMS) is notable for:

    A. Being the MS type featuring the most inflammatory activity

    B. Not featuring periods of remission; patients experience progressive deterioration

    C. Being the most common type of MS

    D. Always leading to cognitive deficits

31. Which of the following statements by a patient with suspected multiple sclerosis indicates an understanding of blood work and the diagnosis of multiple sclerosis?

    A. "A CBC will show an underlying hematologic disorder."

    B. "A TSH will show evidence of thyroid issues."

    C. "A CMP will show a metabolic disturbance."

    D. "No blood test will confirm the diagnosis of multiple sclerosis."

32. Which of the following treatments is matched correctly with the targeted symptom?

    A. Neurontin for fatigue

    B. baclofen for nerve pain

    C. propranolol for tremors

    D. dalfampridine for nystagmus

Lesson 8: Parkinson Disease

33. Common signs of Parkinson disease include all of the following except:

    A. Shuffling/short steps

    B. Bradykinesia

    C. Masked face

    D. Hyperphonia

34. The nurse practitioner is considering a clinical diagnosis of Parkinson disease for her 62-year-old male patient. Which of the following statements would lead to a reconsideration of the diagnosis and a look at alternative diagnoses?

    A. On a smell test, the patient shows signs of hyposmia (reduced ability to smell)

    B. On gait assessment, the patient walks in short shuffling steps

    C. On a levodopa medication trial, the patient shows no improvement in motor function

    D. On a motor assessment, the patient shows resting tremor in one hand

35. The nurse practitioner's 40-year-old patient has a recent diagnosis of early-onset Parkinson disease. The patient's tremor is very mild. Which treatment is the most appropriate for this patient?

    A. Deep brain stimulation (DBS)

    B. levodopa (Larodopa)

    C. haloperidol (Haldol)

    D. ropinirole (Requip)

36. Patient and family education on Parkinson disease may include making the patient and family aware that:

    A. Parkinson treatment will slow and eventually reverse the symptoms

    B. The altered gait and rigidity seen in Parkinson disease necessitates the use of a wheelchair for all patients

    C. Antidepressant medications, specifically SSRIs, can be useful to treat both drooling and depression

    D. The patient is at risk for social isolation, as others may interpret the patient's slowed movements and stony expression for slow thinking and social disinterest

Lesson 9: Myasthenia Gravis

37. Myasthenia gravis occurs when antibodies destroy the _____ receptors at the neuromuscular junction causing _____.

    A. adrenergic; muscle contraction

    B. dopaminergic adrenergic; muscle contraction

    C. acetylcholine; muscle weakness

    D. metabotropic; muscle weakness

38. A patient experiencing unexplained muscle weakness, diplopia, ptosis, and difficulty breathing is to receive a Tensilon test (edrophonium). Which finding is suggestive of myasthenia gravis?

    A. The patient experiences an exacerbation of paralysis

    B. The patient experiences a sense of warmth with facial flushing

    C. The patient reports a ringing in the ears

    D. The patient experiences improved muscle strength

39. A patient diagnosed with myasthenia gravis is discussing her frustration with the muscle weakness associated with the disease, especially in relation to ADLs and exercising. Which statement is the best response by the nurse practitioner?

    A. "It is best to complete the tasks first thing in the morning."

    B. "It is best to complete the tasks mid-afternoon, after you have eaten lunch."

    C. "It is best to complete the tasks in the evening, during the commercials of your favorite shows."

    D. "It is best to complete the tasks at bedtime to relax you before sleeping."

40. A patient is newly diagnosed with myasthenia gravis. Which of the following includes symptoms usually associated with myasthenia gravis?

    A. Bowel and bladder dysfunction and spasticity

    B. Ascending paralysis with ultimate respiratory symptoms

    C. Cogwheel rigidity and loss of coordination

    D. Progressive weakness that is worse at the day's end

Lesson 10: Guillain-Barré Syndrome

41. A family member of a patient with Guillain-Barré syndrome asks about the paralysis associated with the disorder. Which statement by the NP best describes the paralysis?

    A. "The paralysis is temporary; the disease is self limiting."

    B. "The paralysis is progressive and permanent; we can talk about what that looks like for you."

    C. "The disease does not cause paralysis, just a tingling sensation in the lower extremities."

    D. "The paralysis is like chronic fatigue; it gets worse throughout the day."

42. In speaking with a patient with suspected Guillain-Barré syndrome, the nurse practitioner asks if the patient has a history of:

    A. Head injury without follow-up treatment

    B. Damage to the spinal cord

    C. Respiratory illness in the past four weeks

    D. Seizure activity diagnosed at birth

43. Which of the following is accurate regarding the workup of GBS?

    A. An erythrocyte sedimentation rate within normal levels rules out GBS

    B. Electromyography and nerve conduction studies are routinely measured in the workup of GBS

    C. A cerebrospinal fluid (CSF) level with normal protein levels and elevated WBC is suggestive of GBS

    D. MRI is both sensitive and specific for diagnosis of GBS

44. Which of the following is accurate regarding the treatment of GBS?

    A. Patients frequently require treatment for tachycardia; they rarely require treatment for bradycardia

    B. Long-term antihypertensive medications will be part of the treatment plan

    C. Corticosteroids (oral and intravenous) are commonly used as monotherapy

    D. Plasma exchange and IVIG (immunoglobulin therapy) are commonly used to hasten recovery

Lesson 11: Seizure Disorders

45. Atonic seizures are known to typically:

    A. Involve uncoordinated movements/thrashing, thus putting the patient at risk for accidentally hitting nearby objects

    B. Involve muscle weakness/limpness, thus putting the patient at high risk for falls

    C. Last more than five minutes, thus putting the patient at risk for status epilepticus

    D. Involve a loss of awareness resembling daydreaming, thus putting the patient at risk for poor academic performance

46. The nurse practitioner provides instructions for the family of a patient ("Joe") with a seizure disorder. Which of the following statements by a family member suggests further teaching is needed?

    A. "I will not restrain Joe when he is having a seizure."

    B. "I will assist Joe to the floor when he is having a seizure."

    C. "I will turn Joe's head to the side when he is having a seizure."

    D. "I will hold Joe's head to protect it when he is having a seizure."

47. The patient with epilepsy is morbidly obese and lets the nurse practitioner know she is trying to lose weight. The patient states that she is willing to take an anti-seizure medication, but she does not want to take any medication associated with weight gain. The nurse practitioner knows to avoid prescribing:

    A. lamotrigine (Lamictal)

    B. topiramate (Topamax)

    C. phenytoin (Dilantin)

    D. valproic acid (Depakote)

48. The nurse practitioner knows that febrile seizures are most highly associated with which age group?

    A. Newborns

    B. Infants

    C. Young adults

    D. Older adults

49. The nurse practitioner is providing patient education to a newly diagnosed epileptic patient. The nurse practitioner lets the patient know that seizure triggers can include:

    A. Hypersomnolence

    B. Herbal tea

    C. Inadequate insulin

    D. Cigarette use

Lesson 12: Brain Tumors

50. Mr. R. is a 63-year-old patient with a history of hypertension, hyperlipidemia, and lung cancer. He has had a new onset of fatigue, nausea/vomiting, and memory loss for the last two weeks. Which statement is true regarding the patient's symptoms?

    A. The symptoms would be expected based on the patient's age

    B. The symptoms could be related to metastases of lung cancer to the brain

    C. The symptoms could be related to a transient ischemia attack (TIA)

    D. The symptoms could be related to worsening of hypertension

51. Which of the following is not a differential diagnosis for a brain tumor?

    A. Meningitis

    B. Toxoplasmosis

    C. Pseudotumor cerebri

    D. Acute angle glaucoma

52. The purpose of debulking of a brain tumor is to:

    A. Remove all of the tumor

    B. Disrupt cancer cells' ability to multiply

    C. Improve quality and length of life

    D. Prevent further growth of the tumor

53. Following recent eradication of a brain tumor, the nurse practitioner should counsel the patient to:

    A. Report new hearing changes

    B. Follow up yearly

    C. Follow a low-protein diet

    D. Drive with extra caution

54. Which statement is true regarding brain tumors?

    A. Secondary brain tumors are most common in adolescents

    B. High-dose glucocorticoids are used in treatment if lymphoma is suspected

    C. Seizures are the most common symptom associated with a brain tumor

    D. CT scan with contrast is the imaging modality of choice to diagnose a brain tumor

ANSWERS AND EXPLANATIONS

Lesson 1: Cranial Nerve Overview

1. B

These symptoms are characteristic of Bell palsy, which reflects damage to the facial nerve, CN VII **(B)**. CN V (A) is the trochlear nerve, which reflects sensation and motor function of the temporal and masseter muscles. Cranial nerves IX (C) and X (D) innervate the tongue and throat (pharynx and larynx).

2. A

Earlier implementation of treatment is correlated with better recovery of nerve function **(A)**; prednisone is most effective if used within three days of onset of symptoms. Evidence is strong for the use of corticosteroids for patients who present within three days of symptom onset, and the recommended dose is 1 mg/kg/day (to a maximum of 80 mg per day) PO daily for 10 days, making (B) and (C) incorrect answer choices, respectively. Prednisone has anti-inflammatory effects; it does not strengthen the nerve, so choice (D) can be eliminated.

3. D

CN III, IV, VI **(D)** are associated with extraocular movements. CN II (A and B) controls central and peripheral vision and is not involved with EOM. CN V (C) is the trigeminal nerve that controls motor strength of temporalis and masseter muscles and sensation.

4. B

Cranial nerves IX and X **(B)** innervate the tongue and throat (pharynx and larynx). CN XI (A and C) controls neck and shoulder movement. CN XII (D) innervates the tongue, working with speech and swallowing.

Lesson 2: CVA & TIA

5. C

An immediate referral to the ED **(C)** is appropriate for suspected stroke. The etiology of the neurological changes must be determined before giving aspirin (A). This intervention is contraindicated in a patient with a hemorrhage. An echocardiogram (B) is considered when a cardiac source of embolism is suspected and laboratory data (D) are part of the diagnostic process; either of these concerns is second to getting the patient to the ED.

6. A

Ataxia, unilateral facial numbness, headache **(A)** are common signs/symptoms of acute stroke. Slurred speech may be present, but gait may be ataxic and limited orientation is common, not those listed—eliminate (B). Eliminate (C), as facial weakness is generally unilateral, not bilateral; and eliminate (D)—myopia is not common, but unilateral visual changes, such as double vision, are common.

7. C

Arm weakness/pronator drift **(C)** is a common, sensitive test for stroke. It is part of the FAST assessment. An ataxic gait (A) is not specific to stroke. Elevated troponin (B) is seen with cardiac tissue damage. Facial drooping is generally unilateral, not bilateral (D).

8. C

Antiplatelet therapy, clopidogrel **(C)**, is given to prevent new clots from forming. For the patient with uncontrolled blood pressure, a beta-blocker (A) may be used, but is not the first line of defense here. Warfarin (B), an anticoagulant, is usually recommended for the patient with an irregular heart rhythm; we do not have that information in the question stem. Nitroglycerine (D), a vasodilator, is more commonly used for chest pain or angina.

Lesson 3: Dementia/Delirium

9. D

A diagnosis of dementia is not made based on a patient's ability to think objectively without prejudice **(D)**. To make a diagnosis of dementia as per DSM-5 criteria, a decline in memory and a decline in at least one of the following must be present: ability to generate coherent speech and understand spoken or written language (A); ability to recognize or identify objects (assuming an intact sensory function) (B); ability to execute motor activities (assuming intact motor and sensory abilities and comprehension of tasks) (C); and ability to think abstractly, make sound judgments, and plan and carry out complex tasks.

10. C

Donepezil blocks cholinesterase, the enzyme responsible for breaking down acetylcholine. This results in the accumulation of acetylcholine and causes continuous stimulation of the muscles, glands, and central nervous system. It can stabilize cognitive decline **(C)** and help with symptoms, but does not cure, reverse (A), or stop progression. It does not stimulate the release of cholinesterase (B and D).

11. C

Further testing **(C)** is needed, including geriatric-specific assessment tools, imaging, and blood tests. Other causes of mental status changes need to be ruled out. Memory loss is *not* a normal part of aging (A) and is a sign of dementia. Memory impairment with normal functioning (intact activities of daily living) (B) is a characteristic of mild cognitive impairment (MCI). Although women are more likely to develop Alzheimer disease (D), it still occurs in men.

12. B

Leaving the house keys and car keys on a rack by the door **(B)** requires follow-up. A person with dementia and known history of wandering is likely to pick up on recalled cues consistent with leaving the home. Visible keys may cause the person to wander. Motion detectors on doors within the home (A), emergency phone numbers posted on the refrigerator (C), and having a home health aide stay at the home (D) are all safety interventions that should be employed for someone at risk for wandering.

13. B

Maintaining eye contact and a relaxed, friendly approach **(B)** will put the patient at ease. Therapeutic communication is an important intervention for those with dementia. Open-ended questions (A), while usually therapeutic, can be taxing for a patient with dementia. Simple yes or no questions can be easier. Rather than rephrase a statement (C), it is better to restate the phrase (so the patient can hear the same words again and process them). Give the patient time to find words or gestures to finish a statement rather than complete the statement for the patient—it takes time for the patient to process or find words.

14. D

Inattention **(D)** is a distinguishing characteristic of delirium. Diagnosis requires the presence of inattention, acute onset, fluctuating course, and disorganized thinking or altered level of consciousness. Memory impairment (specifically recent) (A), sleep disturbance (B), and permanence (C) are features suggestive of dementia.

Lesson 4: Neurologic Exam

15. C

RAM assesses coordination, a function of the cerebellum **(C)**. Testing the cerebral function (A) includes testing the frontal lobe, parietal lobe, temporal lobe, and occipital lobe; RAM testing is not specific to the cerebral functioning. Testing the deep tendon reflexes (B) involves striking the selected tendon with a hammer. Frontal lobe functioning (D) involves personality, language, mood, and memory, which are not tested with RAM.

16. D

A positive Romberg test is documented when a patient is unable to maintain balance when standing with eyes closed and arms stretched to the front **(D)**. The other three answer choices are not reflective of the Romberg test. Heel to toe (A) walking is a different means of assessing cerebellar motor function. Inability to maintain balance with one foot stretched outward (B) is not reflective of the Romberg test; this would be a test of balance. The ability to maintain upper arms outstretched (C) may be assessed when checking for signs of stroke, and the eyes may remain open in that assessment.

17. C

A rating of 2 **(C)** indicates a normal response. A rating of 0 (A) indicates the reflex is absent. A rating of 1 (B) indicates reflexes are diminished. A rating of 3 (D) indicates a brisk response.

18. B

The heel to toe test assesses coordination **(B)**. An example of a mental status (A) test is the MMSE, which tests orientation, recent and remote memory, concentration, and abstraction detail. Romberg test is used to test motor strength and balance (C). Testing the deep tendon reflexes (D) is done by striking the tendon.

Lesson 5: Headaches

19. B

A secondary headache **(B)** is a headache caused by an underlying organic disease process. Primary headaches (A) have no apparent underlying organic disease process. Tertiary headaches (C) do not exist. Chronic headaches (D) are characterized by their frequency, not underlying pathology.

20. A

A new onset of headache during pregnancy **(A)** is considered a red flag symptom warranting further evaluation by an obstetrics specialist. Diet changes (B), sensitivity to high-pitched sounds (C), and immunization status (D) are not elements that typically trigger or influence headache activity.

21. D

Headache triggered by the Valsalva maneuver **(D)** are considered a red flag symptom because it could be indicative of a Chiari malformation and should be further evaluated by neurology. History of similar headache (A), age younger than 30 (B), and headaches resembling tension headaches (C) are all considered to be low risk.

22. C

Prophylaxis therapy should be initiated in all migraine patients requiring triptan therapy equal to or greater than twice per week. Propranolol 80–240 mg daily **(C)** is a common prophylaxis therapy used in migraine management. Though calcium channel blockers and tricyclic antidepressants are therapies used for migraine prophylaxis, amlodipine (A) and trazodone (B) are not considered first-line therapy. The chronic use of analgesics (D) for migraine activity control is discouraged, since we know its use can trigger "rebound" headaches.

Lesson 6: Meningitis

23. D

The Kernig and Brudzinski tests **(D)** may be positive in the presence of meningeal irritation, such as with meningitis. The Barlow (A), Galeazzi (B), and Trendelenburg (C) tests are used for evaluating development dysplasia of the hip.

24. B

Bacterial meningitis usually presents with rapid onset of fever, headache, and nuchal rigidity **(B)**. The fever is neither intermittent (A) nor low-grade (C). Gradual onset of symptoms (D) is more likely with viral meningitis.

25. C

In the presence of bacterial meningitis, the CSF demonstrates low glucose and high protein **(C)**. The opening CSF pressure in bacterial meningitis is usually high, not low (A). Lymphocytosis (B) is usually associated with viral meningitis, as are normal glucose and protein (D) in the CSF.

26. B

Group B *Streptococcus* **(B)** is not vaccine-preventable. Immunizations are recommended for the prevention of *Neisseria meningitidis* (A), *Haemophilus influenzae* type B (C), and *Streptococcus pneumoniae* (D) infections.

Lesson 7: Multiple Sclerosis

27. C

Multiple sclerosis is best described as an autoimmune disorder typically featuring inflammation of the spinal cord, an inflamed optic nerve, and ataxia **(C)**. Amyotrophic lateral sclerosis (ALS) is described in choice (A), disseminated encephalomyelitis in choice (B), and Guillain-Barré in choice (D).

28. A

This patient's age and ethnicity **(A)** are risk factors for multiple sclerosis. Patients who are between 15–60 years old and Caucasian are at risk, as are females with autoimmune diseases such as hypothyroidism, diabetes, or inflammatory bowel disease. Male gender (B and C) and hypertension (C and D) are not established risk factors for multiple sclerosis.

29. C

About one-half of MS patients eventually experience cognitive deficits **(C)**. Some patients experience progressive deterioration with no remissions (A). Many MS patients maintain the ability to walk, although some need assistive devices (B). MS patients tend to have a shorter life expectancy than people in the general population (D).

30. B

PPMS is notable for patients experiencing progressive deterioration **(B)**. Relapsing-remitting MS is believed to be the MS type with the most inflammatory activity (A) and the most common type of MS (C), not primary progressive multiple sclerosis. Not all MS sufferers develop significant cognitive deficits (D).

31. D

No blood test will confirm the diagnosis of multiple sclerosis **(D)**; this is a correct statement. Blood work is not expected to show an underlying hematologic disorder (A), thyroid issues (B), or metabolic disorder (C).

32. C

Propranolol can be used for tremors **(C)**. Neurontin (A) can be considered for nerve pain. Baclofen (B) may be used for increased muscle tone/muscle spasms. Dalfampridine (D) may be helpful for gait and motor dysfunction.

Lesson 8: Parkinson Disease

33. D

Hyperphonia **(D)** is not common to Parkinson disease; hypophonia (low speaking voice) is common. Gait impairment (A), slowed movement (B), and masked face (C) are all commonly seen in the patient with Parkinson disease.

34. C

If, on a levodopa medication trial, the patient shows no improvement in motor function **(C)**, a diagnosis other than Parkinson disease should be considered. Hyposmia (A), short shuffling steps (B), and resting tremor (D) are all recognized signs of Parkinson disease.

35. D

Ropinirole **(D)** is the most appropriate intervention for this patient, as Requip can treat restless leg syndrome. Deep brain stimulation (A) involves fairly risky surgery and would not be the first choice for mild Parkinson disease. Levodopa (B) would not be first-line in a young Parkinson patient with mild tremor. Levodopa tends to "wear out" in effectiveness in under 10 years. It is preferable to use a different medication while the patient's tremor is still mild. Levodopa can always be introduced later and is generally given in combination with carbidopa to reduce side effects and more effectively pass the blood-brain barrier. Haloperidol (C) is an antipsychotic. No psychosis was reported for this patient. As a first-generation antipsychotic, this medication would be contraindicated in a Parkinson patient. It reduces dopamine even further and could induce an akinetic crisis.

36. D

It is true that the Parkinson patient is at risk for social isolation **(D)**. It is not true that treatment will slow and eventually reverse the symptoms (A); treatment is symptomatic, Parkinson disease cannot currently be cured. It is not true that all patients will need a wheelchair (B), despite the risk of falls. It is not SSRIs (C), but rather tricyclic antidepressants, that will treat both drooling (because of anticholinergic properties) and depression.

Lesson 9: Myasthenia Gravis

37. C

With myasthenia gravis, antibodies destroy or block the receptor sites for acetylcholine at the neuromuscular junction, which prevents the muscle from contracting **(C)**, causing weakness. Adrenergic (A), dopaminergic, and metabotropic (D) receptors are not involved in the pathophysiology of MG.

38. D

Edrophonium (given in the Tensilon test) prevents the breakdown of acetylcholine, which allows more of the neurotransmitter (acetylcholine) to be present at the neuromuscular junction, resulting in improved muscle strength **(D)** if myasthenic crisis is present. If the patient experiences an exacerbation of paralysis (A), a true cholinergic crisis is present. Neither a sense of warmth with facial flushing (B) nor tinnitus (ringing in the ears) (C) occurs.

39. A

Patients with myasthenia gravis tend to have greater muscle weakness as the day progresses (the muscles are tired from use); the best muscle strength is first thing in the morning **(A)**. For that same reason, midafternoon (B), in the evening (C), and at bedtime (D) are not the best options.

40. D

Myasthenia gravis is associated with progressive weakness that is worse at the day's end **(D)**. Bowel and bladder dysfunction and spasticity (A) refer to symptoms of multiple sclerosis. Ascending paralysis with ultimate respiratory symptoms (B) refers to symptoms of Guillain-Barré syndrome. Cogwheel rigidity and loss of coordination (C) refer to symptoms of Parkinson disease.

Lesson 10: Guillain-Barré Syndrome

41. A

The paralysis of Guillain-Barré syndrome is temporary **(A)**. The disease is self-limiting, and treatment is aimed at lessening the severity of the immunity attack and supporting the patient while the body recovers. The paralysis is progressive, but not permanent (B). The disease will ultimately cause temporary paralysis (C); the patient may have a tingling sensation, even after the paralysis resolves. Muscle weakness, not necessarily paralysis, that gets worse throughout the day (D) is suggestive of myasthenia gravis.

42. C

Commonly, a patient with GBS will report a history of respiratory **(C)** or gastrointestinal infection in the previous month. Head injury (A), damage to the spinal cord (B), and seizures (D) are not precursors to the disease.

43. B

Electromyography and nerve conduction studies are routinely measured in the workup of GBS **(B)**. An ESR is used to rule out other diagnoses than GBS (A). CSF with elevated proteins, not normal proteins (C), and normal WBC is suggestive of GBS. MRI is more helpful in excluding other diagnoses than in diagnosis of GBS.

44. D

Plasma exchange and IVIG (immunoglobulin therapy) are commonly used to hasten recovery **(D)**. Arrhythmia management includes atropine for bradycardia; rarely is tachycardia treated (A). It is not long-acting antihypertensives (B), but rather short-acting medications that treat hypertension; hypotension is often treated with fluids. Corticosteroids (C) are not commonly used, as data does not support their efficacy.

Lesson 11: Seizure Disorders

45. B

Atonic seizures typically involve muscle weakness or limpness **(B)**. Uncoordinated movements and thrashing (A) are suggestive of clonic activity. Seizure activity of 5 minutes (C) is a medical emergency; atonic seizures usually last <15 seconds. Loss of awareness resembling daydreaming (D) is common in absence seizure, not atonic seizures.

46. D

While it is appropriate to put a pillow under the head of someone having a seizure, further teaching is needed if the family member plans to *hold* Joe's head to protect it **(D)**. It is true that the family member should not restrain Joe (A), should assist Joe to the floor (B), and should turn Joe's head to the side (C) while he is having a seizure.

47. D

While all four medications listed are anticonvulsant medications, valproic acid (Depakote) **(D)** is the one most associated with significant weight gain. Lamotrigine (A), topiramate (B), and phenytoin (C) are much less likely to have that side effect.

48. B

Infants **(B)** are the most likely to experience febrile seizures. While newborns (A), young adults (C), and the elderly (D) can experience seizures, they tend not to be febrile in nature.

49. D

Nicotine, from cigarette use **(D)** for example, can trigger seizures. Other triggers include inadequate sleep, not hypersomnolence (A); caffeine, not herbal tea (B); and hypoglycemia, from overuse of insulin for example, not inadequate amounts of insulin (C).

Lesson 12: Brain Tumors

50. B

The symptoms could be related to metastases of lung cancer to the brain **(B)**. Lung cancer is one of the most common types of cancer to metastasize to the brain. The symptoms would not be expected based on the patient's age (A). Symptoms of a TIA (C) occur over a short time frame, not two weeks. Nausea/vomiting and memory loss would not be related to worsening of hypertension (D).

51. D

Acute angle glaucoma **(D)** is not a differential diagnosis for a brain tumor. Meningitis (A), toxoplasmosis (B), and pseudotumor cerebri (C) are all possible differential diagnoses.

52. C

The purpose of debulking is to improve quality and length of life **(C)**. A resection is done with the goal of removing all the tumor (A). Tumor-treating fields are used to disrupt the cancer cells' ability to multiply (B). The purpose of debulking is not to prevent further growth of the tumor (D).

53. A

New hearing changes **(A)** can be a sign that the tumor has returned. Initially the patient will have follow-up every two to three months, not yearly (B). There is no reason to follow a low-protein diet (C). The patient will not be able to drive (D) with recent seizure activity.

54. C

Seizures are the most common symptom associated with a brain tumor **(C)**. Secondary brain tumors (A) are most common in older adults. Primary brain tumors are most common in adolescents. High-dose glucocorticoids (B) are contraindicated in suspected lymphoma. CT scan with contrast (D) is used if MRI with contrast is contraindicated; MRI with contrast is the imaging modality of choice.

CHAPTER 12

Psychiatric

LESSON 1: ABUSE

Learning Objectives
- Recognize risk factors and signs of abuse
- Apply screening tools for abuse
- Understand obligation of mandatory reporting

Intimate partners, elders, and children are populations that are vulnerable to abuse. While mandatory reporting does not apply to domestic violence (in general), it does apply to actions against children and elders (*for elder abuse see Chapter 18, Lesson 3*). This lesson will address domestic violence, child abuse, and substance use disorders.

Domestic Violence

Domestic violence (or intimate partner violence) is a pattern of behaviors in which one partner maintains power and control over another partner. These behaviors may include physical harm, sexual violence, emotional abuse, threats, and intimidation.

Consider the holistic needs of a patient. Unconditional support and compassionate inquiry about abuse are important nursing interventions. Both can validate domestic abuse as a healthcare concern. Be aware of how your personal attitude can affect your feelings toward those suffering from abuse.

Risk Factors for Being a Perpetrator of Intimate Partner Abuse
- Teen/young adult
- Low income/economic stressors
- Low educational status
- Unemployment
- Substance abuse
- History of traumatic childhood circumstances, being abused and/or neglected as a child, violence between parents, sexual violence in home
- Stress
- Anxiety
- Belief in strict gender roles

> **Pro Tip**
> - Identify patients at risk and take steps to prevent intimate partner abuse before it begins. This can include interventions like family therapy, teaching social and emotional skills, and utilizing programs aimed at reducing peer violence.
> - Resources for victims of intimate partner abuse/domestic violence include shelters, hotlines, and safe houses. Victims may need to avail themselves of legal support such as restraining orders. For imminent danger, call 911.

Child Abuse

The U.S. Child Abuse Prevention and Treatment Act defines child abuse as "(a)ny recent act or failure to act on the part of a parent or caretaker, which results in death, serious physical or emotional harm, sexual abuse or exploitation, or an act or failure to act which presents an imminent risk of serious harm."

Assessment

In the case of physical abuse, a child may present with suspicious physical injuries that do not match the explanations offered by the parent/caregiver.

Suspicious Physical Injuries
Injuries in symmetrical patterns, such as round scars from cigarette burns
Bruises in the shape of an object, such as a belt buckle
Immersion burns (such as glove and sock burns to hands/feet, which suggest intentional immersion in boiling water)
Multiple fractures in varying stages of healing
Cerebral hemorrhage or loss of consciousness (from shaking)
Repeated visits for medical care for unusual, hard-to-explain sickness in child, such as repeated stomach ailments (may represent Munchausen by proxy)

Table 12.1.1

In general, an abused child can present with physical and psychological symptoms that do not align with normal growth and development.

General Symptoms/Signs of Abuse	
Physical symptoms	Dehydration, malnutrition, hematomas, bruises, cuts, fractures, lacerations, burns
Psychological symptoms	Low self-esteem, anxious behavior, withdrawn behavior, aggressive behavior by child, emotional lability, fearfulness, trying to cover up injuries

Table 12.1.2

Screening Tools

Brief Child Abuse Potential Inventory (BCAP): a short version (31 questions) of the 160-question Child Abuse Potential Inventory (CAP); can be predictive of future abuse

Conflict Tactics Scale Parent to Child (CTS-PC): evaluates the extent to which parents/caregivers use reasoning and nonviolent discipline, psychological aggression, and physical assault in response to a child's behavior

Diagnosis

Below are the legal definitions related to child abuse. A formal diagnosis is made using DSM-5 criteria. Note: the criteria differ slightly from the legal definition of the terms.

Types	General definitions
Neglect	Failure of a parent or other person responsible for the child to provide adequate age-appropriate nourishment, clothing, shelter, medical care, education, or supervision to the point where a child's safety and well-being are threatened with physical or psychological harm
Emotional abuse	Injury to the psychological or emotional stability of the child (e.g., belittling, disparaging, threatening to abandon, etc.) that may cause serious behavioral, emotional, or mental disorders
Sexual abuse	Unwanted sexual activity, with perpetrators using force, making threats, or taking advantage of persons not able to give consent; abuse may be overt (hands on) or covert (implied or suggested rather than physically acted out)
Physical abuse	Non-accidental physical injury of a child (e.g., beating, punching, shaking, choking, kicking, burning, hitting, etc.) by a parent or caregiver—whether or not the injury was intended
Parental substance abuse	Maternal drug and/or alcohol use during pregnancy; direct and indirect effects on a child living with a caregiver (or caregivers) with a substance use disorder
Abandonment	Occurs when a parent (or caregiver) deserts a child without regard for the child's safety and well-being

Table 12.1.3 Definitions of Types of Abuse

Risk factors for child abuse in the home are many: marital discord, domestic violence, substance abuse, nonbiological parent in the home, work stress, inadequate housing, financial hardship, child with a disability, mentally ill parent, parent unfamiliar with normal stages of growth and development, parent who suffered child abuse, and previous visit by Child Protective Services (CPS).

Plan

A nonjudgmental approach helps establish rapport and building trust. The child needs to be interviewed alone (separate from parent/caregiver) if possible. Documentation of the observed interactions between the child and caregiver(s) is important, as is documentation of the physical exam findings (take photographs). For examination purposes in the case of sexual abuse, this needs to be performed by a sexual assault forensic examiner.

Mandatory Reporting

Mandatory reporting is required when an individual knows or has reasonable cause to believe or suspect that a child has been subjected to abuse or neglect.

Treatment

Treatment options exist for both the parent and child.

Parent	Child
Parental education	Cognitive behavioral therapy
Triple P (teaches adaptive—as opposed to maladaptive—parental interventions)	Eye movement and desensitization/EMDR
Systematic Training for Effective Parenting (STEP)	Therapeutic play
Parent-child interaction therapy	School-mediated interventions

Table 12.1.4 Treatment Options

Referrals

A diagnosis or legal charge of abuse requires a multidisciplinary approach. An initial (but unsubstantiated) suspicion of child abuse may lead to a referral to CPS and further investigation. A primary care provider's diagnosis of child abuse would necessitate the referral/subsequent involvement of a psychology or psychiatric specialist. Further, a substantiated charge of child abuse may involve the following:

- Child Protective Services—for continued follow-up
- Social workers
- Family members
- School-based support (such as a school social worker or school nurse)
- Legal services/possible court-mandated requirements for parents
- Local child welfare services

Substance Use Disorders

Substance use–related diagnoses include alcohol, opioids, cannabinoids, sedatives, other stimulants, hallucinogens, tobacco, volatile solvents, and multiple drugs or other psychoactive substances. The diagnostic criteria are relatively consistent for many of the disorders. Patients may be diagnosed with a use disorder (problematic use patterns), withdrawal disorder, or intoxication.

Definitions

- **Binge drinking:** most common pattern of excessive alcohol intake; consumption (5 or more drinks for a man; 4 or more drinks for a woman in the span of 2 hours); the person is not alcohol dependent
- **Delirium tremens:** severe form of alcohol withdrawal; onset of confusion, hypertension, irregular heart rate, fever that can progress to seizure; medical emergency that can be fatal

The role of the healthcare professional can be defined by SBIRT (screening, brief intervention, and referral to treatment). **Screening** refers to a preliminary systematic evaluation of the likelihood that an individual has a substance use condition. **Brief intervention** refers to limited-time effort to provide information, increase motivation to avoid substances, or assist the individual in learning behavioral skills. **Referral to treatment** refers to efforts made to facilitate those whose substance use necessitates additional care.

Assessment

Part of the assessment and diagnosis process is determining the patient's readiness to change:

- **Precontemplation:** patient is not yet considering change or is unwilling or unable to change
- **Contemplation:** patient acknowledges concerns and is considering the possibility of change, but is ambivalent and uncertain
- **Preparation:** patient is committed to and is planning to make a change in the near future, but is still considering what to do
- **Action:** patient is actively taking steps to change but has not yet reached a stable state
- **Maintenance:** patient has achieved initial goals such as abstinence and is now working to maintain gains

Screening Tools

Short screening tools are meant to assess if a longer conversation of use, frequency, risky behaviors, and consequences of substance use is warranted.

CRAFFT 2.0: a series of six questions developed to screen children ages 12–18 for high-risk alcohol and other drug use disorders simultaneously

AUDIT-C: a three-item alcohol use screen that can help identify persons who are hazardous drinkers or have active alcohol use disorders

CAGE AID: a five-question tool used to screen for drug and alcohol use. If a person answers yes to two or more questions, a complete alcohol assessment is advised

Diagnosis

Regardless of the substance, the diagnosis of substance use is based on a pathological set of behaviors related to the use of that substance. A person needs to meet two or more of the criteria to be diagnosed with a substance use disorder. These behaviors include:

- **Impaired control**
  - Using for longer time frame or larger amounts than intended
  - Wanting to reduce use, but not able
  - Spending excessive time getting, using, recovering from use
  - Intense cravings
- **Social impairment**
  - Continued use despite problems with employment or social obligations
  - Continued use despite interpersonal problems
  - Reduced social activities because of substance use
- **Risky use**
  - Uses substances in physically dangerous situations
  - Uses substances knowing it may worsen an existing physical or psychological condition
- **Pharmacological indicators (tolerance and withdrawal)**
  - Needing an increased amount of a substance to achieve the desired effect
  - Physical symptoms with abrupt cessation of the drug

A SBIRT approach can reach patients with a wide range of substance use conditions and provide an appropriate level of care. Early recognition and brief intervention is cost-effective.

Takeaways

- Knowing risk factors for abuse can help alert the nurse practitioner to abuse.

- Suspicion of child abuse carries a mandatory reporting requirement for nurse practitioners.

- With substance use/abuse, the role of the healthcare professional can be defined by SBIRT (screening, brief intervention, and referral to treatment).

LESSON 2: ANXIETY

Learning Objectives
- Identify the signs and symptoms of anxiety disorders
- Interpret screening tools related to anxiety disorders
- Identify appropriate treatment and referrals related to anxiety disorders

Anxiety disorders are the most commonly occurring mental health diagnoses in the U.S. Symptoms of anxiety are commonly experienced, but when symptoms interfere with daily living an anxiety disorder should be considered.

Assessment—Anxiety

Onset of symptoms usually occur before the age of 21 years. Females have a greater prevalence than males, and it is common to have a first-degree relative with an anxiety disorder.

- **Physical symptoms:** tachycardia, hyperventilation, palpitations, chest pain, nausea, vomiting, dizziness, choking sensation, tremors, sweating, tearfulness, appetite changes, sleep disturbance, dry mouth, numbness, muscle tension

- **Psychological/social symptoms:** difficult to control thoughts of worry, restlessness, irritability, concentration issues, derealization, avoidance, fear of leaving home, distorted blame

Anxiety disorders and depressive disorders are often co-occurring conditions. Screen for both for accuracy of diagnosis and treatment.

Diagnosis

DSM-5 criteria for generalized anxiety disorder (GAD) includes excessive anxiety and worry occurring more days than not for the past 6 months, about a number of events or activities, where the individual finds it difficult to control the worry. The anxiety and worry are associated with three or more of the following symptoms:

- Feeling restless
- Easily fatigued
- Difficulty concentrating/mind going blank
- Irritability
- Muscle tension
- Sleep disturbance

Only one symptom is required for children. The symptoms significantly impact social, occupational, or other areas of everyday life and cannot be attributed to the physiological effects of a substance or another medical condition.

Other anxiety disorder diagnoses:

- **Separation anxiety disorder:** anxiety/fear related to being separated from an individual to whom the individual is attached
- **Selective mutism:** failure to speak in situations where there is an expectation to speak, regardless of speaking in other situations
- **Specific phobia:** anxiety/fear related to a particular object or situation
- **Social anxiety disorder:** anxiety/fear regarding a social situation
- **Panic disorder:** panic attacks that are recurrent and unexpected
- **Agoraphobia:** anxiety/fear regarding being unable to escape a place or situation

Screening Tools

Generalized Anxiety Disorder-7 (GAD-7): a seven-item self-report scale that screens anxiety symptoms over the past two weeks and rates symptoms as minimal, mild, moderate, and severe

- Scores of 0–4, minimal
- Scores of 5–9, mild
- Scores of 10–14, moderate
- Scores of >14, severe

Screen for Childhood Anxiety-Related Emotional Disorders (SCARED): a child and parent/guardian self-report to screen for childhood anxiety disorders including general anxiety disorder, separation anxiety disorder, panic disorder, social phobia, and school phobias. This screening scale is for children aged 8–18 years.

- Total score of 25 or higher indicates an anxiety disorder
- Specific anxiety disorders are indicated by questions/scores related to each diagnosis

Plan

Treatment

Evidence-based practice indicates the best outcomes from a combination treatment plan that includes pharmacological intervention and psychotherapy. Neurotransmitters involved in anxiety symptoms are:

- Gamma-aminobutyric acid (GABA)
- Serotonin (5-HT)
- Norepinephrine (NE)
- Dopamine (DA)

First-line medication therapy for anxiety is a selective serotonin reuptake inhibitor (SSRI). The initial phase of identifying the correct medication and dose may take up to 3 months; followed by a maintenance phase of 6–12 months to achieve symptom control. Start with a low dose and increase slowly if symptoms warrant. The choice of medication is based on:

- Medications previously taken, success in treatment, and side effects
- Medications taken by relatives, success, side effects
- Medications currently being taken, potential interactions, other diagnoses
- Medication allergies

Selective Serotonin Reuptake Inhibitors (SSRIs)

- **Citalopram, escitalopram, fluoxetine, fluvoxamine, paroxetine, sertraline:** selectively inhibit serotonin reuptake

Serotonin-Norepinephrine Reuptake Inhibitors (SNRIs)

- **Desvenlafaxine, duloxetine, levomilnacipran, venlafaxine:** inhibit norepinephrine, serotonin, and dopamine

Anxiolytics—non-benzodiazepine

- **Buspirone:** exact mechanism unknown; binds to serotonin and dopamine D2 receptors

Anxiolytics—benzodiazepines

- **Alprazolam, chlordiazepoxide, clonazepam, clorazepate, diazepam, estazolam, flurazepam, lorazepam, oxazepam, temazepam, triazolam:** bind to benzodiazepine receptors and enhance GABA effects

Medication class	Potential common adverse effects	Clinical information
SSRIs	Sexual dysfunction, nausea, diarrhea, insomnia, withdrawal on discontinuation, potential drug interactions, weight gain, agitation, and hyperactivity; fluoxetine is more activating than other SSRIs	Decrease dose/frequency in hepatic impairment; paroxetine must be tapered down due to significant withdrawal potential; risk for serotonin syndrome
SNRIs	Nausea, dizziness, insomnia, sedation, constipation, and sweating; venlafaxine may increase blood pressure	Decrease dose in hepatic and renal failure; must be tapered down due to significant withdrawal potential; prescribe with caution if h/o glaucoma
Anxiolytics: non-benzodiazepines	Insomnia, agitation, and nausea	Avoid use in renal and hepatic severe impairment
Anxiolytics: benzodiazepines	Impairment of psychomotor performance, amnesia, dependence and withdrawal symptoms after long-term treatment; rebound anxiety after short-term treatment	Decrease dose/frequency in hepatic impairment; high potential for misuse/dependency; ideally used only for short periods of time, 2–6 weeks

Table 12.2.1 Medication Therapy for Anxiety Disorders

Benzodiazepines mediate the neurotransmitter GABA and are effective in treating anxiety symptoms, although they also have the potential for abuse/misuse. If a benzodiazepine is prescribed, it should be for a short period of time, 2–6 weeks. Treatment periods of longer duration may result in tolerance, dependence, and withdrawal with discontinuation.

Education

- Medications that affect serotonin tend to increase symptoms of nausea, vomiting, and diarrhea, which may be decreased by eating prior to dosing
- Decrease dose slowly to avoid discontinuation syndrome

> **DANGER SIGN** Serotonin syndrome results from taking medications that affect serotonin, such as migraine rescue medications, certain pain medications, or cough and cold preparations. Serotonin syndrome is a medical emergency—symptoms vary and can include confusion/agitation, headache, dilated pupils, tachycardia, hypertension, sweating, fever, shivering, muscle rigidity, and diarrhea.

Referrals

- Mental health specialist such as a PMHNP or psychiatrist for complicated anxiety, comorbid diagnoses, and treatment failures
- Psychotherapy: cognitive behavioral therapy (CBT)

Assessment—Posttraumatic Stress Disorder (PTSD)

DSM-5 criteria for PTSD involves the exposure to actual or threatened death, injury, or violence in those 6 years of age or older. These exposures can be experienced directly, witnessed, or subjected to repeated/extreme exposures. Exposure can also occur through having knowledge that family members or friends experienced these events. One or more of the following symptoms occur after the event:

- Intrusive memories of the traumatic event that are recurrent and involuntary
- Distressing dreams related to the traumatic event that are recurrent
- Dissociative reactions such as flashbacks
- Internal/external cues related to an aspect of the trauma event with physiological reactions

Patients experience a persistent avoidance of stimuli that is associated with the trauma, negative cognitive/mood changes, and alterations in arousal/reactivity. The symptoms will have been occurring for more than one month. Children less than 6 years of age can be diagnosed with PTSD and are best served in a practice that specializes in children's mental health.

Screening Tools

Primary Care PTSD Screen (PC-PTSD): a four-question screening tool is commonly used; an answer of yes to three or more questions prompts follow-up

Treatment

A combination treatment plan includes pharmacological intervention and psychotherapy.

- SSRI/SNRI for anxiety symptoms
- Mirtazapine, prazosin, propranolol, trazodone to improve sleep and relieve nightmares
- Clonidine and propranolol to decrease hyperarousal
- Carbamazepine and valproic acid to address aggression, impulsiveness, and irritability

Referrals

- Given the complexity of treatment, appropriate referral is needed for patients with PTSD. All children 6 years of age or younger should be referred to a mental health specialist for that age group
- Psychotherapy: cognitive behavioral therapy (CBT), eye movement desensitization and reprocessing (EMDR), and exposure therapy

Takeaways

- Anxiety disorders are common. Screen for physical, psychological, and social symptoms.
- Screening scales such as GAD-7, SCARED, and PC-PTSD assist in diagnosis and treatment progression.
- SSRIs and psychotherapy are first-line treatment.
- Refer complicated patients such as those with comorbid diagnoses and treatment failures.

LESSON 3: DEPRESSION

> **Learning Objectives**
> - Identify the signs and symptoms of depressive disorders
> - Interpret screening tools related to diagnoses of depression
> - Recommend appropriate treatment and referrals related to depressive disorders

Depressive disorders are among the leading causes of death and disability in the U.S. affecting patients across the life span. Almost half of all adults who are depressed will not seek treatment; therefore, nurse practitioners must screen for and treat depressive symptoms to improve patient outcomes.

Assessment

Onset of symptoms can occur at any age and peaks at 20 years of age in the U.S.; females have a greater prevalence than males. It is common to have a first-degree relative with a depressive disorder. Carefully assess patients with an increased risk of relapse:

- Symptoms of suicide ideation, prior suicidal attempts, psychosis
- Ongoing depressive episode of longer than >2 years in duration
- Depressive symptoms occurring before 20 years of age or after 50 years of age
- Lack of symptom relief between episodes of depression
- Persistent symptoms of depression preceding this episode

Diagnosis

DSM-5 criteria for major depressive disorder (MDD) must include at least five of the following symptoms during the same two-week period and represent a change from previous functioning. At least one of the symptoms must be either a depressed mood or loss of interest/pleasure.

- Depressed mood (in children the mood can be irritable)
- Loss of interest/pleasure
- Change in appetite leading to significant weight loss or gain
- Change in sleep, insomnia, or hypersomnia
- Psychomotor retardation or agitation
- Loss of energy, fatigue
- Inappropriate guilt/feelings of worthlessness
- Change in ability to focus/concentrate
- Recurrent thoughts of death, suicide ideation without a plan, a suicide attempt, or a specific plan for suicide

Significant distress or impairment in social, occupational, or other areas of functioning must exist, and the symptoms cannot be attributed to the effects of substance use or a medical condition.

Other depressive disorders:

- **Persistent depressive disorder (dysthymia):** depressed mood occurring more days than not for at least 2 years in adults and at least 1 year in children/adolescents
- **Premenstrual dysphoric disorder:** symptoms of mood lability, irritability, dysphoria, and anxiety occurring during the menstrual phase and relenting at menses
- **Substance/medication-induced depressive disorder:** depressive symptoms that are associated with the ingestion, injection, or inhalation of substances with depressive symptoms persisting after the expected effects of the substance
- **Depressive disorder due to another medical condition:** symptoms of depression that are the direct effect of a medical condition
- **Other specified depressive disorder:** characteristic depressive symptoms are present without meeting the full criteria of a depressive disorder; symptoms are clinically significant; specific reason for not meeting the criteria is given
- **Unspecified depressive disorder:** characteristic depressive symptoms are present without meeting the full criteria of a depressive disorder; symptoms are clinically significant; specific reasons for not meeting the criteria are not given
- **Disruptive mood dysregulation disorder:** chronic, severe irritability with temper outburst occurring three or more times a week in two different settings over the past year that is developmentally inappropriate in children and adolescents

Postpartum Depression

Postpartum depression results in extreme symptoms of depression and anxiety thought to be caused from the rapid changes in hormone levels after giving birth paired with sleep deprivation from being a new mother; it occurs in about 15% of births. The symptoms of postpartum depression are different from baby blues, which occurs in 80% of births, in that the symptoms are severe and interfere with the mother's ability to care for herself or others. If left untreated, the symptoms of postpartum depression can last months to years and interfere with the health of the mother and the growth and development of the infant.

- Screen all mothers—not only at postpartum checks but also at newborn well checks
- Scores of 10 or higher on the Edinburgh Postnatal Depression Scale (EPDS), a 10-item self-report scale, indicate possible depression and warrant further assessment and possible treatment
- Treatment may include psychotherapy, psychopharmaceuticals, and support

Screening Tools

Patient Health Questionnaire (PHQ-9): a 9-item self-report scale that screens, diagnoses, monitors, and measures the severity of depressive symptoms in adults, rating depression symptoms from minimal to severe

PHQ-9: the PHQ-9 modified for use with adolescents aged 11–19 using the same rating scores

- Scores of 0–4, minimal depression
- Scores of 5–9, mild depression
- Scores of 10–14, moderate depression
- Scores of 15–19, moderately severe depression
- Scores of 20–27, severe depression

Beck Depression Inventory: a self-report scale designed for those 13 years of age and older

Center for Epidemiological Studies Depression Scale for Children (CES-DC): a 20 item, self-report scale that screens for depression in children and adolescents. A score of >15 indicates significant depression

Columbia–Suicide Severity Rating Scale (CSSR-S): evaluates suicidal behaviors and ideation in adolescents and adults

Plan

Treatment

Evidenced-based practice indicates the best outcomes from a combination treatment plan that includes pharmacological intervention and psychotherapy. Neurotransmitters involved in depressive symptoms are:

- Serotonin (5-HT)
- Norepinephrine (NE)
- Dopamine (DA)

First-line medication therapy for depression is a selective serotonin reuptake inhibitor (SSRI). If two SSRIs are deemed treatment failures after adequate dose and time, a serotonin norepinephrine reuptake inhibitor (SNRI) is suggested. The choice of medication is based on:

- Medications previously taken, success in treatment, and side effects
- Medications taken by relatives, success, and side effects
- Medications currently taking, potential interactions, and other diagnoses
- Medication allergies

Generally, 4–8 weeks of treatment are needed to assess if the patient is responsive or unresponsive to a medication. Screen for adherence to medication, side effects, and symptom relief or worsening. Common side effects include gastrointestinal disturbance and sexual dysfunction. Treatment should be continued for 6–9 months for patients experiencing a positive response to medications. Compliance is improved with patient teaching regarding length of treatment. Consider maintenance medication if deemed chronic depression. Relapse in symptoms occurs most frequently within the first two months of medication discontinuation.

For SSRIs & SNRIs, see Chapter 12, Lesson 2.

Additional medications include:

Atypical Antidepressants

- **Bupropion:** inhibits the reuptake of norepinephrine, dopamine
- **Mirtazapine:** blocks alpha 2, which increases norepinephrine and serotonin

Serotonin Modulators

- **Trazodone** and **nefazodone:** blocks serotonin
- **Vilazodone:** blocks serotonin reuptake
- **Vortioxetine:** increases release of serotonin, norepinephrine, dopamine, histamine, glutamate, acetylcholine

Tricyclic Antidepressants

- **Amitriptyline, amoxapine, clomipramine, desipramine, doxepin, maprotiline, nortriptyline, protriptyline, trimipramine:** inhibit serotonin and norepinephrine reuptake
- **Imipramine:** serotonin and norepinephrine reuptake inhibitor

Medication class	Potential common adverse effects	Clinical information
Atypical antidepressants	Dizziness, insomnia, paresthesia, and blurred vision	Start with a low dose and increase slowly to avoid adverse effects; avoid bupropion in patients with h/o seizure or eating disorders
Serotonin modulators	Nausea, somnolence, dry mouth, dizziness, constipation, weakness, and blurred vision	Start with a low dose and increase slowly to avoid adverse effects; taper dose over a week before discontinuing
Tricyclic antidepressants	Cardiac effects, blurred vision, constipation, dry mouth, urinary retention, sedation, increased appetite leading to weight gain, confusion, delirium, decreased seizure threshold, sexual dysfunction, diaphoresis, and tremor	Dangerous in overdose due to prolongation of the QT interval leading to arrhythmias and seizures; start with a low dose and increase slowly to avoid adverse effects; taper the dosage to discontinue; do not prescribe with SSRIs or MAOIs

Table 12.3.1 Medication Therapy for Depression

Referrals

- With a diagnosis of depression, consultation and/or referral to a psych/mental health professional should be considered; referral is needed for patients with comorbid diagnoses, treatment failures, chronic depression, and children/adolescents; emergent referral/hospitalization is required for suicidal patients
- Psychotherapy: cognitive behavioral therapy (CBT), interpersonal therapy (IPT), problem solving therapy (PST)

Takeaways

- Depressive disorders are among the leading causes of death and disability in the U.S. Screen all patients for self-harm and suicidal ideation.
- Almost half of all depressed adults will not seek treatment; therefore, screening for depression is important in primary care appointments.
- Screening scales such as PHQ-9, PHQ-A, CES-DC, and CSSR-S assist in diagnosis and treatment progression.
- Medications and psychotherapy are first-line treatment.
- Assess for medication side effects such as sexual dysfunction to promote compliance and recovery.

LESSON 4: EATING DISORDERS

Learning Objectives
- ■ Identify the diagnostic criteria of eating disorders
- ■ Recognize screening tools used to aid in the diagnosis of eating disorders
- ■ Recommend appropriate treatment and referrals related to eating disorders

Eating disorders are characterized by serious disturbances in eating behaviors that result in impairment in physical health and psychosocial functioning. Eating disorders usually begin in adolescence or young adulthood, although cases have been identified in children as well as late onset after 40 years of age. Eating disorder diagnoses are associated with an increased risk of suicide.

> **Pro Tip: Screening Scales for Eating Disorders**
>
> **SCOFF:** clinician-administered questionnaire; two or more "yes" answers require further investigation:
>
> - Do you make yourself **S**ick because you feel uncomfortably full?
> - Do you worry you have lost **C**ontrol over how much you eat?
> - Have you recently lost more than **O**ne stone (14 pounds or 6.35 kg) in a 3-month period?
> - Do you believe yourself to be **F**at when others say you are too thin?
> - Would you say that **F**ood dominates your life?
>
> **Eating Disorder Screen for Primary Care:** clinician-administered questionnaire; two or more abnormal responses require further evaluation:
>
> - Are you satisfied with your eating patterns? (No is abnormal)
> - Do you ever eat in secret? (Yes is abnormal)
> - Does your weight affect the way you feel about yourself? (Yes is abnormal)
> - Have any members of your family suffered with an eating disorder? (Yes is abnormal)
> - Do you currently suffer with or have you ever suffered in the past with an eating disorder? (Yes is abnormal)

Assessment—Anorexia Nervosa

Symptoms must be present for three months to meet the criteria for anorexia nervosa. Female to male ratio is 10:1, and the onset of symptoms is often associated with a stressful event. The outcome is highly variable, and hospitalization is often necessary to stabilize medical complications. Mortality results from medical complications and suicide.

Diagnosis

DSM-5 criteria for anorexia nervosa:

- Restriction of energy intake relative to requirements, which leads to a significantly low body weight related to age, sex, development, and physical health; children/adolescents may fail to gain expected weight or may not maintain developmental trajectory (reaching expected height without gaining expected weight)
- Intense fear of gaining weight or becoming fat, or persistent behavior that interferes with weight gain, such as exercise, while at a significantly low weight
- Disturbance in how the body weight or shape is experienced, unrealistic influence of body weight and/or shape on self-evaluation, and persistent lack of recognition of the seriousness of low weight

Severity rating:

- Mild: BMI ≥ 17 kg/m^2
- Moderate: BMI 16–16.99 kg/m^2
- Severe: BMI 15–15.99 kg/m^2
- Extreme: BMI <15 kg/m^2

Differential Diagnosis

Anxiety disorders, depressive disorders, bipolar disorders, and obsessive-compulsive disorders commonly occur with anorexia nervosa. It is important to treat the underlying mental health disorders as well. Additional differential diagnoses include **medical conditions (GI disease, hyperthyroidism, malignancies, AIDS), schizophrenia, substance use disorders, body dysmorphic disorder, bulimia nervosa, avoidant/restrictive food intake disorder**

Plan

Treatment

Treatment planning should involve an interdisciplinary approach, including nutritional rehabilitation, psychotherapy, monitoring for refeeding syndrome, and other medical complications. Pharmacotherapy is not the initial treatment for anorexia nervosa, although medications may be added to treat comorbid mental health diagnoses.

Referrals

- A diagnosis of anorexia nervosa should prompt referral(s) to providers that specialize in the treatment of eating disorders, including a mental health provider, dietitian, and a medical clinician
- Psychotherapy: cognitive behavioral therapy (CBT), psychodynamic psychotherapy, specialist supportive clinical management, motivational interviewing, family therapy, and cognitive remediation therapy

Assessment—Bulimia Nervosa

Symptoms must be present at least once a week for a period of three months. The onset of symptoms is often associated with a period of dieting or soon afterwards. Multiple stressful events are also associated with the onset of symptoms. The course of illness may be chronic or intermittent, with periods of remission and recurrence. Mortality results from medical complications and suicide.

Diagnosis

DSM-5 criteria for bulimia nervosa:

- Recurrent binge eating, which requires eating within a 2-hour period of time an amount of food that is greater than most people would consume in a similar period of time and setting, as well as a feeling of lack of control over the episode
- Recurrent behaviors that are inappropriate to prevent weight gain such as self-induced vomiting, use of laxatives, diuretics, fasting, and/or excessive exercise
- Binge eating and behaviors to prevent weight gain must occur at least once a week for a period of three months
- Evaluation of self is inappropriately influenced by weight and body shape
- Symptoms do not occur exclusively during episodes of anorexia nervosa

Severity rating:

- Mild: Average of 1–3 episodes per week
- Moderate: Average of 4–7 episodes per week
- Severe: Average of 8–13 episodes per week
- Extreme: Average of 14 or more episodes per week

Differential Diagnosis

Differential diagnoses include **anorexia nervosa binge-eating/purging type, binge-eating disorder, Kleine-Levin syndrome, major depressive disorder with atypical features, borderline personality disorder**

Anxiety disorders, depressive disorders, and bipolar disorders commonly occur with bulimia nervosa. It is important to treat for underlying mental health disorders as well for comprehensive care and recovery.

Plan

Treatment

Evidenced-based practice indicates the best outcomes from a combination treatment plan that includes nutritional rehabilitation, psychotherapy, antidepressants, and monitoring for medical complications. Medications should be initiated with a low dose and increased slowly if needed to reduce adverse effects. Avoid use of bupropion due to risk of seizures in patients with bulimia nervosa.

Generally, 4–8 weeks of treatment are needed to assess if the patient is responsive or unresponsive to a medication. Screen for adherence to medication, side effects, and symptom relief or worsening. Common side effects include gastrointestinal disturbance and sexual dysfunction. Continue medication for at least 6–12 months after response or remission. Duration of treatment is patient-specific.

First-line treatment is an SSRI (fluoxetine). Second-line treatment would be a different SSRI (citalopram, fluvoxamine, sertraline)—*refer to Table 12.2.1 in Chapter 12, Lesson 2.* Third-line treatment is tricyclic antidepressants—*refer to Table 12.3.1 in Chapter 12, Lesson 3.* Additional medications include:

Anticonvulsants

- **Topiramate:** sodium channel modulator

Serotonin Modulators

- **Trazodone:** blocks serotonin receptors and reuptake pump

Monoamine Oxidase Inhibitor (MAOI)

- **Phenelzine:** blocks monoamine oxidase from breaking down serotonin, norepinephrine, dopamine

Medication class	Potential common adverse effects	Clinical information
Anticonvulsant	Weight loss; may exacerbate eating disorder psychopathology regarding body weight	Taper the dosage to discontinue
Serotonin modulator	Nausea, somnolence, dry mouth, dizziness, constipation, weakness, and blurred vision	Do not abruptly discontinue therapy; taper dosage gradually to prevent rebound effect; taper dose over a week before discontinuing to avoid negative effects
MAOI	Monitor for increase in depressive symptoms, suicide ideation	Taper dose gradually to prevent rebound effect; foods containing tyramine must be avoided due to risk of hypertensive crisis

Table 12.4.1 Medication Therapy for Eating Disorders

Referrals

- Bulimia nervosa is best managed by an interdisciplinary care team that specializes in the treatment of eating disorders including a mental health provider, dietitian, and medical clinician
- Psychotherapy: cognitive behavioral therapy (CBT) and family therapy

Assessment—Binge Eating Disorder

Symptoms must be present at least once a week for a period of three months. The onset of symptoms is common in adolescents and college-aged young adults and may occur later in life. Dieting often follows binge eating. Remission rates are higher for binge eating disorders than for anorexia nervosa or bulimia nervosa.

Diagnosis

DSM-5 criteria for binge eating disorder:

- Recurrent binge eating, which requires eating within a two-hour period of time an amount of food that is greater than most people would consume in a similar period of time and a feeling of lack of control over the episode
- Binge eating episodes must include at least three of the following: eating faster than normal; eating until feeling overly full and uncomfortable; consuming large amounts when not hungry; eating alone due to feeling embarrassed about the amount consumed; feeling disgusted, depressed, or guilty after binge eating
- Distress regarding binge eating
- Is not associated with recurrent behaviors to prevent weight gain; does not occur exclusively during anorexia nervosa or bulimia nervosa

Severity rating: same as bulimia nervosa (see above)

Differential Diagnosis

Differential diagnoses include **bulimia nervosa, obesity, depressive disorder, bipolar disorder, borderline personality disorder, anxiety disorder**

Plan

Treatment

Treatment planning will be similar to bulimia nervosa and includes psychotherapy, pharmacotherapy, behavioral weight loss, and monitoring for medical complications. Medications should be initiated with a low dose and increased slowly if needed to reduce adverse effects. Avoid use of bupropion due to risk of seizures.

Medication class	Mechanism of action	Potential common adverse effects	Clinical information/patient education
First-line treatment **selective serotonin reuptake inhibitors (SSRI)**: fluoxetine, citalopram, fluvoxamine, sertraline	*See Lesson 2, including Table 12.2.1*	*See Lesson 2, Table 12.2.1*	*See Lesson 2, Table 12.2.1*
Second-line treatment **Anticonvulsant**: topiramate	*See above, including Table 12.4.1*	*See Table 12.4.1*	*See Table 12.4.1*
CNS stimulant: lisdexamfetamine	Blocks reuptake of norepinephrine and dopamine	Decreased appetite	Take in the morning with or without food due to potential for insomnia if taken later in the day; it is a prodrug and is not active until absorbed and converted in the intestinal tract

Table 12.4.2 Medication Treatment for Binge Eating Disorder

Referrals

- Binge eating disorder also necessitates referral and management by an interdisciplinary care team that specializes in the treatment of eating disorders
- Psychotherapy: cognitive behavioral therapy (CBT), family therapy, and behavioral weight loss therapy

Takeaways

- Eating disorders are associated with an increased risk of suicide; screen at every visit.
- Clinician administered screening scales aid in diagnosis.
- Psychotherapy is the first-line treatment.

LESSON 5: BIPOLAR DISORDERS

Learning Objectives
- Identify the signs and symptoms of bipolar disorders
- Interpret screening tools related to diagnoses of bipolar disorders
- Recommend appropriate treatment and referrals related to bipolar disorders

Bipolar disorder is a mood disorder that is characterized by episodes of mania, hypomania, and depressive symptoms which are often life-threatening. At least 50% of patients who recover from an episode of mania or hypomania experience recurrence within two years. Recurrence is associated with suicide attempts, decreased social/occupational functioning, and cognitive impairment. Treatment resistance increases with each recurrence.

Assessment

The average age of the onset of first manic, hypomanic, or major depressive episode is 18 years for bipolar I disorder. Onset of symptoms can occur at any age, including childhood or 60–70 years of age. Assessment of children and adolescents should be completed by a mental health provider that specializes in this age group, due to the complexity of developmental variations.

- Male to female prevalence is similar
- More than half of manic episodes occur immediately prior to a depressive episode
- Onset of manic symptoms in late mid-life or late-life necessitates evaluation of neurocognitive disorders and substance use/withdrawal
- More common in higher-income countries
- Separated, divorced, or widowed individuals have a higher incidence
- Family history increases risk of development
- Risk of suicide is 15 times greater than the general public

Diagnosis

DSM-5 criteria for bipolar I disorders must include at least one manic episode, a period of abnormal and persistent elevated and expansive mood with increased energy and/or goal distinctiveness. The manic episode must last at least one week, most of the day, for nearly every day. During this period, at least three of the following must be present and represent a change from previous behavior:

- Distractibility
- Excessive high-risk behaviors such as gambling, sexual indiscretion, etc.
- Flight of ideas
- Inflated self-esteem/grandiosity
- Lack of sleep
- Psychomotor agitation or increased goal-directed activity
- Talkative/pressured speech

The symptoms cannot be better explained by another medical condition or substance use. Symptoms of hypomania and/or major depression may be present, but are not required to meet the criteria of bipolar I disorder.

DSM-5 criteria for bipolar II disorder must include at least one current or past hypomanic episode and a current or past major depressive episode. A hypomanic episode differs from a manic episode only in length of time. A hypomanic episode must last at least four consecutive days and occur most of the day for nearly every day. Patients with a diagnosis of bipolar II disorder have never met the criteria for a manic episode, and the symptoms cannot be better explained by another medical condition or substance use.

A major depressive episode requires at least five of the following symptoms occurring during the same two-week period and is a change in level of functioning. Symptoms occur most of the day, nearly every day, and it requires either a depressed mood or loss of interest/pleasure (*refer to Chapter 12, Lesson 3*).

Differential Diagnoses
- **Cyclothymic disorder:** multiple hypomanic symptoms for at least two years in adults and one year in children and adolescents that do not meet the criteria for hypomanic episode; also experiences periods of depressive symptoms that do not meet the criteria for a major depressive episode
- **Substance/medication-induced bipolar and related disorder:** symptoms of elevated, expansive, irritable mood; may or may not exhibit depressed mood; symptoms occurred during or soon after medication or substance ingestion or withdrawal that is capable of producing the symptoms
- **Bipolar and related disorder due to another medical condition:** symptoms of elevated, expansive, irritable mood that is the direct effect of a medical condition
- **Other specified bipolar and related disorder:** symptoms of hypomanic episodes with a duration of two to three days, along with major depressive episodes or hypomania that does not meet the criteria of a hypomanic episode and does not occur along with a depressive episode
- **Unspecified bipolar and related disorder:** characteristic bipolar disorder symptoms are present without meeting the full criteria of diagnosis, symptoms are clinically significant; specific reason for not meeting the criteria may or may not be given

Screening Tools
Young Mania Rating Scale (YMRS): a clinician-administered scale that evaluates symptoms of mania over the previous 48 hours. A score of 12 indicates manic symptoms

Mood Disorder Questionnaire (MDQ): an adult self-report scale that screens for symptoms of mood disorder. A positive screen should be followed by a comprehensive evaluation to determine a diagnosis

Columbia–Suicide Severity Rating Scale (CSSR-S): evaluates suicidal behaviors and ideation in adolescents and adults

Plan

Treatment

Treatment should include pharmacological intervention and psychotherapy. The exact mechanism of action for mood stabilizers is unknown.

First-line medication therapy for bipolar disorder is a mood stabilizer. After the mood is stabilized, depressive symptoms can be treated with a selective serotonin reuptake inhibitor (SSRI); if two SSRIs are deemed treatment failures after adequate dose and time, a serotonin norepinephrine reuptake inhibitor (SNRI) is suggested, and then a medication from the other category if needed (*see Table 12.5.1*). The choice of medication is based on:

- Medications previously taken, success in treatment, and side effects
- Medications taken by relatives, success, and side effects
- Medications currently taking, potential interactions, and other diagnoses
- Medication allergies

Generally, 2–3 weeks of treatment are needed to assess if a patient is responsive or unresponsive to a medication. Screen for adherence to medication, side effects, and symptom relief or worsening. Maintenance medication is recommended for symptom control, and compliance is improved with patient education. Treatment resistance increases with each relapse.

Mood stabilizers

- **Carbamazepine, lamotrigine:** voltage-sensitive sodium channel antagonist
- **Lithium:** alters sodium transport across cell membranes
- **Valproate:** voltage-sensitive sodium channel modulator

Second-Generation Antipsychotics

- **Aripiprazole:** dopamine 2 partial agonist
- **Asenapine, iloperidone, lurasidone, olanzapine, paliperidone, risperidone, quetiapine, ziprasidone:** block dopamine 2, serotonin 2A receptors
- **Brexpiprazole:** serotonin 5-HT1A, dopamine 2 partial agonist, serotonin 5-HT2A receptor+6 antagonist
- **Cariprazine:** dopamine 2, serotonin 5-HT1A partial agonist
- **Clozapine:** dopamine 2, serotonin 2 antagonist, noradrenolytic, anticholinergic, antihistaminic, and arousal reaction inhibitor
- **Pimavanserin:** serotonin 2, 2C receptor inverse agonist/antagonist

First-Generation Antipsychotics

- **Haloperidol, fluphenazine, perphenazine:** blocks dopamine 2 receptors
- **Loxapine:** blocks dopamine 2 receptors, serotonin 2A antagonist

Medication class	Potential common adverse effects	Clinical information
Mood stabilizers	• **carbamazepine:** aplastic anemia, agranulocytosis • **lamotrigine:** serious skin rash • **lithium:** CNS depression, heart failure, hypercalcemia, hypothyroidism, renal effects • **oxcarbazepine:** hyponatremia, dizziness, nausea, vomiting • **valproate:** hepatotoxicity, weight gain, bruising	• **carbamazepine:** monitor CBC; contraindicated in pregnancy • **lamotrigine:** monitor for rash/teaching re: risk for Stevens-Johnson syndrome • **lithium:** monitor level due to a very narrow therapeutic window; monitor thyroid and renal function teaching re: polydipsia/risk for dehydration • **oxcarbazepine:** monitor sodium level • **valproate:** contraindicated in pregnancy; monitor liver function
Second-generation antipsychotics	Metabolic syndrome, hypotension, sedation, dry mouth, constipation, blurred vision, urinary retention, hyperprolactinemia, extrapyramidal symptoms, cardiac effects, cardiomyopathies, cataracts, sexual dysfunction	clozapine and olanzapine have a significantly higher risk for metabolic syndrome; aripiprazole, lurasidone, pimavanserin, and ziprasidone are associated with the lowest risk of metabolic syndrome (monitor for weight changes)
First-generation antipsychotics	Extrapyramidal symptoms, tardive dyskinesia, hyperprolactinemia, neuroleptic malignant syndrome, QT prolongation, metabolic syndrome, dry mouth, constipation, blurred vision, urinary retention, orthostatic hypotension	Avoid use in older adults with dementia

Table 12.5.1 Medication Treatment for Bipolar Disorder

Additional medications may include:

- SSRIs or SNRIs
- Atypical antidepressants
- Tricyclic antidepresants
  - *For the above meds, refer to Table 12.2.1 in Chapter 12, Lesson 2*
- Serotonin modulators: trazodone, nefazodone, vilazodone, vortioxetine; *refer to Table 12.3.1 in Chapter 12, Lesson 3*

Referrals

- Refer patients to a mental health provider due to the need for maintenance medication, high rate of treatment resistance, and potential for suicide
- Emergent referral/evaluation and potential hospitalization is required for patients whose behavior places themselves or others at risk as well as patients who are suicidal
- Psychotherapy: cognitive behavioral therapy (CBT), interpersonal therapy (IPT), problem-solving therapy (PST), mindfulness, stress management

Takeaways

- Mood stabilizers are the first-line medication treatment for bipolar disorder.
- Patients with bipolar disorder have a high rate of relapse.
- Screening tools such as the YMRS and MDQ can assist in diagnosis.
- Always screen for suicidal ideation and behaviors.
- Assess for mania/hypomania as patients usually present for treatment during depressive episodes.

LESSON 6: PSYCHOTIC DISORDERS

Learning Objectives
- Identify the signs and symptoms of a psychotic disorder
- Recognize the risk factors that contribute to the development of a psychotic disorder
- Recommend appropriate treatment and referral for psychotic disorders

Psychosis is a disorder of thought. The most common symptoms of psychosis include hallucinations, delusions, and disorganized thinking and speech. Causes of psychosis include adverse reactions to medications, substance use, and mental health disorders. Schizophrenia will be the focus of this lesson.

Assessment

Schizophrenia is a severe, persistent mental illness that is treatable. Early identification and treatment result in better outcomes.

- Average age of onset of symptoms is 18 years in males and 25 years in females
- Onset of schizophrenia is rare before the age of 10 years and after 40 years

Diagnosis

DSM-5 criteria for schizophrenia—delusions, hallucinations, or disorganized speech—must be present for diagnosis during a one-month period (or longer) for a significant part of that month. Additionally, the patient may exhibit:

- Grossly disorganized or catatonic behavior
- Negative symptoms (diminished/impaired ability to function and express emotion)

The diagnosis of schizophrenia is met when the duration of symptoms lasts for at least six months, level of functioning is below prior levels achieved, and other diagnoses have been ruled out.

Other psychotic disorder diagnoses:

- **Delusional disorder:** one or more delusions for one month without meeting the criteria for schizophrenia
- **Brief psychotic disorder:** sudden onset of delusions, hallucinations, or disorganized speech or behaviors within a two-week period of time
- **Schizophreniform disorder:** diagnostic criteria is identical to schizophrenia, except the duration is 1 month but <6 months
- **Schizoaffective:** symptoms of a psychotic disorder, as well as meeting criteria for major depressive disorder or mania
- **Substance/medication-induced psychotic disorder:** delusions and/or hallucinations resulting from the effects of a substance/medication
- **Psychotic disorder due to another medical condition:** delusions and/or hallucinations resulting from a medical condition and not resulting from a mental health disorder

Risk Factors

An interaction of genetics and the environment appears to increase the risk of developing schizophrenia:

- Family history of schizophrenia
- History of antenatal stress, malnutrition, complicated pregnancy/birth
- Psychosocial factors: childhood trauma, drug use in adolescence/young adulthood

Screening Tools

Abnormal Involuntary Movement Scale (AIMS): a 12-item clinician-administered assessment tool used to monitor early indications and severity of tardive dyskinesia, which can be a side effect of antipsychotic medications used to treat psychotic disorders

Plan

Treatment

Treatment planning should include pharmacological intervention, psychosocial treatments, and coordinated care such as case management, family support, and educational and employment assistance.

Medications used to treat psychotic disorders are antipsychotics. The neurotransmitter involved in psychotic symptoms is dopamine (DA).

Second-Generation Antipsychotics

- **Aripiprazole:** dopamine 2 partial agonist
- **Asenapine, iloperidone, lurasidone, olanzapine, paliperidone, risperidone, quetiapine, ziprasidone:** blocks dopamine 2, serotonin 2A receptors
- **Brexpiprazole:** serotonin 5-HT1A, dopamine 2 partial agonist, serotonin 5-HT2A receptor+6 antagonist
- **Cariprazine:** dopamine 2, serotonin 5-HT1A partial agonist
- **Clozapine:** dopamine 2, serotonin 2 antagonist, noradrenolytic, anticholinergic, antihistaminic, and arousal reaction inhibitor
- **Pimavanserin:** serotonin 2A , 2C receptor inverse agonist/antagonist

First-Generation Antipsychotics

- **Haloperidol, fluphenazine, perphenazine:** blocks dopamine 2 receptors
- **Loxapine:** blocks dopamine 2 receptors, serotonin 2A antagonist

For information regarding adverse effects and clinical information, refer to Table 12.5.1 in Chapter 12, Lesson 5.

Initial response is generally seen within two weeks, but may take six weeks for full result. Monitor weight, lipid profile, glucose, prolactin levels, and liver function tests on the initiation of medications, yearly and more frequently as needed.

Referrals

Refer all patients with psychotic disorders to mental health professionals. Psychotherapy may include individual therapy and social skills training.

Takeaways

- Delusions, hallucinations, or disorganized speech must be present for a diagnosis of schizophrenia.
- Patients with a schizophrenia diagnosis tend to experience comorbid diagnoses of obesity, diabetes, and metabolic syndrome. Screen for and treat for better health outcomes.
- A multi-team approach is required for patients with a diagnosis of schizophrenia. At presentation, if the patient is a threat to themselves or others, then emergent referral and hospitalization is needed.

LESSON 7: NEURODEVELOPMENTAL DISORDERS

Learning Objectives

- Identify the diagnostic criteria for attention deficit hyperactivity disorder, autism spectrum disorder, and tic disorder
- Evaluate screening tools to assist in diagnosis
- Select appropriate treatment for diagnosis

Neurodevelopmental disorders are conditions identified by the DSM-5 as having an onset of symptoms in the early developmental period. These disorders include areas of impairment in personal, social, academic, and occupational functioning and are often co-occurring. Many disorders are classified in areas such as communication, intellect, and motor skills, including attention deficit hyperactivity disorder (ADHD), autism spectrum disorder, and tic disorder.

Attention Deficit Hyperactivity Disorder

An interaction of genetics and the environment increase the risk of developing ADHD.

Approximately 5% of children and 2.5% of adults have a diagnosis of ADHD in most cultures. Academic underachievement, family stress, strained relationships, substance abuse, delinquency, accidental injuries, job failure, and other mental health issues can be the consequences of untreated ADHD.

Diagnosis

DSM-5 criteria for ADHD must include a pattern of inattention and/or hyperactivity-impulsiveness that interferes with development or function. To meet the criteria for either subtype (inattention or hyperactivity/impulsivity), the patient must demonstrate 6 or more symptoms, for at least 6 months, that are inconsistent with developmental level and negatively impact social/academic/occupational success. The symptoms may not be the result of oppositional behavior, defiance, hostility, or not understanding directions.

Inattention	Hyperactivity/impulsivity
Lack of close attention to detail, makes careless mistakes	Fidgets—hands, feet, squirms in seat
Difficulty sustaining attention to tasks/play	Leaves seat when expected to stay seated
Does not seem to listen when spoken to directly	Runs, climbs when inappropriate
Does not follow through, fails to finish schoolwork, chores	Unable to play or participate in leisure activities quietly
Difficulty organizing tasks/activities	Is seen as "always on the go" or "driven by a motor"
Avoids tasks that require sustained mental effort	Talks excessively
Often loses things needed for tasks/activities	Will blurt out answer before the question is completed
Easily distracted by external stimuli	Difficulty waiting in line or for his/her turn
Forgetful in daily activities	Interrupts or intrudes

Table 12.7.1 DSM-5 ADHD Diagnostic Criteria

- Several symptoms must present before 12 years of age
- For adolescents >17 years of age and adults, at least five symptoms of hyperactivity and impulsivity or symptoms of inattention are required
- Symptoms must be present in two or more settings such as home, school, or social settings

Other ADHD Diagnosis
- **Other specified attention deficit hyperactivity disorder:** does not meet criteria for an ADHD diagnosis, even though symptoms are consistent with the diagnosis and cause clinical significance
- **Unspecified attention deficit hyperactivity disorder:** does not meet criteria for an ADHD diagnosis, even though symptoms are consistent with the diagnosis; causes clinical significance; clinician does not specify the reason

Differential Diagnosis

Differential diagnoses include **oppositional defiant disorder, intermittent explosive disorder, other neurodevelopmental disorders, specific learning disorders, intellectual disability, autism spectrum disorder, reactive attachment disorder, anxiety disorder, depressive disorder, bipolar disorder, disruptive mood dysregulation disorder, substance use disorder, personality disorder, psychotic disorder, medication-induced symptoms of ADHD, neurocognitive disorder**

Screening Tools

Vanderbilt Scale: both the parent version and teacher version; must be completed and meet scoring criteria for a positive diagnosis of ADHD

Plan

Treatment

Treatment should include pharmacological intervention, psychosocial treatments, and coordinated care such as case management, family support, and educational and employment assistance. The neurotransmitters involved in ADHD symptoms are:

- Dopamine (DA)
- Norepinephrine (NA)

Medications used to treat ADHD are stimulants (first-line) and non-stimulants (second-line). Because of this, screen all patients for first-degree relatives experiencing sudden death from a cardiac issue 50 years of age or less. An ECG is required and read as normal before stimulants are started in these patients.

Stimulants

- **Methylphenidate, amphetamine:** dopamine reuptake inhibitor

Non-Stimulants

- **Atomoxetine:** norepinephrine reuptake inhibitor

Alpha 2 Agonist

- **Clonidine, guanfacine:** centrally-acting alpha 2A adrenergic receptor agonist

Medication class	Potential common adverse effects	Clinical information
Stimulants	Appetite suppression, insomnia, mood lability, dizziness, rebound, tics, psychosis	Start with a low dose and increase slowly to minimize adverse effects; monitor for diversion and misuse; stimulants can lower the threshold for seizures; not recommended in those with anorexia nervosa; monitor blood pressure throughout treatment
Non-stimulants	Potential increased risk of suicidal ideation	May be less efficacious than stimulants; response time 2–8 weeks; drug holidays are not an option
Alpha 2 agonist	May lead to hypotension and orthostasis	Also treat coexisting conditions such as sleep disorders, tic disorders

Table 12.7.2 Medication Treatment for ADHD

A common side effect of stimulants is appetite suppression, which may lead to weight loss. Educating about healthy, high-calorie snacks can limit weight loss. Monitor height and weight throughout treatment. Monitor symptoms of concentration, impulsiveness, distraction, and hyperactivity to determine treatment response over a 2–4 week period of time.

Referrals

- Refer to mental health providers patients that do not respond to medications; have comorbid symptoms of anxiety, depression, seizure disorders, eating disorders; or have side effects/reactions that are severe
- Many children, especially younger children, may benefit from a referral for behavior modification to build habits of organizational skills

Autism Spectrum Disorder

Autism spectrum disorder (ASD) is a neurodevelopmental disorder that is typically identified in the second year of life. An increase in prevalence in recent years has been attributed to the possibility of an expansion of the diagnostic criteria, an increase in public awareness, and an actual increase in ASD.

It is believed that an interaction of genetics and the environment increase the risk of developing ASD. Risk factors include:

- Brother, sister, family member with ASD
- Born premature or with a low birth weight
- Born to older parents

Diagnosis

DSM-5 criteria for ASD includes persistent deficits in social communication and interactions that occur in multiple settings, such as social-emotional reciprocity and nonverbal communication behaviors. At least two of the following must occur:

- Stereotyped or repetitive movements, use of objects, or speech
- Insistence on sameness, inflexibility, fixed routine
- Restricted, fixated interests that are abnormal in content or level of focus
- Hyper- or hyposensory input

Differential Diagnosis

Differential diagnoses include **selective mutism, language disorders, social communication disorders, intellectual disability, stereotypic movement disorder, ADHD, schizophrenia**

Screening Tools

All children should be screened at the 18- and 24-month well visit and any time a developmental concern is identified.

- **Ages and Stages Questionnaires (ASQ):** a parent-completed screening tool that assesses general development in children 1–66 months. The tool must be purchased
- **Modified Checklist for Autism in Toddlers (MCHAT R/F):** a parent report screen tool for children 16–30 months to identify when a more in-depth screening is indicated. The tool is free to use
- **Screening Tool for Autism in Toddlers and Young Children (STAT):** screens for ASD in children 24–36 months. Training is required to be able to administer and interpret the results

Plan

Referrals

If screening is positive, refer family to a mental health provider, a developmental specialist, and/or a special needs/language specialist for further evaluation and treatment. Applied behavioral analysis (ABA) therapy is used for the diagnosis of ASD and neurodevelopmental delays.

Tic Disorder

Tics are rapid/abrupt/reoccurring motor movement or vocalizations; they occur frequently in childhood and are usually transient. Males are more commonly affected than females, and approximately 3 to 8 per 1,000 school-aged children are affected.

The cause of tic disorders is not known, but it does appear that genetics may play an important role in tic development. Risk factors may include:

- Family history of tic disorder
- Low birth weight
- Complications during birth
- Alcohol and smoking during pregnancy
- Infections

Diagnosis

DSM-5 criteria for tic disorder is categorized into one of the following three diagnoses:

Tourette Syndrome

- Includes both multiple motor and at least one or more vocal tics being present, not necessarily occurring at the same time
- Tics may wax and wane in frequency but have persisted for more than a year since the onset
- Onset before 18 years of age
- Symptoms cannot be attributed to the effects of substance use or another medical condition

Persistent Motor or Vocal Tic Disorder

- One or more motor or vocal tics have been present, but not both motor and vocal
- Tics may wax and wane in frequency but have persisted for more than a year since the onset
- Onset before 18 years of age
- Symptoms cannot be attributed to the effects of substance use or another medical condition
- Criteria has never been met for Tourette disorder

Provisional Tic Disorder

- One or more motor or vocal tics
- Tics have been present for less than a year since the onset
- Onset before 18 years of age
- Symptoms cannot be attributed to the effects of substance use or another medical condition
- Criteria has never been met for Tourette disorder or persistent motor or vocal tic disorder

Other Tic Disorder Diagnosis

- Other specified tic disorder
- Unspecified tic disorder

Differential diagnoses include: **abnormal movements related to other medical condition, substance-induced and paroxysmal dyskinesias, myoclonus, obsessive-compulsive,** and **related disorders**

Screening Tools

There are no screening tools for tic disorders. Diagnosis is made from a complete history and physical examination.

Plan

Treatment

Treatment is based on the severity of the symptoms and the level of interference with daily life. Medication therapy is best coordinated by a mental health provider.

Referrals

Refer to a mental health provider after causes of other medication conditions and effects from substances have been ruled out. Habit-reversal training (HRT) has been shown to decrease the frequency and severity of symptoms.

Takeaways

- A comprehensive evaluation for suspicion of ADHD, ASD, and tic disorders includes physical exam, use of valid screening tools, and screening for concurrent mood and neurological disorders.
- ECG is necessary before starting medications for ADHD for those with a first-degree relative experiencing sudden death from a cardiac issue at 50 years of age or older.
- Screen for ASD at the 18- and 24-month well checkups—earlier if there are developmental concerns.
- Refer for medication management and therapy if tic disorder is severe and interfering with education, home, social interactions, or relationships.

LESSON 8: SUICIDE

Learning Objectives

- Recognize suicidality as a major health concern to be addressed in primary care
- Utilize screening tools for suicidality
- Recognize risk factors for suicidality
- Employ appropriate treatment options for depression/suicidality

In 2013, suicide was the tenth leading cause of death in the U.S., with about 41,000 U.S. deaths attributed to suicide that year. More than 800,000 deaths are attributed to suicide yearly worldwide. Given these statistics, the importance of screening for suicide, within the nurse practitioner's purview, is clear.

Assessment

Assessment cannot occur if providers don't ask. Do not assume patients will overtly express suicidality. Many make vague statements like "Everything sucks" or passive statements such as "I wish I could just stop breathing."

According to one USPSTF study of U.S. primary care providers, possible suicidality was addressed in only 11% of encounters with patients who—unknown to the providers—screened positive for suicidal ideation. Even for patients with more obvious suicide risk—presenting with major depression, adjustment disorder, or requesting antidepressants—only about 36% of U.S. primary care physicians explored the issue of suicidality.

Screening Tools for Suicidality

Suicide Assessment Five-Step Evaluation and Triage (SAFE-T): a five-step evaluation and triage screen to identify risk vs. protective factors, conduct a suicide inquiry, assess risk level and potential interventions, and document a treatment plan

SAD PERSONS scale (SPS): screen features a 10-item mnemonic where each letter corresponds to a risk factor for suicide: Sex, Age, Depression, Previous attempt, Ethanol abuse, Rational thinking loss, Social supports lacking, Organized plan, No spouse, Sickness

- Has proven popular, but its ability to predict suicide and reliability has been questioned

Columbia–Suicide Severity Rating Scale (CSSR-S): evaluates suicidal behaviors and ideation in adolescents and adults

see Chapter 12, Lesson 3, for further information on this scale

Suicide Behavior Questionnaire (SBQ-R): assesses suicide-related thoughts and behavior

- Has been found to have good reliability in a range of adult and adolescent clinical and nonclinical settings

Diagnosis

Consider if any underlying factors could be contributing to depression. These can include:

- Medications or supplements, including but not limited to antimicrobials, antihypertensive, hormones, sedatives, narcotic pain medication
- Substance abuse
- Medical or neurological conditions, including but not limited to multiple sclerosis, stroke, vitamin B12, thyroid disorders, lupus, cancer

Suicide Risk Factors

- **History:** previous suicidal behavior by the patient; FH of suicide
- **Gender:** women are about four times more likely to attempt suicide, but men successfully commit suicide more than four times as often as women—likely related to men's proclivity to choose more violent means for suicidal attempts, such as firearms
- **Age:** suicide is rare before puberty and rates rise with age; though older people attempt suicide less frequently than younger people, they are more successful; those 75 years of age or older manifest suicidal rates three times those of younger patients
- **Race:** two-thirds of suicides are white males; however, other communities (Inuit and Native American) evidence higher rates of suicidality than the national rate
- **Religion:** suicide rates of Roman Catholics are traditionally lower
- **Marital status:** never-married singles attempt suicide at a rate twice that of married individuals; divorce increases suicide risk: divorced males commit suicide at three times the rate of divorced women
- **Physical health:** physical illness is a contributing factor—up to 50% of suicides
- **Mental health:** psychiatric patients have up to 12 times the risk of those without a diagnosed mental illness; it has been estimated that 10% of schizophrenic patients eventually commit suicide
- **Substance abuse:** up to 15% of alcohol-dependent patients commit suicide; the suicide rate for heroin dependent persons is 20 times that of the general population
- **Sudden life stressor:** events such as death or financial/job loss

Plan

Treatment

SSRIs are considered the first-line medication option for depression. Of note, in the first few weeks of treatment (when medication levels are still subtherapeutic), depressed patients may be *more* at risk for suicide.

For suicidal ideation without intent, make a suicide contract for safety. Provide crisis contact information, such as the National Suicide Prevention Line (1-800-273-8255) or the National Suicide Text Hotline (text "CONNECT" to 741741). Have a short-term follow-up plan in place.

Non-Medication Options
Cognitive behavioral therapy
Phototherapy
Vagal nerve stimulation (shows efficacy with epileptic patients displaying depressed mood)
Electroconvulsive therapy (severe depression not responsive to antidepressants; some bipolar patients)
Transcranial magnetic stimulation (TMS) (severe depression not responsive to antidepressants)
Deep brain stimulation (experimental treatment for the most severe forms of depression)
Interpersonal therapy

Table 12.8.1

Referrals

- If suicidal ideation is identified, emergent referral/evaluation and potential hospitalization is needed
- Suicidal patients should be followed by a mental health specialist

Pro Tip

Suicidal behavior disorder and non-suicidal self-injury are now in DSM-5 as "conditions for further study." There are ICD-10 codes for suicidal ideation and suicide attempt; Z91.5 is "personal history of self harm" for non-suicidal self-injury. Suicidal behavior disorder applies to patients who have attempted suicide within the prior 24 months. Non-suicidal self-injury describes self-harm without suicidal intent.

Takeaways

- Potential suicidality is a major health concern that can be addressed in primary care through screening.
- Knowing risk factors for suicidality can assist the provider in diagnosis.
- Suicidal patients typically require hospitalization and should be followed by a mental health specialist such as a PMHNP or psychiatrist.

PRACTICE QUESTIONS

Select the ONE best answer.

Lesson 1: Abuse

1. The nurse practitioner is speaking with a parent who abused her child. Which of the following risk factors would the nurse practitioner expect to find?

   A. Single-parent home situation

   B. History of parental mental illness

   C. Consistent communication patterns

   D. History of a parent having been abused

2. Donna, a 20-year-old single mother, lives in a rundown apartment in a dangerous area of her city. After her 12-hour shift as a cashier, she comes home irritable. She admits she yells, berates, and belittles her 7-year-old son. Lately, she has taken to locking him in the basement when she is too tired. Together, these behaviors may potentially be considered:

   A. Neglect

   B. Physical abuse

   C. Emotional abuse

   D. Not abusive, as she does not hit her child

3. Which of the following may require mandatory reporting from the nurse practitioner?

   A. A withdrawn 5-year-old patient with multiple fractures of varying stages of healing

   B. A 70-year-old patient who states her 40-year-old daughter has been stealing her Social Security check

   C. A 19-year-old still living with his parents who has not completed high school is disruptive, and, according to his parents, is "acting out"

   D. An anxious 29-year-old housewife who states that her husband is "always angry" at her and appears to have caked-on make-up concealing a black eye

4. A patient describes his alcohol use as 2–3 drinks per night, 4–5 nights per week. He has been missing work and family functions because of his drinking. He reports wanting to reduce his drinking, but not being able to. He admits to having a problem and has vague plans to make changes. Which stage of change does this represent?

   A. Precontemplation

   B. Contemplation

   C. Preparation

   D. Action

Lesson 2: Anxiety

5. The diagnostic criteria for generalized anxiety disorder (GAD) include all of the following except:

   A. Irritability

   B. Apprehension

   C. Early morning awakening

   D. Difficulty concentrating

6. Which of the following is commonly reported by individuals with an anxiety disorder?

   A. Muscle tension

   B. Hypersomnolence

   C. Skin rashes such as hives

   D. Constipation

7. When starting therapy with an SSRI for GAD, the nurse practitioner should consider starting with a(n):

   A. SSRI, as the patient will see a decrease in symptoms within two weeks

   B. SSRI, which will not affect any other medications taken

   C. Low dose and slowly increasing the dose if needed

   D. SSRI that is known to be more energizing

8. In assessing a patient for PTSD, you should expect the following to be reported except:

    A. A feeling of detachment

    B. Hyperarousal

    C. Sleep issues

    D. Inability to recall the precipitating event

Lesson 3: Depression

9. Which of the following patients meets the criteria for major depressive disorder?

    A. A 32-year-old female with symptoms of emptiness, lack of pleasure, weight loss, insomnia, inappropriate guilt, and lack of focus nearly every day for the past month

    B. A 32-year-old female with symptoms of a depressed mood for the past two months after losing her job

    C. A 20-year-old male with inability to initiate or maintain sleep and lack of motivation for the past two weeks

    D. A 20-year-old male with symptoms of fatigue, being tired, insomnia, and lack of focus for the past month

10. A diagnosis of major depressive disorder must include either a depressed mood or which of the following symptoms?

    A. Feelings of worthlessness

    B. Loss of interest or pleasure

    C. Sleep issues

    D. Recurrent thoughts of death

11. A 38-year-old male has been taking an SSRI for the past four months for depression. He is experiencing new symptoms of sexual dysfunction and is having difficulty reaching orgasm. You advise him that:

    A. Sexual dysfunction is a common side effect to an SSRI and may not resolve without changing the classification of his medication

    B. Changing to another SSRI will would most likely be beneficial

    C. This is a common side effect to an SSRI, but is only transient and the symptoms will resolve

    D. This is an uncommon side effect to SSRIs, and he will be need to be referred to a urologist

12. You are assessing a 24-year-old female who received a score of 12 on the PHQ-9. According to her questionnaire, the severity of her depression is:

    A. Minimal

    B. Mild

    C. Moderate

    D. Severe

Lesson 4: Eating Disorders

13. Anorexia nervosa must be considered in children and adolescents who:

    A. Fail to maintain the normal developmental trajectory

    B. Lose weight without physiological cause

    C. Think they are overweight despite maintaining a normal BMI

    D. Participate in multiple sports to maintain weight

14. A 20-year-old male is evaluated and reports recurrent episodes of binge eating, vomiting, and the use of laxatives to control weight several times a week for the past three months. The NP determines the criteria for a diagnosis of:

    A. Binge eating disorder is met

    B. Anorexia nervosa with binge-eating/purging type is met

    C. Bulimia nervosa is met

    D. Binge-purge disorder is met

15. When assessing a patient with a diagnosis of anorexia nervosa, it is very important at every encounter to evaluate for:

    A. Associated eating disorders

    B. Suicide ideation, behaviors, and risk factors for self-harm

    C. Family history of eating disorders

    D. Substance use disorder

16. Evidence-based practice treatment for eating disorders include(s):

    A. Medications to decrease symptoms

    B. Therapy to address unhealthy thoughts regarding food and weight in order to decrease symptoms

    C. Strict monitoring of food intake and limiting exercise

    D. A combination of medications, therapy, and nutritional and medical care

Lesson 5: Bipolar Disorders

17. You are evaluating a 20-year-old college student who presents with symptoms of moodiness, not sleeping well, feeling more down than usual. The student asks if he has bipolar disorder. What is true about this patient?

    A. The patient meets the criteria for bipolar disorder, and you start medication

    B. The patient meets the criteria for bipolar disorder, and you refer to a mental health provider

    C. The patient does not meet the criteria for bipolar disorder but does warrant further evaluation

    D. The patient does not meet the criteria for bipolar disorder but does meet criteria for depressive disorder

18. You are concerned your patient is exhibiting possible symptoms of bipolar disorder and need to evaluate further. The best choice of screening tool is:

    A. PHQ-9

    B. GAD-7

    C. MDQ

    D. DAST-10

19. A patient who is new to your practice states she has been treated for bipolar disorder. She requests you continue her current medications, which are lamotrigine, dextroamphetamine, and sertraline. She has current prescription bottles in her name for these medications. Your plan includes a diagnostic assessment and:

    A. Prescribing all three medications, since these medications are evidenced-based practice for bipolar disorder

    B. Not prescribing any medications until you receive her records from previous healthcare providers

    C. Not prescribing any medications and referring her to a mental health provider

    D. Prescribing lamotrigine and sertraline only and referring her for ADHD testing

20. Which of the following are first-line medication treatments for patients with a bipolar disorder diagnosis?

    A. Antidepressants

    B. Mood stabilizers

    C. Anxiolytics

    D. Mood stabilizers and antidepressants together

Lesson 6: Psychotic Disorders

21. The risk of developing schizophrenia is related to an interaction between genetics and environmental factors such as:

    A. Family history, exposure to viruses, and psychosocial factors

    B. Family history, other mental health diagnoses, and home location

    C. Family history, marital status, and nutritional status

    D. Family history, other medical diagnoses, and education level

22. It is important to obtain labs on patients taking atypical antipsychotics:

    A. Prior to initiating medications, every six months, and more frequently if needed

    B. After being on the medication for six months and yearly thereafter

    C. Prior to initiating medications, at three months, six months, yearly, and more frequently if needed

    D. After being on the medication for three months, at six months, and yearly

23. Which of the following is the most appropriate action to take for a 21-year-old male presenting with the symptom of "hearing voices"?

    A. Complete a mental status exam (MSE)

    B. Order labs for substance use

    C. Complete a physical examination

    D. Call the crisis team

24. The Abnormal Involuntary Movement Scale (AIMS) should be administered to:

    A. Patients you suspect are having symptoms of tardive dyskinesia

    B. Patients receiving psychotropic medications

    C. All patients receiving an antipsychotic medication

    D. All mental health patients

Lesson 7: Neurodevelopmental Disorders

25. The nurse practitioner is evaluating a 10-year-old male for ADHD per his parents' and teacher's request. Symptoms include decreased level of focus, impulsivity, and hyperactivity occurring in school. His grades have also declined. With this information, the nurse practitioner will:

    A. Diagnose ADHD and start medications

    B. Diagnose ADHD and refer the family for behavioral modification therapy

    C. Not make any diagnosis, but evaluate further for ADHD

    D. Not make any diagnosis, and refer back to the school guidance department

26. A screening tool that aids in the evaluation and diagnosis process of ADHD in children is the:

    A. Vanderbilt Scale

    B. SCARED Scale

    C. Y-BOCS

    D. YMRS

27. A 9-year-old female is following up with you after starting a trial of a stimulant medication for a diagnosis with ADHD. She has lost 1 pound over the past month, has a decreased appetite, and is doing better in school, but her guardian is concerned about the decrease in appetite. What is your plan of treatment?

    A. Stop the medication since this is not a common side effect to stimulants and reevaluate in one month

    B. Wean off the current stimulant, start another stimulant to minimize weight loss, and reevaluate in one month

    C. Stop the stimulant, prescribe another classification of medication, and reevaluate in one month

    D. Explain that loss of appetite is a common side effect of stimulant medications, help the family identify healthy and calorie-rich snacks, and reevaluate in one month

28. It is important to screen for autism spectrum disorders (ASD) at:

    A. The 18- and 24-month well-child check

    B. Every well-child check

    C. The 18- and 24-month well-child check and any time there is a concern for delays

    D. The 12-, 18-, 24-, and 36-month well-child check

Lesson 8: Suicide

29. Which of the following statements is true about the risk of suicide?

    A. Suicidal patients will present with overt statements about self-harm

    B. A screening tool such as SPS is the primary means of assigning a patient for suicide potential

    C. Married individuals are more likely to attempt suicide than single individuals

    D. Mental illness, including substance use, contributes to suicidality

30. The FNP is asked to evaluate a new patient who presents as clinically depressed. The FNP develops a concern about the patient's risk of suicide based on all of the following factors except:

    A. The patient stating, "Everything is fine"

    B. The patient describing his impulsive nature

    C. The patient's wife sending him to see the NP

    D. The patient having taken fluoxetine for several months

31. Treatment of depression may include all of the following except:

    A. Selective serotonin reuptake inhibitors

    B. Dialectical behavior therapy

    C. Cognitive behavioral therapy

    D. Interpersonal therapy

32. Which of the following patients may be most at risk for a completed suicide?

    A. A 75-year-old recent widower

    B. A 19-year-old female college student

    C. A married mother with financial concerns

    D. A Roman Catholic 22-year-old male

ANSWERS AND EXPLANATIONS

Lesson 1: Abuse

1. D

A history of a parent having been abused **(D)** is a risk; family violence follows a multigenerational pattern. Single-parent homes (A) and a history of parental mental illness (B) are not established risk factors for child abuse. Consistent communication patterns (C) are characteristic of healthy functioning, not a risk for abuse.

2. C

Yelling, berating, and belittling are examples of emotional abuse **(C)**. Neglect (A) is more concerned with the egregious withholding of resources from a child, such as failure to provide adequate medical care. Physical abuse (B) involves physical contact with the child, such as hitting or shaking. It is not accurate to state there is no abuse occurring (D).

3. A

A withdrawn 5-year-old patient with multiple fractures of varying stages of healing **(A)** may require mandatory reporting. While a daughter stealing a Social Security check (B), a 19-year-old son that is acting out (C), and a 29-year-old who appears to be covering a black eye (D) are all concerning and may be legitimately referred to social services, legal services, or psychiatric specialty follow-up, only (A) calls for mandatory reporting.

4. C

A patient who is committed to and planning to make a change in the near future but is still considering what to do represents the stage of preparation **(C)**. Precontemplation (A) means the patient is not yet considering change or is unwilling or unable to change. Contemplation (B) suggests the patient acknowledges concerns and is considering the possibility of change, but is ambivalent and uncertain. Action (D) means taking steps to change but not yet reaching a stable state.

Lesson 2: Anxiety

5. C

Although early morning awakening **(C)** is often experienced by patients with an anxiety disorder, it is not a diagnostic criterion. Irritability (A), apprehension (B), and difficulty concentrating (D) are all diagnostic criteria.

6. A

Muscle tension **(A)** is a commonly reported physical symptom of anxiety. Hypersomnolence (B) can be associated with depression. Hives (C) can be associated with anxiety disorders in some patients, but are not a common finding. Constipation (D) is generally not associated with anxiety; many patients will experience GI symptoms such as nausea and diarrhea.

7. C

Due to side effects and tolerability, it is important to start with a low-dose SSRI and increase slowly if needed **(C)**. Most patients do not see a change in symptoms until 4 weeks, rather than 2 weeks (A). SSRIs can affect other medications (B); therefore, it is always important to consider all patient medications when prescribing a new medication. Patients with anxiety generally do not tolerate medications that are energizing (D) due to symptoms of irritability and sleep disturbances.

8. D

Patients with a diagnosis of PTSD have an ability to recall the precipitating event **(D)**—usually with vivid detail as if they are experiencing the event again. A feeling of detachment (A) and hyperarousal (B) are common symptoms of PTSD, and sleep issues (C) are commonly experienced by patients with PTSD.

Lesson 3: Depression

9. A

Symptoms of emptiness, lack of pleasure, weight loss, insomnia, inappropriate guilt, and lack of focus nearly every day for the past month **(A)**—5 or more of the required 9 elements occurring over the same two-week period, including either depressed mood or loss of pleasure—meet the requirement for MDD. Choices (B), (C), and (D) meet the requirement of depressed mood for the same two-week period, but not the required 5 of 9 elements.

10. B

According to the DSM-5, a patient must experience either a depressed mood or loss of interest or pleasure **(B)** to meet the criteria for major depressive disorder. Feelings of worthlessness (A), sleep issues (C), or recurrent thoughts of death (D) may be elements of a depressive disorder, but are not diagnostic requirements.

11. A

Sexual dysfunction is a common side effect for SSRIs **(A)**. Most patients that experience sexual dysfunction to one SSRI will experience the same side effects to another SSRI; changing (B) will not be beneficial. The side effect of sexual dysfunction is not transient (C) and will be experienced until changes are made. Since sexual dysfunction is a common side effect to SSRIs there is no need for a referral (D); it is best to change the medication.

12. C

A PHQ-9 score of 10–14 indicates moderate depression severity **(C)**. A PHQ-9 score of 1–4 indicates minimal depression severity (A). A PHQ-9 score of 5–9 indicates mild depression severity (B). A PHQ-9 score of 20–27 indicates severe depression severity (D).

Lesson 4: Eating Disorders

13. A

A common symptom of anorexia nervosa in children and adolescents is failure to maintain the developmental trajectory **(A)**. Weight loss (B) must be significant to meet the diagnostic criteria; weight loss alone will not meet criteria. A normal BMI (C) precludes the diagnosis of anorexia nervosa. Participating in multiple sports to maintain weight (D) suggests the child would be overweight without physical activity. This is not a criterion for anorexia nervosa.

14. C

The criteria for a diagnosis of bulimia nervosa is met with this description **(C)**. Binge eating disorder (A) does not include symptoms of vomiting and laxative use to control weight. Anorexia nervosa (B) with binge-eating/purging type requires symptoms of significant weight loss or failure to gain weight in children and adolescents. Binge-purge (D) is a symptom, not a disorder.

15. B

The risk of suicide **(B)** is increased for patients with a diagnosis of anorexia nervosa, and due to lethality must be evaluated at every encounter. Although assessing for associated eating disorders (A) is important at the initial encounter, subsequent assessments will not change the treatment. Asking about family history of eating disorders (C) is an important part of the initial assessment. It is important to assess for substance use (D) at the initial appointment and at any time symptoms are present.

16. D

Evidence-based treatment for eating disorders includes a combination of medications, therapy, nutritional counseling, and medical care **(D)**. Medications (A) are helpful, especially to treat comorbid symptoms of anxiety or depression, but are not the sole treatment. Therapy (B) is an important part of treatment, but not the only treatment. Monitoring of intake and limiting exercise (C) may be a part of the treatment plan, but not the primary intervention.

Lesson 5: Bipolar Disorders

17. C

The patient does not meet the criteria for mania or hypomania, which is a required element of a bipolar disorder diagnosis **(C)**. Knowing this, we can eliminate choices (A) and (B). The given symptoms do not allow for a diagnosis of depressive disorder (D); required is the two-week time frame and additional (5 of 9) characteristics. Further evaluation is needed to determine diagnosis, treatment, and/or referral.

18. C

The Mood Disorder Questionnaire (MDQ) **(C)** is an initial self-report screen to identify symptoms of bipolar disorder. PHQ-9 (A) is a screening tool for depressive symptoms; GAD-7 (B) is a screening tool for anxiety symptoms, and the DAST-10 (D) is a screening tool for drug abuse.

19. D

Lamotrigine and sertraline **(D)** are evidence-based practice for bipolar disorder with depressive symptoms. A thorough diagnostic assessment will provide needed information to ensure the nurse practitioner is prescribing the medications appropriately. Dextroamphetamine is the treatment for ADHD and will often worsen symptoms of bipolar disorder. Therefore, you can omit choice (A). Referring for ADHD testing for confirmation of diagnosis before treatment is the best practice. Lamotrigine and sertraline may be necessary for symptom control, but unless you are certain of an ADHD diagnosis there is no harm in holding the dextroamphetamine until the diagnosis is confirmed. Patients with a diagnosis of bipolar disorder will decompensate quickly if medications for mood stabilization are stopped, and records from previous providers may take weeks to receive (B). Referral to a mental health provider will take time and it is unsafe to remove mood stabilizers in bipolar patients (C).

20. B

Mood stabilizers **(B)** are the first-line medication treatment for bipolar disorder symptoms. Antidepressants (A) may be used to treat depressive symptoms, and anxiolytics (C) may be used to treat anxiety symptoms, but both only after the mood is stabilized. Even though mood stabilizers and antidepressants (D) are often used together in long-term treatment, it is important to stabilize the mood first and start one medication at a time to monitor for symptom response and potential side effects.

Lesson 6: Psychotic Disorders

21. A

Family history, exposure to viruses, and psychosocial factors combined **(A)** are known risk factors to developing schizophrenia. Other mental health diagnoses (B), marital status (C), and other medical diagnoses and educational level (D) are not known risk factors for schizophrenia.

22. C

Labs are needed before initiating medications to establish a baseline, at 3 months and at 12 months, and then, if within normal range, annually and more frequently if needed **(C)**. The second set of labs is taken at three months, not six months (A). Baseline measurements are needed; obtaining labs only after being on medications for six months (B) and three months (D) does not establish baseline measurements.

23. A

Auditory hallucinations ("hearing voices") are a symptom, and no clinical determination can be made from one symptom; further evaluation is needed in the form of a complete MSE **(A)**. Ordering labs (B) may be a part of the assessment, but is not the first action to take. Physical examination (C) may be needed after the MSE is completed. Calling the crisis team (D) is not the first step; complete the MSE first and then determine if the crisis team is needed.

24. C

Due to the increased risk of developing tardive dyskinesia with antipsychotics, AIMS screening is necessary to evaluate risks and benefits in continued treatment with an antipsychotic medication **(C)**. The AIMS will assist in screening before a patient develops full symptoms of tardive dyskinesia (A). Only antipsychotics present an increased risk of tardive dyskinesia, not other psychotropic medications (B). There is no evidence to support screening all mental health patients (D).

Lesson 7: Neurodevelopmental Disorders

25. C

To meet the criteria for ADHD, symptoms must occur in at least two settings; these symptoms only occur in school. Given the above information, further evaluation **(C)** is needed. The reported symptoms do not meet the criteria for ADHD, as they occur in only one context, making (A) and (B) incorrect (even though behavioral modification therapy may help). Referring to the guidance department (D) is not appropriate; further evaluation of the symptoms should be made by a mental health provider.

26. A

The Vanderbilt Scale **(A)** rates symptoms of ADHD in school age through middle school age. The SCARED Scale (B) is an anxiety rating scale for children. The Y-BOCS (C) is a rating scale for symptoms of obsessions and compulsions, and the Young Mania Rating Scale (D) rates mania symptoms.

27. D

Appetite decrease is a common side effect of stimulants that can usually be minimized by adding healthy, calorie-rich snacks **(D)**. You should also always reevaluate. There is no need to stop the medication (A and C) or wean off the current stimulant (B), as appetite decrease is common with stimulants.

28. C

The recommendations to screen for ASD are at the 18- and 24-month well-child check and any time there is a concern regarding development **(C)**. Even though 18 and 24 months are correct in choice (A), it is also important to screen at other appointments if there are developmental concerns.

Lesson 8: Suicide

29. D

It is true that mental illness, including substance use, contributes to suicidality **(D)**. Psychiatric patients have up to 12 times the risk of those without a diagnosed mental illness. Patients do not always present with overt statements (A); vague statements must be addressed as well. Screening tools (B) are one part of an assessment, but not the primary means. Knowing the risk factors and a holistic assessment are equally important. Never-married singles attempt suicide at a rate twice that of married individuals (C).

30. C

The fact that the patient's wife sent him **(C)** is not a concern. At face value, this defines a supportive relationship—a protective factor for suicide. Vague or passive statements such as "everything is fine" (A) do not rule out suicidal ideation. Impulsive nature (B) is a risk for suicide, as is taking an antidepressant (D) (i.e., diagnosis of depression).

31. B

Dialectical behavioral therapy **(B)** is not a first-line therapy for depression. SSRIs (A), CBT (C), and interpersonal therapy (D) are used for depression.

32. A

A 75-year-old recent widower **(A)** is most at risk for a completed suicide. The recent death of a spouse, especially for males, is considered a suicide risk factor. White females (B) may attempt suicide more, but they tend to complete suicide at a rate far less than men. Being married (C) could be considered a protective factor. Being Roman Catholic (D) could be considered a protective factor (as suicide is prohibited in this belief system).

CHAPTER 13

Endocrine

LESSON 1: ADDISON'S DISEASE

Learning Objectives
- Understand the etiology of Addison's disease
- Know the signs and symptoms of Addison's disease
- Be aware of treatment options for Addison's disease

Addison's disease (AD) is a disorder characterized by underproduction of cortisol, along with primary adrenal insufficiency and aldosterone deficiency. About 1 in 100,000 people in the United States suffer from Addison's disease.

To understand AD, it is important to understand how cortisol is produced. The structures involved are the hypothalamus, the pituitary, and the adrenal glands (known jointly as the HPA axis). First, the hypothalamus produces corticotropin-releasing hormone (CRH). Second, CRH stimulates the pituitary gland to produce adrenocorticotropic hormone (ACTH). Lastly, ACTH stimulates the production of cortisol from the adrenal glands.

There are three types of AD:

1. Primary: involves disruption of the functioning of the adrenal gland or destruction of the adrenal gland (which produces hormones)—the "last stop" on the production line

2. Secondary: insufficient pituitary ACTH release with subsequent reduction in hormone production—the "middle stop" of the production line

3. Tertiary: insufficient hypothalamic CRH leading to reduced levels of ACTH; associated with dysfunction on the "first stop" of the cortisol production line

Etiology of Addison's Disease	
Autoimmune Addison's disease	Seen in up to 90% of U.S. cases of AD; caused by a malfunctioning immune system that attacks the adrenal glands
Polyglandular autoimmune (PGA) syndromes	• PGA I: adrenocortical failure occurring simultaneously with candidiasis and hypoparathyroidism • PGA II: autoimmune AD occurring simultaneously with thyroid autoimmune diseases and/or type 1 diabetes mellitus; sometimes additional disorders appear in this syndrome as well, such as myasthenia gravis or celiac disease
Infectious disease	The most common infectious agent causing adrenal disease is tuberculosis (TB); others include cryptococcosis and HIV

Table 13.1.1

Etiology of Addison's Disease (Continued)	
Medications	Include ketoconazole, etomidate, metyrapone
Cancer	Cancer metastasizing from other areas of body (such as breast and lung cancer), causing destruction to the kidneys/adrenal glands
Suppression of the hypothalamic-pituitary-adrenal axis	Typically caused by the administration of exogenous steroids; when suddenly withdrawn, adrenal crisis can erupt

Table 13.1.1

Assessment

Subjective

- Arthralgia
- Fatigue
- Myalgia
- Salt craving
- Anorexia
- Nausea

Objective

- Classic sign: skin bronzing/skin hyperpigmentation, especially in friction-bearing areas such as the knuckles, palmar creases, axilla, and elbows, and also sometimes on the mouth or gums
- Weight loss
- Hyponatremia
- Hyperkalemia
- Vomiting
- Hypotension

Pro Tip
- It can be difficult to pinpoint cases of AD due to vague symptoms, such as weakness or fatigue. These symptoms can be found in conditions as wide-ranging as depression, anorexia nervosa, or hypothyroidism.
- In cases of adrenal gland destruction, >90% of the glands must be destroyed before clinical/laboratory results may register the insufficiency.

Diagnosis

Diagnostic testing	
Morning serum cortisol	Gold standard test; <3 mcg/dL suggests adrenal insufficiency; >18 mcg/dL excludes adrenal insufficiency; 3–18 mcg/dL is inconclusive and suggests further testing is needed
Overnight single-dose metyrapone test	Induces a rapid fall of cortisol, which in healthy patients would cause an increase in CRH and ACTH with a resulting rise in endogenous cortisol; Addison's patients fail to show an increase in cortisol Note: the patient needs close monitoring for hypoglycemia, and the test is contraindicated in patients with epilepsy and coronary disease
Serum electrolytes	Can show hyperkalemia, hyponatremia, and occasionally hypercalcemia
BUN	Sometimes elevated
CBC	May show eosinophilia or anemia
Plasma aldosterone/ plasma DHEAs	Typically suppressed
Plasma renin	Typically elevated
Vital signs	Hypotension
ACTH stimulation	Blood level of cortisol measured before and after administration of ACTH; Addison's patients fail to show the expected rise in cortisol

Table 13.1.2 Diagnostic Testing for Addison's Disease

Differential Diagnosis

Differential diagnoses for AD include **alcoholism, malnutrition, hyperthyroidism, diabetes, eating disorders, occult malignancy, tuberculosis,** and **sarcoidosis**.

> **Pro Tip**
>
> Adrenal crisis: can involve manifestations of shock or kidney failure. Lack of cortisol means that the patient's system fails to mount an appropriate response to a stressor (i.e., surgery).
>
> Symptoms of adrenal crisis include severe leg, back, or abdominal pain, syncope, loss of consciousness, dizziness, vomiting, fatigue, and hypotension. Treatment often involves injectable steroids and should not be delayed. Hospitalization is typically required.

Plan

Treatment

Treatment for Addison's Disease
Adrenal crisis/acute Addison's episode: corticosteroid replacement (with IV fluids for rehydration and glucose for hypoglycemia)
Ongoing treatment: oral glucocorticoid and mineralocorticoid replacement for life
(Careful monitoring is needed, as high doses of steroids can cause edema, hypertension, and hypokalemia—Cushing-like symptoms. Doses are adjusted during times of increased stress. Additionally, long-term steroid use can contribute to the development of osteopenia/osteoporosis, as well as worsening of acid reflux.)

Table 13.1.3

Education

- AD involves lifelong treatment
- Patients should not abruptly stop high-dose corticosteroids
- If symptomatic, patients may need treatment for acid reflux
- All patients (but especially older and/or female patients) should have regular bone density testing

Referral

- For complete workup and treatment, refer to an endocrinologist

Takeaways

- AD can be underdiagnosed. Consider the diagnosis in the case of a patient with multiple correlating symptoms such as fatigue, hypotension, and hyperpigmentation.
- AD features cortisol insufficiency. In contrast, Cushing's syndrome features hypercortisolism.

LESSON 2: DIABETES

Learning Objectives
- Define key characteristics of diabetes
- Identify diagnostic criteria for diabetes
- Select appropriate treatment options for diabetes

About 30 million people in the United States (about 9% of the total population) have the diagnosis of diabetes. Diabetes can be considered a group of related disorders of metabolic function: type 1 diabetes, type 2 diabetes (a combination of insulin resistance, inadequate insulin production, and increased glucagon secretion), and gestational diabetes (which occurs during the second or third trimester of pregnancy). Of the three conditions, type 2 diabetes is the most common, accounting for about 90% of diabetic cases.

Diabetes Type 1	
Etiology	• Autoimmune destruction of insulin-producing pancreatic beta cells • Destruction may be gene-related: some people have altered genetic coding on chromosome 6; their genes code for human leukocyte antigen (HLA) complexes, which may trigger destructive immune reactions • Diabetes 1 may also be triggered by viral infections such as German measles or rotavirus • Some cases of type 1 categorized as idiopathic, with no known cause identified
Average age of diagnosis	Typically <40 years old, with two peak age groups: 4–7 years old and 10–14 years old
Prevalence in U.S.	Up to 3 million people (about 10% of the overall diabetic population)

Screening	Not recommended as:
	  – Condition is either typically diagnosed in childhood or of sudden onset
	  – No current preventative treatment
	
	Note: while screening for type 1 diabetes is not considered cost-effective, clinicians should not fail to diagnose a case if it is suspected

Common signs	Polydipsia, polyuria, polyphagia
Diet	Heart-healthy diet, avoid alcohol or at least use in moderation, always carry a sugar source
Risk factors	Sibling or parent with type 1 diabetes, peak ages as above, more common in people living in cold climates, exposure to a virus
Diabetes type 1 was once called "juvenile diabetes," as it is commonly seen in children. However, this term has fallen into disfavor as it can also occur in adults—e.g., after a viral infection.	

Table 13.2.1

Diabetes Type 2	
Etiology	• Believed to be multifactorial in origin • Features insulin resistance/deficiency with resulting glucose intolerance and hyperglycemia • Genetic predisposition and environmental factors believed to be causative • Lifestyle factors that can contribute include being overweight, poor diet, and lack of exercise
Average age of diagnosis	45–64 years old, but increasing numbers of younger adults/pediatric patients being diagnosed
Prevalence in U.S.	About 30 million
Screening	Yes, based on risk factors (see below)
Common signs	Polydipsia, polyuria, polyphagia
Diet	• Diabetic diet (high nutrient, low fat/carb such as ADA 1800 or ADA 2000) • Maintenance of appropriate weight for height
Risk factors	• Certain ethnic groups: African American, Hispanic, Asian American, Native American, and Pacific Islander • History of type 2 diabetes in first- or second-degree relative or history of gestational diabetes, chronic steroid use, A1C >5.7%, acanthosis nigricans, ≥age 45, nonalcoholic fatty liver disease (NAFLD), overweight, central obesity, dyslipidemia, sedentary lifestyle, polycystic ovary syndrome

Table 13.2.2

Gestational diabetes (GD)	
Etiology	Proposed causes include changes from pregnancy, extra weight from pregnancy, and genetic predisposition
Average age of diagnosis	≥35 years old have an increased risk of gestational diabetes
Prevalence in the U.S.	Exact number is not definitively known, but research suggests 5–18% of pregnant women develop GD
Screening	Typically in second trimester, between 24–28 weeks of pregnancy
Common signs	• There are often no signs of GD; this is why testing is important • Sometimes GD may be identified by the discovery of glycosuria or an abnormally large fetus • Sometimes the pregnant woman may show classic diabetes symptoms such as polydipsia or polyuria • Adverse results of GD can include maternal hypertension/preeclampsia, preterm birth, and fetal macrosomia
Diet	• Pregnant women with GD may need nutritional evaluation • Per the American Diabetes Association (ADA): a GD diet helps maintain maternal/fetal well-being and appropriate maternal weight gain while avoiding hyperglycemia, ketones, and excessive weight gain
Risk factors	Certain ethnic groups (African American, Hispanic, Native American, or Asian), obesity, previous high-birthweight baby, polycystic ovary syndrome, criteria met for prediabetes previous to pregnancy, 1st-degree relative with type 2 diabetes

Table 13.2.3 Gestational Diabetes

Assessment

Subjective

- Polyphagia
- Polydipsia
- Polyuria
- Irritable mood
- Fatigue
- Blurry vision
- Numbness/tingling in extremities

Objective

- Unexplained weight loss
- Hyperglycemia

Sometimes diabetes is discovered during treatment of another condition, often the sequela of the original diabetes. Sequelae are conditions related to poor diabetic control/end-organ damage.

Sequelae of Diabetes
Cardiac: coronary artery disease, atherosclerosis, heart failure, acute myocardial infarction
GI: gastroparesis, intestinal enteropathy (pathology of the intestine), NAFLD
GU: erectile dysfunction, UTI, microalbuminuria, kidney compromise, kidney failure
Immune: slowed wound healing, yeast infection
MS: bone disease
Neuro: diabetic neuropathy, diabetic retinopathy, blurry vision, blindness
Skin: poor wound healing (and diabetic ulcers), yeast infections

Table 13.2.4

Pro Tip

Two potentially life-threatening conditions that may develop secondary to diabetes are diabetic ketoacidosis (DKA) (more common in type 1) and hyperosmolar hyperglycemic non-ketotic syndrome (HHNK) (more common in type 2). Often a precipitating event triggers DKA or HHNK, such as infection (with possible fever/dehydration) or deficient insulin.

DKA is a top cause of mortality in type 1 diabetes. Typical features include:

- Serum glucose level >250 mg/dL
- Dehydration
- Elevated serum ketone levels
- Serum pH <7.3
- Serum bicarbonate level <18 mEq/L
- Kussmaul breathing

HHNK can result in a 5–10% mortality rate. Signs include:

- Dehydration
- Bicarbonate concentration >18 mEq/L
- Serum pH >7.3
- Plasma glucose level of ≥600 mg/dL
- Serum osmolality of ≥320 mOsm/kg
- Changes in consciousness
- Rarely, ketonuria

Treatment involves fluid replacement, identifying and addressing underlying causative factor(s), and reversing acidosis/ketosis.

Diagnosis

It is important to identify patients that are showing early signs of diabetes, known as prediabetes. Caught at an early stage, the condition may be reversible with diet and lifestyle changes.

Prediabetes	
HgbA1c	5.7%–6.4%
Fasting glucose test	100–125 mg/dL
Oral glucose tolerance test	140–199 mg/dL
Without intervention, prediabetes will likely progress to type 2 diabetes within 10 years. The CDC suggests that about 85 million Americans are prediabetic but have not yet been diagnosed.	

Table 13.2.5

Diagnostic Testing

Type 1 and type 2 diabetes:

- Random serum glucose: symptoms of diabetes and a serum glucose level >200 mg/dL on one occasion, or glucose >200 mg/dL on two occasions without symptoms = diabetes
- Hemoglobin A1C level: ≥6.5% on two separate tests
- Fasting plasma glucose level (eight hours of no caloric intake)
    - <100 mg/dL = normal
    - 100–125 mg/dL = prediabetes
    - ≥126 mg/dL on two separate tests = diabetes
- Oral glucose tolerance test: serum glucose measured two hours after a glucose load of 75 grams
    - <140 mg/dL = normal
    - 140–199 mg/dL = prediabetes
    - >200 mg/dL at two hours = diabetes
- Pancreatic auto-antibodies: auto-antibodies to glutamic acid decarboxylase, islet cells, islet antigens, insulin and zinc transporter (ZnT8); if present, suspect autoimmune destruction of pancreatic beta cells, as seen with type 1 diabetes (there is a possibility of false negatives: the absence of pancreatic auto-antibodies does not rule out type 1 diabetes)
- Fasting C-peptide: low or undetectable = no insulin secretion from pancreatic beta cells, as seen with type 1 diabetes or advanced DM

Gestational diabetes:

- 50-g glucose challenge test (GCT)
    - If glucose ≤139 mg/dL at one hour, no additional testing is needed and gestational diabetes is ruled out
    - glucose ≥140mg/dL, a 100-g glucose tolerance test (GTT) is performed
        - GDM is diagnosed if two or more plasma glucose measurements meet or exceed the following thresholds: fasting level of 95 mg per dL, one-hour level of 180 mg per dL, two-hour level of 155 mg per dL, or three-hour level of 140 mg per dL
- Glycosuria cannot be seen as diagnostic for gestational diabetes; about half of pregnant women may suffer from glycosuria at some point in their pregnancy (possibly related to increased glomerular filtration rate)

Pro Tip

About 1 in 5 U.S. teens is obese—a significant risk factor for diabetes. Clinicians should consider testing teens with risk factors.

Patients with metabolic syndrome (*see Chapter 13, Lesson 5*) should be tested for diabetes and encouraged to make lifestyle changes.

Differential Diagnoses

Differential diagnoses include: acromegaly, alcoholism, Cushing syndrome, diabetes insipidus, infection, polycystic ovary syndrome (PCOS), pheochromocytoma.

Plan

Treatment

Treatment for diabetes
Diabetes type 1: lifelong insulin, *see Table 13.2.7 and Chapter 4, Lesson 6*
Diabetes type 2: *see Table 13.2.8 and Chapter 4, Lesson 6*
Gestational diabetes: if mild, may be controlled with diet and exercise; otherwise, may require insulin treatment

Table 13.2.6 Treatment for Diabetes

Insulin types	Onset	Peak	Duration
insulin lispro (Humalog)	5–15 mins	1–2 hours	3–5 hours
Regular insulin	0.5–1 hour	2–4 hours	5–8 hours
NPH	1–2 hours	4–12 hours	18–24 hours
insulin glargine (Lantus)	1–1.5 hours	No peak (delivered steadily)	20–24 hours
Pre-mixed			
Humulin 70/30	30 mins	2–4 hours	14–24 hours
Humulin 50/50	30 mins	2–5 hours	14–24 hours
Humalog 75/25	15 mins	30 mins–2.5 hours	14–24 hours
Novolin 70/30	30 mins	2–12 hours	14–24 hours
Novolog 70/30	10–20 mins	1–4 hours	$\geq$24 hours

Table 13.2.7 Types of Insulin

Antihyperglycemic management of diabetes mellitus	
Step 1: Monotherapy	• biguanide: metformin (Glucophage); contraindicated if eGFR ≤30 • If A1C not at goal after 3 months, move to step 2 (A1C goal for most diabetics is ≤7%)

Step 2: Dual therapy	• Choice based on effectiveness, side effects, likelihood of adherence, cost, risk of hypoglycemia, effect on weight (*see Chapter 4, Lesson 6, for specifics of each medication class*)
	• biguanide + medication from one of the following classes:
	  – Second-generation sulfonylurea: glipizide (Glucotrol), glimepiride (Amaryl)
	  – glucagon-like peptide (GLP-1): liraglutide (Victoza), exenatide (Byetta)
	  – thiazolidinedione (TZD): pioglitazone (Actos)
	  – sodium glucose co-transporter 2 inhibitor (SGLT2 inhibitor): canagliflozin (Invokana), dapagliflozin (Farxiga)
	  – dipeptidyl peptidase 4 inhibitor (DPP-4 inhibitor): linagliptin (Tradjenta), saxagliptin (Onglyza)
	  – alpha glucosidase inhibitor: acarbose (Precose)
	  – non-sulfonylurea secretagogue (meglitinides): nateglinide (Starlix), repaglinide (Prandin)
	  – insulin
	• May start at this step if A1C ≥9%
	• If A1C not achieved after 3 months on two-medication regimen, move to step 3

Step 3: Triple therapy	• Continue with two-class medication regimen + add medication from a different class listed in step 2
	• If A1C goal not reached after three months of triple therapy, then:
	  – If taking oral medications only, add injectable
	  – If taking GLP-1, add basal insulin
	  – If taking titrated basal insulin, add GLP-1 or mealtime insulin
	  – Add TZD or SGLT-2 if not already taking this class for patients that are resistant to other treatment

Step 4: Combination injectable therapy	• biguanide + basal insulin + mealtime insulin + GLP-1 • May start at this step if A1C ≥10% and/or blood glucose >300 mg/dL

Table 13.2.8 Antihyperglycemic Management of Diabetes Mellitus

Education

- Type 1 diabetes

  - Lifelong insulin

  - Signs/symptoms of hypoglycemia (shakiness, sweating, dizziness); always have an available glucose source, such as glucose tablets or fruit juice

  - Signs/symptoms of hyperglycemia (frequent urination, hunger, excess thirst, and fatigue); may need a one-time corrective dose of insulin or a change in overall regimen if the hyperglycemia is ongoing

  - Signs/symptoms of DKA (fruity sweet-smelling breath, nausea/vomiting, abdominal pain) and signs of HHNK (drowsiness, increased thirst, polyuria, and dehydration); both require emergency care

- Type 2 diabetes

  - Maintain good glycemic control to prevent end organ damage and/or progression to insulin use

  - Signs/symptoms of hypoglycemia, hyperglycemia, DKA, and HHNK

- Gestational diabetes
  - Hyperglycemia tends to resolve after pregnancy, but patient is at a higher risk for developing type 2 diabetes later in life
  - Expect daily glucose testing, more frequent prenatal visits, special diet recommendations, and post-pregnancy testing
- All diabetic and prediabetic patients need education regarding healthy diet (American Diabetes Association diet), exercise, lifestyle changes, and smoking cessation (smoking greatly increases the risk of cardiovascular events) to prevent progression of diabetes and end organ damage
- All diabetic patients need yearly dilated eye exams; education to monitor feet for sores, callouses, cuts, or changes in skin; report changes immediately

Referral

- Ophthalmology: diabetic retinopathy, yearly dilated eye exams
- Endocrinology: poor glycemic control
- Gastroenterology: GI sequelae, such as gastroparesis
- Podiatry: diabetic foot ulcers, trimming of nails
- Cardiology: sequelae such as heart failure
- Nephrology: sequelae such as renal compromise/failure
- Nutritionist: diet to maintain glucose control
- Hospitalization: DKA or HHNK

Takeaways

- Recognize signs of DKA and HHNK, as these conditions are life-threatening.
- Identify prediabetic patients and encourage them to make lifestyle changes to avoid developing diabetes.
- If not contraindicated, patients with type 1 or type 2 diabetes should be started on daily aspirin, ACE inhibitor, and statin therapy to prevent sequelae and/or cardiovascular complications.
- Even a small amount of weight loss (about 5–7% of body weight) can help arrest the progression of prediabetes to diabetes.

LESSON 3: CUSHING SYNDROME

Learning Objectives

- ■ Understand the etiology of Cushing syndrome
- ■ Know the signs and symptoms a Cushing patient may exhibit
- ■ Be aware of treatment options for Cushing syndrome

Cushing syndrome is a disorder characterized by the overproduction of cortisol. Cortisol is produced in the adrenal glands after stimulation by adrenocorticotropic hormone (ACTH). Thus, cortisol overproduction can emanate from dysfunction at the level of the adrenal glands (such as an adrenal tumor), dysfunction at the level of the pituitary gland (such as a pituitary tumor), or ectopic production of ACTH (a tumor not at the pituitary, but located somewhere else in the body that has started producing ACTH—a neuroendocrine tumor). High doses or long-term use of oral, injected, or topical steroids can also potentially cause Cushing syndrome.

Assessment

Subjective

- Fatigue

- Bone discomfort

- Depression/anxiety

Objective

Classic signs include new or worsening hypertension, spindly appearing arms and legs with contrasting round red face (e.g., moon face), fat deposits around neck and upper part of back (e.g., buffalo hump), and truncal obesity. Additional signs are:

- Easily bruised, thinned skin; striae on thighs, arms, breasts, and/or abdomen; poor wound healing

- Hyperglycemia

- Infertility/erectile dysfunction

- Hirsutism

- Irregular or absent menses

- Hypokalemia, hypernatremia, and occasionally hypocalcemia

> **Pro Tip**
>
> About 80% of Cushing's sufferers have hypertension.
>
> Pituitary gland tumors are 5 times more likely in women than men.
>
> Addison's disease: a condition where the adrenal glands do not produce enough steroid hormones, resulting in hypocortisolism—essentially the opposite of Cushing syndrome.

Diagnosis

Diagnostic methods include:

- Vital signs (Cushing syndrome is associated with hypertension)

- 24-hour UFC (urinary free cortisol level); most Cushing sufferers have elevated cortisol, but some mild cases may show normal cortisol, thus creating a false negative

- Low-dose dexamethasone suppression testing (LDDST); suppression absent in Cushing syndrome

- Midnight plasma cortisol and late-night salivary cortisol measurements (elevated cortisol levels between 11 PM–12 AM)

- CT scan or MRI (to look at pituitary and adrenal glands to detect changes such as tumors)

- CBC with differential (high WBC/high neutrophil levels sometimes associated with Cushing syndrome)

- Glucose tolerance (Cushing syndrome is associated with hyperglycemia)

- CMP (Cushing syndrome is associated with hypokalemia, hypernatremia, and occasionally hypocalcemia)

> **Pro Tip: Cushing Disease vs. Cushing Syndrome**
>
> Cushing disease is hypercortisolism originating from a benign tumor on the pituitary gland, causing overproduction of adrenocorticotropic hormone (ACTH).
>
> Cushing syndrome is a more general term. It refers to the effects of excessive ongoing hypercortisolism on the body.

Differential Diagnosis

Differential diagnoses for Cushing: **metabolic syndrome, chronic anxiety/depression, PCOS, poorly controlled diabetes, excessive alcohol use (can cause Cushingoid appearance)**

Plan

Treatment

Treatment for Cushing syndrome depends on the cause.

Treatment for Cushing Syndrome	
Surgery	Ideally, complete removal of the mass when a tumor is the underlying cause
Radiation	Applied to any tumor tissue that cannot be excised or if the patient is not an optimal surgical candidate
Medications	• To help reduce excessive cortisol production: metyrapone (Metopirone), mitotane (Lysodren), and ketoconazole (Nizoral) • To help reduce the effects of excessive cortisol (though not actually reducing production): mifepristone (Korlym), a cortisol blocker designed for use in patients who have type 2 diabetes or glucose intolerance
Reducing exogenous steroids	Be aware that steroids cannot be stopped abruptly; these must be tapered slowly, as sudden stoppage could cause adrenal insufficiency

Table 13.3.1

Education

Make patients on long-term steroid therapy aware of the signs of hypercortisolism/Cushing syndrome.

Referral

Given the complexity of the diagnosis, consultation and/or referral to an endocrinologist should be considered. If surgical intervention is needed, then a surgery consultation will be in order.

Takeaways

- Know the hallmark signs of Cushing syndrome: "moon face," "buffalo hump," truncal obesity, and new or worsening hypertension.
- Be on the alert for Cushing signs/symptoms in long-term steroid users.

LESSON 4: HYPOGLYCEMIA

Learning Objectives
- Discuss the most common causes of hypoglycemia
- Identify symptoms of hypoglycemia
- Order the appropriate diagnostic test(s) when hypoglycemia is suspected
- Develop a treatment plan for a patient with hypoglycemia

Hypoglycemia is a clinical syndrome that is classified as a reduction in plasma glucose arising from abnormalities in glucose homeostasis. It is most often seen in patients with diabetes mellitus (DM) and rarely in patients without DM. Diabetics receiving insulin have a more than threefold increased risk of developing hypoglycemia.

In those with DM, all episodes of low plasma glucose with or without symptoms that expose a patient to harm are considered hypoglycemic episodes. For a hypoglycemic disorder to be diagnosed in those without DM, patients must be symptomatic and have a documented low blood glucose level, and the symptoms must be relieved when the plasma glucose is raised (Whipple triad).

The most common causes of hypoglycemia in a patient with DM are insulin overdose, skipping a meal, exercise, or overdosing oral hypoglycemic medication. Other etiologies for those with or without DM include:

- Infection, sepsis
- Critical illness (cardiac, renal, and hepatic diseases; sepsis with multi-organ damage)
- Insulinoma (a tumor in the pancreas that secretes an excessive amount of insulin)
- Idiopathic
- Drug-induced (e.g., insulin, sulfonylureas, salicylates, quinine, pentamidine, sulpha drugs, alcohol)

Pro Tip: Gerontological Considerations

Hypoglycemia in the elderly is associated with various morbidities, which encompass both physical and cognitive dysfunctions. It can lead to disability, frailty, and a poor overall outcome for the patient. Episodes of hypoglycemia can lead to cardiac disturbances and arrhythmias as well as altered mental status contributing to accidents/falls with subsequent injury such as fractures/traumatic head injuries, seizures, coma, and even death.

For individuals over the age of 65 who are otherwise healthy, a goal of HgbA1c <7 is ideal. When comorbidities, frailty, or a shortened life expectancy are present, a more realistic goal may be to decrease the symptoms of hyperglycemia. The elderly are at an increased risk for developing hypoglycemia for a variety of reasons. Predisposing factors include:

- Tight glycemic control
- Poor nutritional intake
- Impaired renal or hepatic function
- Polypharmacy
- Medication noncompliance
- Isolation
- Presence of comorbidities that can mask the symptoms of hypoglycemia (dementia, delirium, CVA, MI, seizures, sleep disturbances)

Assessment

Conduct a thorough history. Determine the patient's current medication regimen and identify if any changes have been made recently. Inquire about alcohol intake, illicit drug use, recent illnesses or surgeries, recent DM diagnosis, activity, and diet, including a 24-hour recall. Ask about endocrine diseases and renal or hepatic failure.

Physical signs of hypoglycemia may be mistaken for other clinical conditions. The elderly tend to exhibit fewer symptoms and at a lower threshold than younger adults.

The normal lower limit for blood glucose is 70 mg/dL. The threshold for the appearance of symptoms is variable, but typically occurs between 50–55 mg/dL.

Physical signs	Symptoms
Tachycardia	Altered mental status (confusion, belligerence, inappropriate behavior)
Diaphoretic, pale, skin with decreased turgor	Headache
Hypothermia	Nausea, vomiting
Hypertension	Fatigue
Tachypnea	Sweating
Dysrhythmias	Shakiness, weakness
Tremors	Anxiety
Seizures	Dizziness
Unconsciousness	Blurred vision
	Paresthesia

Table 13.4.1 Signs and Symptoms of Hypoglycemia

Diagnosis

Rapid diagnosis of hypoglycemia is essential to prevent serious complications. Diagnosis is made by obtaining a blood glucose sample during the event. A value of less than 70 mg/dL is considered abnormal and should be treated in the presence of symptoms. In patients with DM, a value less than 63 mg/dL indicates a need for treatment.

To rule out other causes of low blood glucose, check CBC, CMP, serum insulin, cortisol, TSH, and LFTs. If a blood glucose sample cannot be obtained during a symptomatic episode, an oral glucose tolerance test and/or a 72-hour fasting plasma glucose test can replicate the conditions in which hypoglycemia would be present if a hypoglycemic condition exists.

Differential Diagnosis

Differential diagnoses for hypoglycemia: **postprandial syndrome, medication side effect, psychiatric disease, metabolic disorder, cardiac disease, neurological disease, insulinoma, alcoholism**

Plan

Preventing hypoglycemic episodes is an integral part of the treatment plan. Discuss with the patient each of the following guidelines regarding the management of hypoglycemic disorders:

- Assessment of risk factors and tailoring treatment regimens as appropriate
- Providing patient education and empowerment

- Frequent self-monitoring of blood glucose
- Flexible and rational drug regimens
- Individualized glycemic goals
- Ongoing professional guidance and support
- Prevention of nocturnal hypoglycemia
- Recognition of early signs and symptoms of hypoglycemia
- Prevention of exercise-induced hypoglycemia

In patients with DM who are asymptomatic, but experience a BG of less than 70 mg/dL, defensive actions may be taken. The measurement should be repeated in 15 minutes; driving and other critical tasks should be avoided, and simple carbohydrates can be ingested.

In all symptomatic patients, the quickest, most effective treatment is the ingestion of 15–20 grams of a fast-acting carbohydrate, such as four glucose tablets, one tablespoon of sugar or honey, or 4 ounces of sweetened fruit juice. Once asymptomatic, a long-acting carbohydrate and a protein should be ingested to prevent the recurrence of symptoms.

Treatment for severe hypoglycemic episodes (a blood sugar of ≤30 mg/dL) requires glucagon administration, usually 0.5–1.0 mg SC/IM.

Education

Educate patients to self-recognize hypoglycemic symptoms and perform frequent self-monitoring of blood glucose (SMBG). Educate caregivers and family members to recognize the symptoms of hypoglycemia and how to administer glucagon.

Strenuous activity should be avoided, though routine exercise programs are approved. Patients should check their blood sugar prior to exercising, avoid exercising late at night, and, if taking insulin, avoid exercising during the insulin's peak action time.

Advise patients how to avoid hypoglycemic episodes during sick days. Consuming carbohydrate-rich drinks and other liquids, checking blood sugar at least four times a day, taking diabetes medications as prescribed, and drinking plenty of water can help to reduce the risk of developing hypoglycemia on sick days.

Referral

For complete workup and treatment, refer to an endocrinologist. A dietician can develop an individualized dietary plan that includes frequent meals and snacks, limiting refined carbohydrates, avoiding simple sugars, and increasing protein and fiber.

Takeaways

- The threshold for the appearance of symptoms is variable, but is typically around 50–55 mg/dL.
- Symptoms of hypoglycemia, such as confusion and agitation, may be mistaken for other clinical conditions, such as delirium.
- The most effective treatment for asymptomatic and symptomatic hypoglycemia is 15–20 grams of fast-acting glucose.

LESSON 5: METABOLIC SYNDROME

Learning Objectives

■ Define metabolic syndrome

■ Recognize risk factors for developing metabolic syndrome

■ Identify signs and symptoms characteristic of metabolic syndrome

■ Discuss the five diagnostic criteria that comprise metabolic syndrome

■ Develop a treatment plan for a patient with metabolic syndrome

Metabolic syndrome is associated with insulin resistance, as well as adipose tissue dysfunction. It is a clinical condition in which risk factors for developing diabetes mellitus and atherosclerotic cardiovascular disease coexist. More than one-fourth of adults in the United States meet the diagnostic criteria for metabolic syndrome. Left untreated, it will progress to diabetes mellitus.

Complications of metabolic syndrome include coronary and peripheral artery disease, cerebrovascular disease, left ventricular hypertrophy, heart failure, ischemic stroke, and renal dysfunction. It has also been associated with obstructive sleep apnea and various malignancies.

Risk factors for developing metabolic syndrome include:

- Family history
- Poor diet
- Sedentary lifestyle
- Menopause
- Smoking
- Increasing age
- Obesity, specifically fat that is visceral or intra-abdominal
- Ethnicity (more prevalent in Mexican Americans and African Americans)

Assessment

Subjective

Patients typically present with complaints related to the complications of metabolic syndrome, such as chest pain, dyspnea with exertion, and peripheral neuropathy, or report a history of hyperglycemia, hypertension, or dyslipidemia.

Objective

Truncal obesity is visibly suggestive of the condition; elevated blood pressure is another characteristic. Hypertriglyceridemia, hypertension, hyperglycemia, and reduced HDL are also used for diagnosis. A skin examination may reveal acanthosis nigricans or xanthomas.

Diagnosis

According to the guidelines from the American Heart Association (AHA) and the National Heart, Lung, and Blood Institute (NHLBI), metabolic syndrome may be diagnosed when a patient meets at least three of the following five criteria:

1. Waist circumference >35 in. for women and >40 in. for men; if Asian American, >32 in. for women and >35 in. for men

2. Blood pressure ≥130/85 mmHg

3. Fasting glucose ≥100 mg/dL

4. Triglycerides ≥150 mg/dL

5. HDL-C <50 mg/dL in women and <40 mg/dL in men

Patients with a history of hyperglycemia, hypertension, and dyslipidemia should be screened for metabolic syndrome. CBC, LFTs, renal studies, lipid panel, CMP, and CRP should be drawn if metabolic syndrome is suspected.

Plan

Treatment

The goals of treatment are to correct or eliminate the characteristics that comprise metabolic syndrome. Lifestyle changes, including diet, exercise, and weight loss, are the first steps that must be taken toward treating metabolic syndrome. Suggest diets high in fruits, vegetables, and whole grains, such as the Mediterranean diet or DASH diet. Recommend a minimum of 150 minutes of moderate physical activity per week.

Blood pressure should be less than 140/90 mm Hg in general and less than 130/80 mm Hg in patients who meet criteria for diabetes mellitus. Patients may require an antihypertensive to maintain an ideal blood pressure. Pharmacologic therapy is recommended to treat elevated LDL-C and decreased HDL-C. Hyperglycemia is treated with either insulin or an antidiabetic agent, such as metformin. Encourage smoking cessation, as smoking is a risk factor for developing metabolic syndrome. Treatment of associated conditions, such as obstructive sleep apnea, may improve the symptoms of metabolic syndrome.

Diagnostic criteria	Medication
Elevated blood pressure	ACEI, ARB
Elevated LDL-C	Statin
Decreased HDL-C	Niacin
Elevated triglycerides	Niacin, fibrates, omega-3 fatty acids
Hyperglycemia	Insulin, anti-diabetic agent

Table 13.5.1 Pharmacological Treatment of Metabolic Syndrome

Referral

Refer diabetic patients who meet diagnostic criteria to a dietician and endocrinologist. Refer high-risk patients and those with cardiac symptoms to a cardiologist. With treatment, it is possible to delay or prevent metabolic syndrome from progressing to diabetes mellitus and cardiovascular disease.

Takeaways

- Intra-abdominal, visceral obesity is the most significant risk factor for developing metabolic syndrome.
- Criteria for diagnosis are elevated blood pressure, triglycerides, and fasting blood sugar; decreased HDL-C; and waist circumference.
- Treatment focuses on lifestyle changes and reducing or eliminating the diagnostic criterion using pharmacologic therapy.

LESSON 6: THYROID DISORDERS

Learning Objectives
- Identify signs and symptoms of common thyroid disorders
- Examine the laboratory and radiography procedures essential to the diagnosis of thyroid disorders
- Identify management aspects of common thyroid disorders

Various diseases of the thyroid gland are seen in primary care patients. It is important to know the clinical presentation for each one, as well as the associated laboratory tests, in order to appropriately diagnose and manage the disorders.

Hypothyroidism is a very common disorder in the U.S. and can present across the life span. It results from thyroid gland failure or from surgical removal of the thyroid gland. Symptoms can range from very mild symptoms to severe symptoms that require hospitalization. Chronic lymphatic thyroiditis (Hashimoto thyroiditis), an inflammatory disorder, is the most common cause of hypothyroidism in North America. Subclinical hypothyroidism may also occur.

Hyperthyroidism is less common than hypothyroidism, but is still seen in the primary care setting. Graves disease (an autoimmune disorder) is the most common cause of hyperthyroidism, and toxic multinodular goiter (TMG) is the second most frequent cause.

Thyroid nodules are often noted in the primary care setting and may be asymptomatic or symptomatic (associated with hypothyroidism or hyperthyroidism). They are often noted as an incidental finding on a diagnostic test such as a CT scan or MRI. The majority of thyroid nodules are benign, but in some cases may be malignant (*refer to Chapter 13, Lesson 7, for information related to thyroid cancer*).

Definitions
- **Exophthalmos:** anterior bulging of the eye, outside of the orbit
- **Hypothyroidism:** deficiency of thyroid hormones (T3 and T4)
- **Hyperthyroidism:** excess production of thyroid hormone
- **Thyroid nodule:** a mass within the thyroid gland
- **Thyrotoxicosis:** acute, life-threatening, hypermetabolic state related to excessive thyroid hormone release (also commonly called thyroid storm)
- **Subclinical hypothyroidism:** mild deficiency of thyroid hormones (T3 and T4); results are normal and usually asymptomatic

Assessment

History

Hypothyroidism	Graves disease (hyperthyroidism)	Toxic multinodular goiter (hyperthyroidism)
• Iodine deficiency • Female gender • Age >40 • History of other autoimmune disorders • Chromosome disorders • Radiation exposure • Surgical removal of thyroid gland	• Family history of Graves disease • Female gender • Age 40 • History of other autoimmune disorders • Cigarette smoking • Emotional or physical stress • Pregnancy or recent childbirth	• Female gender • Age >60

Table 13.6.1 Risk Factors for Thyroid Disease

Review of Systems

Hypothyroidism:

- **Constitutional:** weight gain, difficulty losing weight, fatigue
- **GI:** constipation
- **Skin:** dry skin
- **Neuro:** memory issues
- **Psych:** depression
- **Reproductive:** heavy or irregular menstrual periods

Hyperthyroidism (Graves disease, toxic multinodular goiter):

- **Resp:** difficulty swallowing or breathing (TMG)
- **CV:** palpitations
- **GI:** diarrhea
- **Skin:** moist skin
- **Neuro:** nervousness, restlessness
- **Reproductive:** menstrual changes, erectile dysfunction, decreased libido

Diagnosis

Diagnosis of thyroid disorders is based on history and physical examination findings, as well as laboratory and diagnostic testing results. One of the most sensitive tests for thyroid function is thyroid-simulating hormone (TSH). A measure of TSH alone is not sufficient to diagnose hyper- or hypothyroidism. Combining TSH with FT4 accurately determines how the thyroid gland is functioning, and T3 is often added to diagnose hyperthyroidism or determine its severity.

Typical hormone levels:

- TSH: 0.4 and 4.0 mIU/L
- Total T4: 4.6–12 ug/dL
- Free T4 (FT4): 0.7–1.9 ng/dL
- Total T3: 80–180 ng/dL
- Free T3 (FT3): 2.3–4.2 pg/mL

Disorder	Subjective findings	Objective findings	Labs
Hypothyroidism	• Cold intolerance • Irritability • Face puffiness	• Periorbital and peripheral edema • Enlarged thyroid • Bradycardia • Delayed deep tendon reflexes • Thin, brittle nails	• High TSH • Low FT4 • Positive titer antithyroid antibodies (seen with Hashimoto) (normal <1:100)
Hyperthyroidism	• Heat intolerance • Increased sweating • Anorexia • Anxiety • Voice change or hoarseness (TMG)	Generalized: • Diffusely enlarged thyroid • Tachycardia • Atrial fibrillation • Fine, resting tremor • Brisk deep tendon reflexes Graves disease: • Upper eyelid retraction, lid lag, downward gaze, staring appearance • Exophthalmos • Pretibial myxedema • Thyroid acropachy Toxic multinodular goiter: • Stridor • Tracheal deviation • Superior vena cava syndrome	• Low TSH • Low–normal FT4 • High T3 and T4 • Nuclear thyroid scan: diffuse uptake (Graves), nodular uptake (TMN)
Thyroid nodules	• Most often none, unless associated with hypo- or hyperthyroidism • Neck pain or dysphagia (large nodules)	• Possibly visible or palpable • Hoarse voice (large nodules)	• Normal TSH

Table 13.6.2 Diagnostic Findings of Thyroid Disorders

DANGER SIGN Thyroid storm is a potentially life-threatening condition resulting in high-output cardiac failure. Symptoms include sudden onset of hyperthermia, tachycardia, nausea, vomiting, diarrhea, and altered sensorium. Closely monitor, hospitalize if needed, and treat with propylthiouracil.

Plan

Disorder	Treatment	Patient education	Referral
Hypothyroidism	Synthetic levothyroxine at initial doses of 25–75 mcg daily based on age, clinical condition, and other comorbidities; adjust to maintain levels of TSH, FT_4, and FT_3 within reference range	• Instruct lifelong replacement will be necessary • Maintain follow-up every 6–12 months as recommended • Report drug side effects: chest pain, palpitations, tachycardia	• Age <18 years to pediatric endocrinologist • Pregnancy • Significant cardiac disease • Surgical consultation if enlarged thyroid threatens airway
Hyperthyroidism	• propranolol for symptomatic relief until hyperthyroidism is normalized • Thiourea drugs (methimazole, propylthiouracil) • Single oral dose radioactive iodine (RAI-131) (avoid in pregnancy, breastfeeding, or ophthalmopathy)	• Avoid pregnancy until euthyroid • Graves: wear sunglasses, use lubricating eye drops and cool compresses to eyes • After radioactive iodine, avoid pregnant women and children for several days	• Pregnant woman with uncontrolled hyperthyroidism (for fetal surveillance) • Surgery in certain cases
Thyroid nodules	Thyroid ultrasound at baseline, then monitor at least annually	Report new onset of symptoms of hypo or hyperthyroidism or difficulty swallowing	Refer for fine needle aspiration if nodule ≥1 cm with suspicious sonographic characteristics

Table 13.6.3 Treatment and Referral Plan for Thyroid Disorders

Takeaways

- Treatment for hypothyroidism is lifelong, and patients should not change brand of synthetic thyroid hormone.
- Hyperthyroidism is treated with propranolol to manage symptoms until normalized with other treatments such as thioureas.
- Monitor patients with thyroid nodules annually, referring for fine needle aspiration when nodule becomes 1 cm or larger with suspicious characteristics on ultrasound.

LESSON 7: THYROID CANCER

Learning Objectives
- Understand risk factors for thyroid cancer
- Recognize signs and symptoms of thyroid cancer
- Know treatment options for thyroid cancer

Thyroid cancer may present as a thyroid nodule; however, the majority of thyroid nodules are benign on biopsy. In general, patients with thyroid cancer have an excellent prognosis, with five-year survival rates estimated to be as high as 98%.

Assessment

Risk Factors

- A personal history of being exposed to radiation, especially to the head or neck
- FH of thyroid disease/thyroid cancer
- FH of conditions such as multiple endocrine neoplasia or familial medullary thyroid carcinoma
- Inherited genetic predispositions to thyroid conditions, such as familial adenomatous polyposis (FAP predisposes sufferers to the development of polyps), Gardner syndrome (a variant of FAP), and Cowden syndrome (causes benign tissue overgrowth and increased risk of breast, uterine, and thyroid cancer)
- Being female

Subjective

- Pain/discomfort in thyroid area

Objective

- Regional lymphadenopathy
- Dysphonia/hoarseness
- Dysphagia
- Dyspnea
- Hemoptysis
- Presence of a nodule or nodules

> **Pro Tip**
>
> Thyroid nodules are four times more prevalent in women than men, but men have a higher chance of developing *cancerous* thyroid nodules.
>
> A classic presentation of thyroid cancer involves a non-symptomatic nodule found in a female in her 30–50s.
>
> Most thyroid nodules are not cancerous: benign colloid nodules are the most common. Cancerous thyroid nodules are often hard, painful, and large. However, even non-symptomatic nodules can turn out to be cancerous, so all nodules should be evaluated.

Diagnosis

Diagnostic methods may include:

- Fine needle aspiration/biopsy
- TSH testing (T3/T4 levels are usually normal in thyroid cancer, but levels can help in differential diagnosis)
- Thyroid ultrasound
- Laryngoscopy (to check for normal movement of the vocal cords)
- Radioactive iodine uptake (RAIU)

Differential Diagnosis

Differential diagnoses for thyroid cancer: **benign thyroid nodules, parathyroid cancer, goiter, Hashimoto's thyroiditis**

Plan

Treatment

Treatments for thyroid cancer may include:

- Surgical removal of the thyroid gland; includes partial thyroidectomy (such as removal of only one lobe of the thyroid) or total thyroidectomy
- Radioactive iodine ablation
- Removal of regional lymph nodes (if involved by metastasis)
- Chemotherapy
- Antineoplastic medications such as lenvatinib (Lenvima)

> **Pro Tip**
>
> Post-surgery, be on the alert for thyroid storm, hypercalcemia (from accidental damage to the parathyroid glands), vocal cord damage, and damage to the airway (causing dyspnea).
>
> Thyroid storm is a serious condition featuring hypermetabolic symptoms like tachycardia, pyrexia, and malignant hypertension. It can result from thyroidectomy (although historically it is more typically associated with goiter surgery).

Education

Total thyroidectomy as well as radioactive iodine ablation renders the patient unable to create their own thyroid hormones. The patient can expect lifelong supplementation with medication such as levothyroxine (Synthroid).

Referral

At least initially, patients will be referred to endocrinology. Oncology is also typically involved in developing and implementing a treatment plan.

Takeaways

- Post-thyroidectomy, the nurse practitioner should be on the lookout for dyspnea, hoarseness, confusion, muscle weakness, and/or hypermetabolic symptoms, as these may indicate adverse sequelae.
- Post-treatment (such as surgery or ablation), the patient can expect lifelong hormone replacement.

PRACTICE QUESTIONS

Select the ONE best answer.

Lesson 1: Addison's Disease

1. The most common cause of Addison's disease is:

    A. A malfunctioning immune system that attacks the adrenal glands

    B. Metastatic cancer that attacks the kidneys and adrenal glands

    C. Steroid use that leads to the suppression of the hypothalamic-pituitary-adrenal axis

    D. Medication use

2. Which of the following is a sign of Addison's disease?

    A. Glucose intolerance

    B. Hypotension

    C. Acne

    D. Hypertension

3. The gold standard test for Addison's disease is:

    A. Elevated BUN

    B. Elevated plasma renin

    C. Morning serum cortisol

    D. Serum electrolytes (showing hypokalemia and hyponatremia)

4. Which statement is true regarding Addison's disease?

    A. It is easily diagnosed, as its classic signs of hyperkalemia, hyponatremia, hyperpigmentation, and fatigue are readily recognizable

    B. It is difficult to pinpoint due to its vague symptoms, such as weakness or fatigue—symptoms that can be found in conditions as wide-ranging as depression or anorexia nervosa

    C. It is similar to Cushing syndrome, especially because it features hyperglycemia

    D. It only involves the hypothalamus

5. Symptoms of adrenal crisis can include:

    A. Excitability

    B. Hypertension

    C. Severe leg, back, or abdominal pain

    D. Craving of sweets

6. When considering a diagnosis of Addison's disease, potential differential diagnoses include:

    A. Cushing syndrome

    B. Osteoporosis

    C. Depression

    D. Hyperthyroidism

Lesson 2: Diabetes

7. A hallmark sign of gestational diabetes (GD) in the expectant mother is/are:

    A. Glycosuria

    B. Vision changes

    C. Polydipsia

    D. No signs

8. Prediabetic patients can be identified by a fasting glucose blood test of:

    A. <100 mg/dL

    B. 100–125 mg/dL

    C. 126–150 mg/dL

    D. 150–200 mg/dL

9. Peak ages for developing type 1 diabetes include:

    A. 1–2 years old

    B. 10–14 years old

    C. 16–18 years old

    D. Early adulthood

10. Diabetic ketoacidosis is a potentially life-threatening sequela of diabetes. It features:

    A. A plasma glucose level of >600 mg/dL

    B. Serum bicarbonate >15 mEq/L

    C. Dehydration

    D. Serum pH >7.3

11. Differential diagnoses for diabetes mellitus (DM) may include the following except:

    A. Alcoholism

    B. Diabetes insipidus

    C. Polycystic ovary syndrome (PCOS)

    D. Cirrhosis

12. Which might prompt a diagnosis of diabetes mellitus (DM)?

    A. Hemoglobin A1C levels of ≥6.5% on two separate tests

    B. An oral glucose tolerance test of 130 mg/dL

    C. A fasting plasma glucose test of 120 mg/dL

    D. A one-time random glucose test result of 150 mg/dL

Lesson 3: Cushing Syndrome

13. The nurse practitioner knows conditions mimicking Cushing syndrome include:

    A. Anxiety

    B. Hyperthyroidism

    C. Tuberculosis

    D. Metabolic syndrome

14. Medication management options for Cushing syndrome may include:

    A. rifampin (Rifadin)

    B. ketoconazole (Nizoral)

    C. prednisone (Sterapred)

    D. hydroxychloroquine (Plaquenil)

15. Signs and symptoms of Cushing syndrome can include:

    A. Bronzed skin

    B. Weight loss

    C. Orthostatic hypotension

    D. Round face

16. Treatment options for Cushing syndrome can include:

    A. Corticosteroid replacement

    B. Parathyroid gland removal

    C. Propranolol

    D. Tapering off exogenous steroids

17. The nurse practitioner would not expect the Cushing patient to exhibit:

    A. Hyperkalemia

    B. Striae

    C. Hyperglycemia

    D. Hirsutism

18. About 80% of Cushing sufferers have:

    A. Irregular menses

    B. Hypertension

    C. Hypotension

    D. Hypocortisolism

Lesson 4: Hypoglycemia

19. A patient presents with a blood sugar of 51 mg/dL. You would anticipate seeing the following symptoms except:

    A. Slurred speech, unsteadiness, and vomiting

    B. Confusion, syncope, and blurred vision

    C. Seizures, diarrhea, and chest pain

    D. Headache, palpitations, and nausea

20. Diagnosis of hypoglycemia is made by obtaining a blood glucose sample during the event. If a sample can not be taken at that time, which of the following diagnostic tests can be conducted to replicate the conditions in which hypoglycemia would be present?

    A. 12-hour fasting blood glucose

    B. Insulin-induced hypoglycemia test

    C. CT scan

    D. Oral glucose tolerance test

21. The symptoms of hypoglycemia can mimic all of the following serious clinical conditions except:

    A. Myocardial infarction

    B. Transient ischemic attack

    C. Cerebrovascular accident

    D. Cardiogenic shock

22. A 24-year-old patient with diabetes mellitus type 1 presents to the clinic with complaints of a recent severe hypoglycemic episode. Which of the following symptoms would you expect the patient to report?

    A. Anxiety, dizziness, indigestion

    B. Nausea, vomiting, diarrhea

    C. Sweating, shakiness, headache

    D. Confusion, weakness, dry mouth

23. How many grams of fast-acting glucose should a patient ingest to treat asymptomatic and symptomatic hypoglycemia?

    A. 10–15 g

    B. 15–20 g

    C. 20–25 g

    D. 25–30 g

Lesson 5: Metabolic Syndrome

24. To meet diagnostic criteria for metabolic syndrome, a patient's triglyceride level should be greater than or equal to:

    A. 100 mg/dL

    B. 150 mg/dL

    C. 200 mg/dL

    D. 250 mg/dL

25. In addition to waist circumference, blood pressure, triglycerides, and fasting blood sugar, what other lab value is diagnostic criteria for metabolic syndrome?

    A. Albumin

    B. Total cholesterol

    C. HDL-C

    D. LDL-C

26. All of the following are obesity types considered harmful due to a large production of cytokines and likeliness of resulting in metabolic syndrome except:

    A. Gynecoid

    B. Visceral

    C. Intra-abdominal

    D. Central

27. Risk factors for developing metabolic syndrome include all of the following except:

    A. Obesity

    B. Cardiovascular disease

    C. Smoking

    D. Sedentary lifestyle

28. In a patient with metabolic syndrome, a goal blood pressure is equal to or less than:

    A. 120/80

    B. 135/85

    C. 140/90

    D. 150/80

Lesson 6: Thyroid Disorders

29. Which of the following signs and symptoms are consistent with hyperthyroidism?

    A. Brittle nails and constipation

    B. Dry skin and cold intolerance

    C. Edema and weight gain

    D. Diarrhea and weight loss

30. Which of the following is true about initiation of levothyroxine therapy in the elderly?

    A. Response time is much quicker

    B. Levels should be checked in 1 week

    C. Lower doses are required

    D. Higher doses are required

31. Which of the following is the normal laboratory range for thyroid-stimulating hormone?

    A. 0.7–1.9 ng/dL

    B. 0.4–4.0 mIU/L

    C. 4.6–12 ug/dL

    D. 80–180 ng/dL

32. Which of the following is the most sensitive indicator of overall thyroid function?

    A. TSH

    B. Free T3

    C. Thyroxine

    D. Free T4

Lesson 7: Thyroid Cancer

33. After a complete thyroidectomy, a patient complains that she is experiencing muscle twitches, abdominal pain, polydipsia, and polyuria. The nurse practitioner thinks that the patient is experiencing a complication from her surgical procedure. The nurse practitioner believes the patient is suffering from:

    A. Thyroid storm from excessive hormones released during the thyroidectomy

    B. Diabetes insipidus from damage to the hypothalamus during the thyroidectomy

    C. Hypercalcemia from damage to the parathyroid glands during the thyroidectomy

    D. Hypercortisolemia from damage to the adrenal glands during the thyroidectomy

34. The nurse practitioner knows that risk factors for thyroid cancer include all of the following except:

    A. A family history of multiple endocrine neoplasia

    B. Being female

    C. A personal history of being exposed to head or neck radiation

    D. Inherited genetic predisposition to neurological conditions

35. The nurse practitioner is educating a patient on typical expectations status post thyroidectomy. The nurse practitioner makes the patient aware of the need for lifelong:

    A. Antineoplastic medication—such as lenvatinib (Lenvima)—due to a high thyroid cancer recurrence

    B. Hoarseness due to the unavoidable vocal cord damage

    C. Dysphagia due to the unavoidable esophageal damage

    D. Hormone replacement with levothyroxine (Synthroid), as thyroidectomy eliminates the body's ability to produce any thyroid hormone

36. Diagnostic testing for thyroid cancer can include:

    A. T3 and T4

    B. Large needle biopsy

    C. Endoscopy

    D. Neck ultrasound

ANSWERS AND EXPLANATIONS

Lesson 1: Addison's Disease

1. A

A malfunctioning immune system **(A)** is the most common cause of AD. Metastatic cancer to the kidneys and adrenal glands (B), steroid use (C), and medication use (D) are all potential causes of Addison's, but they are not the most common cause.

2. B

Hypotension **(B)** is a sign of Addison's disease. Glucose intolerance (A), acne (C), and hypertension (D) are all signs of Cushing's syndrome.

3. C

The gold standard test for Addison's disease is morning serum cortisol level **(C)**. Elevated BUN (A), elevated plasma renin (B), and serum electrolytes showing hypokalemia and hyponatremia (D) are all possible indicators of Addison's, but they not the gold standard. The results could be indicative of other conditions.

4. B

Addison disease is often missed by clinicians and is difficult to pinpoint due to is vague symptoms **(B)**. Hyperkalemia, hyponatremia, and hyperpigmentation (A) are symptoms of Addison's disease but are not readily recognizable; AD is not easily diagnosed. AD is not similar to Cushing syndrome (C). It could be said they are "opposites." AD features cortisol insufficiency, while Cushing syndrome features hypercortisolism. AD can originate from the hypothalamus (D) or any portion of the hypothalamic-pituitary-adrenal axis.

5. C

Severe leg, back, or abdominal pain **(C)** are symptoms of adrenal crisis. Adrenal crisis is not associated with excitability (A) or hypertension (B) (hypotension is seen). Craving of sweets (D) is not seen with adrenal crisis.

6. D

Hyperthyroidism **(D)** is a potential differential diagnosis for AD. Cushing syndrome (A) features hypercortisolism, not cortisol insufficiency, and would not be a differential diagnosis. Osteoporosis (B) and depression (C) are not potential differential diagnoses.

Lesson 2: Diabetes

7. D

There are often no signs **(D)** of gestational diabetes: that is why maternal testing is needed (especially in patients with risk factors like obesity or a previous high-birthweight baby). Glycosuria (A) can be present in pregnancy without GD. Vision changes (B) can be related to hyperglycemia but could be attributed to many other things and are rarely present with GD. Polyuria (C) is rarely present as a sign of hyperglycemia with GD.

8. B

Prediabetic patients have a fasting glucose of 100–125 mg/dL **(B)**. A result less than 100 mg/dL (A) is a normal result. A result of 126–150 mg/dL (C) or 150–200 mg /dL (D) can be indicative of diabetes.

9. B

The peak age for developing type 1 diabetes is 10–14 years old **(B)** and 4–7 years old. Patients 1–2 years old (A) and 16–18 years old (C) are not the peak age to develop type 1 diabetes. Although type 1 diabetes can develop in early adults (D), there is no "peak" adult age.

10. C

Dehydration **(C)** is a feature of DKA. Dehydration can also be a feature of hyperosmolar hyperglycemic non-ketoacidosis (HHNK), but a plasma glucose greater than 600 mg/dL (A), serum bicarbonate greater then 15 mEq/L (B), and serum pH greater than 7.3 are all hallmarks of HHNK, not DKA.

11. D

Cirrhosis **(D)** is not a differential diagnosis for diabetes. It is typically caused by alcohol abuse or hepatitis B or C, and may cause symptoms such as jaundice. An unrelated liver condition, nonalcoholic fatty liver disease (NAFLD) has been associated with diabetes mellitus. Alcoholism (A) is a differential diagnosis for DM. Diabetes insipidus (B) can cause polyuria and polydipsia, mimicking DM, but this condition does not feature polyphagia and hyperglycemia. PCOS (C) is a differential for DM. The hormonal changes in PCOS can cause insulin resistance and hyperglycemia, thus mimicking DM.

12. A

Two separate Hgb A1c results of 6.5% or above **(A)** would prompt a diabetes diagnosis. An oral glucose tolerance test of 130 mg/dL (B) is normal, not a concern related to diabetes. A fasting plasma glucose test of 120 mg/dL (C) is considered prediabetes. A one-time random glucose test of 150 mg/dL (D) would not be definitive: a diagnosis would require that the patient exhibit signs of diabetes and a serum glucose level greater than 200 mg/dL.

Lesson 3: Cushing Syndrome

13. D

Metabolic syndrome **(D)** shares features in common with Cushing syndrome such as truncal obesity and hypertension. Anxiety (A), hyperthyroidism (B), and tuberculosis (C) share features with Addison's disease.

14. B

Ketoconazole (Nizoral) **(B)** is a medication used for Cushing syndrome. Rifampin (Rifadin) (A) is an anti-tuberculosis medication. Prednisone (Sterapred) (C) is a steroid; the nurse practitioner would want to reduce steroid use, not increase it. Hydroxychloroquine (Plaquenil) (D) is an anti-malarial/antirheumatic medication.

15. D

Moon face (a round face) **(D)** is a hallmark sign of Cushing syndrome. Bronzed skin (A), weight loss (B), and orthostatic hypotension (C) can be signs of Addison's—that is, of hypocortisolism, not hypercortisolism.

16. D

Tapering off exogenous steroids **(D)** is used to treat Cushing syndrome. Corticosteroid replacement (A) is used to treat Addison's disease. Parathyroid gland removal (B) may treat hypercalcemia caused by a parathyroid gland disorder, but it would not help treat Cushing syndrome. Propranolol (C), a beta-blocker, is used to treat hypertension that may be associated with Cushing, but it does nothing for the overproduction of cortisol.

17. A

Hyperkalemia **(A)** is a sign of Addison disease, not Cushing syndrome. Striae (B), hyperglycemia (C), and hirsutism (D) are all potential signs of Cushing.

18. B

About 80% of Cushing sufferers have hypertension **(B)**. While irregular menses (A) is a potential sign of Cushing, only female Cushing sufferers could have irregular menses (thus not 80% of the total Cushing population). Hypotension (C) and hypocortisolism (D) are associated with Addison's, not Cushing.

Lesson 4: Hypoglycemia

19. C

While one may see seizures, diarrhea and chest pain **(C)** are not symptoms typical of hypoglycemia. Signs and symptoms noted in choices (A), (B), and (D) are common in episodes of hypoglycemia.

20. D

An oral glucose tolerance test **(D)** can replicate the conditions in which hypoglycemia would be present and aid in the diagnosis of a hypoglycemic disorder. It is measured after a patient fasts for 8 hours without food/fluid. A 72-hour fasting plasma glucose is used, rather than a 12-hour fasting blood glucose (A). An insulin-induced hypoglycemia test (B) is used to diagnose adrenal insufficiency. A CT scan (C) can diagnose insulinomas, but does not replicate the conditions of hypoglycemia.

21. A

The symptoms of hypoglycemia do not mimic those of myocardial infarction **(A)**, but can be mistaken for a TIA (B), CVA (C), or cardiogenic shock (D).

22. C

Symptoms of hypoglycemia include sweating, shakiness, and headache **(C)**. Indigestion (A), diarrhea (B), and dry mouth (D) are not symptoms of hypoglycemia.

23. B

A patient should ingest 15–20 grams **(B)** of fast-acting glucose to treat hypoglycemia. (A), (C), and (D) are incorrect.

Lesson 5: Metabolic Syndrome

24. B

A triglyceride level $\geq$150 mg/dL **(B)** is a component of the diagnostic criteria for metabolic syndrome. A triglyceride level of 100 mg/dL (A) is within normal levels. Triglyceride levels of 200 mg/dL (C) and 250 mg/dL are greater than diagnostic criteria.

25. C

HDL-C **(C)** is the fifth component that makes up the diagnostic criteria for metabolic syndrome. Albumin (A), total cholesterol (B), and LDL-C (D) are not diagnostic criteria.

26. A

Gynecoid obesity **(A)** is found in the hips and gluteal regions and is less likely to result in metabolic syndrome. Visceral (B), intra-abdominal (C), and central (D) obesity all describe the type of obesity that leads to metabolic syndrome.

27. B

Cardiovascular disease **(B)** is a complication of metabolic syndrome, not a risk factor for its development. Obesity (A), smoking (C), and a sedentary lifestyle (D) are all risk factors for developing metabolic syndrome.

28. C

The goal blood pressure should be $\leq$140/90 **(C)**. Normal recommended blood pressure is 120/80 (A).

Lesson 6: Thyroid Disorders

29. D

Diarrhea and weight loss **(D)** are associated with hyperthyroidism. Brittle nails and constipation (A), dry skin and cold intolerance (B), and edema and weight gain (C) are signs and symptoms of hypothyroidism.

30. C

Lower doses of levothyroxine are required **(C)** in the elderly. Response times are not quicker (A) in the elderly. Levels should be checked in 6–8 weeks, not 1 week (B). Higher doses (D) are not required in the elderly.

31. B

Normal range of TSH is 0.4–4.0 mIU/L **(B)**. Normal free T4 is 0.7–1.9 ng/dL (A). Normal total T4 is 4.6–12 ug/dL (C). Normal total T3 is 80–180 ng/dL (D).

32. A

Thyroid-stimulating hormone (TSH) **(A)** is the most sensitive indicator of overall thyroid function. It provides a sensitive and specific evaluation of circulating free T3 and free T4. Triiodothyronine (T3) (B) is one of two major hormones produced by the thyroid gland; the other is thyroxine (C). Free T4 (D) refers to the amount of circulating thyroxine.

Lesson 7: Thyroid Cancer

33. C

Muscle twitches, abdominal pain, polydipsia, and polyuria are consistent with hypercalcemia **(C)**. Classic symptoms of thyroid storm (A) would include tachycardia, hypertension, and fever. While polydipsia and polyuria and even muscle cramps can occur with diabetes insipidus (B), the hypothalamus is not near the thyroid gland and should not be damaged during a thyroidectomy. The patient's symptoms are not consistent with hypercortisolemia (D); also, the adrenal glands are not near the thyroid and should not be damaged during a thyroidectomy.

34. D

Inherited genetic predisposition to thyroid conditions, not neurological conditions **(D)**, pose a risk of thyroid cancer. A family history of multiple endocrine neoplasia (A), being female (B), and a personal history of being exposed to head or neck radiation (C) are all believed to be risk factors for thyroid cancer.

35. D

Following a thyroidectomy, a patient will need lifelong hormone replacement with levothyroxine (Synthroid) **(D)**, as thyroidectomy eliminates the patient's ability to produce her own. Antineoplastic medication (A) may be a possible treatment, but it would not be lifelong. Lifelong hoarseness (B) and lifelong dysphagia (C) are adverse outcomes that can follow a thyroidectomy, but they are not unavoidable.

36. D

A neck ultrasound **(D)** is used for diagnostic testing for thyroid cancer. T3/T4 (A) levels are usually normal in thyroid cancer, but levels can help in differential diagnosis. Fine needle, not large needle (B), biopsy is used. Laryngoscopy, not endoscopy (C), is used for diagnostic testing.

CHAPTER 14

Hematologic

LESSON 1: ANEMIAS

Learning Objectives
- Define key characteristics of common anemias
- Identify diagnostic criteria for common anemias
- Select appropriate treatment options for common anemias

Anemia is defined as a decrease in red blood cell (RBC) mass or reduced number of circulating RBCs, not just a drop in hemoglobin (Hgb) lab value. Anemia is not a disease, but rather a condition reflective of an underlying, existing problem.

Anemia is discovered and quantified by measurement of RBC count, Hgb concentration, and hematocrit (Hct), yet the lab data must be interpreted cautiously, as it can be affected by changes in plasma volume (i.e., dehydration elevates these levels and increased plasma volume in pregnancy can lower them without affecting the RBC mass).

Assessment

Initially, anemia can go unnoticed. Presentation varies and patients are often asymptomatic unless the Hgb is less than 10 g/dL. Signs and symptoms emerge as the anemia worsens—untreated, reduced oxygenation carrying capacity has consequences.

Detailed questions can help determine the etiology:

- Age, ethnic background
- Females: menstrual history (duration, frequency, flow) and pregnancy (whether patient is currently pregnant or has a history of anemia with any prior pregnancy)
- Jaundice, abdominal pain, change in bowel habits (tarry stools or those indicating malabsorption)
- Fatigue, history of anemia, previous transfusions, rejection as a blood donor
- Changes in body weight (suggestive of malabsorption, wasting disease of infectious, metabolic, or neoplastic origin, thyroid disease)
- Medication (prescription, OTC, vitamin and herbal supplements) and dietary practices/restrictions

Subjective

The patient may report shortness of breath, tachycardia, and irregular heartbeat, which reflect the initial oxygen deficit and the body's attempt to compensate. Other symptoms include fatigue, lightheadedness, dizziness, and decreased exercise tolerance.

Objective

Physical examination may be unremarkable unless the anemia is severe. Patients may present with pallor (conjunctiva or mucous membranes, nail beds, and palmar creases). Gradual onset may lead to functional and cognitive decline, coronary and pulmonary insufficiency; rapid onset (such as blood loss) results in hypovolemia, hypotension, and hypoxia. A rectal and pelvic examination cannot be neglected, because tumor or infection of these organs can be the cause of anemia.

Type/etiology	Distinguishing physical sign
Anemia of chronic disease (ACD) • Decreased RBC production (decreased activity of bone marrow, inadequate erythropoietin production, decreased response to erythropoietin) • Increased RBC loss or destruction	Fatigue, pallor
Iron deficiency anemia (IDA) • Blood loss or poor absorption • Inadequate iron stores	Extreme fatigue, pallor
Vitamin B12 deficiency anemia • Inadequate absorption or poor dietary intake/low levels of B12 • Examples: pernicious anemia, s/p gastrectomy, ETOH abuse	• Smooth, beefy red tongue, often sore • Neurologic changes (paresthesia, weakness, loss of coordination, loss of proprioception)
Folic acid deficiency anemia • Inadequate absorption or poor dietary intake	Sore tongue, cheilosis, and symptoms associated with steatorrhea *Not characterized by neurological changes*
Thalassemia • Abnormal Hgb lead to hemolysis • Risks for alpha thalassemia: Asian, African ancestry • Risks for beta thalassemia: African, Mediterranean, Middle Eastern ancestry	Beta thalassemia major: pallor, weakness, jaundice, organomegaly, poor growth, pubertal delay
Hemolytic anemia • Mechanical causes, infection, autoimmune disease lead to destruction of RBCs in the bloodstream or spleen • Congenital/inherited (e.g., sickle cell) or acquired (e.g., ABO incompatibility) • Consider if abrupt fall in Hgb or significant reticulocytosis • Presence of spherocytosis or RBC fragments on peripheral smear	Icterus, jaundice, dark-colored urine
Sickle cell anemia • Inherited hemolytic anemia • Hemoglobin protein is abnormal, making red blood cells rigid; they clog the circulation because they are unable to flow through small blood vessels	• Fatigue, jaundice, pain crises from vascular occlusion • In infants and toddlers, painful swelling of the feet and hands may be the first indication of the condition
Aplastic anemia • Bone marrow failure leads to destruction or deficiency of blood-forming stem cells in the bone marrow, resulting in an inadequate number of RBCs, WBCs, and platelets • The few cells that are made are normal	• Pancytopenia with symptoms of anemia and thrombocytopenia, recent infections, fever, and skin rashes • For diagnosis, 2 of the following: Hgb <10 g/dL; platelet count <50 × 109/L; absolute neutrophil count <1.5 × 109/L

Table 14.1.1 Type of Anemia, Etiology, and Distinguishing Physical Characteristics

Diagnosis

Anemia is classified by etiology, reticulocyte response, and lab value descriptions.

Etiology

- Blood loss: gastrointestinal bleed, NSAID use, menstrual bleeding
- Decreased production of RBCs: kidney problem, marrow problem (iron deficiency, vitamin deficiency, bone marrow and stem cell problems, sickle cell anemia)
- Destruction of RBCs: hemolysis or bleeding (infection, drugs, toxins, autoimmune attack, HTN, clotting disorders, enlargement of the spleen)

Order a complete blood count, with platelet count with automated differential (includes RBC indices and morphology on manual differential) and a reticulocyte count (percent and number). Adult male and female values are provided below. Pediatric values vary by age.

Hemoglobin, Hematocrit

The ratio of Hgb: Hct is 1:3 (e.g., Hgb 12 g/dL: Hct 36%) and remains relatively consistent, but may be altered with severe fluid volume overload or deficit. African Americans have Hgb levels of 0.5–1 g/dL lower on average:

- Male: Hgb: 14–18 g/dL, Hct: 40–54%
- Female: Hgb: 12–16 g/dL, Hct: 37–48%

Mean Corpuscular Volume (MCV)

MCV is a reflection of RCV size (volume) and is used to define the etiology of anemia. Values are as follows:

- Microcytic: MCV <80 fL (small cell)
- Normocytic: MCV 80–100 fL (normal size cell)
- Macrocytic: MCV >100 fL (abnormally large cell)

Mean Cell Hemoglobin Concentration (MCHC)

The MCHC is the average hemoglobin concentration in the red blood cells. Normochromic refers to normal color when the MCHC is 32–37 g/dL. Hypochromic refers to pale color of the RBC when the MCHC is less than 32 g/dL.

Red Cell Distribution Width (RDW)

The RDW indicates the degree of size variation among circulating RBCs. A value less than 15% is normal. Above 15% can be an early indication of either microcytic or macrocytic anemia.

Reticulocyte Count

The body's normal response to anemia is to create new cells (reticulocytes). The reticulocyte count is a measure of the proportion of immature RBCs in the blood. A value of 1–2% is normal. The absolute reticulocyte count is best used in anemic states.

If anemia is present on CBC and corrected reticulocyte index <2.5, classify by RBC indices.

Anemia is commonly classified according to cell size (normocytic, microcytic, and macrocytic) and cell color (hypochromic or normochromic).

	Normocytic, hypochromic	Microcytic, hypochromic	Macrocytic, normochromic
RBC indices	• Normal MCV, MCHC, RDW • Cells of normal size, normal color, and about the same size	• Low MCV, MCHC, high RDW • Small cells due to insufficient hemoglobin; new cells are smaller than old cells	• High MCV, normal MCHC, high RDW • Large cells with normal hemoglobin; new cells are larger than old cells
Order	• Total iron binding capacity • Serum Iron • Ferritin	• Total iron binding capacity • Serum Iron • Ferritin	• Vitamin B12 • Folate
Test results	• High TIBC • Low iron • Low ferritin	• Low/normal TIBC • Low/normal iron • Normal/high ferritin	• Vitamin B12 <200 pg/mL • Serum folate <2.5 ng/mL
Suggest	Anemia of chronic disease (ACD)	• Inflammation • Chronic disease • Thalassemia: order Hgb electrophoresis to confirm diagnosis	• Deficit B12: may order Schilling test to dx lack of intrinsic factor/pernicious anemia • Folate deficiency

Table 14.1.2 Anemia Type, Description, Additional Tests, and Possible Etiologies

Plan

Treatment

Treatment differs depending on anemia type.

Anemia	Treatment and follow-up
Anemia of chronic disease	• Manage underlying pathophysiology • Recombinant human erythropoietin (epoetin alfa), SQ or IV 3 times a week • Hct increase ~4% in 2 weeks • Iron deficiency anemia often presents as ACD; supplemental iron needed
Iron deficiency anemia	• Elemental iron 300 mg daily, in divided doses • Ferrous sulfate (65 mg elemental iron in 325 mg tablets) is better absorbed than ferrous gluconate • In children <12 years of age, prescribe 3 mg/kg elemental iron (as ferrous sulfate) given once daily with juice, not milk, and not with a meal • Iron stores (serum ferritin): 4–6 months to return to normal levels • Serum iron: reflect recent intake; return to normal earlier than serum ferritin levels • Hgb: return to normal after 2–4 weeks of treatment • Reticulocytosis noted in 3–10 days
Vitamin B12 deficiency anemia	• Vitamin B12 100 mcg/day IM × 7 days, then weekly × 4, then monthly • In oral form, vitamin B12 is inconsistently absorbed • Concurrent iron supplementation as needed • Neurological symptoms (if present <6 months) should resolve
Folic acid deficiency anemia	• Folic acid 0.5–1 mg/day (with usual dose being 1 mg daily) • Treat underlying cause • Preconception counseling • Prenatal vitamin for the pregnant patient

Table 14.1.3 Anemia Treatment and Follow-Up

Anemia	Treatment and follow-up
Thalassemia	• Alpha thalassemia (mild forms) may not require specific treatment, except to manage low hemoglobin levels (as needed) • Beta major (Cooley anemia): long-term transfusion therapy (to maintain the patient's hemoglobin level at 9–10 g/dL), iron chelation, and supportive measures (folic acid replacement and monitoring for complications such as pulmonary hypertension, osteoporosis, bone fractures, poor dentition, and heart failure) • Beta minor: usually requires no treatment

Table 14.1.3 Anemia Treatment and Follow-Up (Continued)

Referral

Certain findings warrant a referral. For example: if anemia is present on CBC and corrected reticulocyte index ≥ 2.5, order a peripheral smear and refer, and, if findings are consistent with a type of anemia that would be beyond the scope of primary care (such as sickle cell anemia or aplastic anemia), seek consultation and/or make the appropriate referral.

Takeaways

- Presentation is highly variable, yet initial symptoms may include shortness of breath, tachycardia, irregular heartbeat, fatigue, lightheadedness, dizziness, and decreased exercise tolerance.
- Anemia is commonly classified according to cell size and cell color.
- Treatment of anemia depends on the underlying etiology.

LESSON 2: LYMPHOMAS

Learning Objectives
- Define key characteristics of lymphomas
- Identify diagnostic criteria for lymphomas
- Select appropriate treatment options for lymphomas

Lymphomas are an assorted family of neoplasms characterized by undisciplined cell reproduction of lymphocytes, a subtype of white blood cells. These neoplasms typically originate in lymph-associated sites such as the thymus, lymph nodes, bone marrow, and the spleen. There are two kinds of lymphoma: Hodgkin lymphoma and non-Hodgkin lymphoma.

Non-Hodgkin lymphoma (NHL) represents a group of more than 60 cancers that account for about 4% of cancers in the United States. About 70,000 adults and children are diagnosed with NHL yearly. Some examples of NHL include: mycosis fungoides, Sézary syndrome, and primary central nervous system lymphoma.

Hodgkin lymphoma (HL) represents a group of six cancers and is much less common than NHL. According to the National Institutes of Health, about 0.2% of men and women will be diagnosed with HL at some point during their lifetime. Fewer than 10,000 new cases are reported in the U.S. each year. It is rare in patients under 5 years old, and is more commonly seen in ages 20–30 and over 55. Classic HL accounts for more than 90% of all cases of HL. Nodular sclerosis is the most common form of classical HL.

NHL and HL have a similar presentation. Differentiating between them requires biopsy and histological examination. NHL can develop from B-lymphocytes or T-lymphocytes; more than 85% of NHL is derived from B-lymphocytes. Histology shows malformed cells called Reed-Sternberg cells and Hodgkin cells in HL. Cells proliferate to crowd out normal white blood cells, leaving the immune system impaired.

Assessment

A number of risk factors and conditions are associated with NHL and HL lymphomas:

- PMH of the following: immune conditions like rheumatoid arthritis, systemic lupus, and sarcoidosis; mononucleosis caused by Epstein-Barr virus; ulcerative colitis
- FH of lymphoma
- Immune suppression/deficiency (such as use of immunosuppressive drugs and HIV)
- Exposure to ionizing radiation associated with NHL

The signs and symptoms of NHL and HL are similar.

Subjective	Objective
• Fatigue • Bone pain • Pruritus	• Typically asymptomatic lymphadenopathy (in areas like axilla, groin, side of neck) • Unexplained weight loss (>10% in 6 months) • Cough • Hepatosplenomegaly • Fever (>100.4°F/38°C) • Night sweats

Table 14.2.1 Subjective and Objective Characteristics of Lymphoma

Pro Tip

The five-year survival rate for HL is around 85% (depending on patient age and metastasis). If HL is localized (has not metastasized), the five-year survival rate is >90%.

Though it has not been established as a cause of HL, Epstein-Barr virus has been associated with nearly half of all cases.

The five-year survival rate for NHL is around 71% (again, dependent on patient age and metastasis). If the NHL is localized, the five-year survival rate is around 83%.

The incidence of NHL has been increasing 1–2% annually since the 1970s.

Diagnosis

Diagnostic methods include:

- Excisional biopsy of an intact node: considered the gold standard; fine needle aspiration or even core biopsies are not considered definitive diagnostically, as they may not offer enough information
- Bone marrow aspiration and biopsy
- CBC with differential: thrombocytopenia, leukopenia, and anemia
- Serum protein electrophoresis: monoclonal immunoglobulin spike is associated with some types of B-cell lymphomas
- Serum lactate dehydrogenase: elevation due to multiple tumors
- Flow cytometry: information about how fast tumors are growing, if from B-lymphocytes or T-lymphocytes
- Serum electrolytes: hypercalcemia or other electrolyte changes
- Uric acid level: elevated due to tumor burden/tumor lysis

- Computed tomography scan
- Positron emission tomography scan
- Chest x-ray
- HIV testing: if a suspected underlying condition

Differential Diagnosis

Differential diagnoses for lymphoma include **mononucleosis, HIV, toxoplasmosis, sarcoidosis, autoimmune disease, another form of cancer (leukemia, small cell lung cancer)**

> **Pro Tip**
>
> Leukemia and lymphoma are both blood cancers. Leukemia (an overproduction of malfunctioning white blood cells) can be differentiated from lymphoma in that leukemia tends to cause petechiae, easy bruising, and easy bleeding due to reduced platelets, and often causes anemia due to reduced red blood cells. *For more on leukemia, see Chapter 14, Lesson 5.*

Plan

Treatment

Treatment Options for Lymphoma
Chemotherapy
Stem cell transplant (from donor or autologous), to reestablish immune function after chemotherapy
Radiation therapy
Immunotherapy, such as monoclonal antibodies
Tyrosine kinase inhibitors (Inhibit cancer growth)
Surgery (rare)

Table 14.2.2

Education

Improved treatments have made both HL and NHL prognoses more favorable. However, patients (especially those who received radiotherapy) should be vigilant for the appearance of secondary cancers (such as breast cancer), cardiovascular complications (due to cardiotoxic chemotherapy treatments), decreased fertility (due to radiation and/or cytotoxic agents), and neurological sequelae (such as memory impairment or progressive multifocal leukoencephalopathy).

Referral

Referral to a hematologist/oncologist is needed (diagnostic and treatment planning as well as long-term surveillance). Cardiology may also be involved if cardiotoxic treatments end up compromising the heart.

Takeaways

- HL and NHL are blood cancers. NHL is more common and has a slightly less favorable overall survival rate than HL.

- Differentiation between the HL and NHL requires histological examination.

- The gold standard for diagnosis in lymphoma is excisional biopsy of an intact lymph node.

LESSON 3: MULTIPLE MYELOMA

Learning Objectives
- ■ Define key characteristics of myelomas
- ■ Identify diagnostic criteria for myelomas
- ■ Be aware of appropriate treatment options for myelomas

Multiple myeloma is the most common malignant tumor originating in bone. It accounts for about 1% of all cancers in the U.S., with an annual incidence of about 4–5 cases per 100,000 people and about 15,000 new cases per year.

Assessment

Risk Factors

- African American (2–3 times more common than Caucasian Americans)
- Increased body mass
- Male (slightly more common than females)
- >65 years of age (<2% of patients are under 40 at diagnosis; only about 10% are under 50)
- Agricultural occupations/exposure to herbicides, working with petroleum products, and/or working with plastics or heavy metals (more studies are needed; these associations are weak)
- Monoclonal gammopathy of undetermined significance (MGUS)—premalignant plasma cell disorder

Pro Tip
While multiple myeloma is the most common bone cancer that originates in bone, the most common malignancies in bone are derived from metastasis—that is to say, from a primary cancer originating elsewhere in the body.

Subjective

- Bone pain
- Loss of appetite
- Fatigue

Objective

- Osteolytic lesions
- Unexplained anemia, leukopenia, and thrombocytopenia (resulting from decreased production of these cells in bone marrow)
- Hypercalcemia (excessive calcium from breakdown of bone)
- Renal insufficiency/kidney failure (excessive proteins produced by myeloma cells and hypercalcemia; calcium crystals overtax and damage the kidneys)
- Weight loss
- Mental confusion (increased viscosity of blood from excess protein may decrease cerebral perfusion)
- Frequent infections (bone marrow dysfunction results in leukopenia)
- Spinal cord compression (if weakened spine collapses and puts pressure on nerves)
- Hepatosplenomegaly

Diagnosis

Diagnostic methods include:

- Magnetic resonance imaging (MRI): visualize osteolytic lesions (>5 mm)
- CT scan: visualize soft tissue changes (Note: contrast dye typically not used to avoid exacerbating kidney failure in an already compromised multiple myeloma patient)
- PET scan: visualize organs and tissues that may be affected
- Bone marrow biopsy: determine how many myeloma cells have infiltrated bone marrow
- Bone x-rays: discover bone damage
- CBC with differential: check RBC, WBC, platelet levels
- CMP: assess electrolyte levels, total protein, albumin, BUN, creatinine, uric acid
- Serum free light chain testing: elevated levels of immunoglobulin light chains expected in multiple myeloma (≥100)
- Quantitative immunoglobulins: check immune system status (deficiency in immunoglobulin levels)
- Serum protein electrophoresis: look for abnormal antibodies, such as monoclonal immunoglobulins or "M proteins"
- Fat pad aspirate: sometimes M proteins deposit in fatty areas of body (amyloidosis)

Differential Diagnosis

Differential diagnoses for multiple myeloma: **osteomyelitis, arthritis (mono/polyarticular), amyloidosis, neuroplastic osteoarthropathy (Charcot joint), avascular necrosis, Paget's disease, stress fracture(s)**

> **Pro Tip**
> The hypercalcemia often experienced by multiple myeloma patients can be mild or severe (>18 mg/dL). Treatment of hypercalcemia can include hydration, corticosteroids, bisphosphonates, or even calcitonin. Severe hypercalcemia may require hemodialysis.

PLAN

Treatment

- Stem cell replacement
- Chemotherapy
- Immunomodulators
- Radiation
- Surgery (usually not curative, but for symptom relief)
- Management of complications and end organ damage

Education

Multiple myeloma patients should be on the lookout for any adverse sequelae and report suspicious symptoms to their provider. Symptoms may include:

- Nausea/vomiting, increased thirst, confusion, constipation, weakness: could indicate hypercalcemia
- Decreased urine output: could indicate worsening kidney function
- Breathing difficulties: could indicate anemia
- Frequent infections: could indicate immune compromise

Patient should also avoid falls or trauma (using assistive devices as needed), as their bones may be weakened and damaged.

Referral

Hematology/oncology, pathology, and nephrology may be involved in the diagnostic and treatment plans for multiple myeloma.

Takeaways

- Multiple myeloma should be considered in patients >65 years old with bone pain or other bone-loss related symptoms (especially in African American patients).
- Providers must be prepared to manage a range of possible sequelae for multiple myeloma patients, including management of anemia, leukopenia, thrombocytopenia, possible hypercalcemia, kidney failure, frequent infections, and neurocompromise.

LESSON 4: THROMBOCYTOPENIA

Learning Objectives

- Define key characteristics of thrombocytopenia
- Identify diagnostic criteria for thrombocytopenia
- Recognize possible causes of thrombocytopenia

Thrombocytopenia is defined as a platelet count that falls beneath the normal range of 150,000–450,000/microL in adults. Thrombocytopenia may result from increased destruction of platelets, decreased production, and sequestration (congregation of the platelets in the spleen, resulting in decreased circulation).

Assessment

Risk Factors/Potential Causative Factors of Thrombocytopenia	
Medication	• quinine (Qualaquin) • rifampicin (Rifampin) • trimethoprim-sulfamethoxazole (Bactrim) • Measles-mumps-rubella vaccine • Heparin-induced thrombocytopenia (HIT): HIT can be mild, with a drop in platelets after heparin initiation with a subsequent return to normal values; it can be serious, in an immune-mediated form where the body forms antibodies against the heparin (Note: a drop in half of the platelet count in a recent heparin patient, even if the value is within normal range, should raise suspicion for HIT)
Underlying medical conditions	• Disseminated intravascular coagulation • Sepsis • Pulmonary embolism • Liver disease • Immune thrombocytopenia: an alteration in immune response leads to this common acquired bleeding disorder (characterized by increased platelet destruction and inhibited megakaryocyte platelet formation) • Mononucleosis • Cytomegalovirus • Aplastic anemia • Systemic lupus • HIV (immune dysfunction is associated with thrombocytopenia in HIV patients, along with other blood cell abnormalities such as anemia) • Bone marrow pathology (any disease that may affect WBC, RBC, and platelets)
Treatment-related	Chemotherapy
Alcohol abuse	In addition to folate deficiency and splenomegaly
Pregnancy	As a component of HELLP syndrome
Splenomegaly	Platelets can congregate in the spleen instead of circulating normally throughout the body

Table 14.4.1

Subjective
- Fatigue
- Dizziness
- Weakness
- Bruising easily

Objective
- Petechiae, often on the lower legs
- Purpura
- Prolonged bleeding from even minor lacerations/cuts
- Menorrhagia
- Tarry stools (or other signs of occult GI bleeding)
- Hematuria
- Jaundice

- Epistaxis (nosebleeds) and/or bleeding gums
- Altered mental status (which may indicate brain bleed)
- CBC (reflecting low platelet values)

> **Pro Tip**
>
> For comparison, having >450,000 platelets/microL is considered thrombocytosis.
>
> Thrombocytopenia is generally a sign of another underlying condition, and is often accidentally discovered through a routine blood draw.
>
> In pregnant women with low platelet counts, providers should be sure to exclude HELLP syndrome, a variant of preeclampsia that features hemolysis, elevated liver enzymes, and low platelet count. Patients with HELLP may exhibit changes in vision, abdominal pain/difficulty breathing from liver distention, hypertension, and proteinuria.
>
> In patients >60 years of age, thrombocytopenia should prompt consideration of underlying bone marrow cancer or lymph-related disorders, such as lymphoma.
>
> Thrombocytopenia combined with fever should prompt a nurse practitioner to ask about recent travel and consideration of rickettsial infections (such as Rocky Mountain spotted fever), Ebola, and mosquito-borne illnesses such as malaria and dengue fever.

Diagnosis

Diagnostic methods include:

- CBC with differential
- Visual examination (may see petechiae, purpura, etc.)
- Blood smear (to examine blood cells microscopically)
- Bone marrow testing
- PT/PTT and INR (to evaluate clotting time)
- CT scan or ultrasound of spleen (to check for abnormalities of spleen and/or liver)

Differential Diagnosis

- Congenital diseases such as May-Hegglin anomaly: autosomal dominant disorder featuring giant, often malformed platelets
- Chronic liver disease: may cause platelet breakdown and platelet sequestration in the spleen so that while the overall number of platelets is normal, many are not circulating
- Pseudothrombocytopenia: an error in lab sampling in which platelets clump together, leading to a lower total count than is actually present
- Hemophilia: genetic disease of abnormal or missing clotting factors

Plan

Treatment

Treatment of thrombocytopenia depends upon the underlying cause. For example, thrombocytopenia caused by alcohol abuse typically reverses itself in a few days after alcohol abstinence. If heparin-induced, cessation of the heparin typically reverses the condition. Even in cases of HIV, once patients are treated with antiretroviral therapy, the incidence of thrombocytopenia decreases. Thrombocytopenia is harder to treat with involved medical conditions, such as disseminated intravascular coagulation (DIC) or sepsis. In some cases, the patient is treated with steroids or platelet replacement.

> **Pro Tip**
> Thrombotic thrombocytopenic purpura (TTP) and idiopathic thrombocytopenic purpura (ITP) are both disorders that involve platelets. In TTP, there is spontaneous platelet aggregation (platelets are overused), and in ITP, there is a failure of the blood to clot (overall failure or simply a delay in clotting). The same symptoms result: easy bleeding and bruising. TTP is treated with blood transfusions; ITP is treated with steroids.

Education

Pregnant patients, patients with HIV, patients undergoing chemotherapy, those taking heparin (especially <10 days initiation), and patients with known alcohol abuse should be advised to report signs of low platelets such as excessive nosebleeds, bruising, or petechial rash.

Referral

Depending on the cause of the thrombocytopenia, various specialists may be involved. These may include hematology (if underlying blood disorder), oncology (if underlying cancer), hepatology (if underlying liver dysfunction), and infectious disease (if underlying HIV infection or other infectious agents).

Takeaways

- Newly discovered thrombocytopenia may be the first sign of an HIV infection; HIV testing may be warranted.
- The mechanism of thrombocytopenia is typically destruction of platelets (such as in DIC) or reduction in platelet formation (such as with aplastic anemia).
- Treatment depends on the underlying cause. Removing an offending cause like medication can help reverse thrombocytopenia. In many cases, thrombocytopenia may be a symptom of a complicated underlying condition such as sepsis, which may involve a multipronged treatment approach.

LESSON 5: LEUKEMIA

> **Learning Objectives**
> ■ Describe the presenting signs and symptoms associated with leukemia
> ■ Distinguish laboratory findings consistent with leukemia
> ■ Identify appropriate treatment options for leukemia

Leukemia is a primary malignancy of the bone marrow in which the normal components are supplanted by abnormal white blood cells. Additionally, the rampant overgrowth of those cells may cause displacement of other blood cells, resulting in pancytopenia and placing the patient at risk for anemia and bleeding.

Leukemia is classified as either lymphocytic or myelogenous. Additionally, each type may occur as either an acute or chronic form of malignancy. Acute lymphoblastic leukemia (ALL) occurs more commonly in children. It is the most common type of malignancy in childhood, with 85% of cases occurring in children between 2–5 years old. In contrast, chronic lymphoblastic leukemia (CLL) mainly affects older adults. While acute myelogenous leukemia (AML) is the second most common type of leukemia in children, with a peak incidence in adolescence, chronic myelogenous leukemia (CML) rarely occurs in children. The average age of CML at diagnosis is 64 years old. Complications of leukemia include metastasis to the bone, central nervous system, or other organs; alterations in childhood growth and development; late effects of neurocognitive function problems; and cardiovascular, ocular, metabolic syndrome, reproductive, or thyroid dysfunction.

Leukemia treatments have advanced significantly over the past 50 years. Survival is dependent upon quick initiation of appropriate leukemia-fighting therapies.

Definitions

- **Absolute neutrophil count (ANC):** a measure of the total number of neutrophils (segmented and banded)
- **Leukocytosis:** increased numbers of white blood cells
- **Lymphoblast:** an immature lymphocyte
- **Myelogenous:** non-lymphocyte white blood cells
- **Neutropenia:** abnormally few neutrophils
- **Pancytopenia:** deficiency of red blood cells, white blood cells, and platelets

Assessment

Subjective

Risk factors	Associated leukemia
Down syndrome, neurofibromatosis, and other genetic syndromes	ALL, AML
Ionizing radiation exposure	ALL, AML, CML
Benzene exposure	AML
Household pesticide in utero and first 3 years of life	Childhood ALL
Prior chemotherapy treatment	Adult ALL
Herbicide (agent orange) exposure	CLL

Table 14.5.1 Risk Factors for Leukemia

Symptoms

- Fever (ALL)
- Lethargy (ALL)
- Bleeding or bruising (ALL, AML)

> **Pro Tip**
> Many patients with chronic leukemia are asymptomatic at the time of diagnosis, with marked leukocytosis being found incidentally when a CBC is drawn for another reason.

Review of Systems

- **Constitutional:** fatigue, malaise (common in acute leukemia, less common in chronic leukemia), weight loss (adult ALL, AML), night sweats (CML), fever
- **Resp:** shortness of breath (ALL, CLL)
- **GI:** abdominal pain, nausea, vomiting (childhood ALL)
- **Neuro:** headache (childhood ALL)
- **MS:** spine or long bone pain (ALL)
- **Immunologic:** recurrent infection (CLL, childhood ALL)

Objective

- Abdominal tenderness (ALL)
- Hepatomegaly (ALL, CLL)
- Splenomegaly (ALL, CLL, CML)
- Lymphadenopathy (ALL, CLL)
- Pallor (ALL)
- Petechiae, purpura, bruising (ALL)
- Salmon-colored or blue-gray papular lesions (AML)
- Subcutaneous nodules (AML)
- Leukocytosis

> **DANGER SIGN** Signs of increased intracranial pressure such as headache, vision changes, or vomiting may indicate central nervous system invasion. Refer to the nearest emergency department for further evaluation and treatment.

Diagnosis

When leukocytosis is noted on a CBC, a repeat CBC is indicated. Predominance of lymphocytes could indicate asplenia or splenic sequestration. Lymphocytosis may also occur with cytomegalovirus (CMV), Epstein-Barr virus (EBV), pertussis, or tuberculosis infection, and they should be ruled out. It is recommended that a peripheral smear be obtained if any of the following are also present:

- WBC count >20,000
- Anemia
- Significantly increased or decreased platelet levels
- Unexplained fatigue, fever, or weight loss
- Lymphadenopathy, hepatomegaly, or splenomegaly

A predominance of atypical lymphocytes may occur with CMV, EBV, or HIV infection. An increase in normal-appearing lymphocytes, lymphoblasts, or other precursor blood cells could indicate the presence of leukemia. Hematology and oncology are generally involved in the diagnosis and treatment of leukemia. They will perform bone marrow aspiration or biopsy and determine the need for cytogenetic testing, flow cytometry with immunophenotyping, and molecular testing (which further delineates the genetic composition of the leukemia, which along with patient age and comorbid conditions will determine the course of treatment).

Plan

Treatment

Treatment Options for Leukemia
Chemotherapy—ALL most often includes several phases: induction of remission, consolidation, and maintenance with CNS prophylaxis provided in all stages; relapses of leukemia often require reinstitution of chemotherapy
Corticosteroids
Immunotherapy (particularly monoclonal antibodies)
Tyrosine kinase inhibitors
Hematopoietic stem cell transplantation
Radiation therapy (CLL)
Splenectomy (CLL)

Table 14.5.2

Education

Educate patients about the importance of a nutritious diet and adequate rest. Patients and their caregivers and close contacts should avoid sick contacts and crowds while receiving chemotherapy. If fever occurs, seek medical attention. If the absolute neutrophil count is low due to chemotherapy, the patient may be at risk for overwhelming infection. Counsel patient to seek support systems of leukemia survivors.

Referrals

All patients with suspected leukemia should be referred to a hematologist/oncologist.

Takeaways

- Acute lymphocytic leukemia is highly treatable when treatment is initiated early; refer patients with suspected ALL to a hematologist/oncologist quickly.
- Patients with chronic leukemia may be asymptomatic upon diagnosis, with leukocytosis being discovered incidentally.
- When leukocytosis is present on the CBC, repeat the specimen and consider other causes such as CMV, EBV, pertussis, or tuberculosis infection.

PRACTICE QUESTIONS

Select the ONE best answer.

Lesson 1: Anemias

1. Folate deficiency anemia causes which of the following changes in the RBC indices?

   A. Normocytic, normochromic

   B. Macrocytic, hypochromic

   C. Microcytic, normochromic

   D. Microcytic, hypochromic

2. Mary, age 30, had a CBC drawn at her last visit. It indicated that she has microcytic hypochromic anemia. Further testing showed iron deficiency anemia. She was treated with ferrous sulfate 325 mg TID. The following month, a CBC was done, with the following results:

   - Hgb 12.5 g/dL (normal (12–16 g/dL)
   - Hct 36% (normal 35–46%)
   - MCV 84 fL (normal 81–96 fL)
   - Ferritin 25 ng/dL (normal 12–156 ng/dL)

   The most appropriate action is:

   A. Cut back on the iron supplement to BID

   B. Perform a fecal occult blood test

   C. Start her on vitamin B12 supplementation

   D. Continue the present course of treatment

3. Martha has a low mean cell volume (MCV), low mean cell hemoglobin concentration (MCHC), and normal red cell distribution (RDW). What should you consider in terms of diagnosis?

   A. Renal disease

   B. Iron deficiency anemia

   C. Thalassemia

   D. Pernicious anemia

4. Vitamin B12 deficiency anemia causes which of the following changes in the RBC indices?

   A. Normal MCV, MCHC, RDW

   B. Low MCV, MCHC, high RDW

   C. Low MCV, MCHC, normal RDW

   D. High MCV, normal MCHC, high RDW

5. Jack is diagnosed with microcytic, hypochromic anemia (low MCV, low MCHC). Iron and iron binding capacity and ferritin labs are ordered. What finding suggests iron deficiency anemia?

   A. Low iron, high TIBC, low ferritin

   B. Low iron, low TIBC, normal ferritin

   C. High iron, low TIBC, high ferritin

   D. Normal iron, normal TIBC, high ferritin

6. You examine a 75-year-old female who presents with history of DM and rheumatoid arthritis. Her DM has been fairly well controlled with insulin. No significant abnormal findings are found on exam. Lab tests reveal:

   - Hgb 10.1 g/dL (normal (12–16 g/dL)
   - Hct 31.3% (normal 35–46%)
   - RBC 3.65 million mm^3 (normal 4.7–6.1 million mm^3)
   - MCV 81 fL (normal 81–96 fL)
   - TIBC 195 mcg/dL (250–450 mcg/dL)
   - Iron 80 mcg/dL (normal 25–170 mcg/dL)
   - Ferritin 25 ng/dL (normal 12–156 ng/dL)

   These values are most consistent with:

   A. Anemia of chronic disease

   B. Iron deficiency anemia

   C. Thalassemia

   D. Pernicious anemia

Lesson 2: Lymphomas

7. The five-year survival rate for lymphoma is:

   A. Higher for non-Hodgkin lymphoma (NHL) than for Hodgkin lymphoma (HL)

   B. Higher for Hodgkin lymphoma (HL) than for non-Hodgkin lymphoma (NHL)

   C. The same for Hodgkin lymphoma (HL) and non-Hodgkin lymphoma (NHL)

   D. Poor, as with all cancers of the blood

8. Lymphoma survivors need to be vigilant for the appearance of adverse sequelae. Which of the following is not an adverse sequela?

   A. Breast cancer

   B. Cardiac failure

   C. Reduced fertility

   D. Frequent infections

9. The gold standard of diagnosis for lymphoma is:

   A. Fine-needle aspiration

   B. Core biopsy

   C. Excisional biopsy of an intact node

   D. Chest x-ray of lymph node sites

10. A definitive sign/symptom associated with Hodgkin lymphoma (HL) is:

    A. Cough

    B. Pruritus

    C. Night sweats

    D. Reed-Sternberg cells

11. Which of the following is not a risk factor/condition associated with lymphoma?

    A. Family history of rheumatoid arthritis

    B. Personal history of ulcerative colitis

    C. Exposure to ionizing radiation

    D. HIV

12. Non-Hodgkin lymphoma (NHL) represents a group of more than 60 cancers. Which of the following is not contained within this group?

    A. Mycosis fungoides

    B. May-Hegglin anomaly

    C. Sézary syndrome

    D. Primary central nervous system lymphoma

Lesson 3: Multiple Myeloma

13. Most bone cancer originates:

    A. From elsewhere in the body (metastasizing from other cancer sites such as the breast)

    B. In the bone itself

    C. As a sequela from bone trauma

    D. From monoclonal gammopathy of undetermined significance (MGUS)

14. Sequelae associated with multiple myeloma include all of the following except:

    A. Osteolytic lesions

    B. Hypercalcemia

    C. Renal failure

    D. Liver failure

15. Multiple myeloma typically affects patients in:

    A. Childhood

    B. Adolescence

    C. Late adulthood

    D. Early adulthood

16. Diagnostic tests for multiple myeloma may include all of the following except:

    A. Bone marrow biopsy

    B. Serum free light chain testing

    C. Serum protein electrophoresis

    D. Peripheral blood smear

17. Hypercalcemia associated with multiple myeloma can cause symptoms such as:

    A. Irritability

    B. Nausea/vomiting

    C. Diarrhea

    D. Decreased thirst

Lesson 4: Thrombocytopenia

18. When calling a patient back regarding a platelet count of 120,000 platelets/microL and a recheck two weeks later of 99,000 platelets/microL, it is most important to do which of the following?

    A. Advise the patient to avoid alcohol

    B. Advise the patient to have platelets rechecked in one month

    C. Obtain a thorough and up-to-date medication list

    D. Inquire if they are bruising more easily than usual

19. Which of the following is not a possible cause of thrombocytopenia?

    A. Cholecystitis

    B. Sepsis

    C. Measles, mumps, and rubella vaccine (MMR)

    D. Mononucleosis

20. Kira is a 55-year-old female with a history of type 2 diabetes and hypertension. Her meds include metformin (Glucophage) 1000 mg BID, glipizide (Glucotrol) 10 mg BID, glargine insulin (Lantus) 20 units subcutaneously, lisinopril (Zestril) 20 mg daily, rosuvastatin (Crestor) 20 mg daily, and sulfamethoxazole-trimethoprim (Bactrim) 400/80 mg once daily. She was recently started on rosuvastatin for cardiovascular protection and Bactrim for recurrent cystitis. The results of recent laboratory tests are as follows: WBC 8.2 cells/mm^3, RBC 4.3 million cells/mm^3, hemoglobin 13 g/dL, hematocrit 42%, platelets 110,000/microL, A1C 6.8, TC 195, TG 110 mg/dL, LDL 75 mg/dL, and HDL 42 mg/dL. Based on the lab results, what would be the next step in the plan of care?

    A. Increase rosuvastatin dose

    B. Discontinue lisinopril

    C. Decrease glipizide dose

    D. Discontinue Bactrim

21. Which of the following is not a sign or symptom of thrombocytopenia?

    A. Jaundice

    B. Tinnitus

    C. Hematuria

    D. Excessive menstrual flow

22. A routine CBC/differential done on a 28-week pregnant patient reveals a platelet count of 97,000/microL. The plan of care for this patient should include:

    A. Immediate referral to the patient's obstetrician, as the low platelet count could indicate HELLP syndrome

    B. Immediate referral to the patient's obstetrician, as the low platelet count could indicate preterm labor

    C. Advising the patient to notify the obstetrician if she develops bleeding gums, nosebleeds, blood in urine, or blood in stool

    D. Discontinuing prenatal vitamins, as the vitamins can cause low platelets

Lesson 5: Leukemia

23. Which of the following is a risk factor for the development of acute lymphoblastic leukemia?

    A. Agent orange exposure

    B. Benzene exposure

    C. Genetic syndrome

    D. Cystic fibrosis

24. A patient has recently been diagnosed with leukemia. Which of the following symptoms would the nurse practitioner expect to see given this diagnosis?

    A. Nausea, headache, and confusion

    B. Petechiae, fatigue, and fever

    C. Abdominal pain, irritability, and psychosis

    D. Hypotension, bradycardia, and weight loss

25. Splenomegaly may be an objective finding with all of the following leukemias except:

    A. Acute lymphocytic leukemia (ALL)

    B. Acute myelogenous leukemia (AML)

    C. Chronic lymphoblastic leukemia (CLL)

    D. Chronic myelogenous leukemia (CML)

26. The family nurse practitioner (FNP) is reviewing a complete blood count (CBC) report, which shows a white blood cell (WBC) count of 19,000 cells/mm^3 for a patient complaining only of fatigue. Upon repeat CBC, the WBC count is 19,700 cells/mm^3. Which lab test should the FNP order next?

    A. Bone marrow aspiration

    B. Blood culture and sensitivity

    C. Epstein-Barr virus titer

    D. Peripheral blood smear

ANSWERS AND EXPLANATIONS

Lesson 1: Anemias

1. C

Folate deficiency anemia presents as microcytic, normochromic (**C**). Normocytic, normochromic cells (A) suggest anemia of chronic disease. Macrocytic, hypochromic (B) is not a normal presentation of anemia. Microcytic, hypochromic (D) suggests iron deficiency anemia or thalassemia, depending on the RDW.

2. D

The normal Hgb/Hct lab values suggest the current treatment is effective. Serum ferritin stores may take 4–6 months to return to normal levels. Thus, continuing the present course of treatment (**D**) is appropriate. There is no indication that the iron supplement should be cut back (A) and no indication of internal bleeding, thus no need for fecal occult blood test (B). There is no need for vitamin B12 supplementation (C).

3. C

Thalassemia (**C**) presents as microcytic, hypochromic, with normal RDW. Renal disease (A) presents as normocytic, normochromic anemia with normal RDW. Iron deficiency anemia (B) presents as microcytic, hypochromic, with elevated RDW. Pernicious anemia (D) presents as macrocytic, normochromic, with elevated RDW.

4. D

Vitamin B12 presents as a macrocytic, normochromic anemia with elevated RDW (**D**). Normal MCV, MCHC, RDW (A) is seen with anemia of chronic disease. Low MCV, MCHC, high RDW (B) is seen with iron deficiency anemia. Low MCV, MCHC, normal RDW (C) is seen with thalassemia.

5. A

Iron deficiency anemia presents with low iron, high TIBC, low ferritin (**A**). Low iron, low TIBC, normal ferritin (B) is seen with thalassemia or inflammation. High iron, low TIBC, high ferritin (C) is the opposite of what is expected. Normal iron, normal TIBC, high ferritin (D) is not a normal combination of labs re: anemia.

6. A

Anemia of chronic disease (**A**) presents as MCV low or normal, serum iron levels low or normal, and ferritin levels high or normal. This is reflected in the lab values. Anemia of chronic disease can be difficult to differentiate from iron deficiency anemia (B), but iron deficiency anemia presents with low MCV, low serum iron levels, and low ferritin levels. Thalassemia (C) presents with low MCV, low or normal serum iron levels, and low ferritin levels; and with pernicious anemia (D), we would expect a high MCV.

Lesson 2: Lymphomas

7. B

The five-year survival rate is higher for HL (**B**) than for NHL (A). The overall five-year survival rate for non-Hodgkin lymphoma (NHL) is about 71%, compared to Hodgkin lymphoma (HL) at about 85%. The survival rates are not the same (C). The five-year survival rate of lymphoma is good, not poor (D), as are the prognoses of many blood cancers. New treatments are extending the survival rates.

8. D

Frequent infections (**D**) are not potential adverse sequelae of lymphoma. Breast cancer (A), cardiac failure (B), and reduced fertility (C) are all adverse sequelae.

9. C

An excisional biopsy of an intact node (**C**) is the gold standard for diagnosis of lymphoma. Fine-needle aspiration (A) and core biopsy (B) are recognized diagnostic options, but they are not definitive. Chest x-rays of lymph node sites (D) may be used as an ancillary tool, but do not offer histological information and are not definitive.

10. D

The presence of Reed-Sternberg cells (**D**) on histological analysis are definitive for Hodgkin lymphoma (HL). Cough (A), pruritus (B), and night sweats (C) are all possible signs of HL, but none are definitive. They could be found in other conditions.

11. A

Family history of rheumatoid arthritis (**A**) is not a risk factor for lymphoma. Personal history of rheumatoid arthritis is a risk factor. Personal history of ulcerative colitis (B), exposure to ionizing radiation (C), and HIV (D) are all risk factors/conditions associated with lymphoma.

12. B

May-Hegglin anomaly (**B**) is not a type of NHL; it is a congenital disease that causes malformed platelets. Mycosis fungoides (A), Sézary syndrome (C), and primary central nervous system lymphoma (D) are all considered forms of NHL.

Lesson 3: Multiple Myeloma

13. A

Most bone cancer originates from elsewhere in the body (**A**). It is the result of metastasis and does not originate in the bone itself (B). The sequela from trauma (C) is not a recognized causal factor for bone cancer. MGUS (D) is a well-known risk factor for multiple myeloma, but not for one cancer overall.

14. D

Liver failure **(D)** is not a sequela of multiple myeloma. Osteolytic lesions (A), hypercalcemia (B), and renal failure (C) are all possible sequelae associated with multiple myeloma.

15. C

Multiple myeloma typically affects patients in late adulthood **(C)**. Multiple myeloma is primarily a disease of older adults. Less than 2% of multiple myeloma patients are under 40 years old. Only about 10% are under 50 years old. It does not typically affect patients in childhood (A), adolescence (B), or early adulthood (D).

16. D

A peripheral blood smear **(D)** is not a diagnostic test used with multiple myeloma; it can be used in the diagnosis of leukemia. Bone marrow biopsy (A), serum free light chain testing (B), and serum protein electrophoresis (C) are all possible diagnostic tests associated with multiple myeloma.

17. B

Hypercalcemia can cause nausea and vomiting **(B)**. It does not cause irritability (A), diarrhea (C), or decreased thirst (D). In contrast, it can cause confusion, constipation, and increased thirst.

Lesson 4: Thrombocytopenia

18. C

In a patient with thrombocytopenia, it is most important to obtain a thorough and up-to-date medication list **(C)**, as medications can sometimes be the cause. When offending agents are stopped, thrombocytopenia often reverses. The patient should be advised to avoid alcohol (A), as alcohol abuse can be a cause. This answer is not inquiring about alcohol use, but simply telling the patient to avoid it. The patient should have platelets rechecked (B), but one month is too long. The platelet count has decreased by 21,000 in two weeks, so more frequent checks are needed. It would be expected for the patient to bruise more easily (D). This answer does not give clues to possible causes.

19. A

Cholecystitis **(A)** is not a possible cause of thrombocytopenia. Sepsis (B), the MMR vaccine (C), and mononucleosis (D) are all possible causes of thrombocytopenia.

20. D

Discontinuing Bactrim **(D)** would be the correct next step in the plan of care. The platelet count shows thrombocytopenia and could be related to recently starting the Bactrim. The lipid panel is normal and does not warrant an increase in the rosuvastatin dose (A). Based on the lab results, there is no reason to discontinue the lisinopril (B). The A1C is showing good control of diabetes, so a decrease in the glipizide dose (C) would be an incorrect action.

21. B

Tinnitus **(B)** is not a sign or symptom of thrombocytopenia. Jaundice (A), hematuria (C), and excessive menstrual flow (D) are all signs or symptoms of thrombocytopenia.

22. A

A low platelet count on a 28-week pregnant patient should prompt immediate referral to the patient's obstetrician, as the low platelet count could indicate HELLP syndrome **(A)**. The low platelet count does not indicate preterm labor (B). Notifying the obstetrician of bleeding gums, nosebleeds, blood in urine, or blood in stool (C) is important, but not the priority. Prenatal vitamins (D) cannot cause low platelets.

Lesson 5: Leukemia

23. C

Having a particular genetic syndrome **(C)** such as Down syndrome or neurofibromatosis is a risk factor for the development of ALL. Agent orange exposure (A) is a risk factor for CLL. Benzene exposure (B) is a risk factor for AML. Cystic fibrosis (D) is not a risk factor for the development of leukemia.

24. B

Leukemia, with its bone marrow involvement, would result in petechiae from low platelet count, fever related to infection given the low number of effective leukocytes, and fatigue from the low hemoglobin **(B)**. A patient may present with nausea, vomiting, abdominal pain, and weight loss, but headache and confusion (A), irritability and psychosis (C), and low blood pressure and heart rate (D) are not common symptoms.

25. B

Splenomegaly is not usually an objective finding with AML **(B)**, whereas it may be present with ALL (A), CLL (C), and CML (D).

26. D

In the instance of persistent leukocytosis without determined cause, the next step would be to obtain a peripheral blood smear **(D)** to further determine the types of white blood cells present. A bone marrow aspiration (A) would be performed by the hematologist or oncologist after referral. A blood culture and sensitivity (B) is not indicated, as the patient has fatigue and no other signs of infection. An Epstein-Barr virus titer (C) is obtained in the instance of mononucleosis-like symptoms and the presence of atypical lymphocytes.

CHAPTER 15

Immune

LESSON 1: INFECTIOUS DISEASE BASICS

Learning Objectives
- Define the chain of infection and the epidemiological triad
- Distinguish subjective, objective, and laboratory findings related to infectious disease(s)
- Identify the appropriate approach to the treatment of fever

Communicable diseases spread via a chain of infection. Stopping the chain of infection is important to the prevention of widespread disease. Infectious disease recognition and treatment are important skills of the family nurse practitioner. Certain groups such as the very young, the very old, and those who are immunocompromised are at significantly increased risk of more severe infection, such as sepsis.

Definitions

- **Chain of infection:** infectious diseases are transmitted when the infectious agent leaves the host or reservoir (through an exit portal) and is then conveyed to another susceptible host via a particular mode of transmission
- **Epidemiological triangle:** this triad consists of the offending agent and an interaction between the host and environment, resulting in disease
- **Incubation period:** the time period between when an individual is exposed to an infectious agent and when symptoms actually begin to appear

Here is an example of the chain of infection:

- A child in day care has diarrhea → the child's diaper is changed on a pad on the floor and the pad is not disinfected → a different child plays on the pad, putting his hands in his mouth afterwards

Assessment

Subjective
Risk factors:

- Very young age
- Day care or school attendance
- Close living quarters: dormitory, jail, barracks, or long-term care facilities
- Immunosuppression
- Known infectious exposure
- Lack of immunization

- In the newborn: maternal infection, prolonged/difficult delivery
- Recent surgery/invasive procedure
- Recent travel

Review of Systems

- **Constitutional:** fever, chills, night sweats, lethargy, malaise, poor infant feeding, poor appetite
- **HEENT:** eye pain/drainage/redness, ear pain or drainage, nasal discharge, sore throat, oral lesions, neck pain or stiffness
- **Resp:** cough
- **GI:** abdominal pain, nausea, vomiting, diarrhea
- **GU:** dysuria, urinary frequency or hesitancy, pelvic pain, vaginal or penile discharges
- **MS:** joint or bone pain
- **Neuro:** headache, dizziness, seizure
- **Skin:** wound drainage, sores, rash, purpura

> **DANGER SIGN** When neurological symptoms accompany any fever, immediate intervention is required.

Objective

Upon physical examination, note presence of symptoms reported by the patient. Note hyperthermia, tachypnea, or tachycardia. For rashes/skin lesions/wounds, note distribution, color/shape, and drainage. Note presence of eye, ear, nares, pharyngeal, or mouth redness. Determine presence of adventitious breath sounds. Note the patient's affect and energy level and, if a child, interaction with the parent or caregiver.

> **Pro Tip**
> Older adults ordinarily have a lower baseline temperature, thus may display less elevation in temperature with the presence of infection.

Laboratory and Diagnostic Testing

The white blood cell (WBC) count can be helpful in the differential diagnosis of an infectious disease. An elevated WBC count may indicate the presence of infection. Upon examination of the differential, the following elevated cell percentages may indicate:

- Banded neutrophils (bands): severe bacterial infection
- Basophils: parasitic infections
- Eosinophils: parasitic infections
- Lymphocytes: viral infection
- Monocytes: severe bacterial infections
- Neutrophils (polys and segs): acute bacterial infection

Culture and sensitivity (C&S) testing is not required for the diagnosis of all infectious disease, but when used may identify the offending microbe as well as narrow the choice of antimicrobial agents. C&S testing may be performed on blood or any type of body fluid. Elevated C-reactive protein (CRP) and erythrocyte sedimentation rate (ESR) levels may be used as adjuncts in the diagnosis of infectious presences. The CRP is a more sensitive indicator than ESR, and moderate to marked elevations in the CRP may indicate bacterial infection.

Diagnosis

The diagnosis of infectious diseases is made based upon the history and physical examination, and at times laboratory testing results. Fever is generally indicative of an infectious process. Pay particular attention to the length of the fever and the timing of associated symptoms. Rapid diagnosis is possible with appropriate consideration of the epidemiological triangle.

Plan

Treatment

Use antipyretics to reduce fever as needed. Lowering the patient's temperature reduces metabolic rate, lessens the perception of other symptoms, and generally results in the individual feeling somewhat better. Acetaminophen and ibuprofen work well in children; use one or the other to avoid the risk of overdose related to differing dosage amounts and dosing schedules. Do not use aspirin in children under 13 years of age to avoid the development of Reye syndrome. Acetaminophen is the preferred agent for fever treatment in older adults, as the side effect profile is preferred over NSAIDs.

The vast majority of infections (particularly respiratory) are viral in nature and require only symptomatic treatment. If a suspected viral infection persists, rather than resolves, within 7–10 days, further evaluation is needed. In the case of suspected or proven bacterial infection, prescribe the narrowest spectrum antibiotic possible in order to decrease the incidence of antibiotic resistance.

Institute transmission-based isolation precautions as appropriate in addition to standard precautions.

Type of precaution (examples)	Measures
Airborne: transmitted by airborne droplet nuclei or dust particles (measles, varicella, tuberculosis)	• Mask or respirator depending upon disease • Negative pressure room if hospitalized
Droplet: transmitted by droplets with close respiratory or mucous membrane contact (influenza, mumps, rubella, group A *Streptococcus*)	Mask within 3 feet of individual
Contact: transmitted by direct or indirect contact (multi-drug-resistant bacteria, respiratory syncytial virus)	Gloves and gown with patient contact

Table 15.1.1 Isolation Precautions

Education

Encourage appropriate immunizations as recommended to avoid infection with vaccine-preventable organisms. Tepid baths may be helpful in the treatment of fever, but be careful of chilling. Alcohol baths are not recommended. Encourage fluid intake to prevent dehydration related to fever (children and older adults in particular are at increased risk). In older adults, adequate protein intake, as well as folic acid, selenium, zinc, and vitamins C, E, B6, and B12 are recommended for the prevention of infection.

Referrals

Urgent referral/emergency room admission for:

- Febrile infant <3 months of age
- Febrile infant or child who is listless
- Any individual with suspected sepsis

Takeaways

- Infants and older adults are at higher risk for serious infection due to differences in their immune function.
- Elevated CRP is a more sensitive indicator of bacterial presence than an elevated ESR.
- Treat suspected or known bacterial infection with antibiotics.

LESSON 2: MISCELLANEOUS INFECTIOUS DISEASE ISSUES

Learning Objectives
- Differentiate clinical manifestations of infectious diseases
- Choose and interpret laboratory/diagnostic testing for infectious diseases
- Describe appropriate treatment and referrals for infectious diseases

Vector-borne diseases and infectious disease-causing agents of bioterrorism may cause significant morbidity and mortality, yet many of these diseases are highly treatable if accurately diagnosed early in the disease process. Vector-borne disease are most often transmitted via mosquito or tick, while bioterroristic infections can be transmitted in a variety of ways.

Mosquito

- Chikungunya (*Aedes aegypti, A. albopictus*)
- Dengue (*Aedes aegypti*)
- Malaria (*Plasmodium falciparum, P. malariae, P. ovale, P. vivax*)
- West Nile virus
- Yellow fever
- Zika virus

Tick

- Lyme (*Borrelia burgdorferi*)
- Rocky Mountain spotted fever (RMSF) (*Rickettsia rickettsia*)

Other

- Ebola virus disease (bat, primate, person-to-person)
- Lassa fever (rat)
- Marburg hemorrhagic fever (person-to-person)

- Rift Valley fever (infected livestock blood and body fluids, mosquito [less frequent])
- Anthrax (*Bacillus anthracis*)
- Botulism (*Clostridium botulinum*)
- Plague (*Yersinia pestis*)
- Smallpox (*Variola major, V. minor*)

Assessment

Mosquito

Determine potential exposure to infectious agents, travel outside of the U.S., and immunization status. Patients with mosquito-borne diseases present with various, nonspecific complaints that may include symptoms like fever, chills, joint/muscle/body pain, weakness, headache, or vomiting. Conjunctivitis is seen only with Zika virus.

> **DANGER SIGN** The patient with a history of mosquito bites who has become ill and develops hemorrhagic manifestations, such as petechiae or purpura, should be referred to the emergency room.

Tick

Persons with tick-borne infection may be asymptomatic or display certain clinical manifestations. Bell palsy can be a complication of Lyme disease.

Clinical manifestations	Lyme disease	RMSF
Fever	x	x
Erythema migrans	x	
Malaise	x	
Muscle aches	x	
Headache	x	x
Maculopapular rash		x
Vomiting, abdominal pain		x

Table 15.2.1 Distinguishing Tick-Borne Diseases

Other

With Ebola and Lassa, Marburg, and Rift Valley fevers, patients can present with fever, headache, muscle pain, or fatigue/weakness. In addition to these, specific to Ebola there can be diarrhea, vomiting, abdominal pain, and bleeding/bruising. Bleeding from gums/eyes/nose is seen with Lassa fever. Maculopapular rash is seen with Marburg hemorrhagic fever; back pain/dizziness with Rift Valley fever.

Clinical manifestations of illnesses caused by agents of bioterrorism are noted below.

Clinical manifestations	Anthrax	Botulism	Plague	Smallpox
Body aches				x
Buboes		x	x	
Chills	x			
Cutaneous eschar	x			
Descending paralysis		x		
Diplopia		x		
Fever	x		x	x
Headache				x
Mediastinitis	x			
Pneumonia/ARDS			x	
Rash (fluid-filled, pustular)				x
Sepsis			x	
Weakness		x		

Table 15.2.2 Distinguishing Illnesses Caused by Agents of Bioterrorism

Diagnosis

Diagnosis of a vector-borne illness may sometimes be based on history and physical examination alone. Laboratory testing that may serve to confirm the diagnosis includes antigen or antibody-specific enzyme-linked immunosorbent assay (ELISA), polymerase chain reaction (PCR), or nucleic acid testing (NAT). There is not a laboratory test for RMSF.

For illnesses caused by suspected agents of bioterrorism, contact the Laboratory Response Network (LRN) for guidance: **https://emergency.cdc.gov/lrn/contact.asp**. Order a CT scan or MRI scan if botulism is suspected to rule out central nervous system causes of paralysis. Additionally, rule out myasthenia gravis with a Tensilon test. Nerve conduction tests and electromyography may also be performed in the diagnosis of botulism. For plague, lymph node (bubo) aspirate may be sent for culture. Sputum culture or bronchial tracheal washing may also be helpful in the diagnosis of plague.

Plan

Treatment

Prescribe doxycycline for anthrax, RMSF, or Lyme disease. Within 48 hours of a concerning tick bite, prescribe a one-time dose of doxycycline 200 mg PO. If Lyme disease is diagnosed within the first 48 hours of the tick bite; the only treatment needed is one dose of doxycycline 200 mg orally. Additionally, anthrax may be treated with a monoclonal antibody. Antitoxins are available for botulism and inhalation anthrax. For plague, prescribe streptomycin, gentamicin, levofloxacin, or ciprofloxacin. The viral illnesses require supportive therapy only, as there are no curative treatments available.

Education

Encouraging rest and increasing PO fluid intake is recommended for all of the miscellaneous infectious disorders. Fever may be treated with antipyretics. If traveling to an endemic country, vaccination is recommended for yellow fever and malaria. To prevent mosquito and tick bites:

- Avoid mosquito-infested or tick-infested areas
- Wear light-colored protective clothing with long sleeves and pants tucked into socks
- Spray or rub on a chemical insect repellant containing DEET, permethrin, or picaridin
- Stay inside at dawn or dusk, when mosquitoes are most active
- Check adults, children, and pets daily for ticks
- Empty water from all potential outdoor vessels to avoid standing-water breeding grounds for mosquitoes

> **Pro Tip: Tick Removal**
> Grasp the tick at the base of head (closest to the person's skin) with fine-tipped tweezers; pull upward steadily. Cleanse the area well.

Referrals

- Complicated cases of vector-borne illness should be referred to the physician or appropriate specialist
- For infections suspicious of agents of bioterrorism, notify the bioterrorism emergency number at the Centers for Disease Control (CDC) Emergency Response Office: (770) 488–7100

Human Immunodeficiency Virus

Human immunodeficiency virus (HIV), the virus that causes AIDS, can be transmitted through sexual intercourse, by contact with contaminated blood, and by HIV-positive women to their infants during pregnancy or birth and when breastfeeding. HIV disease is caused by infection with retroviruses HIV-1 or HIV-2.

Assessment

No physical findings are specific to HIV. A patient with HIV may by asymptomatic or may present with flu-like illness (fever, malaise, and a generalized rash) or generalized lymphadenopathy. AIDS manifests as recurrent opportunistic infections, ultimately resulting in AIDS-associated dementia and HIV wasting syndrome.

Diagnosis

Early diagnosis of HIV is vital to prevent further transmission of the disease and begin prompt treatment. Recommendations from USPSTF, CDC, and ACP are similar, basically suggesting screening of all adolescents and adults at increased risk for HIV and all pregnant women. It is prudent to screen those seeking treatment for sexually transmitted infections and tuberculosis and those with physical findings consistent with HIV.

Rapid-testing kits are available; however, the most common means for diagnosing HIV is with a screening test (ELISA) and then confirmation with a second test (e.g., Western blot assay or similar).

Plan

The CD4 T-cell count is used as reference to the risk of acquiring opportunistic infections. As HIV infection progresses, the number of these cells declines. A normal range for CD4 cells is about 500–1,500. Antiretroviral therapy is started on patients with a CD4 count of 350 cells/μL or below; a CD4 count below 200 cells/μL is considered definitive for AIDS in the United States.

Highly active antiretroviral therapy (HAART) is the principal means of antiretroviral therapy. Treatment recommendations are age-specific. Antiretroviral therapy is started on patients with a history of an AIDS-defining opportunistic disease, a CD4 count of 350 cells/μL or below, those that are pregnant, and those with hepatitis B (HBV) or HIV-associated nephropathy. Along with HAART, prophylaxis for *Pneumocystis jiroveci* is important; trimethoprim-sulfamethoxazole (TMP-SMX; Bactrim) is generally prescribed.

HIV-infected individuals should be screened for common health problems, including diabetes, hypertension, dyslipidemia, osteoporosis, kidney and liver disease, depression, and tuberculosis. All patients should be vaccinated against influenza, pneumococcal infection, varicella, and hepatitis A and B. Consider routine screening for STIs including trichomoniasis, gonorrhea, and chlamydia, depending on the patient's sexual history.

Digital Resources

- HIV and the pregnant woman: consultation/referral with maternal fetal medicine (MFM)/infection disease specialist; for additional treatment guidelines including preconception, antepartum, intrapartum, and postpartum care, go to **https://aidsinfo.nih.gov/guidelines/html/3/perinatal/0**
- Prevention of opportunistic infections is an important aspect of care; additional information can be found at the following links:
  - **www.cdc.gov/hiv/basics/livingwithhiv/opportunisticinfections.html**
  - **https://aidsinfo.nih.gov/guidelines/html/4/adult-and-adolescent-oi-prevention-and-treatment-guidelines/0**

Referral

All new cases of HIV infection require consultation with an infectious disease specialist.

Methicillin-Resistant *Staphylococcus Aureus* (MRSA) Infection

MRSA infection began as a healthcare setting–related infection but is now contracted within the community, resulting in a high community prevalence of MRSA. A penicillin-binding protein encoded by the mecA gene (PBP-2a) permits *S. aureus* to grow and divide despite the use of beta-lactam antibiotics such as methicillin. MRSA infections begin primarily as skin and soft-tissue infections, yet may progress to more invasive infections.

Assessment

MRSA infection can occur in any person, but factors for increased risk include skin compromise (such as with eczema), bare skin contact with surfaces used by others (such as sauna benches and exercise mats), sharing of towels and other personal items, and day care centers. People who are at increased risk include jail/prison inmates and guards, military personnel, adults and children participating in contact sports, and men who have sex with men.

The patient or a child's parent may state a spider bite is present. A red bump or bumps, tenderness (furuncle), or itching (folliculitis) may occur.

Objective findings include:

- Erythema, edema, possible regional lymphadenopathy (cellulitis)
- Erythematous papule(s) or pustule(s) at hair follicle (folliculitis)
- Nodule(s) with larger area of erythema (furuncle)

Diagnosis

Diagnosis is often made solely upon history and physical examination findings. Polymerase chain reaction (PCR) or latex agglutination tests for mecA are diagnostic. Chromogenic agar may be used for rapid culture with results within 24–48 hours. Traditional culture may also be used. Asymptomatic MRSA colonization may be screened for with a culture from the anterior nares.

Plan

Treatment

Incise and drain abscesses. Treat localized infection without systemic involvement with oral antibiotics for 5 days, extending up to 14 days for more severe infections:

- Trimethoprim-sulfamethoxazole (TMP-SMX)
- Clindamycin
- Doxycycline or minocycline (do not use in children <9 years of age)

Reevaluate the patient within 24–48 hours of antibiotic initiation to determine response. To decolonize a MRSA carrier prior to a scheduled surgery, prescribe mupirocin ointment inserted in anterior nares twice daily for 7 days and daily bathing with chlorhexidine gluconate (2% or 4%) for 1 week.

> **Pro Tip**
> Do not use fluoroquinolones to treat MRSA infection of the skin and soft tissue due to the risk of antibiotic resistance.

Education

Handwashing is important in order to prevent the spread of MRSA via skin contact and respiratory secretions (coughing, sneezing). Instruct patients to contact nurse practitioner if not improving or worsening, and to finish entire prescribed course of antibiotics.

Referral

Refer patients with significant skin involvement or systemic illnesses for possible hospitalization and intravenous antibiotic treatment.

Takeaways

- Many of the miscellaneous infectious disorders result in fever and clinical symptoms; be sure to assess for distinguishing signs and symptoms.
- Lyme disease is distinguished from other tick-borne illnesses by the presence of erythema migrans.
- Of the bioterroristic agents, smallpox is distinguished by a fluid-filled rash, progressing to pustules.
- HIV is most often transmitted by sexual, perinatal, and parenteral means.
- MRSA infection may present as cellulitis, folliculitis, or furuncle.

PRACTICE QUESTIONS

Select the ONE best answer.

Lesson 1: Infectious Disease Basics

1. Which of the following white blood cell elevations as noted on the differential is associated with parasitic infections?

    A. Banded neutrophils
    B. Basophils
    C. Lymphocytes
    D. Neutrophils

2. Which of the following patients is at highest risk for significant infection?

    A. 27-month-old with a temperature of 102.7°F (39.3°C)
    B. 4-year-old with a temperature of 102.0°F (38.9°C)
    C. 15-day-old with a temperature of 100.8°F (38.2°C)
    D. 13-year-old with a temperature of 101.9°F (38.8°C)

3. An otherwise healthy adult has a cough, congestion, and fever. The nurse practitioner should be aware that:

    A. A fever of 102.0°F (38.9°C) indicates need for antibiotics
    B. Antibiotics are required for respiratory infections
    C. Acute onset indicates bacterial infection
    D. Respiratory infections are often viral

4. Which of the following white blood cell elevations as noted on the differential is associated with severe bacterial infections?

    A. Eosinophils
    B. Lymphocytes
    C. Monocytes
    D. Neutrophils

Lesson 2: Miscellaneous Infectious Disease Issues

5. Doxycycline is NOT recommended as a treatment for which of the following?

    A. Anthrax
    B. Lyme disease
    C. Rocky Mountain spotted fever
    D. Smallpox

6. The nurse practitioner is assessing a patient who reports new onset of diplopia and inability to move certain muscles. Which diagnosis does this suggest?

    A. Anthrax
    B. Botulism
    C. Ebola virus
    D. Lassa fever

7. Which of the following is not a likely diagnostic test for vector-borne illnesses?

    A. Enzyme-linked immunosorbent assay
    B. Nucleic acid test
    C. Polymerase chain reaction
    D. Tensilon test

8. The nurse practitioner is assessing a patient who presented with fever and rash. The nurse practitioner notes a red circular area with central clearing and concentric circles. What is the likely diagnosis?

    A. Marburg virus
    B. Lyme disease
    C. Rocky Mountain spotted fever
    D. Smallpox

9. The nurse practitioner is caring for a 4-year-old who attends day care and has two 1.5 cm furuncles on the lower extremity. In order to provide coverage for methicillin-resistant *Staphylococcal aureus* (MRSA), which of the following should the nurse practitioner prescribe?

   A. ciprofloxacin (Cipro)

   B. doxycycline (Vibramycin)

   C. minocycline (Minosin)

   D. trimethoprim-sulfamethoxazole (Bactrim DS)

10. A 34-year-old male patient has been diagnosed with HIV. The patient asks why more than one antiretroviral drug is needed. Of the following statements, which is the best reason for using more than one drug class?

    A. More drugs mean more cure

    B. More drugs inhibit viral replication

    C. More drugs prevent drug interactions

    D. More drugs decrease CD4+ T cells

ANSWERS AND EXPLANATIONS

Lesson 1: Infectious Disease Basics

1. B

Elevated basophil counts **(B)** are associated with parasitic infections, as are increases in eosinophils. Elevated bands (A) are associated with severe bacterial infection (as are monocytes), elevated lymphocytes (C) with viral infections, and elevated neutrophils (D) with acute bacterial infection.

2. C

Newborns **(C)** are at the highest risk for significant infection due to their immature immune systems and lack of exposure to infectious agents for development of antibodies. While young children (A and B) may exhibit a high fever with an infection, they are at less risk for severe infections, as their immune systems are more mature. Adolescents (D) have a mature immune system. The height of the fever is not indicative of the severity of the illness.

3. D

The vast majority of respiratory infections are viral **(D)** and require symptomatic treatment only, unless symptoms persist longer than 7–10 days, at which time further evaluation may be necessary. Antibiotics are not prescribed according to height of fever alone (A), nor are they recommended for most respiratory infections (B). Onset (C) is only one component of the history that is used to determine if the infection is likely to be bacterial or viral.

4. C

Elevated monocyte counts **(C)** are associated with severe bacterial infections, as are increases in banded neutrophils. Elevated eosinophils (A) are associated with parasitic infection, elevated lymphocytes with viral infections (B), and elevated neutrophils (D) with acute bacterial infection.

Lesson 2: Miscellaneous Infectious Disease Issues

5. D

Smallpox **(D)** is a viral illness, thus is not treated with an antibiotic. Anthrax (A), Lyme disease (B), and RMSF (C) are caused by bacteria that are susceptible to doxycycline.

6. B

Botulism **(B)** causes descending paralysis and diplopia. Anthrax (A) results from exposure to an agent of bioterrorism. Ebola virus (C) and Lassa fever (D) are hemorrhagic fevers.

7. D

The Tensilon test **(D)** is used in the diagnosis of myasthenia gravis. An enzyme-linked immunosorbent assay (A), nucleic acid test (B), or polymerase chain reaction (C) may be used to identify the offending virus in vector-borne illness.

8. B

A red concentric circle with central clearing is termed erythema migrans and is a key feature of Lyme disease **(B)**. Marburg hemorrhagic fever (A) and RMSF (C) present with a maculopapular rash. A pustular rash occurs with smallpox (D).

9. D

Trimethoprim-sulfamethoxazole **(D)** is recommended for the treatment of MRSA. Ciprofloxacin (A) should not be used in order to avoid resistance development. Doxycycline (B) and minocycline (C) are not routinely recommended for use in children under 9 years of age.

10. B

The advantage of using more than one class of antiretroviral drugs is that viral replication can be inhibited more than one way **(B)**, which makes it difficult for the virus to thrive. A combination of drugs does not necessitate more cure (A); HIV cannot be cured. Combination therapy will not prevent drug interactions (C); monotherapy will minimize that. CD4+ T cell counts increase with therapy, not decrease (D).

CHAPTER 16

Integumentary

LESSON 1: DERMATOLOGY BASICS

Learning Objectives

- Utilize knowledge of basic skin anatomy to assist in assessment and diagnosis of skin conditions
- Effectively categorize skin lesions
- Appropriately diagnose the presenting dermatological condition

Most patients' skin complaints are garden-variety, so much so that non-dermatologists have developed a two-part rule for dermatological care: "If it's wet, dry it, and if it's dry, wet it."

This rule of thumb may work well for some basic conditions, such as applying nystatin powder to macerated yeasty skin folds or applying emollient cream to overly dry skin. But dermatological conditions tend to be more complex than a two-part rule. Working knowledge of the most common basic dermatological conditions is necessary to offer initial treatment and to determine if a given skin disorder is cutaneous (as opposed to representing a superficial symptom of systemic illness) and whether the patient needs referral to specialty care.

Skin Basics

The skin is the largest organ. It provides a protective waterproof covering, safeguards us from infectious organisms, and allows for somatosensory perceptions such as cold, heat, and touch.

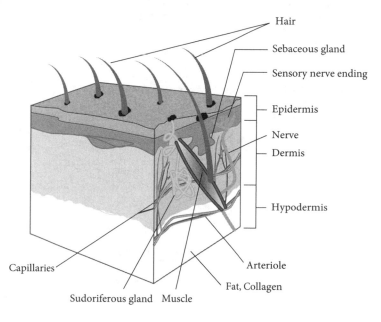

Figure 16.1.1 Anatomy of the Skin

Knowing skin anatomy can help in diagnosis and determining treatment plans for skin problems, specifically knowing if a condition can be treated by the nurse practitioner or if the patient should be referred to a specialist. For example, three related conditions—acne vulgaris, nodulocystic acne, and hidradenitis suppurativa—involve different structures of the skin and different modalities of treatment. Acne vulgaris may be superficial and appropriate for the FNP to treat. Nodulocystic acne is more involved; it can extend into the dermis, cause scarring, and may call for specialized care. Hidradenitis suppurativa can involve sinus tracts of purulent material tunneling deep beneath the skin, and will likely need specialized care.

Common Dermatological Conditions	
Acne	Occurs when hair follicles become clogged with oil and dead skin
Actinic keratosis	Rough, dry scaly patch caused by damage from exposure to ultraviolet radiation
Acrochordon	Small, soft, benign tumor, often associated with obesity; develops in areas where the skin creases (also known as skin tag)
Atopic dermatitis	Dry, pruritic, red rash; may weep and crust over, producing thick plaques of skin (also known as eczema)
Basal cell cancer	Painless raised area of skin; usually develops in sun-exposed areas; may present as sores, growths, bumps, red patches, or scars; may appear shiny with small blood vessels or may present as a raised area with ulceration
Contact dermatitis	Erythemic, pruritic rash or irritation caused by direct contact with a substance (an allergen or irritant)
Callus	Thickened or hardened part of the skin or soft tissue in response to repeated pressure, friction, or irritation
Cherry angioma	Benign tumors, containing an abnormal number of blood vessels (also known as red moles)
Cutaneous candidiasis	Fungal infection causing inflammation, burning, and itching, often in moist skin fold areas (also known as topical yeast infection)
Diaper rash	Sore, erythemic, scaly, and tender skin resulting from yeast infection or contact dermatitis
Keloids	Hypertrophied scar; may be pruritic
Lipoma	Soft tumors made up of adipose tissue
Molluscum contagiosum	Single (or more often several) small, raised, flesh-colored papules with a dimple in the center
Nevi	Birthmark or mole
Onychomycosis	Fungal nail infection; thickened nail with yellow discoloration is common
Psoriasis	Pruritic, erythemic plaque covered with silvery scales
Purpura	Purple-colored spots that do not blanch when pressure applied
Rosacea	Persistent redness (visible blood vessels) in the center of the face
Seborrheic dermatitis	Flaky skin, red scaly patches on scalp, and oily areas of body
Seborrheic keratosis	Brown, black, or tan wart-like lesions; may appear waxy and slightly elevated; common on the face and trunk
Herpes zoster	Painful rash with blisters along an affected dermatome (also known as shingles)
Squamous cell cancer	Thick, rough, scaly patches; elevated growths (similar to a wart); may crust and bleed

Table 16.1.1

Common Dermatological Conditions (Continued)	
Tinea pedis	Foot infection due to dermatophyte fungus (also known as athlete's foot)
Tinea versicolor	Discolored (hypo- or hyperpigmented) patches
Urticaria	Erythemic, raised, itchy welts or wheals (also known as hives)
Verruca vulgaris	Rough surfaced growths caused by some types of human papilloma virus (HPV)
Vitiligo	Lighter patches of skin due to loss of melanocytes (pigmented cells)
Xanthelasma	Yellowish plaques near the inner canthus of the eyelid caused by deposits of cholesterol underneath the skin
Xerosis	Dry skin (may be the result of aging or underlying disease)

Table 16.1.1

Assessment

Subjective

Dermatology often hinges on the clinician's keen eye and knowledge. A thorough exposure history is key for accurate diagnosis of skin lesions.

A patient's rendering of the details relevant to the skin condition may be straightforward: "I was gardening. I accidentally touched a plant with leaf clusters of three—one larger leaf and two smaller leaves off the sides, all with pointed tips. Now I am itchy."

But the nurse practitioner must also be aware that subjective information offered may be tangential or even completely misleading: "The lesion started with a recent spider bite."

Careful questioning and assessment by the clinician may unearth more salient information: the lesion doesn't itch or seem inflamed; it appeared months earlier; it did not improve with steroid application; and it is pearly in appearance. A skin biopsy may then reveal that the lesion originates in the basal cell layer and is in fact basal cell cancer.

Objective

Lesions are generally considered primary or secondary. Primary lesions are either present at birth (such as a birthmark) or caused by disease. Secondary lesions can develop from the original primary lesion or may be caused by the patient (such as the patient scratching poison ivy lesions). Be aware that this distinction is not inviolable: what might be considered a primary lesion in one condition may be considered secondary in another.

Assessment and diagnosis can be aided by precise dermatological descriptors of the kind of lesion presented.

Primary lesion	Description
Macule	A flat (non-palpable) skin lesion <1 cm differing in color from surrounding skin
Patch	A flat (non-palpable) skin lesion >1 cm differing in color from surrounding skin
Papule	A small, raised, often dome-shaped lesion <1 cm in diameter
Nodule	A larger raised palpable lesion >1 cm in diameter
Cyst	An encapsulated lesion filled with liquid or semi-solid material

Table 16.1.2 Dermatological Descriptors—Primary Lesions

Primary lesion	Description
Tumor	A solid lesion, usually >2 cm; it is larger than a nodule and deeper than a plaque (typically extending into the dermis) Note: the term "tumor" in this context does not necessarily imply a cancerous lesion
Plaque	A raised (plateau-like) lesion >1 cm
Vesicle	A raised <1 cm lesion filled with clear fluid (as opposed to purulent material)
Bulla	A raised >1 cm lesion filled with clear fluid
Pustule	A vesicle-like lesion containing pus/purulent material (as opposed to clear liquid)
Wheal	An area of raised edematous skin (also known as hives)
Burrow	An area of tunneled skin caused by a cutaneous insect infestation (such as scabies)
Telangiectasia	Dilated capillaries
Petechiae	Pinpoint-sized skin hemorrhages
Purpura	Larger area of skin hemorrhage (can be palpable or non-palpable)
Ecchymosis	Bruised area of skin

Table 16.1.2 Dermatological Descriptors—Primary Lesions (Continued)

Secondary lesion	Description
Fissure	A linear epidermal crack or tear that can extend to the dermis
Erosion	An area of lost (eroded) epidermal tissue
Lichenification	Thickened, often hyperpigmented skin (typically in areas that have been excessively scratched or rubbed)
Atrophy	Thinned or depressed skin due to loss of underlying dermal or subcutaneous tissue
Excoriation	Broken skin (typically superficial) due to patient scratching

Table 16.1.3 Dermatological Descriptors—Secondary Lesions

Pro Tip

The qualities of skin lesions can be summarized by the acronym **SKIN STATS**: shape, kind (of lesion), impression/appearance, number, size, timeline, arrangement, texture, and section/location on body. Lesion qualities can either rule in or rule out a diagnosis.

Quality	Explanation
Shape	<ul><li>Annular: ring-shaped</li><li>Discoid: disc-shaped</li><li>Targetoid: bull's-eye shaped</li><li>Guttate: teardrop shaped</li><li>Serpiginous: wavy, serpent-like in appearance</li><li>Reticular: net-like in appearance</li></ul>
Kind	<ul><li>Impression/appearance: pink, shiny, flaccid, etc.</li><li>Number: some lesions are unlikely to occur singly or grouped; for example, shingles manifest as multiple grouped vesicular lesions</li><li>Size can lead to a diagnosis; for example, a vesicle is <1 cm and bullae are >1 cm</li><li>Timeline: when the lesion was first noticed; if it changed over time, etc.</li></ul>
Arrangement	<ul><li>Linear: in a line</li><li>Clustered: in a group</li><li>Discrete: occurring singly</li><li>Dermatomal: occurring along a dermatomal zone, as in herpes zoster</li><li>Confluent: lesions that "flow" together</li><li>Exanthematous: widespread rash resembling the rash of measles (also called "morbilliform")</li></ul>
Texture	Palpable (raised), flat, rough, raised, thickened, sandpaper-like, etc.
Location	Focal, regional, or generalized; location can be specified, such as skin folds, groin, scalp, between toes, etc.

Table 16.1.4 Qualities of Skin Lesions

DANGER SIGN

- A lesion that won't heal
- A lesion that reoccurs
- A lesion that grows quickly, changes shape, changes appearance
- For breast tissue, area that appears dimpled/depressed or appears wrinkled (peau d'orange)
- For nails, a dark band of color extending into the cuticle; could be melanoma

---

Case Study

The following provides an example of the diagnostic process and plan in a dermatological case.

A 21-year-old man presents with a two-week history of facial rash. He reports it started as a red, flat lesion that evolved into a "fluid-filled bump" that ruptured, spilling clear fluid that, once dry, left a crust on his skin. He reports itching and burning, but no pain. He tried over-the-counter hydrocortisone cream, with no relief. He has no history of trauma or infection to the area. He reports the area was seemingly intact before the reddened area appeared. He denies fever, weakness, and any other lesions on his body.

On exam, the nurse practitioner finds perioral plaques and papules with an overlying honey-colored crust and an underlying moist erythematic base. Surrounding erythema is minimal.

The most likely diagnosis is impetigo. Given the history and physical, one can rule out acne vulgaris (comedones and pustules, but not plaques) and seborrheic dermatitis (erythematous patches and plaques with greasy, yellow scales).

Treatment includes a topical antibiotic and education to wash the area with antimicrobial soap and avoid touching the area, as well as good hand hygiene.

> **Digital Resource**
>
> The American Academy of Dermatology offers a basic dermatology review here: **www.aad. org/education/basic-derm-curriculum**.

Referral

If the patient desires removal for cosmetic purposes, the patient can be referred to a dermatologist or plastic surgeon. Refer any patient exhibiting a "Danger Sign," as noted previously.

Takeaways

- The acronym **SKIN STATS** can help in classifying lesions. It stands for: shape, kind, impression, number, size, timeline, arrangement, texture, and section/location on body.
- Skin assessment includes assessment of the scalp, oral cavity, and nails.
- In general, the dermatological plan depends on the condition, the level of involvement the patient presents, and the nurse practitioner's expertise.

LESSON 2: DERMATOLOGY/PHARMACOLOGY

> **Learning Objectives**
> - Select topical medications in relation to vehicle, acuity, area affected, frequency of use, and patient age
> - Understand steroid potency/strength
> - Recognize common dermatological medications and their possible adverse effects

Medications that are used for integumentary conditions can be oral or topical agents. Many of these medications are used for conditions that affect other body systems as well. Several are discussed in detail in the lessons of Chapter 4, as mentioned throughout this lesson.

Topical Medication Considerations

> **Pro Tip**
> When considering a topical medication, use the acronym "VALUES"
>
> - **V**ehicle
> - **A**cuity
> - **L**ocation
> - **U**se
> - **A**ge (Ag**E**)
> - **S**trength

Topical drugs are an important part of therapy for dermatologic disease.

- **Vehicle:** delivery system of the medication
  - **Creams:** tend to contain both oil and water, can be soothing, can leave oily residue (hydrocortisone cream for treatment of eczema)
  - **Foams:** easy to apply, dry quickly with little residue (econazole foam for treatment of tinea pedis)
  - **Gels (jelly-like):** can be alcohol- or water-based; tend not to be as occlusive as other vehicles and tend to dry quickly; often useful for hairy areas of body; can be associated with drying, peeling, irritation, erythema (tretinoin gel for treatment of acne)
  - **Lacquer:** Useful for applying to nails; leaves a film residue on treated surface (ciclopirox lacquer for onychomycosis)
  - **Lotions (to be applied on skin):** can be alcohol- or water-based; usually leave less residue, so good for hairy areas; can be associated with skin irritation (clindamycin lotion for treatment of hidradenitis suppurativa)
  - **Oils:** easy to apply, but can leave residue, feel greasy; tend to be less irritating than lotions (fluocinolone oil for scalp psoriasis)
  - **Ointments:** often petrolatum- or propylene-glycol-based; good for dry skin, but can leave greasy residue on clothes/skin; useful for thick lesions, as an ointment is thick and often occlusive; not very effective on hairy areas because it may mat on the hair, not reaching the skin (clobetasol ointment for psoriasis of acne)
  - **Powder:** drying effect, good for macerated skin (ketoconazole 2% powder for tinea versicolor)
  - **Shampoo:** easy to apply, limited time in contact with skin, so reduced chance of side effects such as burning
  - **Spray:** easy to apply, helpful for treating large areas; can accidentally come into contact with mucous membranes or eyes; can have side effects such as burning, stinging, and redness, depending on the formulation (hydrocortisone spray 1% for seborrheic dermatitis)
- **Acuity (severity):** less severe conditions require shorter courses of treatment than more severe conditions
- **Location (affected area):** areas with thicker skin (such as the soles of the feet) can usually withstand stronger topicals than more fragile areas (such as the face)
- **Use (frequency of use):** a less potent medication may be prescribed more frequently than a more potent medication; patient adherence may be less with more frequent dosing
- **Age:** in general, the skin of infants, children, and the elderly is thinner, and they are more prone to adverse effects; caution with prescribing strong occlusive topicals, such as clobetasol ointment
- **Strength** (potency and concentration):
  - **Potency:** high-potency steroids like clobetasol (Temovate) are stronger than weaker steroids such as hydrocortisone (Synacort)
  - **Concentration:** the higher the percentage, the stronger the medication (e.g., hydrocortisone [Synacort] cream 2.5% is stronger than hydrocortisone cream 1%; caution when making concentration comparisons between steroids of differing potencies [e.g., Temovate cream 0.05% is in a higher potency class than hydrocortisone 2.5% cream, so even though the hydrocortisone 2.5% has been prepared at a higher concentration than hydrocortisone 1%, hydrocortisone 2.5% cream is still many times weaker than Temovate cream 0.05%, which is in a higher potency class])

The goal of a topical formulation is to allow sufficient amounts of the active ingredient to be absorbed into the desired skin layers for therapeutic effects.

Steroids

Topical steroids are used for a variety of inflammatory dermatologic conditions. They vary in potency and strength. It is important to consider VALUES when choosing a steroid. The following is a list of steroid classes with a limited list of examples:

- **Super potent**
  - clobetasol propionate 0.05% (Temovate cream/ointment)
  - halobetasol propionate 0.05% (Ultravate cream/ointment)
- **Potent**
  - halcinonide 0.1% (Halog ointment/cream)
  - fluocinonide 0.05% (Lidex cream/gel/ointment)
- **Mid-strength**
  - flurandrenolide 0.005% (Cutivate ointment)
  - mometasone furoate 0.1% (Elocon cream)
  - fluocinolone acetonide 0.03% (Synalar ointment)
- **Mild**
  - fluocinolone acetonide 0.01% (Derma-Smoothe oil, Synalar cream)
- **Low potency**
  - hydrocortisone 2%/2.5% (Nutracort lotion)
  - hydrocortisone 0.5–1% (Cortaid cream/spray/ointment)

Common Dermatological Medications

The following tables offer truncated drug profiles. For complete drug information, consult a medication manual.

Antibiotics	Dermatologic-specific considerations

Oral (*See Chapter 4, Lesson 2, for specifics regarding mechanism of action, side effects/ adverse effects, and prescribing considerations*)
 	
• penicillin: dicloxacillin
• First-generation cephalosporin: cephalexin (Keflex)
• tetracycline: doxycycline, minocycline
• sulfa: sulfamethoxazole/ trimethoprim (Bactrim)
• macrolide: clindamycin
	• dicloxacillin is a narrow spectrum beta-lactam antibiotic used for cellulitis; it inhibits synthesis of the bacterial cell wall:
	  – Side effects/adverse effects: nausea, vomiting, diarrhea, urticaria, rash, hypersensitivity, *C. diff*–induced diarrhea
	  – Pregnancy category B
	  – Can decrease INR, lower seizure threshold; use different agent if MRSA suspected; may reduce effectiveness of oral contraceptives
	• doxycycline used for acne and rosacea, minocycline used for acne; if taking doxycycline or a tetracycline antibiotic, avoid use of retinoids
	• doxycycline, sulfamethoxazole/trimethoprim and clindamycin used for MRSA skin infections; be aware of local resistance

Table 16.2.1 Dermatologic Antibiotics

Antibiotics	Dermatologic-specific considerations

Topical (*See Chapter 4, Lesson 2, for mechanism of action, side effects/adverse effects, and prescribing considerations*)
 	
• mupirocin (Bactroban)
• bacitracin/neomycin/polymyxin B (Neosporin)
• clindamycin (Cleocin T)
• erythromycin
• metronidazole
	• mupirocin used for folliculitis, impetigo
	• bacitracin (polypeptide antibiotic), neomycin, and polymyxin B (aminoglycoside)
	  – bacitracin inhibits bacterial cell wall synthesis, weakens bacterial plasma membrane, is effective against several gram-positive organisms (*see Chapter 4, Lesson 2, for mechanism of other components*)
	  – Used for minor skin infections and excoriation from eczema
	  – Some patients have an allergy to neomycin
	  – Side effects/adverse effects: rash, contact dermatitis
	• Topical clindamycin and erythromycin used in the treatment of acne and can cause skin irritation and dryness
	• erythromycin used for erysipelas (secondary treatment for penicillin-resistant patients)
	• Topical metronidazole used in the treatment of rosacea

Table 16.2.1 Dermatologic Antibiotics (Continued)

Antifungals	Dermatologic-specific considerations
Oral (*See Chapter 4, Lesson 2, for specifics regarding mechanism of action, side effects/ adverse effects, and prescribing considerations*) • griseofulvin (Gris-PEG) • terbinafine (Lamisil) • fluconazole (Diflucan) • itraconazole (Sporanox)	• griseofulvin used for tinea capitis – Side effects: sun sensitivity • terbinafine, fluconazole and itraconazole used for dermatophyte infections including onychomycosis, tinea corporis, tinea barbera, tinea corporis • itraconazole has a **Black box warning** not to use in patients with CHF • fluconazole used for infections caused by candidiasis

Topical
• ketoconazole 2% shampoo, cream or foam (Nizoral)
• terbinafine 1% cream (Lamisil); nystatin 100,000 units/gm powder, ointment or cream; naftifine 1% or 2% cream
• selenium sulfide 1% lotion or 2.5% shampoo
	• ketoconazole is pregnancy category C but negligible absorption expected in topical form; used for tinea corporis, cruris, versicolor, capitis, seborrheic dermatitis
	  – Side effects: burning, alopecia, pruritus, hypersensitivity, angioedema
	  – Caution if allergy to sulfites (cream)
	• terbinafine used for tinea corporis, cruris, and pedis
	  – Available OTC
	  – Side effects: burning, pruritus
	• nystatin topical can be used for all ages
	• selenium sulfide used for tinea versicolor, tinea capitis, seborrheic dermatitis
	  – Side effects: burning, alopecia, hair discoloration
	  – 1% shampoo available OTC as Selsun Blue
	• naftifine used for tinea pedis, corporis, or cruris
	  – Side effects: erythema, burning, pruritus, local irritation, dryness
	• There are several combinations of antifungal and steroid in one product, but caution with the duration because of the steroid component (nystatin/triamcinolone, clotrimazole/betamethasone)

Table 16.2.2 Dermatologic Antifungal Medications

Antiparasitics and antivirals	Dermatological-specific considerations
Antiparasitic • permethrin (Elimite)—topical • ivermectin (Stromectol)—po or topical (*see Chapter 4, Lesson 8*) • spinosad 0.9% suspension (Natroba)	permethrin • Pregnancy category B; not to be used on babies <2 months old; avoid if allergy to chrysanthemums • Adults/children should apply topically from neck down; for infants/babies medication should be applied to the face, neck, and scalp, avoiding the area around the eyes • Pruritus may persist after the treatment, but does not usually indicate treatment failure • May repeat dose after 2 weeks if live mites are seen • Side effects/adverse effects: pruritus, rash, burning, stinging, urticaria, angioedema, anaphylaxis ivermectin used for strongyloidiasis (roundworm), scabies, or pediculosis capitis/pubis • Side effects/adverse effects: edema, pruritis, lymphadenopathy, myalgia, tachycardia, seizures, severe skin reactions • Pregnancy category C; pruritus may persist after treatment, but does not indicate treatment failure; take on empty stomach with water; can affect INR spinosad • Used for treatment of pediculosis capitis in those >6 months • Apply to dry hair and leave on for 10 minutes, then rinse off; does not require removal of nits; may repeat in 1 week if live mites are seen
Antiviral • Topical: penciclovir 1% cream (Denavir) • Oral: acyclovir (Zovirax), valacyclovir (Valtrex) (*see Chapter 4, Lesson 2, for specifics regarding mechanism of action, side effects/adverse effects, and prescribing considerations*)	penciclovir used for herpes simplex 1 • Pregnancy category B • Penciclovir is topical for use on the lips/face; start at onset of prodromal symptoms of herpes labialis Oral antivirals used for herpes simplex 1 or 2, herpes zoster • Dosing varies depending on whether the med is being prescribed for the initial outbreak, recurrence, or suppression

Table 16.2.3 Dermatologic Antiparasitic and Antiviral Medications

Antipsoriatics, antineoplastics, and antirosaceas	Dermatologic-specific considerations

Antipsoriatic
 	
Oral:
• Immunosuppressant: methotrexate (Trexall) (*see Chapter 4, Lesson 10, for specifics regarding mechanism of action, side effects/ adverse effects, and prescribing considerations*)
 	
Topical:
• Vitamin D3 derivative: calcipotriene (Dovonex)
• Corticosteroids: clobetasol (Temovate)
	• methotrexate use is contraindicated with pregnancy and breastfeeding
	• calcipotriene reduces excessive proliferation of skin cells
	  – Pregnancy category C
	  – Avoid in vitamin D toxicity, hypercalcemic patients, or patients taking phototherapy (can cause patients to sunburn more easily); do not apply to face or around eyes; avoid exposing calcipotriene-treated areas to sunlight/sunlamps
	  – Side effects/adverse effects: rash, itching, erythema, xerosis, worsening lesions, hypercalcemia, burning sensation in treated areas

Table 16.2.4 Dermatologic Antipsoriatic, Antineoplastic, and Antirosacea Medications

Antipsoriatics, antineoplastics, and antirosaceas	Dermatologic-specific considerations
Antineoplastic • Antimetabolite: fluorouracil (Efudex, 5-FU) topical • Diclofenac 3% gel	fluorouracil blocks abnormal cell growth used for actinic keratosis (AK) • Pregnancy category X and contraindicated in breastfeeding • Avoid ultraviolet rays, as expected effects of fluorouracil can include redness and peeling (similar to a bad sunburn) • Side effects/adverse effects: tenderness, scaling, blistering, skin rash, itching, erythema, strange taste in mouth, eye irritation, photosensitivity, stomatitis, hematological disorders (such as leukocytosis), ulceration, miscarriage, birth defects, signs of infection (such as fever) diclofenac gel used for treatment of AK; exact mechanism unknown • Caution if renal or hepatic impairment, pregnancy >30 weeks gestation, GI bleeding, or ulceration • Side effects/adverse effects: exfoliation, rash, pruritus, alopecia
Antirosacea Oral: • doxycycline (*see Chapter 4, Lesson 2*) Topical: • metronidazole • Alpha-2 adrenergic agonist: brimonidine (Mirvaso)	brimonidine causes vasoconstriction of blood vessels to reduce erythema in rosacea • Pregnancy category B; use with caution in patients with vascular insufficiency or cardiovascular disease • Side effects/adverse effects: erythema, flushing, burning, skin irritation, contact dermatitis, angioedema, urticaria

Table 16.2.4 Dermatologic Antipsoriatic, Antineoplastic, and Antirosacea Medications (Continued)

Miscellaneous dermatologic medications	Dermatologic-specific considerations
Immune response modifier imiquimod (Aldara)	• Used for actinic keratosis, condyloma acuminata, molluscum contagiosum, verruca vulgaris • Pregnancy category C; contraindicated if immunocompromised or photosensitive • Apply as directed even if lesions appear to be resolved; do not occlude • Discard unused packets of Aldara so that pets or children cannot accidentally ingest the medication • Side effects/adverse effects: redness, swelling, burning, tenderness, induration, burning sensation, weeping skin, fever, myalgia, nausea, chills, fatigue, angioedema, or anaphylaxis
Keratolytic salicylic acid 27.5% solution (Virasal)	• Keratolytic agent used to treat verruca vulgaris and plantar warts • Caution if impaired circulation or diabetes • Side effects/adverse effects: peeling, burning, pruritus, CNS toxicity, metabolic or respiratory alkalosis

Table 16.2.5 Miscellaneous Dermatologic Medications

Miscellaneous dermatologic medications	Dermatologic-specific considerations
Retinoids • tretinoin 0.025%, 0.05%, or 0.01% cream, gel, or solution (Retin-A) • isotretinoin—oral	tretinoin • Used for acne vulgaris and stimulates the turnover of epithelial cells • Caution if sunburn, eczema, or photosensitivity • Side effects: pruritis, blistering, photosensitivity, peeling, erythema isotretinoin • **Black box warning:** extreme risk of teratogenicity; prescribing and distribution limited • Used for severe acne vulgaris that is unresponsive to other treatments • Caution if diabetes, anorexia, psychiatric disorder, obesity, bone metabolic disorder • Side effects/adverse effects: elevated LFT and glucose, weight loss, palpitations, neutropenia, photosensitivity, anemia, epistaxis, psychosis, pseudotumor cerebri, cataracts
Minoxidil 2% or 5% solution	• Used for alopecia by stimulating hair growth • Side effects: skin irritation, pruritus • Can be used for males or females; stop if no hair growth in four months
Immunosuppressants • tacrolimus 0.03% or 0.1% ointment • pimecrolimus 1% cream (Elidel)	• Used for severe atopic dermatitis • **Black box warning:** lymphoma and skin malignancies • Not for use in children <2 years old; use lower strength for 2–5 years old • Do not use for long term • Side effects/adverse effects: flu-like symptoms, fever, asthma, cough, folliculitis, photosensitivity, lymphadenopathy, erythema, skin carcinoma, lymphoma, renal failure, anaphylaxis

Table 16.2.5 Miscellaneous Dermatologic Medications (Continued)

Education

- Use topical antifungal agents for one week after fungus has resolved to prevent recurrence
- Shake suspensions well prior to using
- Use meds as directed and for length of time directed, or complete resolution of dermatologic condition may not occur
- Do not use occlusive dressing over topical steroid medications unless directed
- For medications that can cause photosensitivity: wear sunscreen, hats, long shirts, and pants to prevent sunburn

Takeaways

- When choosing a vehicle, different ones have varying absorption and potency. In order of increasing potency and absorption rate: lotion, cream, gel, ointment.
- When prescribing, specify the tube size (15 gm, 30 gm, etc.) of the topical medication being prescribed. This limits the quantity, such as in the case of topical steroids, so that patients do not overuse the medication and suffer adverse effects.
- Topical steroids can produce systemic effects, especially in children.

LESSON 3: CARCINOMA AND MELANOMA

Learning Objectives

- Differentiate between actinic keratosis, basal cell carcinoma, squamous cell carcinoma, and malignant melanoma
- Identify risk factors for developing each form of skin cancer
- Describe the characteristics of each form of skin cancer, as well as actinic keratosis
- Select the appropriate diagnostic method for each form of skin cancer
- Discuss treatment options for each form of skin cancer, as well as actinic keratosis

Skin cancer is by far the most common form of cancer in United States. More than five million cases are treated each year and one in five adults will be diagnosed with skin cancer in their lifetime. There are three main types of skin cancer: basal cell carcinoma (BCC), squamous cell carcinoma (SCC), and malignant melanoma (MM).

Basal Cell Carcinoma

- Most common form of skin cancer
- Involves the basal cell layer of the epidermis
- Slow-growing, locally destructive carcinoma
- Occurs more often in fair-skinned individuals in sun-exposed areas
- Rarely seen in brown- and black-skinned persons
- Very limited capacity to metastasize
- UV exposure is most significant risk factor, especially prior to age 14

Squamous Cell Carcinoma

- Second most common skin cancer in Caucasians
- Most common skin cancer in African Americans
- Slowly evolving cancer of the epithelial keratinocytes; frequently develops from actinic keratosis
- Low risk of metastasis
- Usually seen on sun-exposed areas; lips of smokers
- Primary risk factors: UV exposure, external carcinogens, HPV virus

Malignant Melanoma

- Most serious form of skin cancer
- Highest potential for metastasis
- Arises from melanocytes
- Primary risk factor is UV exposure, primarily blistering sunburns
- Associated risk factors: family history, fair skin/hair/freckles, tanning bed use

Actinic Keratosis

- Common, precancerous lesion
- Occurs on sun-damaged skin
- Has the potential to develop into SCC over time if not treated

Assessment

Skin cancer type	Subjective	Objective
Basal cell carcinoma	A non healing, painless sore that may bleed	Waxy, pearly, nodule/papule, telangiectasia, central core/depression
Squamous cell carcinoma	A potentially tender, scaly lesion or ulcer that may bleed	Flat or shallow lesion with elevated margins, defined borders, red to opaque; can be ulcerating
Malignant melanoma	A new or changing lesion, most commonly on female's legs and male's back	**A:** Asymmetry **B:** Border irregularity **C:** Color; polychromatic—can be shades of brown, tan, black, blue, red, or white **D:** Diameter >6 mm **E:** Evolving; any change in size, shape, color, elevation, diameter
Actinic keratosis	A scaly, rough patch that peels off and comes back	A scaly, rough macule or patch that is pink/red/white in color

Table 16.3.1 Skin Cancer Assessment

> **Pro Tip**
> Any new, changing, or evolving lesion should be evaluated.

Diagnosis

Differential Diagnosis

Differential diagnoses for BCC/SCC: **eczema, psoriasis, actinic keratosis, seborrheic keratosis, malignant melanoma**

Differential diagnoses for melanoma: **BCC, solar lentigo, hemangioma, melanoma in situ, dysplastic nevus**

Basal cell carcinoma may be diagnosed clinically and confirmed with a shave or punch biopsy. If SCC or MM is suspected, an excisional biopsy should be performed. Shave biopsies may negate the ability to stage an MM, so extra consideration should be taken if MM is suspected. If the patient is clinically symptomatic and MM is suspected, diagnostic imaging should be ordered to evaluate for metastasis. Actinic keratosis is diagnosed clinically.

> **Pro Tip**
> If the diagnosis is in doubt, refer for an excisional biopsy.

Plan

Skin cancer type	Treatment modalities
BCC	Surgical excision with clear margins, electrodesiccation and curettage (ED&C), Mohs; less often: cryotherapy, radiation, photodynamic therapy
SCC	Surgical excision with clear margins, Mohs, topical chemotherapy (such as 5-fluorouracil [Efudex]); less often: radiation, oncology referral
MM	Wide local excision with clear margins and lymph node dissection, oncology referral; adjuvant therapy varies depending on stage; close follow-up
AK	Cryotherapy, topical chemotherapy, topical diclofenac gel, photodynamic therapy; less often: chemical peels, laser therapy

Table 16.3.2 Treatment Considerations for Skin Cancer

Education

Prevention of skin cancer is key. Educate patients on the harmful effects of UV exposure; tell them to minimize their sun exposure, especially between the hours of 10:00 AM and 2:00 PM; instruct them to cover exposed skin and to wear sunblock with an SPF of at least 30 when outdoors. Reapply sunblock every 60–90 minutes while outside, even on cloudy days. Examine skin often, noting any new or changing lesions. A thorough skin examination should be performed by a healthcare provider at least annually.

Referral

Refer the patient with a large or deep tumor, unclear surgical margins, and evidence of nodal or distant metastasis.

Takeaways

- Basal cell carcinoma is a slow-growing cancer; usually a painless, non healing lesion and may be diagnosed clinically.

- Squamous cell carcinoma is a slow growing cancer; usually a tender, flat, or shallow lesion with elevated margins and a tendency to bleed.

- The ABCDEs of skin cancer is a pneumonic used to evaluate a lesion for MM. Excisional biopsy is essential for staging and diagnosis.

- Actinic keratosis is a precancerous lesion—usually a scaly, rough patch that peels off and recurs that can lead to SCC.

LESSON 4: DERMATITIS

Learning Objectives
- Differentiate clinical manifestations of various forms of dermatitis
- Choose and interpret laboratory/diagnostic testing for dermatitis
- Describe appropriate treatment and referrals for dermatitis

Dermatitis refers to an inflammation of the skin. It may occur as a result of allergy (atopic or contact) in areas of increased sebaceous glands (seborrhea) or in the diaper area. Skin dryness is a contributor to atopic dermatitis.

Definitions

- **Atopy:** genetic tendency toward allergic diseases such as asthma, allergic gastroenteropathy, atopic dermatitis, or allergic rhinitis
- **Dennie lines:** a fold or line in the skin below the lower eyelid
- **Satellite lesions:** red maculopapular lesions slightly apart from the main area of the rash

Assessment

Subjective

The health history may include:

- Personal/family history of atopy (atopic dermatitis [AD])
- History of Parkinson disease, CVA, HIV infection, or family history of seborrheic dermatitis (SD)
- Skin contact with an allergen such as a plant, metal, toiletries, cleaning products, or rubber-containing materials (contact dermatitis [CD])
- Symptom remissions and flare-ups (atopic dermatitis, seborrheic dermatitis)

Symptoms

- Pruritus is a hallmark of dermatitis; in atopic dermatitis (also termed eczema), the itching is often intense and followed by scratching; contact dermatitis may also result in intense itching; for seborrheic dermatitis in adolescents and adults, itching may be accompanied by burning; infants with seborrheic or diaper dermatitis do not seem to display behaviors indicating itching
- Rash

Review of Systems

- **Constitutional:** disturbed sleep (from pruritus), diaper-dependent (diaper dermatitis)
- **HEENT:** runny nose (AD), red/itchy eyes with or without clear drainage (AD)
- **Resp:** wheeze or cough (AD)

Objective

Dennie lines may be present in the patient with atopic dermatitis.

Finding	Atopic dermatitis	Contact dermatitis	Seborrheic dermatitis
Skin rash or lesions	Small papules (coalescent) that eventually flake, erythema; may progress to lichenification	Significant erythematous papules (in a pattern matching the exposure, such as linear formation with poison ivy or shape of a ring with nickel)	Erythematous plaques or patches with greasy scale
Area affected	• Infant: cheeks, fronts of arms and legs, scalp • Children: wrists, hands, antecubital and popliteal areas • Adults: antecubital and popliteal areas, posterior neck	Skin: in area(s) of contact	• Infants: scalp (cradle cap), diaper area • Adults: scalp (dandruff), eyebrows, eyelids, nasolabial folds, chin, posterior to ears, upper chest, upper back, axilla, and groin folds

Table 16.4.1 Differentiating Atopic, Contact, and Seborrheic Dermatitis

Diagnosis	Cause	Rash characteristics
Diaper dermatitis	Exposure to urine and feces, moist environment	Red, flat, shiny rash starts in the creases and spreads throughout the diaper area, sometimes with small papules
Diaper candidiasis	Moist environment resulting in overproduction of *Candida albicans*, naturally on skin	Very bright red rash with satellite lesions and possible scaling in the skin folds

Table 16.4.2 Diaper Dermatitis vs. Diaper Candidiasis

Diagnosis

Diagnosis of atopic dermatitis is primarily based upon the clinical manifestations, although serum immunoglobulin E is often elevated. Seborrheic and contact dermatitis, as well as diaper dermatitis/candidiasis, are diagnosed based upon the history and physical examination.

Plan

Diagnosis	Treatment	Patient education	Referral
Atopic dermatitis	• Emollients twice daily or more • Mild disease: lower potency topical corticosteroids 2 times daily • Moderate disease: medium to high potency corticosteroids, 2 times daily, up to 2 weeks, then step back to lower potency OR immunomodulators (tacrolimus, pimecrolimus) 0.1% topical for adults, 0.03% topical for children >2 years of age, applied twice daily • Oral antihistamines are helpful to decrease itching, particularly at bedtime in some patients	• Daily moisturization lotion to face, cream to body; multiple times daily, even when not flared up • Decrease heat in bath/shower, as well as home • Avoid all fragrances in cleansers, moisturizers, soaps, detergents, fabric softeners, dryer sheets	Failure of response to conservative treatment
Contact dermatitis	• Low dose corticosteroids 3–4 times daily OR intermediate dose topical steroids 2 times daily • Oral hydroxyzine or diphenhydramine 4 times daily	• Avoid contact with offending irritant • If known exposure, wash area immediately • Lukewarm oatmeal baths • Calamine lotion after baths	Consult with physician if symptoms worsen despite appropriate treatment

Table 16.4.3 Treatment and Referral Plan for Dermatitis

Diagnosis	Treatment	Patient education	Referral
Diaper dermatitis	Barrier ointment containing vitamins A, D, E, zinc oxide, or petrolatum	• Change diapers frequently • Gently wash the area with soft cloth; avoid harsh soaps and perfumed items • Allow to go diaperless for period of time daily to dry/heal rash • Avoid any type of powder (risk of aspiration/pneumonitis in child)	
Diaper candidiasis	Topical nystatin with diaper changes	As with diaper dermatitis	Persistence despite appropriate treatment
Seborrheic dermatitis	• Infants: daily shampoo with mild baby shampoo, using a soft brush • Toddlers and older: shampoo every other day with a shampoo containing selenium sulfide or ketoconazole; alternatively, shampoo 2 times a week with a coal-tar containing product • Seborrheic blepharitis: warm compresses followed by gentle debridement with cotton-tipped swab and baby shampoo 2 times daily • Consider corticosteroid shampoo or lotion if not improving	Infants: apply petroleum jelly and rub in, about 30 minutes before shampooing to loosen crusts	Dermatologist if fails to improve within 2 weeks with treatment

Table 16.4.3 Treatment and Referral Plan for Dermatitis (Continued)

Takeaways

- Use the pattern of the rash and history to differentiate between types of dermatitis.
- Atopic dermatitis is rare in the diaper area due to moisture presence.
- Dry skin that itches then rashes is likely atopic dermatitis.
- Diaper candidiasis is differentiated from ordinary diaper dermatitis by the presence of satellite lesions.
- Greasy, flaky rash in areas of increased sebaceous glands is likely seborrhea.
- Topical corticosteroids are a choice of treatment for dermatitis, except for in the diaper area.

LESSON 5: INJURY AND WOUNDS

Learning Objectives

■ Differentiate clinical manifestations of injury or trauma

■ Describe appropriate treatment and referrals for injuries to the skin

■ Outline patient education related to the prevention of skin injury

Skin injury may result from minor trauma such as an abrasion or scrape, a bite or sting, thermal injury, or from poor perfusion to a particular area.

Definitions

- **Epibole:** rolled wound edges
- **Hymenoptera:** a large order of stinging insects including wasps, hornets, bees, and ants

Assessment

Subjective

Determine history of the event/injury (insect sting, human or animal bite, sun exposure, thermal injury). For an insect sting, determine any prior sting reaction(s). Note risk factors:

- **Animal bites:** young and elderly
- **Burns:** young and elderly
- **Pressure ulcers:** immobility, acute illness, fecal/urinary incontinence, altered mental status, weight loss, or malnutrition/dehydration
- **Lower extremity ulcers:** diabetes mellitus, arterial or venous insufficiency, peripheral neuropathy, congestive heart failure, hyperlipidemia, obesity, edema, age >65

Symptoms

- Pain, erythema, edema, blistering, and drainage
- Fever
- Difficulty breathing (stings)

Objective

Bites

Type of bite	Objective findings
Cat	Puncture wound, may be deep
Dog	Laceration, abrasion, puncture, possible crush injury
Human	Closed fist wound (hand), laceration, possible crush injury
Rodent	Laceration, abrasion, may be more superficial

Table 16.5.1 Differentiating Findings in Mammal Bites

Burns

Type of burn	Objective findings
Superficial	Dry, erythema, hyperemia, pain, skin blanches easily
Superficial partial-thickness	Clear blisters, wet, weeping skin, erythematous, blanches, painful
Deep partial-thickness	Appears pink to white, does not blanch, painful
Full-thickness	Dark brown or tan, leathery, white with minimal pain
Fourth degree	Extends into muscle, tendon, bone

Table 16.5.2 Objective Findings of Burns

> **Pro Tip**
> Throughout the life span, the palmar surface of the hand and fingers is equal to 1% of body surface area (BSA); use to measure/determine percentage BSA involved for smaller areas.

Stings

Erythema, edema, and rash may be present with hornet/wasp/bee sting. Clusters of papules turning to pustules occur with fire ant stings.

> **DANGER SIGN** Hymenoptera stings may result in anaphylaxis. If patient has symptoms suggestive of laryngospasm or bronchospasm, or reports difficulty breathing, call 911.

Ulcers

Erythema, drainage, and tissue color changes (red, pink, yellow, brown, tan) occur with skin ulcers. Note granulation or necrotic tissue if present. Determine capillary refill and quality of pulses.

Stage	Objective finding
1	Non-blanchable erythema (possibly indurated) with intact skin; not purple or maroon
2	Epidermal or dermal skin loss; pink or red, moist wound bed; no granulation, eschar, or slough
3	Crater-like appearance with full-thickness skin loss, visible fat, granulation tissue, and epibole often present; may have eschar or slough
4	Full-thickness skin and tissue loss with exposure of muscle, bone, and tendons; may have eschar; slough, epibole, or tunneling

Table 16.5.3 Staging of Pressure Ulcers

Diagnosis

Bites, burns, stings, and ulcers are distinguished by the history and physical findings.

Plan

Bites

Treatment

- Culture wound as able
- Cleanse area well with antimicrobial agent; debride as necessary
- Short-term oral prophylaxis with amoxicillin-clavulanate (Augmentin); clindamycin + fluoroquinolone if PCN allergy
- Tetanus prophylaxis

Education

- Keep site clean
- Report redness, swelling, drainage, or increased tenderness to nurse practitioner
- Prevention: do not approach wild animals or animals you are unfamiliar with

Burns

Treatment

Minor burns with the following characteristics may be treated in the outpatient setting:

- An isolated injury not involving the face, hands, perineum, genitalia, or feet
- Not circumferential or crossing major joints
- Partial thickness burns of <5% total BSA in patients <10 years of age or >50 years of age
- Partial thickness burns of <10% total BSA in patients between 10–50 years of age

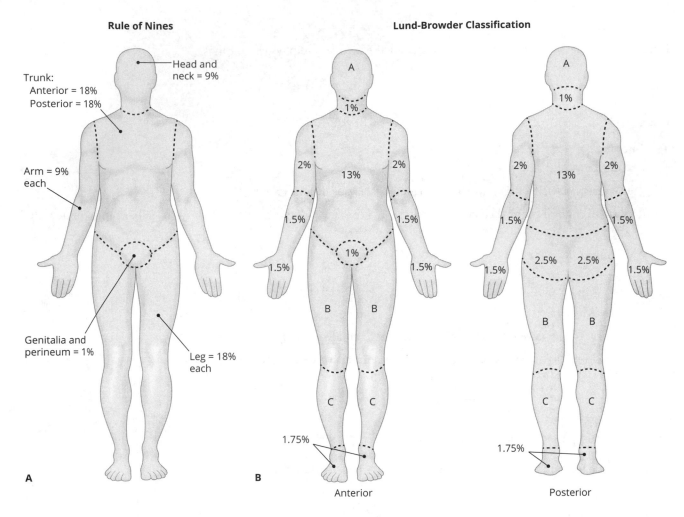

Figure 16.5.1 Estimating Body Surface Area

- Partial thickness burns
  - Cleanse burned area
  - Leave small blisters intact, rupture larger blisters
  - Apply silver sulfadiazine (Silvadene) or mafenide acetate (Sulfamylon)
  - Moist dressing (may use petrolatum gauze)
- Deeper partial thickness burns may benefit from the use of Aquacel Ag or Biobrane

Education
- Notify nurse practitioner if fever, increased pain, or increased redness occur
- Prevention:
  - Set hot water heater no higher than 120 degrees
  - Do not hold children while working with hot items
  - Keep matches, firecrackers, gasoline, and other explosives out of the reach of children
  - Appropriately maintain household smoke alarms

Stings

Treatment

- Diphenhydramine orally every 6 hours or hydroxyzine (Atarax) every 6–8 hours for 24 hours
- Mild anaphylaxis: epinephrine 0.1 mg/kg subcutaneously in children, 0.3 mg intramuscularly in adults

Education

- Ice pack to sting area for 10 minutes
- Avoid disturbing ant hills (ants become aggressive, attacking in swarms when disturbed) and hornet/wasp/bee nests
- Carry EpiPen or EpiPen Jr as prescribed

Ulcers

Treatment

- Diabetic foot and pressure ulcers
  - Obtain culture of drainage if infection suspected
  - Cleanse with normal saline
  - In all instances, change dressing daily and as needed
  - Apply collagenase (Santyl) if debridement needed
  - Use hydrogel if scant drainage present
  - For moderate drainage, apply calcium alginate
- Venous ulcers: for either treatment, apply, then change in 3 days; if tolerating, change weekly
  - Ankle-brachial index (ABI) 0.8–1.0: full compression with Profore
  - Ankle-brachial index (ABI): 0.6–0.8: light compression with Profore Lite **or** apply calcium alginate, wrap with Unna boot (*for more information regarding ABI see Chapter 7, Lesson 9*)

Education

- Do not apply direct pressure to the ulcer site
- Elevate lower extremities as recommended
- Increase protein in diet
- Report changes in the ulcer
- Notify provider for fever or a generalized ill feeling

Referral

- **Bites:** refer all bites to the ears, face, genitalia, hands, and feet; check local authorities for rabies prophylaxis for domestic or wild animal bites
- **Burns:** refer to specialty burn center or emergency room
  - Burns involving >10% BSA (ages 10–50 years) or involving >5% BSA (all other ages)
  - Evidence of inhalation injury
  - Full-thickness burns

- – Facial burns
- – Burns occurring on genitalia or a high-function area such as hand or foot
- – If cosmetic concern
- **Stings:** refer to emergency room if anaphylaxis present
- **Ulcers:** refer/consult wound care specialist if ulcer is extensive or not improving with treatment; refer patients with arterial ulcer or venous ulcer with poor arterial flow to vascular surgeon

Takeaways

- Assess respiratory status in any patient experiencing a sting in order to determine presence of anaphylaxis.
- Treat minor burns in the outpatient setting.
- The ankle-brachial index helps to determine severity of arterial insufficiency in lower extremity ulcers in order for the nurse practitioner to determine treatment or when to refer.

LESSON 6: SKIN INFECTIONS & INFESTATIONS

Learning Objectives
- Differentiate clinical manifestations of bacterial, viral, and fungal skin infections
- Choose and interpret laboratory/diagnostic testing for infectious skin disorders
- Describe appropriate treatment and referrals for skin infections

Skin infections often present with rash and itching. The majority of bacterial skin infections result from group A *Streptococcus* and varicella infection in the past (herpes zoster). Viruses and fungi also cause infections in the skin and result from exposure to those pathogens or overgrowth of resident microbes. The exception is herpes zoster, which results when the dormant virus is reactivated in a reaction to stress or illness.

Definitions
- **Herald patch:** ovoid 2- to 5-centimeter pink, finely scaled lesion with slightly elevated border occurring on the trunk, neck, upper arm, or thigh with pityriasis rosea
- **Kerion:** abscess caused by a fungal infection evidenced by edematous, painful, and boggy plaque on the scalp

Assessment

Subjective
Determine history of the following:

- Varicella infection in past (herpes zoster)
- History of lymphedema, venous insufficiency, obesity, immunosuppression (cellulitis, erysipelas)
- Exposure to pets (tinea, larva migrans)

Symptoms
- Pruritus (herpes zoster, tinea, lice, scabies, possibly mild with pityriasis rosea)
- Erythema
- Rash
- Skin lesion (warts, cellulitis, erysipelas, herpetic whitlow, paronychia)
- Tingling or burning (herpetic whitlow and herpes zoster [before rash starts], burning with tinea pedis)
- Crawling sensation in scalp (lice)

Review of Systems
- **Constitutional:** fever, chills, fitful sleep (scabies)
- **HEENT:** runny nose (impetigo), gingivostomatitis in thumb-sucker (herpetic whitlow)
- **Skin:** genital herpes simplex virus infection (herpetic whitlow), nails break and split (onychomycosis)

Diagnosis

Diagnosis of skin infections and infestations is generally based upon the history and physical examination. Laboratory testing may include:

- Tzanck smear, which shows giant multinucleated cells with herpes zoster
- KOH prep, which demonstrates hyphae with fungal infections
- Bacterial cultures of drainage, which may be used to accurately identify the offending bacteria and determine antibiotic sensitivity

Bacterial skin infections	Objective findings
Carbuncle	Cluster or coalescence of inflamed hair follicles with purulent drainage
Cellulitis	• Erythema, edema, heat, and/or pain (deeper skin and subcutaneous tissue) anywhere on body, but more common on extremities • Preseptal (periorbital) cellulitis: ocular pain, eyelid edema, and erythema (more common in children) • Orbital cellulitis: same as preseptal with addition of proptosis; pain with eye movements, ophthalmoplegia, diplopia
Erysipelas	Red, raised area with sharply demarcated borders
Folliculitis	Blocked hair follicle, small pustules in any hair-bearing area
Furuncle (boil)	Painful, well-circumscribed, inflammatory nodule surrounding a hair follicle
Impetigo	• Vesicles with honey-colored crusting on erythematous base on exposed areas of body, mostly face and extremities, most common in toddlers and preschoolers • Bullous impetigo: flaccid blisters with clear yellow fluid, when ruptures leaves a thin, brown crust • Ecthyma: punched-out ulcerative lesions with raised violet-colored edges (more common on extremities)
Paronychia	• Painful edema and erythema of nail folds, arising rapidly; usually involves one fingernail or an ingrown toenail • Blanching of soft tissue when pressure applied to tip of affected nail

Table 16.6.1 Differentiating Bacterial Skin Infections

Viral skin infections	Objective findings
Herpes zoster	Clustered vesicles on an erythematous base; unilateral and following a dermatome
Herpetic whitlow	Swollen, painful lesion with ulceration on an erythematous base on a finger or a thumb; most often occurring in children
Pityriasis rosea	Herald patch followed by smaller pink, round, or oval scaly lesions on trunk and proximal extremities; often in "Christmas tree" pattern on back; usually spares face, scalp, distal extremities
Verrucae (warts)	Flesh-colored, single papules with irregular and scaly surfaces and possible black pinpoint dots found anywhere on the body, but most commonly hands and feet (only plantar is painful)

Table 16.6.2 Differentiating Viral Skin Infections

Fungal skin infection	Objective findings
Onychomycosis	Opaque white or silvery nails that become thickened, brittle, dull, and yellow to dark brown or blue in color; affecting toenails more often than fingernails
Tinea barbae	Annular lesions with raised erythematous borders and central clearing with broken hairs; inflammatory pustules (may be draining); kerion-like plaques—occurs only in hairy regions of face and neck
Tinea capitis	Annular, scaly plaques on the scalp with central hair breakage resulting in black dots; kerion may be present
Tinea corporis	Pruritic, annular or oval, erythematous, scaling patch, with central clearing and a raised border
Tinea cruris	Starts with erythematous patch on proximal medial thigh partial; central clearing and slightly elevated; demarcated border with possible tiny vesicles; spreads from center outward and to perineum, perianal, gluteal cleft, and buttock areas, with scrotal sparing
Tinea pedis	Pruritic, erythematous lesions with scaling or ulceration between the toes OR diffuse hyperkeratotic eruption (extremely pronounced creases with scaling) covering soles, medial, and lateral aspects of foot
Tinea versicolor	Many small, annular, discrete macules on chest, back, upper arms; may be scaly; are either hypo- or hyperpigmented

Table 16.6.3 Differentiating Fungal Skin Infections

Parasitic infestation	Objective findings
Cutaneous larva migrans (hookworm-related)	A "creeping" eruption; erythematous cutaneous track (linear or snakelike) that migrates
Pediculosis capitis (lice)	Visualization of nits clinging to hair shafts close to scalp, or live lice; possible excoriation of scalp, occipital, or cervical lymphadenopathy
Scabies	Curving S-shaped burrows, especially in-between fingers; lesions are vesiculopapular in nature in infants and young children

Table 16.6.4 Differentiating Parasitic Infestations

Plan

Disorder	Treatment	Patient education	Referral
Carbuncle, furuncle, folliculitis	• Carbuncle: PO doxycycline or cephalexin • Furuncle: incision and drainage for large boils not opening with warm compress treatment • Antibiotics only for extensive boils • Folliculitis: topical mupirocin or clindamycin • Extensive involvement may require oral doxycycline or cephalexin	All: • Good handwashing • Wash linens, towels, underwear in hot water • Do not share towels and washcloths Folliculitis: benzoyl peroxide wash of affected area Furuncle: • Warm compresses to allow to open • Do not squeeze or pop	Extensive involvement or not improving with appropriate treatment
Cellulitis, erysipelas	• PO cephalexin; trimethoprim-sulfamethoxazole if MRSA suspected • Preseptal: PO clindamycin OR trimethoprim-sulfamethoxazole PLUS amoxicillin, amoxicillin-clavulanate, cefpodoxime, or cefdinir	Cellulitis: • Keep affected area raised • Keep clean and dry • Notify office if not improving within 3 days	• Refer for hospitalization (for IV antibiotics): moderate to severe cases, age <1 year, poor response to treatment, purulent wound near eyelid • Refer to ophthalmology or otolaryngology if orbital cellulitis suspected
Impetigo	• Limited: topical mupirocin TID or retapamulin BID for 5 days • Extensive or not responding to topical, or ecthyma: dicloxacillin or cephalexin • MRSA confirmed or suspected: PO doxycycline (>8 years of age), clindamycin, or trimethoprim-sulfamethoxazole	• Gentle washing of crusted lesions • Good handwashing • Clean household surfaces well • Wash linens, towels in hot water; dry on high heat • Do not share personal items • Always use disposable tissue to blow the nose • Avoid scratching area of impetigo to avoid self-inoculation • May return to school 24 hours after beginning antibiotic treatment with draining lesions covered	Refer to physician for incomplete resolution with appropriate treatment or for complications

Table 16.6.5 Treatment and Referral Plan for Bacterial Infections

Burns et al, 2017; Cash & Glass, 2017

Disorder	Treatment	Patient education	Referral
Paronychia	• With full purulent area, loosen cuticle from nail with a no. 11 blade, allowing escape of exudate • Neosporin or mupirocin following soaks • If unresponsive to above, PO dicloxacillin or cephalexin • Cover for MRSA if high prevalence in area (see impetigo)	• Frequent warm soaks with antiseptic • Clip nails straight across • Wear wide-toed shoes	If recurrent, refer for surgical removal of lateral nail

Table 16.6.5 Treatment and Referral Plan for Bacterial Infections (Continued)

Disorder	Treatment	Patient education	Referral
Herpes zoster (shingles)	• famciclovir, valacyclovir, or acyclovir; start within 72 hours for best effect and decrease in severity of outbreak • Pain relief: lidocaine 5% gel	• Avoid pregnant women, immunocompromised individuals, and non-immunized children, as the rash is contagious to them • Post-herpetic neuralgia may occur and can last for at least a month after the rash is healed	Refer if involves a facial or ocular dermatome
Herpetic whitlow	• Burow's solution compresses TID • Dry dressing between compresses • PO acyclovir if immunocompromised	• Rest and elevate the affected digit • NSAID for pain	Refer if severe infection
Pityriasis rosea	• None needed • If pruritus present: tepid oatmeal baths, calamine lotion, medium potency topical corticosteroids, or antihistamines may be helpful	• Rash spontaneously resolves within 6–12 weeks • Keep the body cool • Avoid sunlight if it worsens the rash	

Table 16.6.6 Treatment and Referral Plan for Viral Infections

Burns et al, 2017; Cash & Glass, 2017

Disorder	Treatment	Patient education	Referral
Verruca vulgaris (warts)	• salicylic acid paints BID for 4–6 weeks • salicylic acid plasters applied for 3–5 days to plantar wart, then remove; soak 45 minutes and file dead skin off (3–6 weeks) • retinoic acid gel 0.025% to 0.05% 2 times daily to flat warts • Cover with duct tape 12 hours per day; soak 45 minutes and file dead skin off 6 days in a row • cantharidin 0.7% apply with toothpick, cover with tape 24 hours (plantar and periungual only) • podophyllum 25% in benzoin; apply with toothpick; wash off in 4 hours; reapply in 1 week • imiquimod cream applied daily for 1–2 months • If available, apply liquid nitrogen 20–45 seconds (especially for plantar warts) every 2–4 weeks until wart is gone	• Spread through contact • Warts resolve spontaneously, usually within 2 years • Take care to apply treatments only to wart, avoiding healthy tissue • When filing after treatment, either discard disposable emery board or cleanse reusable nail file with alcohol after each use • Expect blister to form 2 days after cantharidin or cryotherapy	Refer for cryotherapy if needed

Table 16.6.6 Treatment and Referral Plan for Viral Infections (Continued)

Pro Tip

Shingles may be prevented with herpes zoster vaccination (*see Chapter 3, Lesson 4*).

Disorder	Treatment	Patient education
Onychomycosis	• Oral agents are often more effective than topical if the nail is thickened: itraconazole, terbinafine, or fluconazole on a pulse cycle; prescribe to take 1 week of the month (2 cycles for fingernails, 3 cycles for toenails) • If issues such as liver toxicity or drug interactions with oral antifungals, use urea gel to improve penetration of topical amorolfine, ciclopirox, efinaconazole, or tavaborole • Refer for surgical nail removal if oral/topical therapy unsuccessful	• Keep feet clean and dry • Wear flip flops in showers away from home • Do not share nail tools
Tinea barbae and tinea capitis	Tinea barbae: • Pulse itraconazole or fluconazole over a 4–6 week period • Long-term once or twice weekly topical selenium sulfide, ketoconazole, or ciclopirox may help to prevent recurrence Tinea capitis: • griseofulvin PO for 6–12 weeks OR terbinafine PO for 4–6 weeks	Both: • Avoid sharing shaving tools • Ensure tools (e.g., barber scissors, razors, etc.) are sterilized Tinea capitis: • Take griseofulvin with fatty food to improve its efficacy
Tinea corporis and tinea cruris	• Topical terbinafine or naftifine once or twice daily for 1–3 weeks • Extensive involvement or failed topical therapy: PO terbinafine for 1–2 weeks, or PO itraconazole for 1 week	Tinea corporis: • Keep skin clean and dry • Do not share unwashed clothing • Have pet evaluated by vet if it has a rash or patchy hair loss Tinea cruris: • Wear cotton underwear • Avoid tight-fitting clothing • Use desiccant powder daily in inguinal area
Tinea pedis	• Topical antifungal twice daily until 7 days after symptoms cleared	• Keep feet clean and dry • Rinse feet with water and vinegar, drying well • Wear flip flops in showers away from home • Wear clean cotton socks, changing frequently • Use antifungal powder on feet
Tinea versicolor	• selenium sulfide 1% lotion or 2.5% shampoo; apply from neck to knees; leave in place for 10 minutes, then rinse—do once daily for 2 weeks, OR • ciclopirox solution daily • Older adolescents and adults: may use ketaconazole 2% shampoo (as above with selenium) or antifungal creams (if not widespread) twice daily for 2–4 weeks • If severe, may use Diflucan weekly × 2–3 doses	• Do not share towels and washcloths • Wash towels, washcloths, and linens in hot water • Sun exposure makes appearance of hypopigmented areas more prominent • Repigmentation takes several months

Table 16.6.7 Treatment and Referral Plan for Viral Infections

Burns, et al, 2017; Cash & Glass, 2017

Infestation	Treatment	Patient education
Cutaneous larva migrans	Oral ivermectin once daily for 2 days or albendazole daily for 3 days	• Take antihistamines if desired for pruritus • Notify FNP if dry cough develops (may indicate pulmonary involvement)
Pediculosis capitis	Pediculicide such as permethrin or pyrethrin with piperonyl butoxide	• Remove nits with fine-toothed comb from hair (1-inch sections, pay special attention behind ears and to nape of neck) • Inform family, friends, school, and day care contacts • Wash sheets, towels, clothing, headwear • Store other fabric items (decorative pillows, stuffed animals) in secured plastic bags/trash bags for 2 days • Soak brushes and combs • Vacuum house well • Parent to recheck daily at home • May return to school after pediculicide treatment
Scabies	• 5% permethrin applied from neck down at bedtime; rinse off after 8–14 hours, repeat in 1 week • Extensive case: ivermectin, 1 dose every week for 2–3 weeks	• Additional persons needing treatment: everyone living with the patient, recent sexual partner(s) • Use pramoxine lotion or antihistamine as needed to control pruritus • Wash all linens, towels, and clothing in hot water • Vacuum house well; store other fabric items in secured plastic bags/trash bags for 7 days • May return to day care, school, or work the day after treatment

Table 16.6.8 Treatment Plan for Skin Infestations

Burns, et al, 2017; Cash & Glass, 2017

Takeaways

- Initial treatment for carbuncle, impetigo, and paronychia is topical antibiotics, while oral antibiotics should be used for cellulitis.

- Starting antiviral treatment early in the course of herpes zoster (shingles) helps to decrease its severity.

- Always prescribe oral antifungals for tinea capitis and tinea barbae. Other forms of tinea are treated with topical antifungals.

LESSON 7: ACNE & ROSACEA

Learning Objectives
■ Differentiate clinical manifestations of rosacea and various stages/forms of acne
■ Describe patient education for the management of acne and rosacea
■ Delineate appropriate treatment and referrals for acne and rosacea

Acne and rosacea may both have a negative impact upon self-esteem. Acne vulgaris is a disorder of the sebaceous glands, with *Propionibacterium acnes* contributing to the inflammatory process. Acne generally begins in adolescence and can be influenced by hormonal changes, hot/humid weather, and particular medications (halides, hydantoin derivative, lithium, rifampin). The presence of acne-like lesions in the newborn period is termed neonatal acne.

Acne rosacea (commonly called rosacea) is an anomaly in vascular function bringing about recurring episodes of dilation with flushing of the face. This leads to an inflammatory cascade, resulting in papules and pustules.

Definitions

- **Closed comedones:** closed clogged hair follicles (whitehead)
- **Open comedones:** clogged hair follicles which are open, being exposed to air causing blackening (blackhead)

Assessment

Review of Systems

- **Constitutional:** flushing, particularly with exposure to hot/spicy foods, hot or cold environments, or sunlight
- **Endocrine:** hormonal changes (adolescence, menstruation, pregnancy, perimenopause)
- **Psychiatric:** self-consciousness or decreased self-esteem

Symptoms

- **Acne:** oily skin, pimples, and blemishes on face, jaw, upper body
- **Rosacea:** facial redness, small blemishes, frequent episodes of flushing

Diagnosis

Objective finding	Acne vulgaris	Acne rosacea
Age	Adolescence through fifth decade	More often in middle-aged females
Skin tone	Any	More often in fair-skinned
Skin disruptions	Papules, pustules, with inflammation dependent upon severity of acne; possible painful nodules and cysts	Central face/chin/forehead erythema/telangiectasia; small superficial papules, pustules, or nodules
Comedones	Yes	No
Conjunctivitis	No	Possible

Table 16.7.1 Differentiating Acne Vulgaris and Rosacea

Neonatal acne can be seen in newborns at 3–4 weeks of age. Presents as mildly inflammatory small papules and pustules. Comedones are absent.

The American Academy of Dermatology has not recommended a specific classification system for acne (based upon the available, current evidence). However, it is helpful to systematically classify acne:

- **Mild:** noninflammatory, open and closed comedones are present
- **Moderate:** inflammatory, blemishes are increased in number, small papules and pustules are present
- **Severe:** inflammatory, a significantly increased number and severity of blemishes
- **Cystic:** painful nodules and cysts are present on the face, jaw, and/or upper body

Plan

Treatment, Education, and Referral

Acne Vulgaris

- Treatment includes topical benzoyl peroxide every evening (start with 2.5%, may increase to 5%, then 10% if needed); topical clindamycin or retinoid may be added if the area is inflamed; oral doxycycline or minocycline may be used in moderate to severe acne, limited to a 3-month treatment period; for severe acne, scarring, or cystic, prescribe isotretinoin; for post-inflammatory dyspigmentation, use topical azelaic acid as an adjunct

- Educate the patient to wash face twice daily with mild cleanser and use noncomedogenic sunscreen and oil-free moisturizer as needed for dry skin; advise the patient to expect a worsening of skin appearance prior to actual improvement, and resultant dryness; for female patients taking isotretinoin, stress the importance of using two forms of reliable contraception and avoiding pregnancy

- Consult with physician if treatment is unsuccessful after 10–12 weeks or if acne is severe (refer to dermatology)

Rosacea

- Treatment can be topical (metronidazole, clindamycin, sodium sulfacetamide, azelaic acid) and/or oral forms (doxycycline); refractory cases may benefit from isotretinoin

- Educate the patient to avoid triggers, use daily sunscreen, wear protective clothing and hats when outdoors, and use a mild cleanser

- Refer the patient with persistent redness for laser therapy

Neonatal Acne

- There is no treatment

- Educate the parent to wash the infant's face twice daily with clear water

- Refer the infant with persistent or worsening acne beyond newborn period

---

Digital Resource

When prescribing isotretinoin, refer to the iPledge website at **www.ipledgeprogram.com** for important safety information regarding serious adverse effects. Prescribers, patients, and pharmacists must comply monthly with this program in order for the prescription to be filled.

Takeaways

- Noninflammatory acne (mild) may be treated with monotherapy of benzoyl peroxide.
- Inflammation, papules, and pustules distinguish mild acne from moderate to severe acne.
- Rosacea presents with redness in the central face and possible small papules and pustules, but no comedones.

LESSON 8: MISCELLANEOUS DERMATOLOGY ISSUES

Learning Objectives

■ Differentiate clinical manifestations of various dermatologic issues

■ Choose and interpret laboratory/diagnostic testing for various dermatologic issues

■ Describe appropriate treatment and referrals for a variety of dermatologic issues

There are various issues that may affect the skin including alopecia, areata, cysts, hidradenitis suppurativa, psoriasis, subungual hematoma, and urticaria.

Assessment

Subjective

Determine history of psoriasis, atopic disease (urticaria), obesity, and smoking (hidradenitis suppurativa), and assess for risk factors for dermatologic issues. Common risk factors include stress, use of antimalarial drugs, beta-blockers, lithium, nonsteroidal anti-inflammatory drugs, sudden withdrawal of potent topical or systemic corticosteroids, local trauma, HIV infection, alcohol or tobacco use, and antecedent streptococcal infection (child or young adult).

Symptoms

- Rash
- Skin bump(s)
- Pruritus (psoriasis, urticaria)
- Sudden hair loss
- Nail pain (subungual hematoma)

Review of Systems

- **Resp:** difficulty breathing (urticaria)
- **MS:** joint pain or swelling (psoriasis)
- **Psychiatric:** increased stress level (alopecia areata, psoriasis)

Objective

Disorder	Objective findings
Alopecia areata	Round or oval patches of complete or near complete hair loss; fine new hair growth may be seen
Cyst	Skin-colored nodule; may have a central punctum; may be fluctuant (fluid can vary from serous to purulent)
Hidradenitis suppurativa	Inflammatory, tender, or deep-seated nodules, coalescing into tracts; enlarging into painful abscesses (releases malodorous, purulent drainage when ruptured) located in apocrine gland–bearing areas along the inframammary fold in women; tend to be recurrent/chronic

Table 16.8.1 Objective Findings of Dermatological Disorders

Disorder	Objective findings
Psoriasis	• Discrete pink plaques with silvery scale • Possibly pruritic, typically on elbows, knees, scalp, and buttocks; in diaper area of infants • Positive Auspitz sign (punctate bleeding after removing scale) • Stippled or pitting nails • Koebner phenomenon: an isomorphic response (psoriatic lesions occur in areas of local injury such as scratches, surgical scars, or sunburns)
Subungual hematoma	Maroon, black discoloration of nail
Urticaria	Hives; circumscribed, raised, erythematous with central pallor; may be round, oval, snake-shaped; may be accompanied by angioedema of face, lips, extremities, and genitals

Table 16.8.1 Objective Findings of Dermatological Disorders (Continued)

> **DANGER SIGN** Angioedema may occur with urticaria. Carefully assess airway if mouth is involved.

Diagnosis

Diagnosis of these dermatological disorders is based upon the subjective and objective findings. Helpful laboratory tests include:

- Antistreptolysin O titer (if recent strep infection and initial onset of psoriatic lesions)
- Eosinophilia occurs with urticaria
- Skin biopsy may be performed by dermatologist to verify diagnosis of alopecia areata

Plan

Alopecia Areata

- **Treatment**
  - Minoxidil 5% cream twice daily
  - Anthralin: leave on 20–60 minutes, then wash off
  - Children: topical lower potency corticosteroid
- **Education**
  - Reassure patient they did not cause hair loss (it is an autoimmune response, worsened with stress)
  - Stress management techniques such as yoga, meditation, tai chi, exercise
  - Hide hair loss with hairstyle change or by wearing a wig or other head covering
  - Join a support group
- **Referral**
  - Adults to dermatology for intralesional corticosteroid injections

Cyst

- **Treatment**
  - Incision and drainage
  - PO doxycycline, minocycline or cephalexin
  - Kenalog injection

- **Education**
  - If I&D performed, keep site clean and dry
  - If packing placed during I&D, advance/remove as directed
- **Referral**
  - Refer to dermatology if large cyst or recalcitrant/recurrent

Hidradenitis Suppurativa

- **Treatment**
  - Topical clindamycin
  - Oral doxycycline or minocycline
  - Resorcinol 15% cream: apply thin layer to nodule twice daily
- **Education**
  - Weight loss and smoking cessation are encouraged
  - Healthy diet
  - Cleanse with antibacterial soap
- **Referral**
  - Refer to dermatology if it continues to recur or there is significant scarring

Psoriasis

- **Treatment**
  - Keratolytic agents (salicylic acid)
  - Topical steroids, medium to high potency for short period (plaque resolution), then change to lower potency 3–4 times per week to maintain remission
  - Coal tar preparations, especially shampoo (may not be well accepted by patients due to messiness and odor)
  - Corticosteroid resistant: calcipotriene (Dovonex) twice daily up to 8 weeks, avoiding face and skin folds or anthralin (Drithocreme); use short-term (avoid sunlight)
- **Education**
  - Use emollients
  - Avoid harsh soaps/exfoliants, scrubbing, skin dryness
  - Sunlight exposure benefits some patients
  - Oatmeal baths to loosen scale
  - Apply coal tar products at bedtime, allow to stay on 15 minutes, then rinse off
  - Manage stress
- **Referral**
  - If involvement >20% of body, refer for phototherapy; ultraviolet A light exposure is associated with increased skin cancer risk
  - With refractory cases, refer to rheumatologist (may need biologic therapy, cyclosporine, methotrexate, or systemic retinoids)
  - If extensive, arthritic, or inflammatory disease, refer to rheumatologist

Subungual Hematoma

- **Treatment**
  - Nail trephination: make one or more holes in the area of the nail hematoma with a portable cautery device or heated 18-gauge needle, ensuring hole is large enough to drain the hematoma
- **Education**
  - Soak affected nail bed with antiseptic soap three times daily until drainage has stopped
  - Monitor for signs of infection
- **Referral**
  - Nail injuries that involve lacerations or a crushing fracture of the distal phalanx should be referred to an orthopedist

Urticaria

- **Treatment**
  - Discontinue offending allergen
  - Antihistamines
  - Avoid heat
  - Oral corticosteroids
  - Epinephrine is first-line treatment of anaphylaxis
- **Education**
  - Avoid triggers such as food allergies, insect stings, medications, contact with known allergens
- **Referral**
  - If symptoms are present >6 weeks duration

DANGER SIGN   Stevens-Johnson syndrome is a medical emergency.

- May have prodrome (usually 1–3 days): high fever, sore throat, chest pain, cough, diarrhea, vomiting, and/or arthralgia
- Blistering with widespread mucosal involvement of eyes, nose, mouth
- Rash: erythematous macules on head/neck, spreading to trunk and extremities
- Blisters form within hours; rash may become hemorrhage and is confluent

---

Takeaways

- Cysts can be distinguished from hidradenitis suppurativa by the presence of a punctate head.
- Key diagnostic factors for hidradenitis suppurativa are recurrence and location in apocrine gland-bearing areas.
- A classic presentation of psoriasis is distinct pink lesions with silver plaques on extensor surfaces, like elbows.

PRACTICE QUESTIONS

Select the ONE best answer.

Lesson 1: Dermatology Basics

1. A 19-year-old patient was seen by the nurse practitioner to get refills for her asthma and hay fever medications. At that visit, the patient shows the NP a "rash" behind her knees and in her antecubital areas. When asked what else has changed in her routine, the patient tells the NP she started playing soccer and is taking a hot shower before heading home after practice each day. Based on the patient's symptoms, the care plan may include:

   A. Washing as usual and using soothing oatmeal lotion on affected areas

   B. Avoiding foods with peanuts

   C. Avoiding overly hot baths

   D. Advising to stop scratching the areas so the rash will go away

2. The nurse practitioner's 65-year-old patient is homeless and has been staying in a local shelter. He complains of pruritus on his ventral wrists and in the webbed areas of his fingers. The nurse practitioner examines his wrists. The most likely description of his lesions is:

   A. Multiple well-demarcated plaques with overlying silvery-white scale

   B. Erythematous papules with coalescing/edematous plaques (wheals)

   C. Multiple erythematous vesicles and papules with accompanying silvery linear burrows and secondary excoriations

   D. Expanding circular red rash with central clearing

3. A mother has brought in her 7-year-old son for examination. According to the mother, the boy has been feeling "under the weather" and has had a mild temperature, mild sore throat, and an on-and-off headache for a week. While her son states he feels better and his fever and sore throat are now gone, he still looks "feverish" to the mother, as the skin on his cheeks has turned bright red as if he were slapped. What is the likely cause of his condition?

   A. Child abuse

   B. Toxoplasma gondii

   C. Coxsackievirus

   D. Parvovirus B19

4. A few months after entering a nursing home, the 75-year-old patient has developed a painful vesicular rash in a dermatomal distribution on her right chest and an additional forehead rash. The nurse practitioner suspects _____ and will seek a referral to a _____.

   A. herpes simplex; dermatopathologist

   B. herpes zoster; ophthalmologist

   C. shingles; infectious disease specialist

   D. crusted scabies; wound specialist

5. The patient has greasy yellow flakes on her scalp and behind her ears. The patient says she washes her hair weekly. The nurse practitioner recommends that the patient change her hair care regimen. She believes the patient is suffering from _____ and may benefit from the daily use of _____.

   A. seborrheic dermatitis; ketoconazole shampoo (Nizoral)

   B. scalp psoriasis; ingenol mebutate (Picato)

   C. head lice; permethrin cream (Elimite)

   D. alopecia; clobetasol propionate spray (Clobex)

6. The patient shows the nurse practitioner a lesion on his third finger, right hand. It is a 1 cm, dome-shaped verrucous papule with small black punctate spots. The patient is to be referred to dermatology. Treatment for his lesion may include daily application of:

   A. mupirocin (Bactroban)

   B. salicylic acid (Durasal)

   C. ammonium lactate (Lac-Hydrin)

   D. calamine lotion

Lesson 2: Dermatology/Pharmacology

7. A new patient complains of new itchy "bumps" in her genital area. After consulting the Internet for advice, the patient applied a small amount of vinegar to each lesion to help identify their cause. She found this produced acetowhite changes on the surfaces of the lesions. The nurse practitioner visualizes flesh-colored papules with a cauliflower appearance in the patient's genital area and determines that the lesions are most likely:

   A. Herpetic whitlow and can be treated with a course of acyclovir

   B. Molluscum contagiosum and can be treated with applications of Canthacur

   C. Condyloma acuminatum and can be treated with a course of imiquimod (Aldara)

   D. Verruca vulgaris and can be treated with cryotherapy

8. A patient suffering from psoriasis is concerned about possible adverse effects from steroid overuse. The nurse practitioner knows adverse effects can include all of the following except:

   A. Striae

   B. Hypopigmentation

   C. Thinning skin

   D. Hyperpigmentation

9. A patient does not want to continue ciclopirox nail lacquer 8% (Penlac) for onychomycosis and wants to know what treatment might be most effective. Which of the following would the nurse practitioner likely prescribe?

   A. terbinafine (Lamisil) 250 mg by mouth once daily for six weeks

   B. Vicks VapoRub applied nightly to each affected nail

   C. ciclopirox (Loprox) cream applied nightly

   D. doxycycline (Vibramycin) 40 mg orally daily for 6 weeks

10. A 5-year-old patient has mild eczema on her cheeks. Her mother prefers to use a leftover prescription for topical clobetasol cream 0.05% (Temovate) instead of going to the pharmacy for a new prescription. The nurse practitioner uses the following elements to determine if this medication can be used except:

    A. Patient's age

    B. Expiration date of the medication

    C. Location of the condition

    D. Severity of the condition

Lesson 3: Carcinoma and Melanoma

11. A 58-year-old African American male presents to the clinic with complaints of a non-tender sore on his upper lip that appeared approximately two months ago. PMH is non-contributory, though he has a 30 pack-per-year smoking history. Upon examination, the FNP notes a slightly elevated, erythematous plaque with well-defined borders and no telangiectasias. The suspected diagnosis is:

    A. Basal cell carcinoma

    B. Squamous cell carcinoma

    C. Actinic keratosis

    D. Psoriasis

12. A 28-year-old female presents to the clinic for an annual skin examination. The nurse practitioner notes a mole on the patient's left leg that is dark brown, circular, slightly raised, and 8 mm in diameter. The nurse practitioner is most concerned about which characteristic?

    A. Diameter

    B. Color

    C. Shape

    D. Slight elevation

13. If malignant melanoma is suspected, which of the following diagnostic methods should be utilized?

    A. Shave biopsy

    B. Fine-needle biopsy

    C. Punch biopsy

    D. Excisional biopsy

14. Mohs surgery, a technique in which a lesion is excised and examined under a microscope to determine if the edges are free from cancer, is an appropriate treatment option for which of the following lesions?

    A. Basal cell carcinoma

    B. Malignant melanoma

    C. Actinic keratosis

    D. Seborrheic keratosis

15. A 31-year-old female presents to the clinic with concerns about a mole on her back that seemed to "appear overnight." Upon further investigation, you learn that her father has a history of squamous cell carcinoma, she had several blistering sunburns as a teenager, and she wears sunblock with SPF 20 most days. Upon physical exam, you note that she is fair-skinned, blonde, and blue-eyed. Which of the following risk factors is most concerning for malignant melanoma?

    A. Family history of squamous cell carcinoma

    B. Blistering sunburns as a teenager

    C. Use of 20 SPF sunblock

    D. Fair-skinned, light eyes/hair

Lesson 4: Dermatitis

16. Which of the following is not a common irritant in contact dermatitis?

    A. Perfumes

    B. Cotton

    C. Plants

    D. Nickel

17. Where does seborrheic dermatitis most frequently occur?

    A. Scalp

    B. Dorsa of feet

    C. Antecubital spaces

    D. Lower legs

18. Which of the following is true regarding contact dermatitis?

    A. Continued exposure to the irritant is allowable

    B. Medication can control the response to continued irritant exposure

    C. Oatmeal baths and calamine lotion can be helpful

    D. Baths may worsen the response to the irritant and should be avoided

19. Which of the following best describes atopic dermatitis?

    A. Furuncles and carbuncles in clusters with redness

    B. Redness with significant scaling, yet well-tolerated

    C. Dry skin with pruritic rashes, related to a fungus

    D. Dry, pruritic skin with rashes, related to allergy

20. When prescribing a shampoo for seborrheic dermatitis, the FNP should ensure the shampoo includes which of the following ingredients?

    A. griseofulvin

    B. Neosporin

    C. Perfume

    D. selenium sulfide

21. Which of the following is NOT recommended for the treatment of atopic dermatitis?

    A. Repeated moisturizing with lotion to face and cream to body

    B. Twice daily antihistamine cream to affected areas

    C. Fragrance-free detergent, fabric softener, and dryer sheets

    D. Unscented, sensitive-skin Dove soap or Cetaphil cleanser

Lesson 5: Injury and Wounds

22. Which of the following is the preferred choice when prescribing an antibiotic for an adult patient with a human or animal bite?

    A. amoxicillin (Augmentin) clavulanate

    B. cephalexin (Keflex)

    C. doxycycline (Vibramycin)

    D. trimethoprim-sulfamethoxazole (Bactrim DS)

23. The nurse practitioner in the clinic is treating a patient with painful, blistering burns on the left third, fourth, and fifth fingers, extending slightly onto the dorsa. What is the appropriate plan?

    A. Apply silver sulfadiazine cream (Silvadene) to the blisters

    B. Refer for burn specialty care

    C. Open the blisters and apply antibiotic cream

    D. Use a nonadherent dressing to wrap loosely

24. Which of the following is not considered a predisposing factor for the development of lower extremity ulcers?

    A. Young age

    B. Diabetes mellitus

    C. Venous insufficiency

    D. Obesity

25. Which clinical manifestation is characteristic of fire ant stings?

    A. Round, bluish colored papules

    B. Single, large bull's-eye rash

    C. Honey-colored crusting on an erythematous base

    D. Groups of red spots with blisters on top

26. Which medication is appropriate for preventing burn wound infection?

    A. Oral erythromycin

    B. Oral moxifloxacin

    C. Topical corticosteroid

    D. Topical silver sulfadiazine

27. The nurse practitioner caring for an older adult has noted a pressure ulcer exhibiting full-thickness skin loss with a crater-like appearance. The nurse practitioner documents this ulcer as which stage?

    A. Stage 1

    B. Stage 2

    C. Stage 3

    D. Stage 4

Lesson 6: Skin Infections & Infestations

28. The FNP is assessing a teen boy's scalp and notes black dots in a quarter-sized circular pattern. This finding is indicative of:

    A. Melanoma

    B. Early onset male pattern baldness

    C. Tinea capitis

    D. Alopecia areata

29. Which of the following is the best definition of impetigo?

    A. Noncontagious bacterial infection affecting the skin's subcutaneous layers

    B. Noncontagious bacterial infection affecting the epidermal superficial layers

    C. Contagious bacterial infection affecting the skin's subcutaneous layers

    D. Contagious bacterial infection affecting the epidermal superficial layers

30. A 72-year-old presents with a painful rash. The FNP notes a 3-inch strip of vesicles wrapping slightly around the left torso, which is indicative of:

    A. Cellulitis

    B. Erysipelas

    C. Herpes zoster

    D. Impetigo

31. Which condition is associated with a herald patch?

    A. Tinea corporis

    B. Pityriasis rosea

    C. Carbuncles

    D. Impetigo

32. Which of the following is the best description of paronychia?

    A. Swollen, red, painful

    B. Swollen, blue, painful

    C. Painful redness without swelling

    D. Swollen, red, painless

33. The FNP is caring for several individuals with skin infections. Which individual is most likely to have impetigo?

    A. 17-year-old team athlete

    B. 27-month-old in day care

    C. 45-year-old landscaper

    D. 78-year-old in long-term care

34. The FNP student recalls that onychomycosis is an infection of the toenail or fingernail and recognizes that the infection is caused by a:

    A. Bacteria

    B. Fungus

    C. Parasite

    D. Virus

Lesson 7: Acne & Rosacea

35. Which description of clinical manifestations best characterizes acne vulgaris?

    A. Blackened skin on certain body parts

    B. Comedones, papules, pustules

    C. Widespread facial redness

    D. Pruritus, erythema, flakiness

36. Which medication classification is commonly used to treat rosacea?

    A. Antibiotics

    B. Antifungals

    C. Non-steroidal anti-inflammatory drugs

    D. Corticosteroids

37. Moderate acne is best classified by which of the following?

    A. Closed comedones

    B. Inflammation and occasional papules/pustules

    C. Open comedones

    D. Cysts and nodules

38. Which of the following individuals is most likely to experience rosacea?

    A. 5-year-old Caucasian male

    B. 14-year-old African American male

    C. 48-year-old Caucasian female

    D. 69-year-old African American female

39. The nurse practitioner is prescribing monotherapy for a patient with mild acne. Which product will be prescribed?

    A. benzoyl peroxide (Benzagel)

    B. isotretinoin (Accutane)

    C. Topical retinoid (Retin A)

    D. Regular facial moisturizer

40. Which of the following statements regarding rosacea is incorrect?

    A. The cause is unknown

    B. Rosacea may cause dry, red eyes

    C. A biopsy is necessary for diagnosis

    D. A cure does not exist

Lesson 8: Miscellaneous Dermatology Issues

41. A patient presents with patches on both elbows that are not improving, despite use of a topical steroid cream. They are nonpruritic, pink, sharply demarcated papular plaques with a silvery scale. What is the nurse practitioner's diagnosis of this condition?

    A. Eczema

    B. Psoriasis

    C. Rosacea

    D. Xerosis

42. Which treatment recommendation would the nurse practitioner make for the patient diagnosed with alopecia areata?

    A. Begin daily meditation, yoga, or tai chi practice

    B. Take vitamin D; 2000 international units daily

    C. Stop wearing restrictive headbands and hats

    D. Shampoo with an organic, dye-free product

43. Which of the following laboratory findings would be consistent with the diagnosis of urticaria?

    A. Hyphae on KOH prep

    B. Neutropenia

    C. Decreased erythrocyte sedimentation rate

    D. Eosinophilia

44. A patient has psoriasis on both arms. What is the most appropriate treatment recommendation?

    A. Tumor necrosis modulators

    B. Psoralen with ultraviolet A light therapy

    C. Medium-potency topical corticosteroids

    D. Anthralin or calcipotriene

45. Trephination is used to treat which of the following disorders?

    A. Subungual hematoma

    B. Hidradenitis suppurativa

    C. Psoriasis

    D. Urticaria

46. A patient presents with a painful, pimple-like rash in her axilla. She states she has had this once or twice before. What is the most likely diagnosis?

    A. Acne vulgaris

    B. Folliculitis

    C. Hidradenitis suppurativa

    D. Urticaria

ANSWERS AND EXPLANATIONS

Lesson 1: Dermatology Basics

1. C

The patient manifests all three conditions of the atopic triad: eczema, asthma, and hay fever. This fact, and the fact that her symptoms appeared after her new habit of taking hot showers, points to the correct answer **(C)**, avoiding overly hot baths. The oatmeal lotion (A) will help relieve itching from eczema or psoriasis, but washing as usual permits the patient to continue the hot showers that would aggravate her symptoms. Avoiding foods with peanuts (B) supposes the patient has a food allergy; there is no evidence for this. The patient won't stop scratching (D) simply based on advice to do so. It is true that eczema is often described as the "itch that rashes," that is to say, the patient is likely causing excoriations from scratching. However, providing a solution (avoiding overly hot baths) is a better option.

2. C

Pruritus on the ventral wrists and in the webbed area of the fingers is likely scabies, which may be described as multiple erythematous vesicles and papules with accompanying silvery linear burrows and secondary excoriations **(C)**. Multiple well-demarcated plaques with overlying silvery-white scale (A) describes psoriasis. Erythematous papules with coalescing/edematous plaques (wheals) (B) describes hives. An expanding circular red rash with central clearing (D) describes erythema migrans.

3. D

Parvovirus B19 **(D)** is the infectious agent associated with fifth disease. There is no evidence of child abuse (A). Toxoplasma gondii (B) is associated with toxoplasmosis and coxsackievirus (C) is associated with hand, foot, and mouth disease.

4. B

A painful vesicular rash in a dermatomal distribution on her right chest and an additional forehead rash provides a classic description of herpes zoster **(B)**. An ophthalmology referral is warranted due to the risk of herpes zoster ophthalmicus. The lesions are described as dermatomal, and, in the older population, are associated with herpes zoster (a recurrence of chickenpox), not herpes simplex (A), and the nurse practitioner would not refer the patient to the dermatopathologist (who would be examining biopsies on the microscopic and at the molecular level). Shingles (C) is another name for herpes zoster, but the nurse practitioner would not need to refer the patient to infectious disease. The rash described does not fit a description of crusted scabies (D); also, a wound specialist is not typically warranted for this condition.

5. A

Greasy yellow flakes on the scalp and behind the ears is a classic description of seborrheic dermatitis **(A)**, and the treatment described—ketoconazole shampoo—is a standard treatment. Psoriasis (B) is usually plaque-like; also, ingenol is not a treatment for psoriasis. There is no evidence of infestation/lice (C). The description provided does not match the symptoms of alopecia (hair loss) (D).

6. B

Daily application of salicylic acid **(B)** describes standard treatment for verruca vulgaris. Mupirocin (A) is a topical antibiotic. Ammonium lactate (C) is common for hyperkeratotic skin, but it will not cure verruca vulgaris. Calamine lotion (D) is a medication used to treat mild pruritus.

Lesson 2: Dermatology/Pharmacology

7. C

The description of the lesions represent condyloma acuminatum **(C)**, and imiquimod is used as a treatment. Herpetic whitlow (A) is by definition located on the hand. Molluscum contagiosum (B) is caused by poxvirus and typically affects children 1–10 years old. It would unlikely be confined to the genital area. Verruca vulgaris (D) is not commonly seen in the genital area.

8. D

Hyperpigmentation **(D)** is not an adverse effect of a topical steroid. Striae (A), hypopigmentation (B), and thinning skin (C) are adverse effects of topical steroids.

9. A

Research indicates that oral antifungal medications like terbinafine **(A)** are the most effective treatment for onychomycosis. These medications interact with many other medications and can be hepatotoxic. They require patients to avoid alcohol, have liver function testing, and avoid sun exposure. There is a small body of research indicating that daily application of Vicks VapoRub (B) successfully eliminates fungal nail infections, but these results do not show as much efficacy as oral medications. Ciclopirox cream (C) has not been found to be effective in treating onychomycosis, as it does not absorb into the nail. Doxycycline (D) is an antibiotic, not an antifungal.

10. B

While the expiration date **(B)** would be important information, it is not an element to consider in choosing a topical medication. The elements to consider are included in the acronym **VALUES**: Vehicle, Acuity/Severity, Location, Use, agE, and Strength. The patient's age (A), location of the condition (C), and the severity of the condition (D) are all part of the elements.

Lesson 3: Carcinoma and Melanoma

11. B

Squamous cell carcinoma **(B)** is the most common skin cancer in African Americans and often appears on the lips of smokers. A slightly elevated red plaque with well-defined borders is characteristic of squamous cell carcinoma. Basal cell carcinoma (A) is less common in African Americans and is often described as a nonhealing sore. It is usually a raised nodule or papule with telangiectasias and bleeding. Actinic keratoses (C) are often tender and bleed. Squamous cell carcinoma can resemble psoriasis (D), though this patient has no history of psoriasis and the mouth would be an unusual place for psoriasis to develop.

12. A

The most concerning characteristic is the large diameter **(A)**. Any mole >8 mm should be evaluated. The color (B) and shape (C) are normal. A mole with elevation (D) should be evaluated, but the large size is more concerning.

13. D

If malignant melanoma is suspected, a total excisional biopsy **(D)** should be done so staging is possible. Shave biopsies (A) are done for benign moles. A fine-needle biopsy (B) and punch biopsy (C) are not appropriate on lesions suspected of malignant melanoma.

14. A

Mohs is frequently used to treat basal cell carcinoma **(A)** and squamous cell carcinoma. Malignant melanoma (B) is treated with wide local excision. Actinic keratosis (C) is treated with topical agents. Seborrheic keratosis (D) is treated with cryotherapy or curettage.

15. B

The most significant risk factor for developing malignant melanoma is a history of blistering sunburns **(B)**. A family history of melanoma, not squamous cell carcinoma (A), is a risk factor. Sunblock with an SPF of 30 is recommended, but using an SPF of 20 (C) does not increase one's risk of developing malignant melanoma. Fair skin, light eyes, and hair (D) do increase an individual's risk for developing malignant melanoma.

Lesson 4: Dermatitis

16. B

Cotton **(B)** is not usually an offender resulting in contact dermatitis. Common irritants include chemicals such as those found in perfumes (A), cosmetics, personal care, and cleaning products; poison ivy/oak/sumac (C); and metals (D).

17. A

The most common location of seborrheic dermatitis is on the scalp **(A)**, as in cradle cap in infants and dandruff in adolescents and adults. Additional locations include the ears, eyebrows, eyelids, face, upper chest, upper back, axillae, and genital area. The dorsa of the feet (B), antecubital spaces (C), and lower legs (D) are not common locations for seborrhea.

18. C

Oatmeal baths and calamine lotion **(C)** are used to calm and soothe itchy, painful, irritated skin. Continued exposure to the irritant (A) is not advised. Medications (B) are not routinely used to control irritant response; rather, avoiding exposure to the offending substance is advised. Baths (D), particularly oatmeal baths, can be helpful in soothing the skin.

19. D

Atopic dermatitis is the "itch that rashes" and is related to allergens **(D)**. Though it may become secondarily infected, it is not characterized by furuncles/carbuncles (A). It is also not characterized by scaling (B), nor does it result from a fungus (C). Atopic dermatitis is not well-tolerated (B); on the contrary, the pruritus can be extremely bothersome.

20. D

Selenium sulfide **(D)** is one of the important active ingredients in dandruff shampoos. Certain dandruff shampoos include an antifungal in their formulation (ketoconazole or clotrimazole), but griseofulvin (A) is an oral medication. Neosporin (B) is an antibiotic and is not prescribed for seborrhea. In general, perfumes (C) should be avoided in persons with skin conditions.

21. B

Antihistamine creams **(B)** are generally not helpful in atopic dermatitis, though systemic antihistamines may control the response to allergens or triggers. Continual moisturizing (A) is the main focus in the prevention and treatment of atopic dermatitis flares. All products coming into contact with the skin via the clothes (C) or directly (D) should be fragrance-free.

Lesson 5: Injury and Wounds

22. A

Amoxicillin clavulanate (Augmentin) **(A)** is the preferred antibiotic for animal and human bites. Cephalexin (B) is not an appropriate first choice, as it is used primarily for bacterial infections of the respiratory tract, middle ear, skin, bone, and urinary tract. In the case of penicillin allergy in the child under 8 years and pregnant women, doxycycline (C) is an acceptable alternative. In the child younger than 8 years, trimethoprim-sulfamethoxazole (D) is acceptable in the penicillin-allergic patient.

23. B

Burns involving a high-function area such as the hand or foot should be referred to a burn specialty center, rather than treating them in an outpatient setting **(B)**. It is not appropriate to treat this burn in the outpatient setting, so applying Silvadene (A), antibiotic cream (C), or a dressing (D) are not correct choices.

24. A

Young age **(A)** is not considered to be a risk factor for the development of lower extremity ulcers. Predisposing factors include diabetes mellitus (B), venous insufficiency (C), obesity (D), coronary artery disease, peripheral neuropathy, age over 65 years, edema, hyperlipidemia, arterial insufficiency, and congestive heart failure.

25. D

Groups of red (often small) spots with blisters on top of each spot **(D)** are characteristic of fire ant stings. Bluish colored papules (A) do not occur with fire ant stings, nor does a single, large bull's-eye rash (B) (which occurs with Lyme disease). Honey-colored crusting on an erythematous base (C) occurs with impetigo.

26. D

For the prevention of infection in burn wounds, it is appropriate to utilize a topical medication with antimicrobial properties **(D)**. Oral antibiotics (A and B) would be appropriate for treatment, rather than prevention of infection in a burn wound. Topical corticosteroids (C) do not have antimicrobial properties.

27. C

The stage 3 pressure ulcer **(C)** has a crater-like appearance with full-thickness skin loss, possibly with fat exposure. A stage 1 ulcer (A) is indicated when non-blanchable erythema and possibly induration are present on intact skin, while stage 2 pressure ulcers (C) may have blisters with epidermal or dermal skin loss. A stage 4 pressure ulcer (D) has full-thickness skin and tissue loss with exposure of muscle, bone, and tendons.

Lesson 6: Skin Infections & Infestations

28. C

The black dot sign is indicative of tinea capitis **(C)**. The black dots occur in the areas of fungal infection due to the hair breaking off. It is not a sign of melanoma (A) or male pattern baldness (B). Alopecia areata (D) results in round patches of hair loss, but not with black dots.

29. D

Impetigo is a contagious bacterial infection (usually *Streptococcus* or *S. aureus*) affecting the superficial layers of the epidermis **(D)**. Thus, it is not noncontagious (A and B). Impetigo is not an infection of the subcutaneous layers of the skin (C).

30. C

Herpes zoster **(C)**, most often seen in older adults, is very painful and presents as a unilateral strip of vesicles following a dermatome. Cellulitis (A) presents with erythema and edema in a particular area, usually with an entry point. Erysipelas (B) presents as a demarcated reddened skin rash. Impetigo (D) is characterized by honey-colored crusting on an erythematous base.

31. B

Pityriasis rosea **(B)** is a self-limited viral infection that begins with a single oval or round, pink, scaly patch with a raised border (herald patch) on the trunk, upper arm, neck, or thigh before progressing to the classic Christmas tree pattern on the trunk. Tinea corporis (A) is a fungal infection characterized by a pink annular patch with a scaly raised border and central clearing. A carbuncle (C) is a cluster of boils, infected with bacteria, deep within the skin. Impetigo (D) is characterized as an erythematous lesion with a honey-colored crust.

32. A

Paronychia is an infection of the tissue surrounding the nail and presents with painful erythema and edema **(A)**. It does not cause blueness (B). It results in edema, so is not without swelling (C), and is quite painful, not painless (D).

33. B

Impetigo occurs most commonly in toddlers **(B)**. It is not most frequent in adolescents (A), and rarely occurs in adults (C) and older adults (D).

34. B

Onychomycosis is a fungal **(B)** infection of the nail, more commonly the toenail. It is not an infection caused by bacteria (A), a parasite (C), or a virus (D).

Lesson 7: Acne & Rosacea

35. B

Acne vulgaris is characterized by open and/or closed comedones, papules, and pustules **(B)** and may also include cysts or nodules. It is not blackened skin (A). Facial redness may be associated with rosacea (C). Pruritus, erythema, and flaking (D) commonly occur with atopic dermatitis.

36. A

Topical antibiotics such as metronidazole and oral low-dose doxycycline **(A)** are commonly used for rosacea treatment. Azelaic acid also seems to have antimicrobial properties. Antifungal agents (B) and non-steroidal anti-inflammatory drugs (C) are not commonly used to treat rosacea. If corticosteroids (D) are recommended, only low-potency should be used on the face.

37. B

In addition to open and closed comedones, moderate acne features increased numbers of blemishes, mild inflammation, and occasional papules/pustules **(B)**. In mild acne, closed comedones (A) (blackheads) and open comedones (C) are present without inflammation. The key feature of cystic acne is large blemishes on the face, jaw, and/or upper body, which include painful cysts and nodules (D).

38. C

Rosacea may occur in any individual, but it most often affects fair-skinned females of middle age **(C)**. Fair-skinned children (A) are not the most affected group, nor are dark-skinned individuals (B and D).

39. A

Initial monotherapy for the treatment of mild acne is benzoyl peroxide **(A)**. Isotretinoin (B) is reserved for moderate-to-severe acne. A topical retinoid (C) may be added to therapy if needed in the future. Facial moisturizers (D) do not treat acne.

40. C

The clinical manifestations are used for determining the diagnosis; a biopsy is not needed to diagnose rosacea **(C)**. A familial link to rosacea seems to exist, but the cause remains unknown (A). In addition to facial skin redness, rosacea may cause dry, irritated, red eyes (B). While there is no cure (D), control and management are possible through treatment.

Lesson 8: Miscellaneous Dermatology Issues

41. B

The description of the lesions and their location are typical of psoriasis **(B)**. Eczema (A) is an atopic condition resulting in extreme pruritus and a flaking rash. Rosacea (C) is noted by reddening on the face with tiny papules and/or pustules. Xerosis (D) is a term used to refer to very dry skin.

42. A

Implementing a stress reduction practice such as meditation, yoga, or tai chi **(A)** would be most appropriate, as it is thought that alopecia areata may be triggered by stress. Vitamin D (B), not wearing hats or headbands (C), and changing shampoo (D) are not treatment recommendations for alopecia areata.

43. D

As with other type I hypersensitivity problems, eosinophilia **(D)** is present with urticaria. Hyphae on KOH prep (A) is diagnostic of fungal infection. Neutropenia (B) does not typically occur with urticaria, nor does decreased erythrocyte sedimentation rate (C).

44. C

Treatment with medium-potency topical corticosteroids **(C)** until the psoriatic plaques resolve is most appropriate. Tumor necrosis modulators (A) are reserved for severe recalcitrant psoriasis. Psoralen with ultraviolet A light therapy (B) would be more appropriate for generalized psoriasis, yet bears skin cancer risk. Anthralin and calcipotriene (D) are significantly expensive, so are reserved for corticosteroid-resistant cases.

45. A

Trephination refers to the creation of a small hole; in the case of subungual hematoma **(A)**, the small hole is created in the nail to allow release of blood and decrease associated pain with its accumulation. Trephination is not utilized to treat hidradenitis suppurativa (B), psoriasis (C), or urticaria (D).

46. C

The presentation of a painful, pimple-like rash in an apocrine gland-bearing area is characteristic of hidradenitis suppurativa **(C)**. Acne vulgaris (A) presents with pimples occurring on the face, neck, upper back, and chest. Folliculitis (B) may occur in any area with hair follicles. While urticaria (D) may recur dependent upon allergen exposure, it presents as hives—not pimples.

PART THREE

Pediatrics to Geriatrics

CHAPTER 17

Medical Issues for Infants, Children, and Adolescents

LESSON 1: CONGENITAL DISORDERS

Learning Objectives
- Identify clinical manifestations of various congenital disorders
- Choose and interpret laboratory/diagnostic testing used for differentiating congenital disorders
- Differentiate appropriate treatment and referrals related to congenital disorders

Congenital disorders are present from birth but may not be recognizable until later in childhood. Some of these disorders result from chromosomal abnormalities, but many of them do not have a particular causative factor. The nurse practitioner must be able to recognize these disorders to ensure early and appropriate treatment is instituted.

Definitions
- **Autosomal dominant inheritance:** a gene on a non–sex chromosome is affected in one parent, allowing inheritance of the disorder in the child
- **Early intervention:** federally funded program disseminated via individual states to provide infants and children with developmental delays with the services needed to maximize their development in the early years
- **Facies:** appearance of the face typical of a condition
- **Monosomy:** 1 less chromosome is present (resulting in 1 when there should be 2)
- **Trisomy:** 1 extra chromosome is present (resulting in 3 when there should be 2)

Congenital Physical Disorders

Physical disorders may develop in the fetus for a variety of reasons. Some of these are readily visible at birth, while others may not become apparent until later.

Congenital Lacrimal Duct Obstruction

Nasolacrimal duct obstruction occurs in a large number of newborns. Tearing or discharge of one eye is (usually) noted early in life. The lower lid may be slightly reddened. Diagnosis is made by history and physical examination, but a culture of the drainage may rule out infection. Teach parents to clean the eye area with a moist cloth, moving outward. Nasolacrimal duct massage may allow opening of the duct for drainage. Antibiotic ophthalmic medication is prescribed only when an infection is present. If unresolved by several months of age, refer to pediatric ophthalmology.

Congenital Heart Disease

- **Assessment**

  - Tiring with nursing or bottle feeding (ventricular septal defect [VSD])

  - Poor growth (VSD)

  - Frequent squatting (tetralogy of Fallot)

  - Delay in developmental milestones

  - In the initial newborn period: cyanosis, positive pulse oximetry screen

  - After the initial newborn period:

    - Murmur or click, clubbing (VSD)

    - Observed cyanosis (tetralogy of Fallot and others)

    - Discrepancy in upper vs. lower extremity blood pressure (coarctation of the aorta)

    - Weaker lower extremity pulses as compared to upper extremity pulses (coarctation of the aorta)

    - Edema

    - Crackles (with heart failure in VSD)

- **Diagnosis**

  - Differential diagnoses: **ASD, VSD, PDA, aortic stenosis, pulmonic stenosis, MVP, coarctation of the aorta, transposition of the great vessels**

    - Diagnosis made by echocardiogram, ECG, cardiac MRI (evaluated by pediatric cardiologist)

- **Treatment**

  - Support families in complying with medication, feeding regimen, and postoperative care as applicable

  - Continue routine health promotion activities

  - Monitor for infection

- **Education**

  - Weigh child weekly

  - Effects on growth and development are variable

  - Provide frequent rest periods as needed

  - Monitor for infection

- **Referral**

  - Pediatric cardiologist and/or pediatric cardiothoracic surgeon

  - The Children's Heart Association or the Children's Heart Foundation for support

---

Pro Tip

Perform newborn pulse oximetry screening for critical congenital heart disease.

After 24 hours of age and prior to discharge, screen the alert newborn utilizing pulse oximetry on the right hand (preductal) and either of the lower extremities (postductal) simultaneously or in direct sequence. For results <95%, refer to the screening algorithm available here: **www.cdc.gov/ncbddd/heartdefects/hcp.html**.

Developmental Dysplasia of the Hip

- **Assessment**
  - Family history
  - History of breech birth
  - Lopsided walking (in the child)
  - Unequal thigh skin folds
  - Unequal knee height in supine with knees bent (positive Allis sign)
  - Positive Barlow or Ortolani maneuver
  - Trendelenburg gait (older child)
- **Diagnosis**
  - By hip ultrasound
- **Treatment**
  - Support family compliance with use of Pavlik harness if ordered or in postoperative care if surgical correction occurs
- **Education**
  - Must wear harness 23 hours per day—monitor for skin breakdown
- **Referral**
  - Pediatric orthopedic surgeon

Genitourinary Defects

- **Assessment**
  - Observable physical disorder
  - Recurrent UTI or UTI symptoms
  - Incontinence in toilet-trained child
  - Labial adhesions (female)
  - Hypospadias or epispadias (male)
  - Palpable mass (hydronephrosis)
- **Diagnosis**
  - Renal-bladder ultrasound or CT scan reveals hydronephrosis on the site of obstruction
- **Treatment**
  - Antibiotic treatment for current UTI (prophylaxis may also be needed in particular cases)
  - Support postoperatively
- **Education**
  - Monitor for fever, flank pain, and other signs of urinary tract infection
- **Referral**
  - Pediatric urology

Fetal Alcohol Spectrum Disorder

Exposure to alcohol in utero can have a number of negative impacts on the developing fetus. Clinical manifestations include poor growth (in utero and after birth), microphthalmia, micrognathia (upper), microcephaly, flattened philtrum, thin upper lip, single palmar crease, hypotonia, and poor coordination. A varying degree of cognitive, motor, language, and/or psychosocial delay also occurs, including the possibility of intellectual disability. Refer the infant or child to early intervention or special education as needed. Refer to pediatric cardiology if an associated CHD is present, such as VSD or aortic septal defect.

Genetic Syndromes

Down Syndrome (Trisomy 21)

- **Cause**
  - Three chromosomes present on #21; more frequent in maternal age >35 years
- **Assessment**
  - Depressed nasal bridge
  - Flattened facies
  - Single palmar crease
  - Hyperflexibility and joint laxity
  - Low-set and/or abnormally shaped ears
  - Upward slanted eyes and epicanthal folds
  - Tongue protrusion
  - Some degree of intellectual disability
  - Associated with cardiac defects, vision/hearing impairment, intestinal malformations, frequent infections, increased risk of thyroid disease and leukemia
- **Treatment**
  - Focus on treating associated health issues
  - Thyroid testing at age 6 months, 12 months, and annually
  - Cervical x-ray at age 3–5 years to screen for atlantoaxial instability
- **Education**
  - Regular diet and exercise
  - Follow up with early intervention, therapy, and education as recommended
- **Referral**
  - Geneticist
  - Pediatric ophthalmologist by age 6 months
  - Cardiology for echocardiogram to rule out congenital heart disorder
  - Other specialists as needed depending upon associated disorders
  - Early intervention
  - Down syndrome support group

Fragile X Syndrome

- **Cause**
  - Mutation of FMR1 gene on X chromosome (males more severely affected than females)
- **Assessment**
  - Problems with sensation, behavior, or emotion in young child may be the first signs
  - Delayed developmental milestone attainment

- Ranges from subtle learning disabilities to intellectual disability
- Characteristic features become more obvious with age: prominent forehead, prominent jaw, large protruding ears, elongated face, overly flexible fingers, flat feet, large testes (after puberty)

- **Treatment**
  - Supportive treatments for developmental issues
- **Education**
  - Expect a normal life span
  - Follow up with early intervention, therapy, and educational assistance as recommended
- **Referral**
  - Geneticist
  - Early intervention
  - Educational assistance as needed
  - The National Fragile X foundation for support

Klinefelter Syndrome

- **Cause**
  - Male with one or more additional X chromosomes
- **Assessment**
  - Lack of development of secondary sex characteristics
  - Gynecomastia
  - Decreased facial and pubic hair
  - Underdeveloped testicles
- **Treatment**
  - Testosterone therapy to promote muscular development and increase strength (may also have positive self-esteem and concentration effects)
- **Education**
  - Should have normal intelligence with possibility of learning disabilities
  - Infertility will occur
- **Referral**
  - Geneticist
  - The American Association for Klinefelter Syndrome for support

Marfan Syndrome

- **Cause**
  - Mutation in fibrillin-1 gene (autosomal dominant inheritance)
- **Assessment**
  - Joint laxity and hypotonia
  - Tall stature
  - Long, slender limbs; long, narrow face
  - Minimal subcutaneous fat
  - Delayed achievement of fine and gross motor milestones

- **Treatment**
  - Use specialized chart for growth evaluation
  - Monitor for orthopedic issues such as pectus excavatum/carinatum or acetabulum abnormalities, pes planus, or scoliosis
  - Medication as needed for hypertension
- **Education**
  - Family members should be tested
  - Avoid intense exercise until cleared by cardiologist
  - Seek immediate medical care for difficulty breathing (risk of pneumothorax)
  - Follow up with specialists as recommended
- **Referral**
  - Geneticist
  - Annual ophthalmology exam for ectopia lentis (lens displacement)
  - Cardiology to evaluate aortic root dilation/aneurysm and mitral valve prolapse

Turner Syndrome (Monosomy X)

- **Cause**
  - Part or all of one X chromosome missing on the sex chromosome (affects females only)
- **Assessment**
  - Short stature, slow growth
  - Webbed neck
  - Low posterior hairline
  - Wide-spaced nipples
  - Amenorrhea
  - Lack of secondary sex characteristic development
  - Some perceptual and social skill difficulties
- **Treatment**
  - Growth hormone administration to promote increased stature
- **Education**
  - Should have normal intelligence with possibility of learning disabilities
  - Infertility will occur
- **Referral**
  - Geneticist
  - Turner Syndrome Society of America for support

Down syndrome, Fragile X syndrome, Klinefelter syndrome, Marfan syndrome, and Turner syndrome are diagnosed by cytogenic testing (chromosome analysis).

Takeaways

- Many genetic syndromes may be suspected based on physical findings, but must be verified with chromosomal analysis.
- Screen newborns prior to discharge for critical congenital heart defects.
- Signs and symptoms of congenital heart defects past the newborn period include cyanosis, squatting, tiring with feeding, poor growth, and delayed development.

LESSON 2: INFECTIOUS DISORDERS

Learning Objectives

- Identify clinical manifestations of various infectious pediatric disorders
- Choose and interpret laboratory/diagnostic testing used for differentiating pediatric infectious disorders
- Differentiate appropriate treatment and referrals related to pediatric infectious disorders

Infants and young children are more susceptible to infection than other individuals due to their lack of exposure for resistance development (humoral immunity) and immature immune responses. Thus, young children experience significant numbers of infectious disorders. Many may be preventable by immunization.

Definitions

- **Coryza:** inflammation of nasal mucous membranes
- **Exanthem:** a widespread rash
- **Humoral immunity:** the development of antibodies to specific antigens

Acute Febrile Illness

No matter the cause (bacterial, viral, or otherwise), immunocompetent children are apt to run a fever when experiencing an infectious process. In many (if not most) cases, a source for the fever is either found by history and physical examination or revealed with laboratory testing. Most fevers are viral in nature. Occasionally, an infant or young child (age 3–36 months) presents with a fever for which a source cannot be determined.

The concern is occult bacteremia, which is suspected with fever >102.2°F (39°C) and absence of source per history/physical examination/laboratory finding in a child with a white blood cell count ≥15,000/µl. Those children should be referred to the physician/emergency department and potentially treated for bacteremia.

Older children with fever and a likely cause should be treated for the cause (if non-viral) and have their fever managed as needed. Antipyretics can make children more comfortable, increase their likelihood of being able to continue to take oral fluids, and decrease the risk of dehydration. Either acetaminophen or ibuprofen may be used to manage fever, but should not be used together. The recommended doses are acetaminophen 10–15 mg/kg every 4 hours as needed, or ibuprofen 4–10 mg/kg every 6–8 hours as needed.

Pro Tip

Aspirin is contraindicated for the treatment of an acute febrile illness in children due to the risk of development of Reye syndrome.

Infectious Respiratory Disorders

Disorder	Subjective	Objective
Bronchiolitis	• Nasal drainage • Poor feeding • Fatigue	• Cough; may be tight, paroxysmal • Large quantity clear nasal drainage • Wheezing • Tachypnea, nasal flaring, intercostal/suprasternal retractions • Decreased oxygen saturation in some infants • Hyperinflation on chest x-ray
Bronchitis	• History of mild URI symptoms • Fever	• Hacking cough • Coarse rales • Unlabored respirations
Croup	• Fever	• Paroxysmal barking cough • Inspiratory stridor • Suprasternal retractions • Mild dyspnea
Neonatal chlamydial pneumonia	• Nasal congestion • Eye drainage, redness	• Usually no or minimal fever • Staccato cough, paroxysmal • Rales, no wheezing • Liver/spleen easily palpable secondary to hyperinflated lungs
Pneumonia	• Recent URI • Onset may be sudden or gradual	• Productive cough • Tachypnea • Adventitious breath sounds without wheezing

Table 17.2.1 Assessment of Infectious Respiratory Disorders

Neonatal chlamydial pneumonia may be diagnosed if conjunctivitis is present (chlamydial ophthalmia neonatorum). Culture or nucleic acid assay tests positive for *Chlamydia trachomatis*. Diagnosis of bronchiolitis, bronchitis, and croup is based on history and physical examination, though further testing may confirm the diagnosis.

- **Bronchiolitis:** nasal pharyngeal washings positive for respiratory syncytial virus (RSV)
- **Bronchitis:** a chest x-ray may show diffuse alveolar hyperinflation and increasing perihilar markings
- **Croup:** lateral neck x-ray may be obtained to rule out epiglottitis if suspected

Disorder	Treatment	Family education
Bronchiolitis	• Nasal or nasopharyngeal suctioning • Elevate the head of the crib • Oral or intravenous hydration	• Antipyretics for fever or comfort • Cough may persist for several weeks after infection resolves
Bronchitis	Supportive care; expectorants are helpful in some children	• Do not give cough suppressants
Croup	• Exposure to cool air most helpful (steam and humidification not harmful, but no evidence they work) • Racemic epinephrine aerosolized helps with stridor but may have rebound effect • dexamethasone 0.6 mg/kg once, either orally or intramuscularly	• Keep the child quiet; minimize crying • Allow child to sit up in parent's arms if desired

Table 17.2.2 Treatment of Infectious Respiratory Disorders

Disorder	Treatment	Family education
Neonatal chlamydial pneumonia	erythromycin 50 mg/kg/day in 4 divided doses, orally for 2 weeks	• Good handwashing • Finish entire antibiotic course
Pneumonia	• May need inpatient treatment/O$_2$ • PCN or azithromycin • Supportive care	• Good handwashing • Discuss importance of vaccinations (influenza, pneumonia)

Table 17.2.2 Treatment of Infectious Respiratory Disorders (Continued)

Encourage adequate fluid intake for all infants with conditions above, and encourage the parents to call the office if respiratory distress begins to occur. Emergent referral is needed if the infant has an acutely ill appearance or respiratory distress with tachypnea, significant retractions, and poor oral intake.

Kawasaki Disease

Kawasaki disease is an acute systemic vasculitis occurring mostly in younger children. Mild to moderate anemia is present early in the illness, and significant thrombocytosis develops later. A high fever of at least 5 days duration is a key feature. Additional subjective findings include chills, malaise, headache, irritability, abdominal symptoms, and joint pain. Diagnosis is based on fever criteria as noted above and the presence of at least four of the following:

- Diffuse, erythematous, polymorphous rash
- Edema, erythema, desquamation, and tenderness of the feet and hands
- Bilateral conjunctivitis without exudate
- Strawberry tongue, erythematous/edematous pharynx, or fissure/swollen lips
- Cervical lymphadenopathy

Treatment should be coordinated with a specialist and includes aspirin and intravenous immunoglobulin. Educate parents about the importance of ongoing follow-up with the cardiologist. Referral to the pediatric cardiologist for an echocardiogram is warranted due to the risk from myocarditis and later development of coronary artery aneurysm.

> **Pro Tip**
> Aspirin use in children is appropriate with a diagnosis of Kawasaki disease or juvenile arthritis due to proven benefit in these conditions.

Mumps

Mumps is caused by paramyxovirus and spread by infected droplets, resulting in fever and parotitis. Orchitis may occur in prepubertal boys, possibly leading to some testicular atrophy. The communicable period is 1–7 days prior to onset of symptoms until 4–9 days after parotid swelling occurs. Treatment is supportive (antipyretics and analgesics).

Osteomyelitis

Osteomyelitis is a bacterial infection of the bone (most often a long bone) and surrounding soft tissue. Subjective findings include possible fever, history of impetigo or infected wound, irritability, pain, and activity level changes, with refusal to walk if in a lower extremity. Objectively, decreased range of motion may occur, as well as local warmth and tenderness. Changes may be seen on ultrasound, CT scan, or MRI. WBC count is elevated, as are ESR and CRP. Refer to the pediatric orthopedic surgeon for a bone biopsy for accurate identification of the infectious organism. Treatment usually involves 6 weeks of antibiotic therapy.

Viral Exanthems

Disorder	Characteristics
Fifth disease	• Low-grade fever, headache • Mild respiratory symptoms • Rash appears: "slapped cheeks," then on trunk, spreading to lacy rash on extremities—possibly pruritic (spares palms and soles) • Joint edema or tenderness
Measles	• Recent international travel • Fever, cough, coryza, conjunctivitis • Rash appears 3–4 days after above occurs • Maculopapular rash, spreading downward and outward • Koplik spots (bright red spots with blue-white centers on buccal mucosa)
Roseola	• High fever for 3–5 days • Rash appears 12–24 hours after fever resolution • Pinkish red, flat, or raised rash, blanches
Rubella	• Low-grade fever • Pink to red rash beginning on face, spreading head to foot; mildly pruritic • Rash disappears in the same order it appears • Lymphadenopathy in older children • Polyarthralgia common in adolescents
Varicella	• Fever, malaise, anorexia, abdominal pain, headache precede rash by 1–2 days • Rash begins on face, scalp, trunk, with intense pruritus • Erythematous macules evolve to pustules, then vesicles that rupture then scab • Lesions present on body in various stages

Table 17.2.3 Characteristics of Viral Exanthems

Diagnosis of the viral exanthems is based upon the history and physical examination. Laboratory testing is rarely needed.

> **DANGER SIGN** Maternal rubella can result in miscarriage, congenital malformations, or fetal death. Ensure all children are appropriately immunized.

Immunize against childhood diseases as recommended. Treatment of the viral exanthem is supportive in nature. Recommend comfort measures such as antipyretics, antipruritics, and analgesics (if joint pain present) as needed. Teach parents about the communicability period for a diagnosed viral exanthem. Pregnant women should avoid exposure to children with human parvovirus (fifth disease). Refer patients who are immunocompromised or are not improving.

Disorder	Communicability period
Fifth disease	Uncertain, but no longer contagious after onset of the rash
Measles	1–2 days before symptom onset to 4–6 days after rash appears
Roseola	Unknown, but most likely contagious prior to onset of symptoms
Rubella	7 days before to 7 days after the rash's onset
Varicella	1–2 days before onset of rash until all vesicles crusted over

Table 17.2.4 Communicability Period of Viral Exanthems

Takeaways

- A careful history related to prodromal symptoms (if any), fever history, and onset of rash and how it spread are the key to the diagnosis of the viral exanthems.
- Croup may be distinguished from bronchiolitis by its characteristic barking cough and presence of stridor.
- Children with suspected Kawasaki disease should be referred to pediatric cardiology, and those with suspected osteomyelitis to pediatric orthopedics.

LESSON 3: MISCELLANEOUS PEDIATRIC DISORDERS

Learning Objectives

■ Identify clinical manifestations of miscellaneous pediatric disorders

■ Choose and interpret laboratory/diagnostic testing used for differentiating miscellaneous pediatric disorders

■ Differentiate appropriate treatment and referrals related to pediatric miscellaneous disorders

A variety of miscellaneous disorders may affect children. Management of certain disorders in children varies as compared with management in adults.

Definitions

- **Amblyopia:** "lazy eye"; decrease in visual acuity in one eye as compared with the other eye
- **Chorea:** involuntary, random jerking movements
- **Erythema marginatum:** red, ring-like rash occurring on trunk and proximal extremities
- **Esotropia:** non-paralytic deviation of one or both eyes inward
- **Exotropia:** non-paralytic deviation of one or both eyes outward
- **Hirschberg corneal light reflex:** note the location on pupil of a shined light, or how ambient light reflects off the cornea—in a negative test, the light appears symmetrically on both cornea/pupils; in a positive test, the appearance is asymmetric
- **Hyperbilirubinemia:** total serum bilirubin level >5 mg/dL (86 μmol/L) in the newborn

Neonatal Jaundice

Newborns are particularly predisposed to the exhibition of jaundice due to their high red blood cell counts at birth, immature livers, and, to a lesser extent, the presence of an enzyme in breast milk inhibiting the action of glucuronyl transferase. Common risk factors include ABO or Rh incompatibility, cephalohematoma, poor feeding, and prematurity. Total bilirubin ≤5 mg/dL is considered normal in the newborn. Bilirubin peaks at 3–4 days of age in the healthy term infant.

Jaundice appears first on the skin of the face and then spreads down the body; eventually the sclerae become icteric. All term newborns over 24 hours of age displaying jaundice should have total serum bilirubin (TSB), blood type, and Coombs evaluated.

> **DANGER SIGN** Jaundice exhibited in the first 24 hours of life is more likely to be pathologic rather than physiologic in nature. Refer to the pediatrician or neonatologist.

Institute phototherapy for the following infants:

- Infant 25–48 hours old; total serum bilirubin ≥15 mg/dL
- Infant 49–72 hours old; total serum bilirubin ≥18 mg/dL
- Infant >72 hours old; total serum bilirubin ≥20 mg/dL

Encourage frequent feeding (breast or formula). Educate families that physiologic jaundice usually resolves within a few days and has no lasting effects. Refer infants whose bilirubin level does not decrease despite appropriate therapy to the physician.

> **Digital Resource**
>
> To quickly assess the risks of hyperbilirubinemia development in newborns >35 weeks gestational age, use the online calculator BiliTool: **www.bilitool.org**. Enter the age of the infant in hours and the total bilirubin. BiliTool provides the level of risk according to age and lab values and makes recommendations for follow-up (lab recheck, phototherapy).

Strabismus

Strabismus is a deficit in muscle coordination leading to esotropia or exotropia, resulting in an inability of the optic axes to be focused on the same object. In the young child, it affects equality of visual acuity development resulting in amblyopia.

Parents may note the infant or child has crossed eyes or a lazy eye. Objectively, when the cover/uncover test is performed, the eye drifts out of position while the eye is covered and snaps back quickly when uncovered. The Hirschberg corneal light reflex test is positive, and the extraocular movements may be affected.

Proper alignment of the eyes is required for vision to develop equally in the early years of the child's life. Commonly, the eye with stronger muscles is patched in order to strengthen the muscles of the weaker eye. Support parents in their efforts to comply with patching if prescribed. Occasionally, eye muscle or laser surgery is required. Refer the following patients to the pediatric ophthalmologist for further evaluation and treatment:

- Infants ≥3 months of age with strabismus who do not track well
- Any child after 1 year of age with strabismus

> **DANGER SIGN** Amblyopia: a positive Hirschberg reflex is a sign of amblyopia in the developing child, even without the presence of strabismus. Refer these children to pediatric ophthalmology. Test visual acuity beginning at 3 years with an appropriate screener.

Lead Poisoning

Lead poisoning is particularly concerning in the developing child. Lead occurs in paints manufactured before 1978 (paint chips, lead-contaminated dust), lead pipes (contaminated water), herbal remedies (greta, azarcon), and select imported products (toys). Due to their development stage, young children put everything in their mouths, increasing the risk for lead ingestion. Lead can also be found in dust in older homes undergoing renovation. Blood lead levels increase the most rapidly from 6–12 and 18–24 months of age.

Most children have low lead exposure or chronic exposure and are asymptomatic. Thus, it is important to appropriately screen young children for blood lead levels. Determine whether child is low-risk or high-risk using these questions as recommended by the Centers for Disease Control and Prevention (CDC):

- Does the child live in or regularly visit a house with peeling or chipping paint built before 1960?
- Does the child live in or regularly visit a house built before 1960 with recent, ongoing, or planned renovation or remodeling?
- Does the child have a brother or sister, housemate, or playmate being followed or treated for lead poisoning (blood lead $\geq$15 µg/dL)?
- Does the child live with an adult whose job or hobby involves exposure to lead?
- Does the child live near an active lead smelter, battery recycling plant, or other industry likely to release lead?

Signs/symptoms of lead poisoning: lag in growth and development, learning disabilities, irritability, weight loss/anorexia, abdominal pain, constipation

Recommendations for testing/treating are based upon lead levels.

Blood lead level (mcg/dL)	Recommended action
<5	Retest in 6 months if child is high-risk, otherwise repeat test annually
5–14	• Repeat test in 1–3 months to ensure level is not rising • Educate parents to decrease child's exposure to lead • Provide nutritional counseling related to calcium and iron
15–44	• Confirmatory repeat test within 1–4 weeks • Educate parents to decrease child's exposure to lead • Repeat test every 3 months until result is <5
45–69	• Confirmatory repeat test in 2 days • Ensure lead removed from home • Consult with toxicologist—provide chelation with succimer 10 mg/kg orally, 3 times daily for 5 days, then 2 times daily for 14 days
$\geq$70	Hospitalize and refer management to experienced toxicologist

Table 17.3.1 Recommended Actions According to Blood Lead Level

Hypertension

Screen blood pressure annually in all children 3 years of age and older. Use the National Heart, Lung, and Blood Institute's (NHLBI) blood pressure tables for children and adolescents, using height, age, and gender to determine blood pressure percentile: **www.nhlbi.nih.gov/health-pro/guidelines/current/hypertension-pediatric-jnc-4/blood-pressure-tables**.

Stage	BP and percentile per NHLBI table
Normal	<90th percentile for gender, age, and height
Prehypertension	BP ≥120/80, yet <95th percentile for gender, age, and height
Stage 1 hypertension	≥95th and <99th percentile for gender, age, and height on 3 separate occasions
Stage 2 hypertension	>99th percentile + 5 mm Hg for gender, age, and height on 3 separate occasions

Table 17.3.2 Stages of Pediatric Hypertension

All children should participate in physical activity daily. Recommend a DASH-style eating plan for children 10 years and older with prehypertension or hypertension. Consider management of pediatric hypertension in collaboration with the pediatrician or pediatric cardiologist.

Dyslipidemia

Screening for dyslipidemia in younger children is based upon risk factors. Educate families of overweight children to increase child's daily physical activity and decrease intake of nutrient-poor foods. Refer children with documented dyslipidemia to a nutritionist for diet management. Statins are not used in children less than 10 years of age. For children 10 years and older, collaborate with the pediatrician or pediatric cardiologist for medication management.

Universal screening is recommended for children ages 9–11 years of age. Screen those aged 2–8 years and those aged 12–18 years if risk factors are present:

- Close family member with MI, CABG/stent/angioplasty, angina, stroke at age <55 years in males, <65 years in females
- Parent with total cholesterol >240 mg/dL
- Child has diabetes, hypertension, BMI ≥95th percentile for age and gender, moderate- or high-risk medical condition, or smokes cigarettes

Rheumatic Fever

Acute rheumatic fever (ARF) may develop as a sequela to group A streptococcal (GAS) infection, usually about 2–4 weeks after the infection. ARF causes chronic damage to the heart and valves in addition to affecting the joints, skin, subcutaneous tissue, and central nervous system.

ARF is diagnosed based on the revised Jones Criteria. Either two major criteria, or one major and two minor criteria plus evidence of preceding GAS infection, or two minor criteria plus evidence of preceding GAS infection, must be present for diagnosis.

Major criteria	Minor criteria
• Carditis • Chorea • Erythema marginatum • Migratory polyarthritis • Subcutaneous nodules	• Arthralgia • Elevated ESR or CRP • Fever • Prolonged PR interval

Table 17.3.3 Revised Jones Criteria

Prescribe antibiotics for eradication of GAS infection. Anti-inflammatory medications help with arthritis symptoms. Refer to the pediatric cardiologist for echocardiogram and ongoing follow-up related to heart and valve involvement (which varies per individual). Prevention of secondary attacks of rheumatic fever is achieved with prophylactic monthly intramuscular injections of penicillin G benzathine until age 21 years.

Diabetes Mellitus

Historically, children were only diagnosed with type 1 diabetes (insulin-dependent). With the rise in overweight and obese children, type 2 diabetes is now recognized at younger ages. In children, prediabetes exists if fasting blood glucose is >100 mg/dL, or two-hour postprandial glucose is 140–199 mg/dL, or Hgb A1c is 5.7–6.4%. Type 2 diabetes is confirmed as a diagnosis when fasting blood glucose is >126 mg/dL, or a random serum glucose is >200 mg/dL, or Hgb A1c is ≥6.5%.

Metformin (for type 2 diabetes) is the only oral hypoglycemic agent approved by the FDA for use in children. Due to children's ongoing nutritional needs in relation to growth and development, refer all children with diabetes to a pediatric dietician and pediatric endocrinologist for further management. As the primary care provider, collaborate with these specialists and provide needed family support.

Pubertal Alterations

Puberty may either be precocious (early) or delayed. Precocious puberty refers to the development of secondary sex characteristics earlier than usual (before the age of 8 years in girls, 9 years in boys). In girls, the cause is usually unknown, while in boys it is most often related to a CNS abnormality. Delayed puberty refers to delayed secondary sexual characteristic development and most often results due to constitutional delay. Delayed puberty is further defined as having no clinical features of puberty by age 13 years in girls and age 14 years in boys, or as puberty not being achieved within five years of the initial signs of secondary sex characteristic development.

Refer children with precocious or delayed puberty to the pediatric endocrinologist for further evaluation and possible hormone treatment.

Adolescent Idiopathic Scoliosis

Scoliosis refers to a lateral curvature of the spine extending 10 degrees. Adolescent idiopathic scoliosis is the most common type, and the degree tends to worsen quickly during rapid growth. Early screening for and detection of scoliosis is important for promoting best outcomes. Screen girls at ages 10 and 12 and boys at age 13–14.

Subjective findings include recent growth spurt and physical changes related to pubertal development. Pain is not a common finding. Objective findings may include one or more of the following: single scapular prominence, uneven shoulder heights, uneven waistline curve, unilateral rib hump, or abnormalities in the spinal curve. A scoliometer provides a gross measure of the angle of trunk rotation, while spine x-rays (AP and lateral, standing) provide a more accurate reading of the degree of curvature (via the Cobb angle).

Treatment of scoliosis includes ongoing observation, bracing, or surgery. Counsel families about the importance of continued follow-up. Refer to the pediatric orthopedic surgeon, for further evaluation and potential treatment, patients who have:

- Scoliometer angle of trunk rotation $\geq$7 degrees if BMI <85th percentile for age, and $\geq$5 degrees if BMI is $\geq$85th percentile for age
- Cobb angle 20–29 degrees in premenstrual girls, or boys 12–14 years old
- Cobb angle >30 degrees or progression of >5 degrees in any child

Takeaways

- Screen for risk factors for neonatal jaundice, evaluate bilirubin levels, and institute phototherapy as appropriate according to the newborn's age and lab results.
- Ensure all children with amblyopia and/or strabismus are referred to the pediatric ophthalmologist in order to maximize visual acuity development in early childhood.
- Follow the NHLBI guidelines for screening and evaluation of blood pressure in children.

PRACTICE QUESTIONS

Select the ONE best answer.

Lesson 1: Congenital Disorders

1. The nurse practitioner notes a single palmar crease on a young infant. This finding is likely to be associated with which disorders?

    A. Down syndrome and Turner syndrome

    B. Down syndrome and fetal alcohol spectrum disorder

    C. Klinefelter syndrome and Turner syndrome

    D. Fetal alcohol spectrum disorder and Klinefelter syndrome

2. While examining a child, the nurse practitioner notes decreased blood pressure and weakness in the lower extremities as compared to the upper extremities. What is the likely explanation?

    A. Ventricular septal defect

    B. Tetralogy of Fallot

    C. Normal expectation

    D. Coarctation of the aorta

3. At the two-week visit, the nurse practitioner notes clear drainage from the right eye with mild lower lid redness. Which treatment is appropriate?

    A. Oral antibiotics

    B. Topical antibiotics

    C. Nasolacrimal duct massage

    D. Referral to ophthalmology

4. Upon examination of a 2-month-old, the nurse practitioner notes a positive Barlow sign and a positive Ortolani sign. Which diagnostic test is appropriate?

    A. Hip ultrasound

    B. Renal-bladder ultrasound

    C. Hip CT scan

    D. Abdominal CT scan

Lesson 2: Infectious Disorders

5. Which rash is characteristic of varicella?

    A. Polymorphous rash

    B. "Slapped cheek" and lacy rash

    C. Vesicular lesions in various stages

    D. Koplik spots

6. A 3-year-old with a history of impetigo has a low-grade fever. His mother states he is not running around like his usual self. Upon physical examination, the 3-year-old is guarding his left upper leg. The WBC and CRP are elevated. The child should be referred to which of the following specialists?

    A. Physical therapist

    B. Occupational therapist

    C. Rheumatologist

    D. Orthopedist

7. A 4-year-old has a five-day history of high fever and a rash. Which set of additional signs would be necessary for a diagnosis of Kawasaki disease?

    A. Strawberry tongue, scarlatina-form rash on trunk, pharyngitis

    B. Hand desquamation, conjunctivitis, strawberry tongue

    C. Football-shaped lesions on hands, feet, and buccal mucosa

    D. Vesicular lesions in various stages, headache

8. Which complication may occur with mumps?

    A. Orchitis

    B. Osteomyelitis

    C. Myocarditis

    D. Aortic aneurysm

Lesson 3: Miscellaneous Pediatric Disorders

9. For which of the following children should universal dyslipidemia screening be performed?

   A. 20-month-old

   B. 6-year-old

   C. 10-year-old

   D. 16-year-old

10. Which of the following newborns warrants intervention with phototherapy?

    A. 12 hours old, total bilirubin 1.5 mg/dL

    B. 36 hours old, total bilirubin 16 mg/dL

    C. 60 hours old, total bilirubin 17 mg/dL

    D. 72 hours old, total bilirubin 12 mg/dL

11. Which of these girls should be referred to the orthopedic surgeon for evaluation of scoliosis?

    A. Preteen with BMI of 82nd percentile for age and scoliometer angle of trunk rotation of 6 degrees

    B. Preteen with BMI of 87th percentile for age and scoliometer angle of trunk rotation of 4 degrees

    C. 12-year-old with Cobb angle 22 degrees who has not reached menarche

    D. 17-year-old with Cobb angle 24 degrees who reached menarche at age 13

12. A 30-month-old child has a positive Hirschberg reflex. What is the best action taken by the nurse practitioner?

    A. Refer to the pediatric ophthalmologist

    B. Recheck the reflex again in 6 months

    C. Refer to a local optometrist

    D. Document as normal in the record

ANSWERS AND EXPLANATIONS

Lesson 1: Congenital Disorders

1. B

A single palmar crease may be found in the child with Down syndrome and fetal alcohol spectrum disorder **(B)**. It is not a usual finding with Turner syndrome (A and C), nor Klinefelter syndrome (C and D).

2. D

With coarctation of the aorta **(D)**, decreased lower extremity BP and weaker lower extremity pulses are expected findings due to the nature of the defect. They are not associated with ventricular septal defect (A) or tetralogy of Fallot (B), nor are they expected normal findings in a child (C).

3. C

Unilateral, clear eye drainage in the young infant is likely nasolacrimal duct obstruction for which nasolacrimal duct massage **(C)** is the appropriate initial treatment. Oral antibiotics (A) are not indicated, and topical antibiotics (B) would be indicated for purulent drainage, not clear. Referral to ophthalmology (D) would only be indicated for the older infant with continued, unresolved nasolacrimal duct obstruction.

4. A

A positive Barlow and Ortolani sign are suspicious of developmental dysplasia of the hip (DDH), for which an ultrasound **(A)** is the initial diagnostic test. A renal-bladder ultrasound (B) would be ordered for suspected genitourinary defect. Neither hip CT (C) nor abdominal CT (D) would be indicated for suspected DDH.

Lesson 2: Infectious Disorders

5. C

Presence of vesicular lesions in various stages **(C)** is the hallmark of varicella infection. A polymorphous rash (A) is characteristic of Kawasaki disease, while "slapped cheeks" and a lacy rash (B) occur with fifth disease. Koplik spots (D) are specifically characteristic of measles.

6. D

The clinical picture is one of suspected osteomyelitis, so the child should be referred to the pediatric orthopedist **(D)** for a biopsy or aspiration. Neither physical therapy (A) nor occupational therapy (B) are appropriate referrals in this case. Rheumatology (C) would be an appropriate referral for arthritis.

7. B

Hand desquamation, conjunctivitis, and strawberry tongue **(B)** are consistent with Kawasaki disease. Pharyngitis, strawberry tongue, and scarlatina-form rash on trunk (A) are consistent with group A streptococcal infection. Football-shaped lesions on hand, feet, and buccal mucosa (C) occur with hand, foot, and mouth disease. Vesicular lesions in various stages (D) are the hallmark of varicella infection.

8. A

Orchitis **(A)** may occur as a complication of mumps and may lead to some degree of testicular atrophy. Osteomyelitis (B) is a bacterial infection of the bone and surrounding soft tissue. Myocarditis (C) and aortic aneurysm (D) are potential complications of Kawasaki disease.

Lesson 3: Miscellaneous Pediatric Disorders

9. C

Universal lipid screening is recommended for all children ages 9–11 years **(C)**. Lipid screening is not recommended for children under 2 years of age (A). When particular risk factors are present in children ages 2–8 years (B) or 12–18 years (D), lipid screening is then recommended, but it is not a universal recommendation.

10. B

Infants 25–48 hours old with total serum bilirubin ≥15 mg/dL **(B)** need phototherapy. Infants less than 24 hours old who are not jaundiced (A) do not require photo therapy. Infants 49–72 hours old need phototherapy for bilirubin >18 mg/dL, thus a 60-hour-old with bilirubin 17 mg/dL (C) and 72-hour-old with bilirubin 12 mg/dL (D) do not require phototherapy.

11. C

Premenstrual girls with Cobb angle 20–29 degrees **(C)** should be referred to the orthopedic surgeon. A preteen with BMI of 82nd percentile for age and ATR 6 degrees (A) does not meet the criteria for referral: BMI <85th percentile, ATR ≥7 degrees. A preteen with BMI of 87th percentile for age and ATR 4 degrees (B) does not meet the criteria for referral: BMI ≥85th percentile, ATR ≥5 degrees. Premenstrual girls with Cobb angle 20–29 degrees are referred, thus the postmenstrual girl (D) does not meet the criteria.

12. A

A positive Hirschberg reflex is indicative of amblyopia (unequal visual acuity between eyes) and requires referral to the pediatric ophthalmologist **(A)**, as visual acuity is currently in development and must be preserved. Thus, rechecking in 6 months (B), referring to optometry (C), and documenting the finding as normal (D) would not be appropriate actions.

CHAPTER 18

Elderly

LESSON 1: PHYSIOLOGICAL CHANGES

Learning Objectives

- Recognize the social/developmental theories outlining expected changes in the elderly
- Understand how body systems are affected by aging
- Anticipate meaningful interventions that help the elderly manage age-related changes

By 2030, 20% of Americans will be 65 or older. Expected changes of aging include physiological slowing, decreased mobility, psychological stressors (isolation or the death of a spouse or significant other), and lifestyle changes (downsizing financially or adjusting to life in senior housing). Nurse practitioners are in a position to educate, equip, and support seniors as they navigate the challenges of aging.

The Framingham Heart Study (originally designed to study cardiac issues) has followed generations of Americans across the life span and provides support for the contention that seniors who are socially connected and engaged are healthier. In addition, researchers argue that even mild depression appears to reduce immunity and lower resistance to cancers and infections.

Older adults have atypical presentation of acute illness. Knowing normal changes of aging will aid in differentiating true pathology from expected, age-related physiological changes. Subtle changes from a patient's baseline may be the first indicator of disease or disability.

Social and Developmental Theories

Social and developmental theories can pinpoint changes expected for senior populations.

Social and Developmental Theories on Aging	
Erikson's developmental stages	Ego integrity vs. despair: this stage involves either coming to terms with and feeling satisfied about life's work, or alternatively, succumbing to despair, dissatisfaction, and a sense of failure
Roger Gould: transformations in adult development	Posits that the older adult tends to mellow and become more accepting and tolerant
Daniel Levinson: seasons of life	Physiologic changes and personality are interrelated; midlife changes will also bring midlife crises for many adults
Robert Peck: developmental tasks	Three major developmental challenges that can either be successfully navigated or handled maladaptively: • Redefinition of self vs. preoccupation with work role • Body transcendence vs. body preoccupation • Ego transcendence vs. ego preoccupation

Table 18.1.1

Physiological Changes in the Elderly: Implications for Practice

Physiological Changes in the Elderly	
Nervous system—sensorineural	• Slowed motor reaction and memory decline; forgetfulness of both near and remote memory, coupled with awareness of memory decline, is associated with normal memory loss; Alzheimer disease, on the other hand, is marked by loss of near memory while maintaining preservation of remote memory (in initial stages); dementia is not considered normal aging • Loss or reduction in sense of smell and taste; seniors can fail to recognize spoiled food or may over-spice food to compensate for reduced sensory inputs • Sensorineural hearing loss associated with aging (presbycusis) gradually affects the ability to hear high-pitched sounds; hearing loss secondary to overuse of ototoxic medications such as NSAIDs is another potential problem (note: buildup of cerumen will impair hearing; this possibility should be ruled out as a potential cause) • Hardening of the lens (presbyopia), cataracts, increased intraocular pressure; loss of overall visual acuity, loss of night vision; more likely than the general population to have long-standing (and therefore more deleterious) conditions such as glaucoma, diabetic retinopathy, and macular degeneration
Mental health	• 1 in 5 elderly may experience depression, while about 1 in 10 experience anxiety • Dementia, often coupled with corresponding behavioral changes, is now estimated to affect about 1 in 8 Americans >65 years old • Suicide is the cause of approximately 14 of every 100,000 deaths of those >65 year old • Appropriate mental health screens are an important part of eldercare
Cardiac	• Reduced cardiac efficiency and myocardial contractility, a lower maximum heart rate, and diminished cardiac output are typical • Decreased overall perfusion has "downstream" effects such as poor skin healing and inefficient distribution of nutrients and ingested medication • Aging vasculature can result in chronic conditions such as systolic hypertension

Table 18.1.2

Physiological Changes in the Elderly (Continued)	
Pulmonary	• Pulmonary function declines with age; changes in lung compliance reduce oxygen–carbon dioxide exchange • The diaphragm weakens and results in reduced residual capacity • While these changes may not result in shortness of breath during daily activities, the underlying reduction in function can make the older adult more vulnerable in cases of respiratory insult, such as pneumonia
Gastrointestinal	• The sedentary lifestyle of seniors can lead to constipation or even gastroparesis • Loss in underlying muscle strength can reduce peristalsis, making food absorption less efficient • Reduced GI efficiency can lead to poor absorption of nutrients; GI slowing can also lead to reduced drug clearance, which can lead to an increase in adverse medication effects and even medication toxicity • Decreased salivation contributes to dry mouth; side effects of certain medications lead to dry mouth • Changes in dentition or post-stroke dysphagia can predispose the older patient to aspiration pneumonia and malnutrition
Musculoskeletal	Bone loss (such as osteopenia or osteoporosis), loss of muscle mass, balance difficulties, postural instability, kyphosis, and gait changes (lead to increased risk for falls), loss of stature, and arthritis are some of the musculoskeletal issues that occur in the elderly
Endocrine	More likely to have long-standing diabetes, and thus more dangerous end-organ damage such as peripheral neuropathy or diabetic retinopathy
Genitourinary	• Men can experience benign prostatic hypertrophy (and resulting urinary retention) and impotence • Women can experience incontinence, vaginal dryness, and dyspareunia • Renal blood flow declines progressively with age, which can result in decreased excretion of medications
Integumentary	Hair loss, thinning skin, slower wound healing, sun damage (solar lentigines, skin cancer—especially if fair-skinned or history of sunburn), xerosis, senile purpura, and easy bruising (especially if taking NSAIDs)

Table 18.1.2

Takeaways

- Social/developmental theories can help the nurse practitioner anticipate age-related changes in senior patients and implement appropriate supportive measures/interventions.
- Physiological changes associated with aging affect every body system. The nurse practitioner should be aware of these changes and adjust treatment and interventions accordingly.

LESSON 2: RISK FACTORS

Learning Objectives
- Identify risk factors that can cause illness or injury in the elderly population
- Discuss the nurse practitioner's role in addressing risk factors in the elderly

A risk factor is anything that increases the chance an individual may develop an illness or injury. The elderly population faces a greater number of risk factors due to a decline in their overall health and their mental and physical capabilities, among other things. It is important for the nurse practitioner to identify potential and actual risk factors in the elderly population to prevent illness and injury.

Medication Complications

Polypharmacy

Polypharmacy is defined as both the simultaneous use of multiple medications to treat the same ailment, as well as the use of multiple medications. It occurs frequently in the elderly, often due to the increased number of comorbidities. In all likelihood, each comorbidity is managed by a different provider, each who prescribes medications. When a patient has more than one ailment that is being concurrently treated, the risk of polypharmacy goes up. Polypharmacy poses a risk to the patient in that the medications can interact with each other, producing bothersome side effects or dangerous adverse effects. When more than one medication is prescribed for the same ailment, the intended effect is magnified, which can over treat the issue and lead to complications.

Noncompliance and Nonadherence

It is important to note the difference between noncompliance and nonadherence. Noncompliance with medications and medication regimens occurs when a patient deliberately or intentionally refuses a medication or regimen. Nonadherence is unintentional refusal by the patient, such as when they are confused, overwhelmed, or simply do not understand the medication, dosing, or regimen.

Noncompliance with medications in the elderly is common, with studies estimating a rate as high as 57% and an average of 45%. Multiple factors can influence a patient's decision or ability to take medication, which may include age-related physical changes, undesirable side effects, complicated medication schedules or packaging, and financial constraints.

If a medication is causing undesirable side effects, the risk for noncompliance increases. Quality of life is an important consideration, especially in the elderly. If a medication is detracting from one's quality of life, a patient may choose to stop taking the medication.

If the patient's medication schedule is too complicated, such as numerous medications and/or dosing regimens at frequent or unusual times, the risk for noncompliance increases.

It has been well documented in the literature that the high cost of medications places a burden on the elderly and is frequently the leading cause of medication noncompliance. The patient may skip doses to save money.

Nonadherence often results from normal, age-related physiological changes that interfere with a patient's ability to take their prescribed medication. If patients are hard of hearing, they may not hear the instructions given by their provider. If their vision is poor, they may not be able to read the packaging directions. Arthritis can hinder the ability to open packaging. A decline in cognitive functioning can affect a patient's ability to understand a medication regimen and lead to them forgetting to take the medication or even taking too much.

Falls

- Prior history of a fall is perhaps the greatest risk factor
- Orthostatic hypotension
- Decreased mobility, altered gait
- Use of assistive devices: cane, walker, crutches, wheelchair
- Lack of assistive devices: shower chair or bar, cane, walker
- Medications: psychotropics, cardiovascular, hypoglycemics, insulin
- Environmental factors: rugs, cords, decreased lighting, unsafe footwear
- Poor eyesight or hearing
- Prolonged bedrest

- Medical conditions: dehydration, osteoporosis, osteoarthritis, rheumatoid arthritis, aortic stenosis, diarrhea, Parkinson disease, dementia, cerebrovascular accident
- Decreased reflexes

Driving

For many, driving is a sign of independence. Thus, it may be difficult for an aging person to give up this skill, even if their ability to drive safely has declined. Cognitive changes, diminishing vision, impaired hearing, decreased reflexes, decreased attention span, and/or reduced strength, coordination, and flexibility can all impair a patient's ability to drive a vehicle safely.

Pressure Ulcers

A pressure ulcer is an injury to the skin and underlying tissue caused by prolonged pressure. Damage can range from superficial to devastating injury, with lifelong complications. Risk factors for pressure ulcers include bed rest, decreased mobility, malnutrition, smoking, use of a wheelchair, incontinence, dehydration, decreased mental awareness, decreased sensory perception, and medical conditions such as diabetes mellitus and dementia.

Infections

Infections occurring in the elderly, such as influenza and pneumonia, are responsible for a significant increase in this population's rates of morbidity and mortality. A decreased immune system response, the presence of comorbidities, and group living conditions can all increase an elderly person's risk of developing an infection. UTIs are common and often related to catheter use. Skin infections, often caused by *Staphylococcus* bacteria, are easily acquired due to the decreased integrity of the skin.

Depression and Suicide

It is estimated that in the elderly population, as many as 1 in 5 are depressed. Declining health, loss of loved ones, feelings of loneliness, and fear of becoming a burden can contribute to the development of depression. Sadly, elderly men have the highest rate of suicide, at 47 per 100,000. Risk factors for depression and suicide in the elderly include:

- Increasing age, especially > age 85
- Race (Caucasian)
- Sex (male > female)
- Marital status (divorced, widowed)
- Previous psychiatric disorder
- Social isolation
- Misuse of alcohol, medications, drugs
- Declining health
- Financial issues
- Chronic pain
- Loss and grief
- Family discord

The Nurse Practitioner's Role

The nurse practitioner plays an important role in identifying risk factors that may cause harm to older adults, as well as in preventing these risk factors from causing harm.

Medications

Address polypharmacy and medication noncompliance and nonadherence by performing a medication reconciliation during each visit. Review medications with the patient. Ask open-ended questions, such as, "What do you take for your high cholesterol?" Remain nonjudgmental and ask about adherence.

Assess vision, hearing, bilateral upper extremity strength, and hand dexterity to identify potential barriers to medication adherence.

When prescribing a medication, carefully review the scheduling regimen to make sure it isn't too complicated or difficult for the patient to implement. Review potential side effects and encourage the patient to call the nurse practitioner if side effects occur. Be sure to assess the patient's use of OTC and/or herbal supplements—either can add another level of complexity to the patient's medication regimen, as well as the potential for adverse effects. Consider the cost of the medication when prescribing it. Consult Beers criteria when prescribing to determine if the medication is appropriate for the elderly population.

Falls

Conduct a fall risk assessment during each office visit. A fall risk assessment tool, such as the Johns Hopkins Fall Risk Assessment Tool, can be used to assess a patient's future risk for falls. Perform the Timed Up and Go test (TUG) to assess a patient's gait. The TUG test consists of a patient standing up from a sitting position, walking 10 feet, turning around, walking back to the chair, and finally, sitting down again. During the test, observe the patient's gait, postural stability, use of arms, stride length, and sway.

Driving

When discussing driving safety, include the patient's family if possible, as the topic impacts more than just the patient. If risk factors are identified, suggestions for improvement can be made, unless it is determined that it is unsafe for the patient to continue to drive. Actions that can enhance safety include a vision and hearing screening; exercises to increase strength, flexibility, and coordination; and a thorough medication review. If cognitive changes exist, the decision to recommend that the patient stop driving should be made in collaboration with the patient and their family.

Pressure Ulcers

The rate of pressure ulcers can be decreased by conducting a thorough skin assessment at every visit, identifying breakdown early, and implementing a rigorous treatment plan. Assessing a patient's smoking history, mental status, hydration and nutrition status, continence, and mobility are all part of the history and physical process. If identified, stage the pressure ulcer on a I–IV scale and treat accordingly.

Infections

The elderly are at a high risk for acquiring an infection. It is important to identify the signs and symptoms of common infections such as influenza, skin infections, UTIs, and pneumonia. Assess the patient's vaccination status at each visit and encourage them to get the appropriate vaccines. Catheter use should be discouraged unless necessary, and the length of use should be minimized.

Depression and Suicide

Discuss mental health and use appropriate screening tools at every visit. If risk factors are identified, offer mental health services such as referral to psychiatry and grief counseling. Antidepressants, psychotherapy, and electroconvulsive therapy have proven beneficial in elderly patients with depression.

Takeaways

- Polypharmacy and noncompliance are common medication risk factors in the elderly that can cause significant morbidity and mortality.

- Falls pose a serious health risk to the elderly population and can be prevented by using a fall risk assessment tool or the TUG test.

- Unsafe driving is a potentially serious problem for the entire community and should be addressed at every visit.

- Pressure ulcers can cause significant morbidity, but are preventable by using comprehensive assessment skills and rigorous early treatment.

- Infections contribute to high cost, morbidity, and mortality in the elderly, though efforts like meticulous hand hygiene, vaccinations, early identification of symptoms, and early treatment can reduce the impact they have on patients and the healthcare system.

LESSON 3: ABUSE & END OF LIFE

Learning Objectives
- Recognize risk factors and signs of elder abuse
- Be able to educate patients on end-of-life care issues

Most caregiving to elders is provided informally by family members who are not trained to handle the emotional and physical demands. These informal caregivers—who number about 44 million and are mostly women—provide about 75% of eldercare. The vast majority of it is unpaid.

Elder Abuse

As many as 1 in 10 elders (those over 65) are abused, yet as few as 1 in 23 instances are reported.

Types of abuse	Signs and symptoms
Physical abuse	Bruises and fractures at various stages of healing, cuts and lacerations, sprains, broken or lost equipment (such as broken glasses or missing walker), unexplainable injuries, and sudden changes in behavior
Emotional/psychological abuse	Causes emotional distress, agitation, emotional withdrawal, changes in behavior, depressive symptoms, regressive behavior
Sexual abuse	Signs of sexual abuse can include genital bruising, unexplainable vaginal/rectal bleeding, diagnosis of STIs in an elder, soiled underclothing

Table 18.3.1 Types of Elder Abuse

Types of abuse	Signs and symptoms
Neglect	Messy or unkept appearance, weight loss, bedsores, missing or broken eyeglasses, dentures, etc.
Financial abuse	Withdrawal from bank account that the elder cannot explain, legal documents that are changed or have disappeared, missing financial statements, unpaid bills, utilities shut off, signatures that appear to be forged

Table 18.3.1 Types of Elder Abuse (Continued)

Risk Factors for Abuse of Elders

- Substance abuse in the home
- Caretaker or relative with poor coping mechanisms or without knowledge of how to care for elderly
- High level of financial or emotional dependence of the elder
- Depression
- Lack of support and/or caregiver role strain

The Nurse Practitioner's Role

State laws differ in regards to mandatory reporting requirement for elder abuse; most statutes refer to a vulnerable adult—one who, because of physical or mental disability or dependency on institutional services, is vulnerable to maltreatment.

> **Digital Resource**
>
> State statutes and mandatory reporting laws can be found here: **www.justice.gov/elderjustice/elder-justice-statutes-0**.

It is often difficult to identify abused adults since few elders will overtly state that they are being abused. Some reasons may include:

- Fear of reprisal
- Physical dependency on the caretaker (such as for patients with poor mobility)
- Economic dependence on the caretaker
- Worries about incriminating a family member
- Loss of abode (some abused elderly do not own their own homes)
- Fears of being placed in a nursing home

> **Pro Tip**
> - Disabled patients or patients suffering from dementia may be unable to clearly articulate abuse.
> - Social isolation makes elders more vulnerable to abuse.

The nurse practitioner who suspects elder abuse must speak up. Resources for victims of elder abuse include state adult services and ombudsmen. For seniors in immediate danger, the clinician should contact 911.

End of Life

Advance Care Planning

Advance care planning is a process that supports the patient in understanding and communicating personal values, life goals, and preferences of future medical care. This process requires clear communication between patient, family members, and healthcare providers. This process may include advance care directives, but the main goal is that the patient receives care that aligns with his or her preferences.

A growing and important movement in the U.S. has been addressing and providing for end-of-life care. Three important provisions that have been identified are advance care directives, hospice care, and palliative care.

Advance Care Directives

Most clinicians are familiar with DNR ("do not resuscitate") orders and the nurse practitioner's legal obligation to fulfill patient requests in that regard. But not as many clinicians are familiar with the legal background of patient self-determination.

The Patient Self-Determination Act, part of the Omnibus Budget Reconciliation Act of 1990, reinforced the concepts that patients should be provided education explaining their right to make decisions regarding healthcare, including the right to refuse treatment; promoted the promulgation of advance directives made effective upon incapacitation of the patient; and encouraged the reduction of end-of-life treatment costs by identifying unwanted and unnecessary care.

To that end, the case was made for advance directives that went beyond the traditional DNR (which withheld unwanted medical care such as cardiopulmonary resuscitation) and allowed for patients to address their end-of-life needs more comprehensively.

Advance care directives are documents completed by a person who has the capacity to make an informed decision about treatment decisions should he or she in the future be unable to make such decisions. Advance care directives are legal tools directing decision-making and/or appointment of a surrogate agent. The most common advance directive documents are:

- **Durable Power of Attorney for Health Care (DPAHC)**: legal document authorizing another person to make medical decisions on the patient's behalf in the event the patient loses decisional capacity
- **Living will (LW)**: document summarizing a person's preferences for future medical care
- **Physician Orders for Life-Sustaining Treatment (POLST)**: defines specific care to be administered or withheld; this document is considered medical orders; they are portable across healthcare settings (i.e., by paramedics, in residential care facilities, etc.)

> **Digital Resource**
>
> The Center for Disease Control and Prevention (CDC) offers continuing education to providers on advance care planning here: **www.cdc.gov/aging/advancecareplanning/about.htm#More2**.

Hospice vs. Palliative Care

Both hospice and palliative care provide compassionate care to patients with life-limiting illnesses. Many patients, families, and providers equate these services to pain and symptom relief at end of life, but the scope of palliative care is much broader. Palliative care includes symptomatic relief from chronic and life-threatening diseases, regardless of whether the illness is terminal or not.

Hospice	Palliative
Pain and symptom relief	Pain and symptom relief
Compassionate comfort care (as opposed to curative care) for people facing a terminal illness	Compassionate comfort care that provides relief from the symptoms and physical and mental stress of a serious or life-limiting illness
Prognosis ≤6 months	At any stage of disease: diagnosis, during curative treatment and follow-up, and at the end of life
Does not continue life-prolonging medication	Continues life-prolonging medication
Excludes curative treatment	Same time as curative treatment

Table 18.3.2 Hospice vs. Palliative Care

Takeaways

- Be vigilant for signs of abuse in the elderly and aware of the resources. Understand that a patient may not be forthcoming with information. Know the mandatory reporting laws.
- POLST defines specific care and carries within it physician orders that are portable across healthcare settings.
- Palliative care provides symptom relief at any stage of a disease. Hospice has a goal of comfort care at end of life.

PRACTICE QUESTIONS

Select the ONE best answer.

Lesson 1: Physiological Changes

1. The nurse practitioner knows that _____ is not a normal physiological change that occurs in the elderly.

   A. dementia

   B. loss of muscle mass

   C. reduced cardiac function

   D. loss of visual acuity

2. A 75-year-old patient believes she has suffered neurosensory hearing loss. After examining the patient, the nurse practitioner makes the patient aware that her condition is reversible and does not represent loss of sensory function. The NP is referring to which condition?

   A. Hyposmia

   B. Ageusia

   C. Cerumen impaction

   D. Presbycusis

3. The cardiac changes associated with normal physiological aging can have effects across the body systems. Which result below is not normally expected?

   A. Poor skin healing

   B. Reduced cardiac ejection fraction

   C. Increased blood pressure

   D. Multiple-infarct dementia

4. The nurse practitioner knows that the musculoskeletal changes associated with normal physiological aging do not lead to:

   A. Altered posture/gait

   B. Vestibular dysfunction

   C. Loss of stature

   D. Increased risk for fall

5. Gastrointestinal changes associated with aging can lead to less efficient emptying of the bowel. This can likely cause:

   A. Diarrhea

   B. Aspiration pneumonia

   C. Reduced drug clearance

   D. Odynophagia

Lesson 2: Risk Factors

6. Medication nonadherence in the elderly is often caused by all of the following except:

   A. Undesirable side effects

   B. Diminished hearing

   C. High cost of medication

   D. Decline in cognitive function

7. The greatest risk factor for a fall in the elderly population is:

   A. Diminished lighting

   B. Poor eyesight

   C. A personal history of a previous fall

   D. Osteoporosis

8. Certain medical conditions can place an elderly patient at risk for a fall. These conditions include all of the following except:

   A. Dementia

   B. Constipation

   C. Dehydration

   D. Aortic stenosis

9. Which of the following risk factors increases an elderly patient's risk for developing a pressure ulcer?

    A. Use of a walker

    B. Sleep apnea

    C. Alcohol use

    D. Smoking

10. Fall risk assessment tools can be used to assess an elderly patient's risk for falls. The FNP can perform the Timed Up and Go (TUG) test. Which of the following accurately describes the TUG?

    A. Ask the patient to walk 10 feet in a straight line with arms stretched out from their body at shoulder height

    B. From a standing position, ask the patient to walk 15 feet, turn, walk back, and then sit down in a chair

    C. Ask the patient to stand from a sitting position, walk 10 feet, turn, walk back to the chair, and sit down

    D. From a sitting position, ask the patient to stand, walk 15 feet, turn, walk back to the chair, and sit down

Lesson 3: Abuse & End of Life

11. When describing palliative care to an elderly patient, which statement best describes the treatment option?

    A. Palliative care is focused on care and comfort, not cure

    B. Palliative care focuses on symptom relief, but only at the end of life

    C. Palliative care is paid for by Medicare Part A, Medicaid, and insurance

    D. Palliative care may include curative treatment

12. What statement about advance care directives (ACDs) is incorrect?

    A. An advance care directive is related to end-of-life care

    B. A living will is more legally binding than a POLST

    C. An advance care directive describes what medical interventions one does and does not want

    D. An advance care directive defines the individual who is chosen to make healthcare decisions

13. Studies indicate that only 1 in 23 cases of elder abuse are reported. What is one possible reason for this finding?

    A. The elder may worry about incriminating a family member

    B. The mandatory reporting requirement for adults only begins at age 75

    C. Many elders have dementia and may not realize they are being abused

    D. Cases of children's abuse are more important

14. Which form of elder abuse is incorrectly matched with its description?

    A. Self-neglect: when the elderly fail to take precautions to preserve their own health and safety

    B. Sexual abuse: nonconsensual sexual contact

    C. Neglect: the unlawful appropriation or use of another's property for one's own benefit

    D. Physical abuse: intentionally inflicted physical harm, such as bruising, lacerations, fractures, or broken bones

15. An example of an advance care directive is the designation of which of the following?

    A. Funeral director

    B. Primary care provider

    C. Healthcare advocate

    D. Guardian of trust

ANSWERS AND EXPLANATIONS

Lesson 1: Physiological Changes

1. A

Dementia **(A)** is not a normal change in the elderly. Loss of muscle mass (B), reduced cardiac function (C), and loss of visual acuity (D) are all normal physiological changes known to occur in the elderly.

2. C

Cerumen impaction **(C)** refers to a buildup of ear wax, a common reason for decreased hearing in the elderly. It is reversible and does not represent a neurosensory loss since the auditory nerve is not affected. Hyposmia (A) is a decreased ability to smell and represents neurosensory loss. Ageusia (B) refers to a decreased ability to taste. Presbycusis (D) is gradual, age-related sensorineural hearing loss affecting the ability to hear high-pitched sounds.

3. D

Multiple-infarct dementia **(D)** is not a result of normal physiological aging. It is a kind of vascular dementia caused by repeated strokes. Reduced circulation/tissue perfusion leads to slow and poor skin healing (A) and is a normal physiological change with aging. Reduced cardiac ejection fraction (B) is expected because the heart muscle becomes weaker with age and cannot pump blood as efficiently. Increasing blood pressure (C) can be associated with normal physiological aging, as the vasculature becomes less compliant (stiffer), causing pressured blood flow.

4. B

Vestibular dysfunction **(B)** is not caused by musculoskeletal changes. It is associated with dysfunction in the inner ear causing problems with balance and spatial orientation. Altered posture/gait (A), loss of stature (C), and increased risk for fall (D) are all musculoskeletal changes associated with aging.

5. C

Inefficient emptying of the bowel can lead to reduced drug clearance **(C)** and even toxic buildup of medication in the elderly. Less efficient emptying would lead to constipation, not diarrhea (A). Slowed bowel clearance could potentially lead to gastric reflux, but aspiration pneumonia (B) would not be a likely result unless vomiting was a secondary symptom. Odynophagia (D), or pain on swallowing, and reduced efficiency in emptying the bowel are not typically related.

Lesson 2: Risk Factors

6. A

Medication nonadherence is not related to undesirable side effects **(A)**, but is often associated with diminished hearing (B), the high cost of medications (C), and decline in cognitive function (D). Medication nonadherence is unintentional refusal by the patient. Undesirable side effects would likely lead to medication noncompliance, a deliberate or intentional refusal of a medication or regimen.

7. C

The greatest indicator of a fall is a personal history of a previous fall **(C)**. Diminished lighting (A), poor eyesight (B), and osteoporosis (D) are all risk factors associated with falls, but are not the leading cause.

8. B

Constipation **(B)** does not increase the risk for a fall, though diarrhea does. Dementia (A), dehydration (C), and aortic stenosis (D) are all medical conditions that can increase a person's risk for falls, especially in the elderly.

9. D

Smoking **(D)** increases a person's risk for developing a pressure ulcer due to vasoconstriction, which decreases the circulation of blood and oxygen to the wound. Use of a wheelchair, not a walker (A), also increases the risk. Sleep apnea (B) and alcohol use (C) are not associated with the development of pressure ulcers.

10. C

The Timed Up and Go test consists of asking the patient to stand from a seated position, walk 10 feet, turn, walk back to the chair, and sit down **(C)**. Answers (A), (B), and (D) do not accurately describe the TUG test.

Lesson 3: Abuse & End of Life

11. D

Palliative care may include curative treatment **(D)**. This makes choice (A) incorrect. Palliative care focuses on symptom relief at all stages of the disease, not just at the end of life (B). Palliative care is primarily paid for by traditional insurance and self-pay, but Medicare Part B offers some palliative care benefits and Medicaid covers palliative care in some states. Medicare Part A (C) pays for hospice, not palliative care.

12. B

It is incorrect that a living will is more legally binding than a POLST **(B)**. A living will is a document summarizing a person's preferences for future medical care. A Physician Orders for Life-Sustaining Treatment (POLST) defines specific care to be administered or withheld; this document is considered medical orders. An advance care directive relates to end-of-life care (A), describes what medical interventions are and are not wanted (C), and defines the individual who is chosen to make healthcare decisions (D).

13. A

Many elders are abused by family members, but fail to report it. Even though the family member may mistreat the elder, the elder may still wish to protect that family member from criminal prosecution **(A)**. Mandatory reporting requirements for adults is not age-dependent (B), but rather related to vulnerability. Most elders do not have dementia, making choice (C) incorrect. Cases of child abuse are concerning (D), but older adults are also vulnerable and should be protected.

14. C

Neglect is not the unlawful appropriation or use of another's property for one's own benefit **(C)**; that statement defines exploitation. Neglect is better described as caretakers entrusted with the care of an elder failing to provide the resources to preserve the elder's health and safety. Desertion of an elder by a family member or caretaker is abandonment. Choices (A), (B), and (D) are all correctly matched with their descriptions.

15. C

A healthcare advocate **(C)** may be designated in an advance care directive. A funeral director (A), PCP (B), and guardian of trust (D) are not examples of people designated in an advance care directive.

PART FOUR

Professional Practice and Advanced Practice Considerations

CHAPTER 19

Professional Practice

LESSON 1: HIPAA/PRIVACY

Learning Objectives

- Understand common terms and rules associated with HIPAA
- Identify the importance of maintaining privacy
- Recognize implications for utilizing HIPAA in everyday practice scenarios

Definitions

- **Protected health information (PHI):** identifiable health information that is transmitted or held by a covered entity or its business associate; PHI can include demographic data; payment data; or past, present, and future health data
- **Covered entity (CE):** healthcare providers who submit electronic transmissions of any health information subject to HIPAA (e.g., nurse practitioners, medical doctors, medical clinics, nursing homes, pharmacies, dentists, etc.), health plans, and healthcare clearinghouses
- **Business associate (BA):** associate of CE that assists CE with healthcare functions and activities
- **National provider identifier (NPI):** (*see Chapter 19, Lesson 6*)
- **Employer identification number (EIN):** also known as tax identification number, a number assigned to a business by the Internal Revenue Service

HIPAA

The purpose of the Health Insurance Portability and Accountability Act (HIPAA) of 1996 is to set up national standards for electronic healthcare transactions and code sets (ICD 10, CPT codes), provide unique health identifiers (NPI and EIN), and provide for the security of health information. The HIPAA law is Public Law 104–191 and contains the Privacy Rule, Security Rule, Enforcement Rule, and Breach Notification Rule.

- **Privacy Rule:** provides standards for a person to control and understand how health information is used; covered entities are subject to the Privacy Rule; implemented and enforced by the Office of Civil Rights; failure to comply with the Privacy Rule can lead to civil or criminal action; includes electronic, written, and oral health information
- **Security Rule:** provides standards to maintain confidentiality, integrity, and security of an individual's health information and how it is used by covered entities; this rule is enforced by the Office of Civil Rights and is specific to electronic health information
- **Enforcement Rule:** provides standards for compliance, investigations, impositions of civil penalties, and hearing procedures
- **Breach Notification Rule:** provides standards for notifying individuals, the media, and the Secretary of Health and Human Services when a breach of PHI has occurred

Covered entities and their business associates are required to comply with HIPAA. A BA must have an arrangement or written contract with a CE that establishes the BA's job function and its need to protect privacy and security of PHI.

A few of the more common implications are listed below. For additional information, visit the Health and Human Services website (**www.hhs.gov/hipaa/for-professionals/index.html**).

Common Practice Implications of HIPAA
• Every reasonable effort should be made to allow for privacy and confidentiality when speaking with other providers, nurses, and ancillary personnel about a patient, whether that occurs over the phone or in person. Only information necessary to treat the patient appropriately should be shared
• Patients have the right to specify how messages are left. Messages may be left for a patient on an answering machine or with a family member if permitted by the patient. The message should be brief and limited and not disclose any PHI
• It is permissible to have a sign-in sheet for patients and to call patients by name in the waiting room. Information that is not necessary to the sign-in process should not be accessible to others
• PHI can be disclosed to another provider for the purpose of treatment
• Reporting suspected abuse or neglect to the appropriate agency does not violate HIPAA
• When disposing of PHI, no certain method is preferred. Safeguards must be used to limit prohibited or unintentional use or a breach of PHI
• Elementary and secondary schools are not a CE. Health information that is obtained by schools is part of a student's education record and is covered by the Family Educational Rights and Privacy Act (FERPA)
• Immunization records may be given to a school without written consent as long as immunizations are required for school enrollment
• Release of PHI for workers' compensation cases varies by state. A patient may not refuse to disclose information pertaining to a workers' compensation case if the state allows workers' compensation access to those records

Table 19.1.1

Privacy

Maintaining privacy and confidentiality of PHI is essential and required by law. The Office of Civil Rights is responsible for investigating complaints, providing education, and performing compliance reviews regarding HIPAA. The Office of Civil Rights works with the Department of Justice for criminal violations of HIPAA.

Complying with the Privacy Rule
• To comply with the Privacy Rule, a practice is required to: – Secure PHI – Have a designated employee in charge of ensuring privacy practices are followed – Provide employee training regarding HIPAA – Have privacy practices in place – Give patient's information about their rights under HIPAA and information about how their PHI is used
• A patient should be given a notice of CE privacy practices before the first encounter with that patient, and the patient should provide written acknowledgment of those practices
• The privacy practices should be displayed in an accessible, prominent location in the practice
• Patients should be notified of accessibility of privacy practices at least once every 3 years
• If there are changes in privacy practices, the revised document should be made available to the patient before the first encounter after a change has occurred
• Patients have the right to determine how their health information is shared, as long as their request complies with federal and state laws (treatment of minors, emancipated minors, workers' compensation)
• If a breach of PHI occurs, individuals and the Secretary of Health and Human Services (HHS) must be notified within 60 days. The Secretary is notified through the HHS website. If the breach affects more than 500 individuals, then media outlets must be notified. BAs are responsible for maintaining their own privacy and security and for making appropriate notifications regarding breaches of PHI

Table 19.1.2

Takeaways

- HIPAA is a public law that includes the Privacy Rule, Security Rule, Enforcement Rule, and Breach Notification Rule.
- PHI that is necessary to treat a patient may be shared with other treating providers.
- If a patient is an immediate danger to themselves or others, PHI is needed to ensure safety may be shared.
- The Privacy Rule applies to written, electronic, and oral PHI. The Security Rule applies to electronic PHI.

LESSON 2: MALPRACTICE

> ### Learning Objectives
> ■ Understand the elements of a malpractice claim
> ■ Differentiate between types of malpractice insurance policies
> ■ Identify ways to minimize risk of a malpractice claim

As the nurse practitioner workforce has grown, so have the number of malpractice claims involving nurse practitioners. Nurse practitioners are gaining increasing levels of autonomy with medically complex patients, and with this responsibility comes added risk. It is of vital importance to be adequately protected from malpractice claims.

Definitions

- **Medical malpractice:** action or inaction by a medical professional that results in patient injury or death
- **Negligence:** unintentional failure to perform an act that a reasonable person would or would not perform; negligence does not always equate to malpractice

In order to prove malpractice, the following must be present:

- **Duty of care:** established by the provider-patient relationship (could be established inside or outside an office visit or with an individual who is not formally a patient)
- **Breach of the standard of care:** lapse in the care that a reasonable and similarly situated professional would provide
- **Injury:** the individual must have an injury (malpractice cannot be claimed without injury)
- **Proximal cause:** the provider's conduct must have caused an injury that constituted a breach in the standard of care

Considerations

The highest payouts for malpractice claims often come from the areas of neonatology, obstetrics, and geriatrics. Claims are often based on failure to diagnose, improper management, delay in diagnosis, not recognizing complications, wrong medication, improper performance, or lack of monitoring. Primary care and family practice claims may involve failure to order a test or labs, or failure to address results.

The National Council of State Boards of Nursing (NCSBN) maintains nurse practitioners are responsible to protect the individuals they care for and themselves by practicing within the scope of practice as mandated by state statutes, rules, and regulations.

> **Pro Tip: Avoiding Malpractice Claims**
> - Keep accurate and complete documentation
> - Communicate with patients
> - Adhere to the nurse practitioner scope of practice
> - Stay up-to-date and use evidence-based practice
> - Be knowledgeable and comply with your state's Nurse Practice Act
> - Ensure clinical training and certifications are current
> - Follow up on unresolved issues, diagnostic testing that has been ordered, and referrals—always close the loop

Malpractice Insurance

Malpractice insurance is essential to have in the medical profession. Employers may provide coverage to their employees, but it is important to know the details and exclusions of that policy to determine if an individual policy is needed. Consider the financial amount of coverage; make sure policy limits will be adequate. Policies may not cover volunteer work, moonlighting, or self-employment. When choosing an individual policy, make the same considerations. In addition, make sure the insurance broker is registered in the state and has a good financial rating by contacting the National Association of Insurance Commissioners.

- **Claims-based policies:** malpractice insurance that covers claims made during the time coverage is active (once the policy has expired, there is no coverage)
  - Employer-based policies are often claims-based
- **Tail coverage:** insurance that can be purchased at the end of a claims-based policy to extend coverage for claims that may be filed after the fact
  - Employers may provide tail coverage that can be purchased after employment to extend the coverage
  - Tail coverage is usually 150–200% higher than the claims policy
  - Coverage should be continued until the statute of limitations has run out on any possible case that could occur from previous employment; statute of limitations varies from state to state and can often be prolonged for neonatal, obstetric, and pediatric cases
- **Occurrence-based policies:** coverage for any claim that is made during the time coverage was in effect, regardless of whether the policy is still in effect at the time of the claim

National Practitioner Data Bank

The National Practitioner Data Bank (NPDB) is a federal web-based collection of reports on medical malpractice payments and adverse actions of healthcare practitioners, providers, and suppliers. The goal of the NPDB is to improve the quality of healthcare, prevent fraud and abuse, and protect the public. Some organizations that can access the NPDB include state boards, health plans, hospitals, professional societies with peer review, and healthcare entities. They can report and query the NPDB, and it can be used for licensing, hiring, and credentialing. An individual is notified if a report is made against them on the NPDB. A self-query can be done for a fee. This information is not available to the public.

> **Digital Resource**
> NPDB can be accessed here: **www.npdb.hrsa.gov/index.jsp**.

Takeaways

- An occurrence-based policy is usually the most comprehensive type of malpractice policy.
- Minimize risk of malpractice by appropriate communication and collaboration, compliance with policies and procedures, thorough documentation, and follow-up on referrals and unresolved problems.

LESSON 3: MEDICARE/MEDICAID

Learning Objectives
- Understand the main provisions and purpose of Medicare and Medicaid
- Be able to educate patients on Medicare and Medicaid provisions

Government-supported health insurance was first seriously pursued during the Truman administration. It had multiple opponents, including the American Medical Association (AMA), who felt such programs socialized medicine. No clear action was taken during Truman's term, but in July 1965, under Johnson's administration, U.S. Social Security legislation was amended and Medicare and Medicaid were born.

Medicare covers 1 out of 6 Americans (some may have dual coverage with Medicaid): 31% enrollees report cognitive or mental impairment, 17% are under age 65 with permanent disability, 13% are over age 65, and 5% are in long-term care facilities.

Medicaid covers 1 in 5 Americans. About 14% are disabled, 9% are elderly, 43% are children, and 34% are adults. In terms of actual expenditure, 40% of Medicaid dollars are spent on the disabled, 21% on the elderly, 19% on adults, and 19% on children. It is estimated that one-third of Medicaid dollars go toward paying for long-term care spending. Additionally, 50% of U.S. births are paid for by Medicaid.

Medicare

Initially, Medicare (also known as Title XVIII) was comprised of two parts:

- **Part A:** hospital insurance for the elderly
- **Part B:** supplemental medical insurance

Over time, provisions were added to Medicare. In 1972, individuals younger than 65 years of age with permanent disabilities, diagnoses of end-stage renal disease, or other eligibility for Social Security Disability Insurance (SSDI) were allowed access to Medicare funding. Requirements stipulate that recipients must be U.S. citizens or continuous permanent legal U.S. residents for 5 years, with an additional stipulation that either the proposed recipient or spouse has paid Medicare taxes for at least 10 years.

As it stands now, **Medicare Part A** covers most medically necessary hospital, home health, skilled nursing facility, and hospice care.

Medicare Part B covers doctor visits, surgeries, some preventive care, durable medical equipment, hospital outpatient services, diagnostic tests/testing, psychiatric care, and some home health and ambulance services. Patients pay monthly premiums for Medicare Part B.

Medicare Part C—known today as Medicare Advantage—launched in 1997 as part of the Balanced Budget Act to reduce Medicare spending by more than 100 billion dollars. The concept was that privately run medical groups (overseen by the government) could provide cheaper, more efficient care, and sometimes expand options for enrollees.

The private insurers of **Medicare Advantage** (i.e., HMOs and PPOs) are required to offer at least the same coverage as the original Medicare coverage (Part A and Part B). Enrollees in Medicare Advantage often pay a premium (in addition to the Part B premium) to include additional benefits such as dental care. Out-of-pocket expenses for Medicare Advantage can be less than that of a combination of traditional Medicare Parts A and B.

The Medicare Prescription Drug, Improvement, and Modernization Act was passed in 2003, creating a new Medicare component called **Medicare Part D** to provide prescription drug coverage. Enrollees pay monthly premiums for Medicare Part D.

Medicaid

Legislation amending Social Security (specifically Title XVIII) led to the creation of the Medicaid program in 1965. Under Medicaid, the federal government grants states matching funds (Title XIX) to provide healthcare for the indigent and, under specific eligibility considerations, other vulnerable groups.

Originally, Medicaid covered:

- Pregnant women and children <6 years of age with family incomes at or below 133% of the federal poverty line (FPL)
- Children 6–18 years of age with family incomes at or below 100% FPL
- Parents and caretaker relatives meeting eligibility for welfare
- Blind, elderly, and disabled people who qualified for Supplemental Security Income (SSI)

Extensions of Coverage

CHIP

The 1997 Children's Health Insurance Plan (CHIP) covers children (and some pregnant women) in households that make too much to qualify under Medicaid but too little to afford private insurance. This program permits enrollees who earn up to 200% of the federal poverty level. It is estimated that about 9 million U.S. children and 370,000 pregnant women are covered under CHIP. Recently, federal funding was available for this program through September 2017. While the program's future was uncertain through the end of 2017, Congress passed a budget agreement in February 2018 to fund CHIP for another 10 years.

ACA

The Affordable Care Act (ACA) has three goals:

1. Make insurance more affordable/available—tax credits lower costs for households with incomes between 100–400% of the FPL
2. Expand Medicaid coverage for adults with income <138% of the FPL (not all states have expanded their Medicaid programs)
3. Encourage implementation and utilization of healthcare design, which is aimed at lowering costs

See Chapter 19, Lesson 7, for more information regarding the ACA.

Digital Resource

It is useful to know if your low-income patient lives in a state with Medicaid expansion. Visit the following site for a list of Medicaid expansion states: **http://familiesusa.org/ product/50-state-look-medicaid-expansion**.

Mandatory Medicaid Coverage

- Inpatient hospital care
- Outpatient hospital services
- EPSDT: Early and Periodic Screening, Diagnostic, and Treatment services
- Nursing facility services
- Home health services
- Physician services
- Rural health clinic services
- Laboratory and x-ray services
- Family planning services
- Nurse midwife services
- Certified Pediatric and Family Nurse Practitioner services
- Freestanding birth center services (when licensed or otherwise recognized by the state)
- Outpatient hospital care
- Transportation to medical care
- Tobacco cessation counseling for pregnant women

Non-Covered (Optional) Services

- Dental
- Prosthetics
- Eyeglasses
- Respiratory Services
- Hospice

Looking to the Future

Currently Medicare has about 55 million enrollees and Medicaid has about 74 million. The Centers for Medicare and Medicaid Services (CMS) estimate about 11.4 million individuals are dual-enrollees—simultaneously enrolled in Medicare and Medicaid. But the U.S. population is aging. It is expected that by 2060, there will be 98 million Americans over age 65, comprising nearly 1 out of 4 Americans. With this change, enrollment in both Medicare and Medicaid will only increase.

Takeaway

These changes suggest that clinicians can expect to be catering to a population that may be sicker, poorer, more vulnerable, and less mobile. Clinicians should continue to advocate for policies that are advantageous to their patients as the healthcare system navigates through these transitions.

LESSON 4: NURSING ETHICS

Learning Objectives

- Define nursing ethics
- Recognize the importance of nursing ethics
- Be able to implement ethical nursing practice

Nurse practitioners work within an ethical domain, the provider-patient relationship, in which the provider is powerful and the patient is vulnerable. Nurse practitioners generally work without direct supervision, handle very private aspects of the patient's life, and care for individuals who may fail to advocate for themselves, as they are ill.

On the local level, ethical nursing care is guided by the state Board of Nursing, the nurse's work setting (such as a hospital or nursing home), and professional nursing organizations. But the practice of nursing is increasingly complex and can present the novice (and even the experienced) nurse clinician with ethical dilemmas.

Examples of ethical dilemmas in nursing	Possible solutions
The NP wants to provide patient-centered care but works in a correctional facility where he/she has been notified general safety takes precedence over patient-centered care.	The NP may consider meeting with correctional supervisors to identify methods by which patient-centered care can be instituted without compromising safety.
Nursing staff is restricted from using a cell phone in patient areas, but the NP has a sick child at home and wants to check on the child's condition.	The NP could notify the babysitter to call the clinic at a certain time, then notify front-desk staff to page him/her when the babysitter calls.
The NP works for a drug-rehabilitation program. On one hand, patient-centered ideals remind the NP that "pain is subjective." On the other hand, the NP has a moral and ethical responsibility to help the patient get through physical withdrawal to reach a goal of sobriety.	The NP can call a team meeting with others, including the on-staff pain specialist, psychiatrist, mental health technician, and patient, to determine how to address the patient's pain while also helping the patient wean off pain meds.
The NP has noticed that colleagues are posting pictures of patients on social media without patient permission.	The nurse practitioner should notify the supervisor/office manager. This is a HIPAA violation, as well as ethically unsound. *See more on safeguarding privacy in Chapter 19, Lesson 1.*

Table 19.4.1 Ethical Dilemmas in Nursing

Definitions

Key ethical concepts related to patient care/clinical practice:

- **Autonomy:** the patient's right to make decisions about his or her own care
- **Beneficence:** to do good or promote the good of others; demonstrating kindness/generosity
- **Competence:** indicates that the patient is able to make decisions; compromised cognition (found in conditions such as dementia or schizophrenia), sedation, and delirium are all conditions that may lead to a finding of *in*competence
- **Confidentiality:** adhering to rules that safeguard patients' personal health information
- **Fidelity:** maintaining caring commitment, displaying honest conduct, and keeping promises made to the patient
- **Informed consent:** involves discussion/education regarding risks and benefits of testing, procedures, medications, or other treatment; the patient must be mentally competent and able to understand and communicate with the clinician for informed consent to be valid
- **Justice:** presumes that patients have an equal right to healthcare—even disadvantaged patients
- **Nonmaleficence:** do no harm
- **Paternalism:** the opposite of autonomy—not allowing patients to determine or make healthcare choices on their own
- **Veracity:** involves telling the truth to patients; not misrepresenting facts

The American Nurses Association Code of Ethics

The Code of Ethics for Nurses with Interpretive Statements (The Code) is a guide for nurses in providing ethically (as well as medically) competent care. Topics include:

- Respect for human dignity and promotion of social justice (reflecting the larger mission of promoting equal healthcare for all)
- Understanding the nurse-patient relationship (and its professional boundaries)
- Respecting patient wishes (including the right to refuse treatment)
- Protecting patient privacy (from the basics like closing the privacy curtain to more complex issues regarding refraining from disseminating patients' personal information, except for on an as-needed basis)
- Promoting patient safety
- Advocating for patients (for example, in cases of questionable practice or impaired colleagues)
- Showing sound nursing judgment (not only in the nurse's own actions, but in terms of delegation or assignment of duties)
- Maintaining nursing competence (through continuing education and keeping up-to-date with evidence-based practice)
- Advocating for patients in policy and research arenas
- Maintaining the integrity of the nursing profession

> **Digital Resource**
>
> - The ANA offers continuing education on nursing ethics. Find more information here: **https://learn.ana-nursingknowledge.org/products/Code-of-Ethics-An-Overview**. (This CE offering will expire 10/2019.) For a full catalog, visit here: **https://learn.ana-nursingknowledge.org/catalog?pagename=Continuing-Education**
> - The International Council of Nurses also provides ethical guidelines here: **www.icn.ch/publications/position-statement**

Bodies of nursing (such as the ANA) acknowledge that nurses may find themselves with "conflicting values" and complex ethical choices that they have to balance with the demands of everyday practice in a typically high-volume, high-pressure environment.

Takeaways

In general, nurses can successfully provide ethical care if they stay true to the basics:

- Provide patient-centered nursing.
- Treat patients the way they would want themselves or their loved ones to be treated.
- Provide safe, competent care.

LESSON 5: NP SCOPE OF PRACTICE

Learning Objectives

■ Know the organizations/governmental bodies that define nurse practitioner scope of practice

■ Understand why scope of practice for NPs varies state-by-state across the U.S.

■ Be alert for ongoing policy changes affecting NP scope of practice

NP Scope of Practice

The nurse practitioner scope of practice can be defined in two ways: legal/definitional scope of practice and functional limits to scope of practice—that is, limits that are not based on legal confines but nevertheless restrict nurse practitioner action.

There are two national organizations that grant the FNP board certification status: American Nurses Credentialing Center (ANCC) and American Academy of Nurse Practitioners (AANP).

The AANP has created a classification system to define NP scope of practice across the 50 states (for more information, go to **www.aanp.org/legislation-regulation/state-legislation/state-practice-environment**):

- **Full practice:** NP can independently evaluate and diagnose patients, order and interpret diagnostic tests, and begin and manage treatments, including prescription medications

  Examples of practice requirements from Nevada, a "full practice" state:

  - Nurse practitioners with <2000 hours of NP practice or <2 years of practice who wish to be able to prescribe Schedule II controlled substances must have a prescribing protocol signed by an MD, with a copy kept on file with the state BON

  - NPs with >2000 hours of nurse practitioner practice or >2 years of practice are not required to maintain a collaborative agreement/practice protocol

  - For prescribing privileges, the NP must complete an application with the state BON. Once the NP's APRN license is issued and the NP is deemed qualified for prescribing privileges, the board will notify the Board of Pharmacy of the NP's eligibility. The NP must then apply for prescribing privileges with the Board of Pharmacy

  - To prescribe controlled substances, the NP must apply with the Board of Pharmacy and the Drug Enforcement Administration (DEA)

- **Reduced practice:** NP needs a collaborative agreement "with an outside health discipline" to be able to provide patient care. The collaborative agreement may limit the scope or setting of practice

  Examples of practice requirements from New York, a "reduced practice" state:

  - New York does not technically require the nurse practitioner to pass a national certifying exam, although it is listed as one pathway to recognition as an NP in the state

  - NPs need a written collaborative agreement *and* a written practice protocol on file with NYSED in order to practice

  - NPs with >3600 hours of qualifying nurse practitioner practice experience can opt out of the collaborative agreement/practice protocol confinement and register for independent practice

  - For full prescriptive ability, the NP must obtain a National Provider Identifier (NPI), a DEA number, and an official NYS prescription form or authorization to prescribe controlled substances

- **Restricted practice:** NP is not able to provide patient care without supervision, delegation, or team management by an outside health discipline

  Examples of practice requirements from California, a "restricted practice" state:

  - Nurse practitioners are required to have MD supervision to prescribe medications, diagnose, and treat patients

  - For prescription privileges, the nurse practitioner must fill out a separate application order to furnish (prescribe) drugs and devices to patients called a Nurse Practitioner Furnishing Number application. The NP then obtains a DEA number in order to prescribe controlled substances

Interestingly, the Veteran's Administration (VA) allows full scope of practice in any state the nurse practitioner practices, with the exception of one element: the nurse practitioner must follow the relevant state laws regarding prescribing and administering controlled substances.

State Requirements

To be certified as an advanced practice nurse (APN or APRN) in any state, a provider must hold a valid license as a registered nurse in that state and have been awarded a master's, postgraduate, or doctoral degree from an FNP program. Most states require the provider to pass/maintain a national board certification in order to be licensed as an APN.

Digital Resource

Specific requirements to work as an NP vary by state and are defined by each state's Nurse Practice Act (NPA) and the state's BON. Use the Nurse Practice Act Toolkit at **www.ncsbn.org/npa-toolkit.htm** to locate state-specific nurse practice acts and contact the BON.

NP Prescription Privileges

Nurse practitioners can prescribe medications, including controlled substances, in every state. Some states require MD supervision and written protocols. Laws vary by state regarding which scheduled medications the NP is allowed to prescribe. Rules also vary regarding the NP's ability to dispense, administer, or procure medications, so familiarize yourself with the relevant state laws.

Organizations That Help Define NP Scope of Practice

The National Organization of Nurse Practitioner Faculties (NONPF) is a U.S.-based organization with a global footprint that seeks to establish nurse practitioner competencies on the national and international level for primary care nurse practitioners, acute care nurse practitioners, etc.

The American Association of Colleges of Nursing (AACN) works to establish nursing education standards, support nursing policy and research, and assist schools in carrying out those standards.

Pro Tip

To bill Medicare, the nurse practitioner must have an NPI number and national certification. Once the nurse practitioner has Medicare billing privileges, the nurse practitioner can bill Medicare directly or may have an authorized organization (such as the nurse practitioner's place of work) bill on his or her behalf.

For more information on obtaining an NPI number see Chapter 19, Lesson 6. For more on billing Medicare, see Chapter 19, Lesson 3.

Age Considerations Can Limit NP Scope of Practice

Another limitation on scope of practice can present itself if the specialty the nurse practitioner has chosen has an age restriction. FNPs are prepared, by virtue of their family practice focus, to practice across the life span.

Other nurse practitioners may have restrictions on practice due to their educational population focus. For example, a geriatric nurse practitioner cannot take an NP job providing pediatric care even if he or she has years of pediatric nursing experience as a registered nurse. Setting of practice is a bit different. An FNP could reasonably see patients in an acute care setting such as a hospital, given the medical concerns are those commonly seen in primary care (e.g., minor injuries, otitis media, sprains). If the FNP was expected to provide care for unstable, complex patients, the FNP would be practicing outside of the individual's scope of practice.

> ### Pro Tip
>
> NPs should beware of signing employment contracts that legally bind them to perform tasks that they are legally prohibited from performing due to scope or practice limitations.
>
> An example might be an adult nurse practitioner signing a work contract that stipulates (perhaps in fine print) that the NP accepts children's appointments. The nurse practitioner is then put in an untenable position. Should the NP fail to meet the employer's stipulations, the NP is in violation of contract, but by meeting the employer's stipulations, the NP is violating scope of practice as stipulated by the BON.

Scope of Practice Self-Restriction

The nurse practitioner can also self-restrict his or her role of practice. Many new nurse practitioners are cautious, careful to take on roles suited to their personal training, their comfort level with given populations, and their certification. For example, the FNP is technically qualified to treat across the life span. But if the FNP's only experience with pediatrics was during clinical rotation, the FNP may self-select to treat only adults.

To illustrate this point further, some FNPs work in dermatology. While an FNP is not restricted from performing dermabrasion, for example, it is unlikely the FNP received hands-on practice in dermabrasion technique during clinical rotations. Most nurse practitioners would require further training and might avoid performing the procedure until they were able to have further specialized training.

One last example could be described as a form of "functional limitation." Is a nurse practitioner required to obtain a DEA number if that nurse practitioner never intends to prescribe controlled substances? The answer is no. However, functionally speaking, the nurse practitioner might be hard-pressed to find an employer who will hire an NP who does not have a DEA number. An FNP without a DEA would never be able to prescribe an Ativan or Tylenol 3, for example. Also, many pharmacies use clinicians' DEA numbers to get reimbursement for prescriptions.

Takeaways

- The nurse practitioner should be aware that scope of practice changes occur constantly.
- Visiting the websites of the relevant state nursing board, organizations like the American Nursing Association, or certifying organizations such as ANCC or AANP is a good way to stay aware of scope of practice updates.

LESSON 6: NPI NUMBER

Learning Objectives
- Define National Provider Identifier (NPI)
- Understand purpose of an NPI
- Recognize how to obtain an NPI

Definition

- **Enumerator:** one who takes a census or gathers information

National Provider Identifier

The National Provider Identifier (NPI) is a 10-digit unique number that is used to identify providers. The NPI Final Rule was published in January 2004 to establish the NPI as the standard to identify providers. Covered entities use the NPI for financial and administrative transactions under HIPAA. If a provider is not a covered entity, he or she needs an NPI for pharmacy claims. The only time an NPI is not required is for a sole practitioner who accepts cash as the only form of payment. Failure to obtain an NPI for covered entities is an act of noncompliance.

Application for an NPI is only done once. It is free to obtain, and the application can be completed in three different ways:

1. Online through the National Plan and Provider Enumeration System (NPPES) website (*see link below*); this is the most efficient and fastest way to apply; select "Create or Manage an Account"
2. Through an Electronic File Interchange (EFI), which is an organization that applies for an NPI on behalf of the provider
3. Via paper application (CMS-10114) mailed to NPI Enumerator in Fargo, ND; this form can be downloaded from the Center for Medicare and Medicaid Services (CMS) website

Once the application for an NPI is submitted, it is placed in a queue to be reviewed by the enumerator. The application is either denied, returned for being incomplete/needing more information, or approved and the NPI administered. NPI information must be kept up-to-date and it is the responsibility of the provider to ensure accuracy. There is a 30-day window to make changes on the NPPES website for any changes in the NPI information. An NPI is deactivated if a provider goes out of business or dies; this NPI will never be used by another provider, and it can be reactivated if the provider begins practicing again. An individual NPI will never change. A group practice can have a separate NPI for the practice, and if an individual leaves that practice, they will no longer be associated with the group NPI.

Digital Resource

- For general NPI information: **www.cms.gov/Regulations-and-Guidance/Administrative-Simplification/NationalProvidentStand/**
- To apply electronically: **https://nppes.cms.hhs.gov/#/**
- To apply in writing, there application available at: **www.cms.gov/Medicare/CMS-Forms/CMS-Forms/downloads/CMS10114.pdf**

NPI Enumerator contact information:

NPI Enumerator

P.O. Box 6059

Fargo, ND 58108-6059

1-800-465-3203

customerservice@npienumerator.com

LESSON 7: THE AFFORDABLE CARE ACT/HEALTH POLICY

Learning Objectives

■ Understand the provisions of the Affordable Care Act (ACA)

■ Be able to educate patients on ACA provisions

Few pieces of American legislation have been as sweeping and as controversial as the Affordable Care Act (ACA). About 50 million Americans (nearly 1 in 6) were uninsured in 2010. Healthcare costs were rising alarmingly, swallowing 18% of the U.S. gross national product. And while Americans could boast of easier access to specialists, experts noted that in other measures, such as preventative care and access to primary care, Americans lagged behind.

Over the years, there have been many attempts to address healthcare coverage in the United States. The Social Security Amendments of 1965 paved the way for the programs known as Medicare and Medicaid. Another legislative effort allowed for the 1997 Children's Health Insurance Plan (CHIP), covering children whose families made too much to qualify under Medicaid but were still uninsured.

At the state level, Massachusetts experimented with providing universal health insurance coverage in 2006. It surprised naysayers by succeeding in reducing costs, increasing efficiencies, and eventually extending health insurance to more than 98% of its residents.

The Affordable Care Act

The Affordable Care Act was modeled after the Massachusetts legislation, with an intent to provide universal healthcare. It became law in March 2010. Key provisions include:

- Broadened access to insurance
- Increased consumer protections
- Focus on prevention and wellness
- Improved quality and system performance
- Increased healthcare workforce
- Addressing rising healthcare costs

Digital Resource

Detailed information regarding the ACA can be found using the following links:
- **www.ncsl.org/portals/1/documents/health/hraca.pdf**
- **www.healthcare.gov/glossary/affordable-care-act**
- **www.hhs.gov/healthcare/about-the-aca/index.html**

Considerable opposition to ACA remains, even as it has succeeded in providing access to health coverage for an estimated 20 million previously uninsured Americans. Critics panned it as extending Medicare/Medicaid-like coverage, stating that it would prove expensive and untenable over time.

Pros and Cons of the Affordable Care Act	
Pros	**Cons**
Before ACA, many insurers were engaging in questionable practices such as increasing premiums, denying coverage to patients with pre-existing conditions, and imposing annual or lifetime caps on members.	Initially, the ACA appears to punish middle-income recipients. They get caught in the gap where subsidies phase out. (However, some experts believe that as health insurance is more universally adopted, costs will even out.)
The ACA retained many qualities of the already tried-and-true Massachusetts healthcare experiment: consumer choices, health exchanges, and private insurance.	Some experts have noted that ACA bronze plans with low premiums are essentially catastrophic coverage; they are not offering meaningful everyday care.
The ACA includes provisions that address healthcare waste, such as overtreatment and fraud, saving millions.	Some experts think that the ACA will cost $1.76 trillion by 2022, causing an increase in the U.S. debt burden.
Most observers agree that healthcare costs slowed since ACA's enactment.	While healthcare costs have slowed, some critics attribute the slowdown to the recession, not ACA savings.
The individual mandate (the requirement for individuals to either pay a penalty or pay for health insurance) is usually not onerous.	Even though most agree the penalty is not onerous, some critics feel no one should be penalized for *not* enrolling in healthcare. They feel it is a personal choice and not something that should be mandated. (The individual mandate was repealed in 2017 and will become effective in 2019.)
Obtaining insurance though ACA exchange allows for job mobility, since insurance is not tied to an individual employer. This can encourage entrepreneurship.	The ACA has been accused of introducing a "family glitch." Americans who have an employer offering ACA-compliant *individual* health insurance but not *family* insurance are not eligible for ACA.
Despite the improved landscape for job mobility, the ACA did not reduce labor participation as some critics had warned.	The ACA's success was somewhat dependent on the success of its Medicaid expansion provisions. But the Supreme Court made expansion voluntary: individual states can decide to accept Medicaid expansion or forgo it. For this reason, some experts believe ACA is underfunded and attempts to cover more persons than is fiscally wise.
The ACA is projected to cost $200 billion less than first projected for the 2015–2019 period. This directly contradicts others who state it will increase debt burden. (If Massachusetts is a reliable model, it seems more likely that the ACA will rein in costs, rather than increase them.)	Maternity was supposed to be covered under ACA. But pregnancy was not included as a "qualifying event" for which potential members could enroll outside of the yearly enrollment period.

Table 19.7.1

Pros and Cons of the Affordable Care Act (Continued)	
Pros	**Cons**
Healthcare coverage brought increased financial stability for millions of households.	The ACA has enrolled up to 10 million fewer participants than projected. (Some observers attribute this to partisan bickering, wherein states politically opposed to the ACA placed barriers to the enrollment process.)
Early data suggests enactment of the ACA helped reduce nosocomial infections and hospital readmits.	ACA was originally touted as permitting everyone to keep the insurance they had previous to its enactment. This turned out not to be true. A small percentage (5% or so) lost their plans because their plans did not meet ACA standards. (Some could argue that this was *not* actually a "con," but rather a "pro," because it forced insurers to improve some plans, for example, by removing annual lifetime caps.)
Insurance companies were banned from restricting health insurance due to pre-existing conditions. (Insurance companies tended to either drop patients with such conditions or raise their premiums to unaffordable levels.)	
ACA capped patients' out-of-pocket annual/lifetime expenditures.	
ACA extended healthcare coverage for young people (still dependent on their parents' coverage) through age 26.	

Table 19.7.1

The ACA was introduced in a particularly fraught political climate. For this reason, it remains on shaky ground and may be repealed or purposely underfunded.

Takeaways

For many Americans, the ACA offered three substantial improvements to healthcare:

1. Preventing healthcare insurers from denying insurance to Americans due to pre-existing conditions.
2. Capping out-of-pocket expenditures.
3. Extending healthcare coverage for young people (still dependent on their parents' coverage) through age 26.

LESSON 8: REIMBURSEMENTS AND MEDICAL CODING

Learning Objectives
- Define the difference between ICD 10 and CPT coding
- Utilize documentation to determine appropriate CPT coding
- Recognize how reimbursement for services is determined

Medical Coding

Medical diagnosis coding is based on the 10th revision of the International Statistical Classification of Diseases and Related Health Problems (ICD 10). This international system of classification uses alphanumeric codes that give diagnoses and major symptoms a corresponding classification. The purpose of using ICD 10 in diagnosis is for uniformity; tracking of epidemiologic, quality, morbidity, and mortality data; and billing purposes. The World Health Organization publishes, edits, and updates the classification of diseases.

Current procedural technology (CPT) codes are given to procedures, evaluations, surgeries, and tests performed on a patient. CPT codes are revised annually and are a product of the American Medical Association. They describe an interaction between a provider and a patient as a 5-digit code. CPT and ICD 10 codes give a picture of the patient's visit. Together, the codes describe what was done and why it was done.

The nurse practitioner is responsible for ensuring the diagnosis and pertinent symptoms given to the patient are coded correctly. Documentation must be appropriate for the level of care provided. The words "normal," "abnormal," and "regular" should never be used as standalone descriptors in documentation. Likewise, if a particular portion of an exam or test is deferred, it should be noted why it was deferred. The codes are sent to insurance companies to request payment for services. If a test or procedure was done, a corresponding diagnosis code to support the reason for doing the test must be included.

Take the example of a 17-year-old male complaining of sore throat, fever, myalgia, and cough. A rapid strep test and rapid influenza test are performed. The patient is diagnosed with acute streptococcal tonsillitis (J03.00). To have the rapid influenza test covered by insurance, there needs to be a diagnosis code to justify this test (fever R50.9 or myalgia M79.1). The diagnosis J03.00 will cover the rapid strep test, and the rapid strep test and rapid influenza test each have a CPT code.

Billing Medicare for an evaluation and management (E/M) service or office visit requires a CPT code that best represents:

- New or established patient
- **History:** chief complaint (CC), history of present illness (HPI), review of system (ROS), past medical family (PMH) and social history (SH)
  - **Problem-focused visit:** CC, brief HPI
  - **Expanded problem-focused visit:** CC, brief HPI, problem-pertinent ROS
  - **Detailed visit:** CC, extended HPI, problem-pertinent ROS including a review of a limited number of additional systems, PMH, FH, and/or SH directly related to the patient's problem
  - **Comprehensive visit:** CC, extended HPI, ROS that is directly related to the problem(s) identified in the HPI plus a review of all additional body systems, complete PMH, FH, and SH
- Exam (number of body systems examined)
- Medical decision making (risk, complexity)
- If the visit is a preventative/wellness visit, codes different from those listed below are used. The codes for preventative/wellness are determined by age of patient

If a patient visit is primarily spent in counseling, the visit is coded based on the amount of time spent with the patient. Documentation must support the amount of time spent, and the amount of time must be included as well.

New patient visit code	Component	Number of body systems examined	Difficulty in decision making	Time (used as an average)
99201	Problem-focused history	1 body system	1 diagnosis, minimal risk, straightforward complexity decision making	10 minutes
99202	Expanded history	2–7 body systems (limited exam)	1–2 diagnoses, minimal-to-low risk, straightforward complexity decision making	20 minutes
99203	Detailed history	2–7 body systems (extended exam)	1–2 diagnoses, low-to-medium risk, low complexity decision making	30 minutes
99204	Comprehensive history	8 body systems	2+ diagnoses, moderate risk, moderate complexity decision making	45 minutes
99205	Comprehensive history	8 body systems	3+ diagnoses, extensive-to-high risk, high complexity decision making	60 minutes

Table 19.8.1 Coding a New Patient Visit

Established patient	History	Exam	Medical decision making	Time (used as an average)
99211	None	None	Used for minimal services to an existing condition where the provider does not have to see the patient (e.g., nurse-only visit for injection)	5 minutes
99212	HPI (1–3), problem-focused history	1 body system	1 diagnosis, no data, low risk, straightforward complexity	10 minutes
99213	HPI (1–3), ROS (1), expanded history	2–7 body systems	1–2 diagnoses, limited data, low risk, low complexity	15 minutes
99214	HPI (4+), ROS (2–9), PMFSH (1), detailed history	2–7 body systems	2+ diagnoses, moderate data, moderate risk and complexity	25 minutes
99215	HPI (4+), ROS (10+), PMFSH (2), comprehensive history	8 body systems	2+ diagnoses, extensive data and high risk, high complexity decision making	40 minutes

Table 19.8.2 Coding an Established Patient Visit

Two of the three key components—history, exam, and medical decision making—must be addressed in order to select the appropriate evaluation and management (E&M) code. Look at the above example for the patient diagnosed with acute streptococcal tonsillitis. If he were an established patient, the following would be documented for the visit:

- **HPI:** throat with sharp (quality) pain; worse with swallowing and better with acetaminophen and salt water gargles (modifying factors); symptoms started 3 days ago (timing) = 3 HPI
- **ROS:** constitutional: fever; HEENT: sore throat, runny nose, pain with swallowing = 2 ROS
- **Exam:** general: well-developed, well-nourished, no acute distress; HEENT: bilateral TMs clear without effusion, pharynx and tonsils edematous and injected, no exudate bilateral nares erythematous, no drainage; neck: bilateral anterior shotty, tender cervical lymphadenopathy; CV: RRR without murmur; resp: bilateral breath sounds clear = 5 body systems

- **Diagnosis:** acute streptococcal tonsillitis, fever = 2 diagnoses
- Visit code for this patient is 99213 (expanded history, 2–7 body systems, 1–2 diagnoses, low risk, low complexity)

To obtain appropriate reimbursement when coding for a visit if an additional procedure or service occurs as part of the same visit, the nurse practitioner needs to include a **modifier code** (2-digit codes that "modify" the service rendered). For example, a patient presents for an evaluation of a new skin lesion, and the nurse practitioner performs a punch biopsy as a part of the visit. The 25 modifier code will be included (this modifier indicates that a distinct, separate service is performed by the same provider on the same day of the other service).

Electronic medical records will often suggest or automatically assign a visit code based on the documentation, but ultimately the responsibility for correct coding lies with the provider of services.

Reimbursement

Coding and reimbursement go hand in hand. Visits must have the correct diagnosis, procedure, and exam codes. The documentation must support the codes. Proper coding allows for correct reimbursement for services, and reimbursement is determined by third-party payers (Medicare, Medicaid, private insurance) based on the resource-based relative value scale (RBRVS). The RBRVS places a value on services, taking into account the amount of work done by a physician for the service, the practice expense, and malpractice expense in performing the service. The practice and malpractice expense are adjusted based on geographical location, and nurse practitioners are typically reimbursed at 85% of the allowed amount. Medicare often serves as a benchmark for private insurers to determine their payment, and they contract with providers to pay a certain amount for services. The provider's fee is usually higher than the agreed upon amount, but providers will accept the lower rate to be included as a preferred provider on the insurance plan. Private insurance often pays 105% of the E&M visit, 110% of office procedures, and 115% of surgical procedures of what Medicare pays. This type of payment is known as fee for service.

Another type of payment called value-based payment (VBP) is based on the quality of care given, rather than the quantity. VBP looks for certain measures to be obtained and documented during patient visits and/or hospitalizations. Medicare is leading the way with VBP, and there have been frequent changes regarding the best way to proceed with this type of payment. At this time, it is not readily utilized, but there is movement to change payment based on quality measures.

> **Pro Tip**
> Medicare allows for "incident-to" billing. In these instances, Medicare will pay 100% of the physician fee schedule (compared to 85%) even though the service is rendered by an advanced practice provider rather than the physician. However, there are stringent guidelines in order to qualify for incident-to billing. For more information, go to **www.cms.gov/ Regulations-and-Guidance/Guidance/Manuals/downloads/clm104c12.pdf**.

Takeaways

- Medicare is the driving force behind documentation requirements, coding, and reimbursement. Most private payers use Medicare as a benchmark.
- There must be adequate documentation and appropriate ICD 10 code(s) to support the billed CPT code(s) and procedure(s) performed on patients.
- Documentation must address varying elements (history, exam, medical decision making, and/or time) in order to justify the level of E&M coding billed.

PRACTICE QUESTIONS

Select the ONE best answer.

Lesson 1: HIPAA/Privacy

1. All of the following are rules included in HIPAA except:

    A. Privacy Rule

    B. Breach Notification Rule

    C. Health Insurance Rule

    D. Security Rule

2. What is a covered entity under HIPAA?

    A. A medical office that files electronic insurance claims

    B. A public school system that requires immunizations for entry into school

    C. A gym that has clients fill out a health questionnaire prior to joining

    D. A nursing school that provides free blood pressure screenings to the public

3. The goal of the Privacy Rule is to:

    A. Allow for a patient's privacy when performing sensitive procedures

    B. Protect an individual's personal health information

    C. Protect a patient's right to decline treatment

    D. Allow an individual to make a decision about their healthcare at the end of life

4. Which of the following does not represent protected health information?

    A. Address, surgical history, phone number

    B. Diagnosis, medication list, billing and payment information

    C. Patient's smoking status, laboratory results, psychiatric record

    D. Review of systems for a particular visit, student's immunization record held by the school, family history

5. Which action would be a violation of HIPAA rules?

    A. Giving lab results to a patient's girlfriend because she said the patient told her to call and get them

    B. Discussing the treatment plan with another provider who a patient has seen in consultation

    C. Reporting child abuse to the Department of Child Services without the parent's consent

    D. Calling a patient by name in the waiting room

Lesson 2: Malpractice

6. Which of the following statements is true?

    A. The NP previously worked for a company from 1/2014–1/2018. She had a claim-based malpractice policy through this employer. She is covered for a malpractice claim that occurred 12/2017 even though she no longer has this policy and does not have tail coverage

    B. The NP is preparing to retire and decides he will not need tail coverage for his claims-based malpractice policy because he will no longer be in practice

    C. The NP had an occurrence-based policy from 3/2012–4/2018. She is covered for a malpractice claim that occurred 2/2014, even though she is no longer employed and no longer has coverage

    D. The NP had a claims-based policy with a previous employer for 11/2008–11/2018. He starts a new job on 2/2019 and obtains an occurrence policy that starts 2/2019. He is covered for a malpractice claim that occurs 1/2019

7. Which of the following is not a way to prevent a malpractice claim?

    A. Delegate interpretation of lab results and patient callback to nursing staff

    B. Document that a patient was called back about test results and told to repeat testing in three months

    C. Manage hypertension based on the latest evidence-based recommendations

    D. Understand and follow the state's Nurse Practice Act

8. Which of the following is not needed to establish a malpractice case?

    A. An injury

    B. A duty to provide care

    C. A standard of care that was not followed

    D. Documentation that is not complete and accurate

9. Which of the following criteria must be present for medical malpractice to occur?

    A. Breach of standard of care, injury, proximal cause

    B. Negligence, duty of care, proximal cause

    C. Incomplete documentation, poor communication, injury

    D. Duty of care, lack of evidence for practice, injury

Lesson 3: Medicare/Medicaid

10. Which of the following is true about Medicaid and Medicare?

    A. Medicare and Medicaid only cover Americans over 65 years old

    B. Medicare Part B covers most prescription costs

    C. Medicaid is a program in which the federal government gives states matching funds to cover healthcare services

    D. Medicare and Medicaid can expect a decline in enrollment numbers since the number of elderly is expected to decrease by 2050

11. Recent laws have allowed for Medicaid expansion, permitting more Americans to be eligible for health services. What is true regarding Medicaid expansion?

    A. It allowed more people to qualify under income alone (at generally 138% of the federal poverty level)

    B. It created Medicare Part E, which expanded eligibility to those 60 or older, even without disabilities

    C. It reduced drug copays to no more than $10 per prescription

    D. It extended coverage to all permanent U.S. residents, even those who were permanent residents for fewer than five years

12. Medicaid pays for nearly one-half of:

    A. Long-term care in the U.S.

    B. Births in the U.S.

    C. Hospice care

    D. Respiratory care

13. Which Medicare type is not correctly matched with its description?

    A. Medicare Part A: hospital insurance for the elderly

    B. Medicare Part B: supplementary medical insurance

    C. Medicare Part C: also known as Medicare Advantage; involves privately run medical groups providing Medicare services

    D. Medicare Part D: provision of dental services

14. Which of the following is covered by Medicaid?

    A. Eyeglasses

    B. Respiratory services

    C. Inpatient hospital care

    D. Hospice

Lesson 4: Nursing Ethics

15. The nurse practitioner is often called upon to advocate for vulnerable patients. The nurse practitioner can expect to fulfill this role:

    A. Only when the ombudsman is not available

    B. Only in cases where patients who do not have family members available to weigh in on their care

    C. For all patients

    D. Only in situations where the patient is confused or unable to make decisions

16. Which of the following is not an example of an ethical dilemma?

    A. Nursing staff is restricted from using a cell phone in patient areas, but the nurse practitioner wants a cell phone handy to return calls to patients

    B. The nurse practitioner has prescribed an asthma inhaler for her patent, and the patient has decided to purchase the generic version instead of the brand name because it is cheaper

    C. The nurse practitioner wants to provide patient-centered care but works in a facility where general safety takes precedence over patient-centered care

    D. The nurse practitioner has noticed that colleagues are taking photos to post on social media without patient permission

17. Which of the following is not an example of patient-centered ethical nursing care?

    A. Providing for patient safety and maintaining an appropriate nurse-patient relationship

    B. Providing for patient privacy and respecting patient wishes

    C. Providing evidence-based nursing care and advocating for personal vacation time

    D. Respecting patient dignity and advocating for patients in the policy and research arenas

18. Which of the following is an example of nonmaleficence?

    A. A nurse practitioner who has been seeing a long-time dialysis patient makes sure to remember the patient's birthday and helps staff arrange to have a sugar-free birthday cake waiting for the patient in the dayroom for after treatment

    B. A patient calls the nurse practitioner and informs her that she is not going to go through with scheduled gallbladder surgery. She tells the nurse practitioner she would prefer to wait and see if taking ursodiol (Actigall) might help. After making sure that the patient clearly understands the pros and cons of this decision, the nurse practitioner respects the patient's choice

    C. Staff in a nursing home contact the nurse practitioner, stating that a patient who recently began taking an antibiotic has developed signs of angioedema. The nurse practitioner orders the staff to withhold the medication

    D. A nurse practitioner works in a gynecology clinic that predominantly serves teens. The nurse practitioner has noticed that at-risk teens are not receiving equal access to services because they mostly go to a school across town and can't make it to the clinic before closing time. The nurse practitioner shifts the start time at the clinic so that the at-risk teens have equal access to clinic appointments

19. Ethical nursing care considerations should take into account:

    A. Hospital rules

    B. Concern of what one's nursing colleagues will think

    C. Nursing actions that might result in punishment

    D. Human rights overall

Lesson 5: NP Scope of Practice

20. Which definition is correctly matched with the AANP classification defining the NP scope of practice?

    A. Full practice: the nurse practitioner can independently evaluate/diagnose patients and order/interpret diagnostic tests

    B. Reduced practice: the NP is not able to provide patient care without supervision, delegation, or team management by an outside health discipline

    C. Restricted practice: the NP needs a collaborative agreement "with an outside health discipline" to be able to provide patient care

    D. Temporary practice: the NP can independently evaluate/diagnose patients and order/interpret diagnostic tests between the time of graduation and the time of passing the certification exam

21. The Family Nurse Practitioner might be exceeding scope of practice if he or she:

    A. Chooses to work in a non-acute family care clinic based in a hospital

    B. Opens an independent practice in a full-practice state

    C. Chooses to see only patients whose primary diagnoses are psychiatric in nature and is primarily prescribing psychiatric medications

    D. Writes prescriptions without the co-signature of an MD

22. An FNP has decided to work in dermatology and has been made aware that suturing wounds may be part of the job description. A colleague advises that suturing is outside the scope of practice for an FNP because it is "associated with surgery and thus involves acute care." Which is the best response?

    A. Suturing is always outside the FNP scope of practice because most FNP programs do not teach this skill

    B. Many NP schools teach suturing, and NPs can also take continuing medical education for further training on suturing. It is within the FNP scope of practice as long as the FNP is trained in and competent with this skill

    C. Only physician's assistants and MDs are allowed to suture

    D. Only MDs are allowed to suture

23. The two national organizations that are permitted to grant FNP board certification status are:

    A. The American Nurses Credentialing Center (ANCC) and the American Nurses Association (ANA)

    B. The American Academy of Nurse Practitioners (AANP) and the nurse practitioner's local state board of nursing

    C. The American Nurses Credentialing Center (ANCC) and the American Academy of Nurse Practitioners (AANP)

    D. The American Academy of Nurse Practitioners (AANP) and the National Council of State Boards of Nursing (NCSBN)

24. States that authorize full practice authority for an FNP are indicating that the FNP can:

    A. Evaluate and diagnose patients, order and interpret diagnostic tests, and initiate and manage treatment

    B. Evaluate and diagnose patients and order and interpret diagnostic tests, but may need oversight to initiate and manage treatment

    C. Evaluate and diagnose patients, but may need oversight to order and interpret diagnostic tests and to initiate and manage treatment

    D. None of the above: there is no true "full practice authority" for FNPs as they must work under the supervision of an MD

Lesson 6: NPI Number

25. Which statement is true regarding the NPI?

    A. An NPI must be renewed every five years

    B. Once issued, an NPI never changes

    C. A provider can only apply for an NPI by paper application

    D. NPI stands for National Provider Indicator

26. Which organization is responsible for issuing an NPI?

    A. Department of Health and Human Services

    B. State Medical Examiner

    C. National Insurance Regulator

    D. Center for Medicare and Medicaid Services

Lesson 7: The Affordable Care Act/Health Policy

27. The Affordable Care Act (ACA) introduced major healthcare reforms, but did not provide for:

    A. Coverage to patients with pre-existing conditions

    B. Capping of patients' out-of-pocket expenditures

    C. Single-payer healthcare

    D. Coverage of young people (dependents still on their parents' healthcare plan) through age 26

28. Which is not a provision of the Affordable Care Act?

    A. It monitors for fraud and healthcare waste

    B. It ties health insurance coverage to employment with certain employers

    C. It allows for a penalty to be levied against persons who choose to be uninsured

    D. It prevents healthcare companies from dropping patients with pre-existing conditions or raising their premiums

29. Before the Affordable Care Act was enacted, the number of Americans estimated to be without healthcare coverage was:

    A. 10 million

    B. 20 million

    C. 30 million

    D. 50 million

30. The Affordable Care Act helps make healthcare affordable to lower-income patients by:

    A. Allowing health insurance companies to charge more for patients with pre-existing conditions, thus evening out the costs for all

    B. Providing subsidies that help cover the cost of health insurance for lower-income patients

    C. Relegating all lower-income patients to low-cost "bronze" plans

    D. Encouraging lower-income patients to seek emergency room care for routine healthcare needs

31. The Affordable Care Act provision restricting health insurers from denying coverage or increasing insurance premiums to persons with pre-existing conditions applies to all of the following situations except:

    A. A 25-year-old woman who is 32 weeks pregnant and applying for insurance during open enrollment

    B. A 30-year-old man who is self-employed with a private insurance plan purchased through a local insurance carrier, now newly diagnosed with diabetes

    C. A 25-year-old man applying for coverage under his parent's insurance plan who does not live with his parents

    D. A 43-year-old woman who tested positive for BRCA 1 mutation last year and is now applying for insurance through a new employer

Lesson 8: Reimbursement and Medical Coding

32. Which of the following is true regarding diagnosis coding?

    A. As long as CPT codes are documented, diagnosis codes do not need to be included

    B. Coding should follow ICD-9 guidelines

    C. Coding should be accurate and thorough and should explain the patient encounter

    D. Coding for a patient visit is the responsibility of the billing department

33. CPT codes for an evaluation and management (E&M) visit are based on documentation of:

    A. HPI, exam findings, diagnosis, and time spent with the patient

    B. HPI, ROS, exam findings, and diagnosis

    C. Patient's demographic information, HPI, PMFSH, and diagnosis

    D. HPI, exam findings, insurance information, diagnosis, and treatment plan

34. Reimbursement for services by private insurance companies is based on reimbursement by:

    A. Blue Cross; Blue Shield

    B. Medicaid

    C. Health Maintenance Organizations

    D. Medicare

35. Which of the following is false regarding reimbursement?

    A. Nurse practitioners are typically reimbursed at 85% of physician rates

    B. Diagnostic testing will always be reimbursed as long as the reason for testing is documented in the plan of care

    C. Rates of reimbursement for Medicare are based on RBRVS

    D. Private insurance typically reimburses an E&M visit at 105% of what Medicare pays

ANSWERS AND EXPLANATIONS

Lesson 1: HIPAA/Privacy

1. C

The Health Insurance Rule **(C)** is not a rule under HIPAA. The Privacy Rule (A), Breach Notification Rule (B), and Security Rule (D) are all rules under HIPAA.

2. A

A covered entity is a healthcare provider that submits HIPAA transactions, health plans, or healthcare clearinghouses. A medical office that files electronic insurance claims **(A)** would fall under this definition. In these scenarios, a public school system that requires immunizations for entry (B), a gym that has clients fill out a health questionnaire (C), and a nursing school that provides free blood pressure screenings (D) do not fall under the definition of a covered entity.

3. B

The goal of the Privacy Rule is to protect personal health information **(B)**. Allowing for a patient's privacy when performing sensitive procedures (A) is a part of the practice, but is not a goal of the Privacy Rule. A patient's right to decline treatment (C) is a right, but not a goal of the Privacy Rule. Allowing an individual to make decisions about healthcare at the end of their life (D) is part of an advance directive, not part of the Privacy Rule.

4. D

A student's immunization record held by the school **(D)** is part of his or her educational record and is not protected health information. The review of systems and family history would be protected. Address, surgical history, phone number (A); diagnosis, medication list, billing and payment information (B); patient's smoking status, laboratory results, and psychiatric record (C) are all examples of protected health information.

5. A

Lab results are protected health information and can only be given to a patient and those they have designated. Giving the girlfriend lab results because she said the patient told her to call **(A)** does not make her a designated representative. HIPAA allows discussion regarding a patient's PHI between treating providers (B), as long as that information is needed by both providers in the treatment. There is a duty to report suspected child abuse to the appropriate department without consent (C), and it does not violate HIPAA rules. HIPAA allows patients to be called by name (D) and for a sign-in sheet to contain a patient's name. No other identifying information should be made public.

Lesson 2: Malpractice

6. C

The NP with the occurrence-based policy **(C)** is covered for a malpractice claim that occurred 2/2014, which was during the time of coverage. The NP who previously worked for a company from 1/2014–1/2018 (A) is not covered for a claim that occurred 12/2017 because her claims-based policy is no longer in effect, and she did not purchase tail coverage. The NP preparing to retire (B) will need tail coverage until the statute of limitations has run out on all possible cases from the time he was practicing. The NP with a claims-based policy from a previous employer (D) is not covered for a claim that is made before his occurrence policy goes into effect.

7. A

Delegating the interpretation of lab results and patient callback **(A)** can lead to incorrect interpretation of the results, as well as inappropriate follow-up for patients. This can be a basis for a malpractice claim. Documenting that a patient was called back (B) and told when to follow up is thorough documentation. Thorough documentation decreases the risk of a malpractice claim. Managing hypertension based on the latest evidence-based recommendations (C) is proper practice and will decrease the risk of malpractice. Understanding the state's Nurse Practice Act (D) and following that act will decrease the risk of a malpractice claim.

8. D

Documentation that is not complete and accurate **(D)** will make it difficult to defend against a malpractice case. However, it is not needed to establish a case. In order to have a malpractice case, there must be an injury (A), a duty to provide care (B), and a lapse in the standard of care (C). In addition, the lapse in the standard of care must be what caused the injury.

9. A

Medical malpractice requires that breach of standard of care, injury, proximal cause **(A)**, and duty of care be present. Negligence (B) results in harm or death to a patient, but it is not a criterion for medical malpractice. Incomplete documentation and poor communication (C) are actions that could bring about malpractice, but do not need to be present for it to occur. Lack of evidence for practice (D) is not required for medical malpractice, but may contribute to it.

Lesson 3: Medicare/Medicaid

10. C

Medicaid is a cost-sharing program (federal and state) to provide healthcare for the poor and certain vulnerable populations, so choice **(C)** is correct. Medicaid covers individuals other than those over the age of 65 (A). For example, Medicaid can cover children in poor families and disabled persons. Medicare Part D, not Part B (B), provides prescription coverage. The U.S. is expecting its aging population to increase, not decrease (D), which will likely swell the Medicaid/Medicare enrollment numbers.

11. A

Potential enrollees in Medicaid now may qualify under income alone **(A)**, typically up to 138% of the federal poverty level. There is no Medicare Part E (B), and even if there were, it would not be part of Medicaid expansion. Medicaid expansion did not create new rules on medication co-pays (C) and did not extend coverage to all permanent residents (D).

12. B

Nearly one-half of U.S. births **(B)** are paid for by Medicaid. Medicaid does not pay for one-half of long-term care services in the U.S. (A); it pays only for one-third. Medicaid does not generally cover hospice (C), though hospice is covered by Medicare. Medicaid does not typically cover respiratory care (D).

13. D

Medicare Part D covers prescriptions, not dental services **(D)**. It is true that Part A provides hospital insurance for the elderly (A), Part B provides supplementary medical insurance (B), and Part C involves privately run medical groups providing Medicare services (C).

14. C

Inpatient hospital care **(C)** is a mandatory service of Medicaid. Eyeglasses (A), respiratory services (B), and hospice (D) are not typically covered by Medicaid.

Lesson 4: Nursing Ethics

15. C

The nurse practitioner should always advocate for the welfare of all patients **(C)**. All patients are vulnerable: they are sick, and their daily routine has been interrupted and replaced by a medical routine that often asks for passivity and compliance. While the ombudsman is an additional advocate for patient rights (such as in filing a grievance), the ombudsman's presence or absence (A) does not abrogate the nurse practitioner's obligation. Family members can be helpful in advocating for patients, but their absence or presence (B) does not abrogate the nurse practitioner's obligation. While confused patients (D) or those with dementia are especially vulnerable, they are not the only patients who need advocacy.

16. B

Having a patient purchase the generic version of a drug **(B)** is not an ethical dilemma. Typically, generics are as effective as brand name. Additionally, the patient has the right to choose the generic version. Wanting a cell phone when it is not allowed (A) could present an ethical dilemma; the nurse practitioner is obligated to observe hospital rules and privacy concerns. Wanting to provide patient-centered care in a facility that stresses general safety (C) could present an ethical dilemma, in that the safety rules of a correctional facility can override the typical parameters of patient-centered care. Taking pictures of patients with plans to post on social media (D) is a HIPAA violation and may pose an ethical dilemma; the nurse practitioner is obligated to stop the action by reporting the staff to the supervisor.

17. C

While providing evidence-based nursing care is ethically sound, advocating for personal vacation time **(C)** is a workforce issue related to the nurse's own needs, not the patient's. Providing for patient safety (A), patient privacy (B), and patient dignity (D) are all reasonable examples of patient-centered ethical nursing care.

18. C

Nonmaleficence is to, essentially, "do no harm." To demonstrate nonmaleficence, clinicians should avoid acts of commission that might harm a patient, such as ineffective or harmful treatment. Stopping the medication after a patient develops signs of angioedema **(C)** is an example of nonmaleficence. Making arrangements to present a patient with a birthday cake (A) is not an example of nonmaleficence, but could be an example of beneficence—compassionate action toward others. Accepting the patient's decision about surgery after educating about risks and benefits (B) is not an example of nonmaleficence, but could be an example of respecting patient autonomy—the patient's right to make decisions about his/her own care. Changing work hours to meet the needs of patients (D) is not an example of nonmaleficence, but could be an example of seeking justice; in this case, the nurse practitioner is trying to provide equal access to healthcare for disadvantaged teens.

19. D

Ethical nursing care considerations should take into account human rights overall **(D)**. Taking into account hospital rules (A) and what one's nursing colleagues might think (B) are not related to nursing ethics. Nursing actions that might result in punishment (C) may be illegal actions, but that does not mean that they are also unethical. In sum, choices (A), (B), and (C) do not take into account the nurse-patient relationship and the obligations that go with that relationship.

Lesson 5: NP Scope of Practice

20. A

Full practice states the NP can independently evaluate and diagnose patients, order and interpret diagnostic tests **(A)**, and begin and manage treatment, including prescription medications. Reduced practice (B) requires the NP have a collaborative agreement "with an outside health discipline" to be able to provide patient care. Restricted practice (C) prohibits the NP from providing patient care without supervision, delegation, or team management by an outside health discipline. Temporary practice (D) is not a classification of practice.

21. C

An FNP primarily prescribing psychiatric medications and seeing patients whose primary diagnoses are psychiatric **(C)** could be construed as practicing as a Psychiatric Mental Health NP, not as an FNP, and thus exceeding scope of practice. It is allowable for an FNP to see non-acute patients in a family clinic (A), even if the clinic is based in a hospital—role, not setting, determines scope of practice. It would not be exceeding scope of practice for an FNP to open his or her own practice in a full-practice state (B). In fact, the FNP could potentially open his or her own practice in a reduced- or restricted-practice state, but the NP would generally face more obstacles and need proof of MD oversight. The FNP is independently licensed to write prescriptions without the co-signature of an MD (D), although some states require a collaborative agreement with an MD.

22. B

Suturing is actually taught by many FNP programs **(B)**. However, not all FNPs wish to practice suturing, as it requires multilayered knowledge: an understanding of underlying anatomy, wound care techniques, the ability not to introduce functional limitations (such as too-tight sutures that restrict joint movement), and the ability to produce a pleasing cosmetic result (i.e., minor scarring as opposed to major scarring). Suturing is within the FNP scope of practice, not outside (A); many NP programs teach this skill, although not every FNP may wish to suture.

FNPs are allowed to suture, not just physician assistants (C) and MDs (D).

23. C

The ANCC and the AANP **(C)** are currently the only entities that grant national certification for the FNP. The ANA (A) is a professional organization for nurses, but it does not grant FNP certification. The local state board of nursing (B) grants licensure, not certification. The National Council of State Boards (NCBSN) (D) is a consortium of nursing boards and does not grant FNP certification.

24. A

Full practice authority for an FNP implies that the FNP can evaluate and diagnose patients, order and interpret diagnostic tests, and initiate and manage treatment **(A)**. Choices (B) and (C) both imply some element of restricted practice. FNPs are independently licensed and do not need oversight to diagnose and treat (D). This description is more applicable to the status of physician assistants. All physician assistants must be supervised by an MD.

Lesson 6: NPI Number

25. B

An NPI is issued once, and it stays with that provider as long as they practice **(B)**. It will never be reissued to another provider. The NPI does not have to be renewed (A). Once it is obtained, the number is with the provider as long as they practice. An NPI application can be made online or by paper application (C). NPI stands for National Provider Identifier (D).

26. D

The Center for Medicare and Medicaid Services (CMS) is responsible for issuing an NPI **(D)**. The Department of Health and Human Services (A) and State Medical Examiner (B) are not responsible for issuing an NPI. The National Insurance Regulator (C) is a fictitious organization.

Lesson 7: The Affordable Care Act/Health Policy

27. C

The ACA did not provide for single-payer healthcare **(C)**. It allowed marketplaces and private plans to co-exist. The ACA included a provision to prevent health insurance plans from denying coverage to patients with pre-existing conditions (A), for capping of patients' out-of-pocket expenditures (B), and for allowing parents to extend coverage of their young adult children through age 26 (D).

28. B

The ACA does not tie health coverage to employment **(B)**. The ACA does include a provision to monitor for fraud and healthcare waste (A). It does allow for a penalty to be levied against persons who choose to be uninsured (C), and it prevents health insurance companies from dropping patients with pre-existing conditions or raising their premiums (D).

29. D

Roughly 1 out 6 Americans (~50 million Americans) **(D)** was uninsured before the ACA was enacted. After its enactment, about 1 in 11 Americans still remains uninsured.

30. B

The ACA provides for subsidies to cover the cost of health insurance for lower-income patients **(B)**. The ACA stipulates that health insurance companies cannot charge more for patients with preexisting conditions (A). Lower-income patients can pick from any plan in their area's health marketplace (C), and the ACA does not encourage lower-income patients to seek emergency room care for routine needs (D). In fact, the ACA contains provisions intended to lower healthcare costs by reducing fraud and healthcare waste.

31. B

The individual with a private insurance plan with a new diagnosis of diabetes **(B)** does not fall under the ACA preexisting condition provision. The preexisting coverage rule does not apply to "grandfathered" individual health insurance policies. A grandfathered individual health insurance policy is a policy that you bought for yourself or your family (e.g., an individual market plan). The ACA provision on preexisting conditions precluded health insurance agencies (group plans) from excluding or charging higher premiums to patients regardless of disability, psychiatric history, medical history, and genetic predisposition; therefore, pregnant women (A) or BRCA 1 mutation status (D) would not preclude these individuals from being able to obtain coverage in a group plan. Children can join or remain on a parent's plan even if they are not living with their parents (C).

Lesson 8: Reimbursement and Medical Coding

32. C

That coding should be accurate and thorough and should tell a story of why the patient was seen **(C)** is a true description regarding coding. Diagnosis codes must always be documented for a patient visit, making (A) incorrect. Coding should follow ICD-10 guidelines, not ICD-9 guidelines (B). Coding a patient visit is the responsibility of the provider who performed the exam, not the billing department (D).

33. B

Documentation of HPI, ROS, exam findings, and diagnosis **(B)** are all used to code an E&M visit. In addition, PMFSH and plan documentation are assessed when coding appropriately. Time spent with patient (A) is documented when a provider is billing based solely on time spent with the patient in counseling. The patient's demographic information (C) is not utilized to determine correct coding and neither is insurance information (D).

34. D

Medicare **(D)** serves as a benchmark that most private insurance companies utilize to determine reimbursement.

35. B

Diagnostic testing **(B)** will not be reimbursed if diagnosis codes are not documented that support the reason for testing. Choices (A), (C), and (D) are true statements.

CHAPTER 20

Care of Diverse Populations

LESSON 1: CULTURAL COMPETENCY AND HEALTH-RELATED BEHAVIORS

Learning Objectives

- Describe cultural competence and how it applies to practice
- Recognize barriers to culturally congruent care
- Explore causes of health disparities among populations

As the population in the United States continues to become more diverse, it is essential to understand cultural and religious differences and the effects they have on patient care. Cultural competence is the process in which a health professional continually strives to act respectfully, sensitively, and professionally within cultural context.

Cultural competence involves self-examination of one's own cultural healthcare beliefs, values, and professional background. It also involves conducting an assessment of relevant cultural information and having a desire to *want to* engage in a process of meeting the patient's individual cultural needs, as opposed to *needing to* engage. Cultural competence does not imply expertise, but rather knowing that differences exist and understanding the need to appreciate that aspect of our patients.

The American Nurses Association (ANA) is the professional organization responsible for articulating the social relationship between the nursing profession and society. There are three documents which elucidate this social contract:

- The definition of nursing
- The Nursing Code of Ethics
- The Scope and Standards of Nursing Practice (NSSP)

The ANA added Standard 8: Culturally Congruent Practice to the third edition of the NSSP. This standard emphasizes the importance of unique health concerns and approaches in special groups.

> **ANA Definition of Nursing**
>
> Nursing is the protection, promotion, and optimization of health and abilities; prevention of illness and injury; facilitation of healing; alleviation of suffering through the diagnosis and treatment of human response; and advocacy in the care of individuals, families, groups, communities, and populations.

Application of Standard 8 to Nursing Practice

ANA Standard 8 contains a total of 20 competencies regarding culturally congruent care. There are 13 competencies specific to registered nursing practice, an additional 5 specific for graduate-level nursing practice, and 2 more for the practice of the advanced practice registered nurse.

Standard 8: Culturally Congruent Practice and Associated Competencies	
Competencies for the registered nurse	1. Demonstrates respect, equity, and empathy in actions and interactions with all healthcare consumers 2. Participates in lifelong learning to understand cultural preferences, worldview, choices, and decision-making processes of diverse consumers 3. Creates an inventory of one's own values, beliefs, and cultural heritage 4. Applies knowledge of variations in health beliefs, practices, and communication patterns in all nursing practice activities 5. Identifies the stage of the consumer's acculturation and accompanying patterns of needs and engagement 6. Considers the effects and impact of discrimination and oppression on practice within and among vulnerable cultural groups 7. Uses skills and tools that are appropriately vetted for the culture, literacy, and language of the population served 8. Communicates with appropriate language and behaviors, including the use of medical interpreters and translators in accordance with consumer preferences 9. Identifies the culturally specific meaning of interactions, terms, and content 10. Respects consumer decisions based on age, tradition, belief and family influence, and stage of acculturation 11. Advocates for policies that promote health and prevent harm among culturally diverse, underserved, or underrepresented consumers 12. Promotes equal access to services, tests, interventions, health promotion programs, and enrollment in research, education, and other opportunities 13. Educates nurse colleagues and other professionals about cultural similarities and differences of healthcare consumers, families, groups, communities, and populations
Additional competencies for the graduate-level registered nurse	1. Evaluates tools, instruments, and services provided to culturally diverse populations 2. Advances organizational policies, programs, services, and practices that reflect respect, equity, and values for diversity and inclusion 3. Engages consumers, key stakeholders, and others in designing and establishing internal and external cross-cultural partnerships 4. Conducts research to improve healthcare and healthcare outcomes for culturally diverse consumers 5. Develops recruitment and retention strategies to achieve a multicultural workforce
Additional competencies for the advanced practice nurse	1. Promotes shared decision-making solutions in planning, prescribing, and evaluating processes when the healthcare consumer's cultural preferences and norms may create incompatibility with evidence-based practice 2. Leads interprofessional teams to identify the cultural and language needs of the consumer

Table 20.1.1

The ANA specifically addresses main populations that have unique health concerns regarding healthcare access, communication, education, treatment paradigms, and outcomes. They have developed specific resources and tools for the following populations:

- Those suffering from mental health disorders
- The elderly
- LGBT individuals and communities
- Obese individuals
- Racial and ethnic minority groups

Digital Resource

ANA Diversity Awareness Page

www.nursingworld.org/practice-policy/innovation-evidence/clinical-practice-material/diversity-awareness/

Barriers to Culturally Congruent Care

Cultural Knowledge and Bias of the Healthcare Professional

The first step in developing a culturally congruent practice is a self-assessment to determine one's cultural competence and/or bias. The ANA provides access to a cultural competence self-assessment from Georgetown University, which can be accessed online (**https://nccc.georgetown.edu/assessments**). The Cultural Competence Health Practitioner Assessment (CCHPA) is a strength-based model that is conducted in a nonjudgmental, safe environment to determine competencies across linguistics, specific healthcare issues, and cultural norms specific to various populations. It addresses potential bias of the healthcare practitioner and provides additional resources based on strengths and areas to develop.

Language and Linguistics

One of the most basic barriers to culturally competent care is language. According to the Centers for Disease Control (CDC), almost 19% of the U.S. population speaks a language other than English at home.

Title VI of the federal Civil Rights Act of 1964 states that the denial or delay of medical care due to language barriers is discrimination. Therefore, any medical facility receiving federal reimbursement for healthcare services (Medicaid or Medicare) must provide language assistance to patients with limited English proficiency. Additionally, the Joint Commission requires that interpretation and translation services be provided as necessary.

Nonverbal communication is equally important. Everyday gestures may by perceived as rude in other cultures. Consider eye contact, touch, and personal space.

Pro Tip

Ethnicity and culture are similar but different terms.

- **Ethnicity**: based on a group with similar traits (language, heritage); more context-specific than culture
- **Culture**: the milieu in which one lives (social, religious)

Ethnopharmacology

Ethnopharmacology is another barrier to culturally congruent care and encompasses:

- Genetic influences on the effect and metabolism of medications (pharmacogenomics)
  - Pharmacogenomics: identifies the individual genetic determinants of drug activity so that therapy can be tailored to the individual patient; the concepts of ancestral race and ethnicity have a strong influence on the understanding of population-level differences in drug response; understanding the degree to which pharmacogenomic data reveals that polymorphisms among genotype frequency often differs significantly among populations that are categorized by ethnicity and continental origin
  - Reduced response to ACE inhibitors, angiotensin II receptor antagonists, and beta-blockers in African Americans
  - G6PD deficiency among those of Mediterranean and African descent, which leads to greater incidence of hemolytic reactions to medications such as antimalarial medications and sulfa drugs
  - Increased incidence of severe skin reactions due to carbamazepine, which is associated with the presence of HLA-B*15:02 in patients of Asian heritage
  - Other ethnic groups with the presence of multiple functional copies of the gene encoding at CYP2D6 who experience the excessive conversion of codeine into morphine
- Use of traditional or herbal treatments by various ethnic groups: many medicines and treatments have their basis in plant-based pharmacology, and traditional and herbal treatments are becoming better understood; various populations may utilize alternative treatments, and these treatments may impact Western medicine in terms of drug-drug interactions and patient adherence

> **Digital Resource**
>
> NIH Center for Complementary and Integrative Health: **https://nccih.nih.gov**

Perception of Disease

Various ethnic groups have differences in the way they understand the etiology of a certain disease state or injury that will affect their approach to treatment. These culture-bound syndromes can be prominent features in the health concerns of many ethnic groups. For example:

- Cambodians may ascribe headaches, chest pain, palpitations, shortness of breath, and insomnia to koucharang, or "thinking too much"
- In some Hispanic cultures, the "mal de ojo" (evil eye) of a stranger's attention causes illness in children
- Some religious groups believe that disease, death, or injury is a spiritual punishment

Genetic Predisposition to Disease

Consider a patient's genetic predisposition to disease.

- **Cardiovascular disease**: more frequently encountered in ethnic minorities (though not statistically significant); high in African Americans, Native Americans
- **Diabetes**: prevalence is greater in men than women, African Americans, Pacific Islanders, Native Americans
- **Cancer**: African Americans and ethnic minority groups are underrepresented in research; actual numbers are greater than what the research states
- **Mental health**: perceived differently in various ethnic groups; risk factors are different related to discrimination, socioeconomics, availability to healthcare services

Health Disparities among Populations

Access to care, prevalence of disease or injury, and temporal relations are areas where health disparities exist along ethnic or population group lines.

- Access to care: special populations may have a cultural bias against Western medicine, lack of transportation or finances to pay for care, or a fear of accessing the healthcare system due to concerns over arrest and deportation

- Prevalence of disease or injury: certain populations may be at greater risk of diseases or injury (e.g., the LGBT community has a much higher incidence of suicide and assault; recent immigrants have a higher incidence of PTSD, malnourishment, and nonhealing injuries). *See Chapter 3 for more information on these issues*

- Temporal relations: other cultures often have a varying priority or concept of time orientation and may be more past, present, or future-oriented; this can lead to issues with punctuality for clinic visits and frustrations between the patient and the provider

Safe and effective care depends on the cultural competence of the provider. Align the treatment plan to accommodate the cultural needs of the patient. Take the time to understand the unique needs of the patient.

Takeaways

- To be a true patient advocate, one needs to be culturally aware.
- Complete self-assessment of knowledge and bias. Identify specific areas of strengths and areas which need additional development.
- Utilize validated tools and resources to decrease language and cultural misunderstandings and promote cultural awareness and sensitivity.
- Listen to the patient's perspective about their understanding of their health concerns and treatment options.
- Compare the similarities and differences in cultural approaches to treatment.
- When disagreements occur, recognize the differences may be cultural, and do not devalue the patient's view.
- Compromise approaches to diagnosis and treatment and teach from evidence-based knowledge. If a patient's self-treatment is not harmful, promote and integrate this into the overall care plan. If the patient's self-treatment is harmful, explain harm and suggest alternatives.

LESSON 2: SOCIAL DETERMINANTS/INFLUENCES ON HEALTH

Learning Objectives
- List social determinants of health
- Describe the effects of these social determinants on health
- Identify strategies to decrease health disparity

Health risks and health are affected by the places and conditions in which people live their lives—home, school, work, and play spaces—and include social engagement within these spaces. Health disparity exists when individuals are disadvantaged in one or more of these areas. The interplay between these areas is complex, and while a single answer for curing health disparity does not exist, the nurse practitioner must be aware of, screen for, and intervene in these factors.

Definitions
- **Built environment**: man-made environments providing the setting for how people live
- **Health disparity**: health differences closely associated with environmental, social, and/or economic disadvantage
- **Health equity**: the pursuit of the highest standard of health for all people

Social Determinants of Health

Social determinants of health may be referred to as the environmental circumstances and foundations that affect health in general. They are a reflection of the social factors and physical conditions experienced by individuals, families, and populations, rather than a function of race and ethnicity. Inequality in social determinants of health leads to health disparity and impacts morbidity and mortality rates. The social determinants include economic stability, neighborhood and built environment, education status, access to nutritious food, social and community context, and health. Healthy People 2020 has multiple objectives related to the social determinants of health.

Economic Stability

Economic stability is influenced by employment and income, expenses, debts, and support for money-earning efforts such as child care and transportation. When families are experiencing economic instability, its members are more likely to experience alterations in physical and mental health. Economic stability also has a direct effect on housing available to individuals and/or families.

Neighborhood and Built Environment

Neighborhood and built environment can affect health in a positive manner. Safety, walkability, availability of transportation, access to quality/nutritious food, and the presence of parks, playgrounds, libraries, and recreation centers are important components related to neighborhood quality. Homelessness and housing quality may contribute to disparities in health as well. For example, in low-income communities, safety and security of the home, sanitary conditions, and access to electricity and running clean water may be limited and thus contribute to poorer health outcomes.

Education

Early childhood education leads to increases in literacy rates, academic success, and school completion. Vocational training leads to the potential for a higher income. Children born to parents of a lower educational attainment level are more likely to live in an environment that results in less income and more stress and barriers to health, which often lead to a shorter life expectancy.

Access to Nutritious Food

Many adults and children suffer from food insecurity due to inadequate access or economic instability. For example, consider the patient who does not have access to a car and the nearest grocery store is a mile from his or her home. This problem is compounded by the lack of/limited availability of healthy food options within stores in impoverished communities. Programs exist that assist with hunger such as the Special Supplemental Nutrition Program for Women, Infants, and Children (WIC) and the Supplemental Nutrition Assistance Program (SNAP), yet these entitlement programs are limited to those of very low income.

Social and Community Context

The social and community context refers to the individual's integration into the social fabric of his or her environment, which includes community interaction, support systems, and social integration. Advantaged social groups enjoy better health and lower health risks than those who have consistently been exposed to discrimination and social disadvantage.

Health and Healthcare

Having health insurance, whether public or private, does not guarantee access to adequate healthcare. Despite enactment of the Affordable Care Act and the availability of programs such as Medicare, Medicaid, and state Children's Health Insurance Programs, large numbers of Americans of all ages do not have access to health insurance coverage. The cost for this coverage is prohibitive for many working individuals. Healthcare providers choose which insurance programs they will participate in, thereby limiting choices for many individuals and families. This may lead to quality of care issues. Access to insurance does not always equate to adequate access to healthcare. Additional barriers to seeking healthcare include personal belief systems, transportation issues, financial issues (such as co-pays required to be collected at the time of the visit or deductibles that must be met), scheduling conflicts, and concerns with provider's cultural competency and language spoken.

Decreasing Health Disparity

Nurse practitioners in all settings are in a prime position to increase health equity and decrease health disparity. Look beyond individual behaviors or factors. Ask specific questions about social support, occupation, income, housing, food, and access to transportation. Become familiar with government programs designed to decrease health disparities. Know local private and community resources available in the area, and refer patients to these resources as needed. When following up with patients and planning ongoing treatment, reassess social determinants of health. Advocate for needed programs at the community level, and support needed policy changes at the state and federal levels.

Takeaways

- Social determinants of health have a significant impact on health disparities.
- Economic stability, neighborhood and built environment, education level, access to nutritious food, and social or community support have a greater impact on health than individual behaviors alone.
- Nurse practitioners may assist individuals by assessing for social determinant issues and then referring patients for appropriate assistance.

PRACTICE QUESTIONS

Select the ONE best answer.

Lesson 1: Cultural Competency and Health-Related Behaviors

1. Standard 8 of the ANA Scope of Practice and Standards of Care addresses culturally congruent care. Culturally congruent care considers all of the following except:

   A. Linguistics and language translation

   B. Ethnopharmacology and pharmacogenetics

   C. The notion that Western medicine has superior science and should be adhered to when caring for patients from all ethnically diverse backgrounds

   D. Culture-bound syndromes and alternative approaches to disease etiology and treatment options

2. A 65-year-old female of Korean descent presents to the clinic with symptoms of a urinary tract infection. The woman is a recent immigrant from Korea and is accompanied by her nephew who is in the room to translate for her. The nurse practitioner provides culturally competent care for this patient in all of the following ways except:

   A. Telling the nephew to leave the room unless a HIPAA form has been signed

   B. Providing written information to the patient about her health concerns and treatment in Korean

   C. Using a translation app to allow the patient to talk into the app and translate her health concerns into English and vice versa

   D. Offering the patient a toll-free phone number to Korean translators

3. Which of the following, as defined by the American Nurses Association, is not a main population group with unique health concerns?

   A. Elderly patients

   B. Obese patients

   C. Transgender patients

   D. Female patients

4. Which of the following statements is false regarding culturally congruent care?

   A. To provide competent care, it is important to understand one's own cultural biases and competencies

   B. It is permissible to delay medical care until a translator can be located for a patient that does not speak English

   C. In caring for special populations and making follow-up plans, it is important to recognize special populations may have difficulty with transportation for follow-up appointments

   D. It is important to listen to a patient's perspective and understanding of their health concerns

Lesson 2: Social Determinants/Influences on Health

5. All of the following are considered to be social determinants of health except:

   A. Built environment

   B. Education level

   C. Race and ethnicity

   D. Social context

6. Why must the nurse practitioner consider the social determinants of health?

   A. In the United States, all people are treated equally

   B. Considering these factors is the right thing to do

   C. Negative social determinants decrease the cost of healthcare

   D. Social determinants affect a wide range of health and quality-of-life outcomes

7. The nurse practitioner's role related to the social determinants of health is best described by which of the following actions?

   A. Focus on individual behavior to impact health and wellness

   B. Encourage people to take responsibility for their own health behaviors

   C. Assess and intervene for the root causes of disease and health disparities

   D. Lecture people about how to change wrong health behaviors to right behaviors

8. Which of the following is a strategy to decrease barriers to healthcare access?

   A. Limited office hours

   B. Provider cultural competence

   C. Only accepting commercial insurance

   D. Collecting co-pays at the visit

ANSWERS AND EXPLANATIONS

Lesson 1: Cultural Competency and Health-Related Behaviors

1. C

Culturally congruent care does not include the notion that Western medicine has superior science **(C)**. It does include linguistics and language translation (A), ethnopharmacology and pharmacogenetics (B), and culture-bound syndromes and alternative approaches to disease and treatment options (D).

2. A

In some cultures, younger family members consider it an honor to care for older family members. This should not be assumed either way. Telling the nephew to leave the room **(A)** may cause the patient to become fearful. The nephew should not be dismissed from the room without first attempting to consider his role and presence with the patient and observing their interaction. By providing written information (B), using a translation app (C), and offering the patient a toll-free number for a translator (D), the patient's resources and health literacy are increased.

3. D

According to the ANA, female patients **(D)** are not considered a main population with unique health concerns. However, elderly (A), obese (B), and transgender patients (C) all have unique health concerns.

4. B

It is unlawful to delay medical care **(B)** for a patient that does not speak English. Regarding culturally congruent care, it is important to understand cultural biases and competencies (A), recognize special populations may have difficulty with transportation (C), and to listen to a patient's perspective and understanding (D).

Lesson 2: Social Determinants/Influences on Health

5. C

Race and ethnicity **(C)** are not considered to be social determinants of health, as they are fixed characteristics that cannot be influenced. Neighborhood and built environment (A), education level (B), and social context (D), along with economic stability, food, and health and healthcare are the social determinants of health.

6. D

The social determinants of health affect a wide range of outcomes and risks **(D)**. Health disparities continue in the U.S. and affect a large number of people; thus, not all people are treated equally (A). While considering these factors is the right thing to do (B), the correct response is more specific. Lastly, negative social determinants do not decrease the cost of healthcare (C)—they increase its cost.

7. C

In order to have an impact on the social determinants of health, the nurse practitioner must assess and intervene for the root causes of disease and health disparities **(C)**. Focusing on individual behavior (A) and encouraging individual responsibility for health behavior (B) will not have an overall impact on health disparities. Lecturing people about behavior change (D) is not the most effective means of communication; it is more effective to engage the individual in the change process.

8. B

Provider cultural competence **(B)** may assist with decreasing barriers to healthcare access. Limiting office hours (A), not accepting public insurance (C), and having a reputation that the patient must pay at the visit (D) are barriers for certain individuals.

CHAPTER 21

Translational Science/ Evidence-Based Practice

LESSON 1: EVIDENCE-BASED PRACTICE

Learning Objectives
- Define the purpose of evidence-based practice and its critical features
- Describe the six steps of evidence-based practice
- Critically appraise research literature to appropriately integrate evidence into clinical practice

Evidence-based practice (EBP) is a core competency among nurse practitioners. The foremost objective of EBP is to identify the best evidential findings of populations that can be used in making decisions within individual patient care. Evidence-based practice does not produce new research, rather it implements clinical findings from prior research and applies it to form individual treatment plans.

Definitions
- **Clinical significance**: refers to the practical importance of the intervention and whether it can be quantified using effect and Number Needed to Treat (NNT)
- **Confidence interval (CI)**: discloses sampling error; represents the range of values within which the parameter is expected to fall, within a certain degree of confidence (CI%)
- **Likelihood ratio (LR)**: a measurement reflecting a finding's diagnostic significance
- **Odds ratio (OR)**: a relative measure of effect; a comparison between the intervention group and to the non-intervention or control group
- **Sensitivity**: the ability of a test to detect true positives
- **Specificity**: the ability of a test to detect true negatives

Hierarchy of Evidence

Given the independent role of nurse practitioners in diagnostic decision making, testing, and treatment, it is imperative that nurse practitioners are able to find evidence and interpret data in order to answer clinical questions. Aligning a clinical question with the best study design yields the most reliable and precise intervention. Study designs are rated according to level or strength of evidence. The level or strength of evidence is typically portrayed in an evidence-based pyramid hierarchy.

Level	Study design	Design definition
Level I (strongest level)	Systematic review (SR) Meta-analysis of randomized controlled trials (RCTs) Clinical practice guidelines (CPGs) based on SR	Typically focuses on a specific clinical topic and question; involves extensive literature search; studies are then reviewed, assessed, and summarized according to predetermined criteria of the clinical question Statistically combines the results of multiple studies and thus carries "more weight" than a single study on the topic Recommendations based on evidence from a systematic review and a synthesis of the related published research findings; created by a panel of experts
Level II	RCT	Methodologies reduce bias via randomization and blinding; outcomes compared between intervention and control groups
Level III	Controlled trial *without* randomization	Lack of randomization weakens strength of findings; cannot reliably predict the same outcome in a different patient population
Level IV	Case controlled Cohort studies	Retrospective study in which the researcher is seeking to identify patterns among patients, risk factors, and conditions Two groups (cohorts) of patients: one group will have condition and/or receive treatment over a set period of time, compared to another group without condition and/or no treatment
Level V	Single descriptive or qualitative studies	Case report of a collection of information of a single patient or case series of several case reports; neither include control groups for comparison
Level VI (weakest)	Expert opinion	Expert opinion reflects clinical experiences, expertise, and judgments that may come from a variety of sources

Table 21.1.1 Hierarchy of Evidence

Evidence-Based Practice Steps

There are six steps involved in the process of evidence-based practice:

1. Compose a clinical inquiry or guiding question
2. Perform a literature search for the best evidence
3. Critically assess and synthesize the evidential findings
4. Implement and integrate evidence into daily clinical practice
5. Evaluate patient outcomes before and after implemented practice change
6. Disseminate the outcome

Step 1: Compose a Clinical Inquiry

Construct a well-written and well-defined clinical guiding question. The most common format to organize clinical inquiry components is known as PICO:

- **P**: patient, population, or problem of interest
- **I**: intervention or indicator (a prognostic factor) being considered
- **C**: comparison among interventions or between a control
- **O**: outcome to be measured

Step 2: Perform a Literature Search

Consider these four criteria when choosing information resources:

1. **Soundness of evidence-based approach:** identify the study design that best answers the clinical question (the hierarchy of evidence details the reliability of findings—*see Table 21.1.1*)

2. **Comprehensiveness and specificity:** assess the resources' relevance to the clinical practice or patient population involved in the clinical inquiry question

3. **Ease of use:** each database has its own nuances of use, and learning its protocols and/or features improves efficiency in the search

4. **Availability:** multiple databases exist

Most clinicians rely on filtered resources, which are databases composed of pre-appraised and synthesized literature reviews that make recommendations for clinical practice.

Filtered resources	Website	Cost
ACP Journal Club	**www.acponline.org**	Subscription fee
ACP PIER	**www.pier.acponline.org**	ACP member fee
Bandolier	**www.medicine.ox.ac.uk/bandolier/**	Free
Cochrane Library	**www.thecochranelibrary.com**	Free abstracts
DynaMed	**www.ebscohost.com/dynamed**	Subscription fee
MedlinePlus	**www.nlm.nih.gov/medlineplus/**	Free
National Guideline Clearinghouse	**www.guideline.gov**	Free
National Institute of Health and Care Excellence (NICE)	**www.nice.org.uk**	Free
Turning Research Into Practice (TRIP)	**www.tripdatabase.com**	Free
UpToDate	**www.uptodate.com/contents/search**	Subscription fee

Table 21.1.2 Online EBP Filtered Database Sources

Step 3: Assess and Synthesize the Evidence

There are three essential components of evidence appraisal: **validity, study results,** and **applicability**.

The assessment of **validity** is aimed at identifying biases or confounding variables that could influence the strength of the study's findings. It is also an evaluation of the scientific methods used by researchers to obtain the study results.

Questioning the **study results** refers to appraisal of the study's reliability and clinical significance. Within this assessment, it is critical to understand the distinction between *statistical* significance and *clinical* significance. Statistical significance relays that a difference in outcomes exists between the control and intervention groups. The clinical significance highlights the magnitude of this difference. To measure clinical significance, elements of effect size, such as number needed to treat (NNT), number needed to harm (NNH), and confidential interval (CI), should be noted.

In the third component, the evidence is evaluated in its **applicability** to the practice population. The study subjects are compared to the known patient population in demographics, disease severity, risk factors, and comorbidities. Other considerations of applicability may include the study's reproducibility potential and benefit vs. risk analysis.

In **synthesizing the evidence**, the nurse practitioner determines whether to accept or reject the evidence and judges whether or not the evidence helps to answer the clinical inquiry.

Step 4: Integrate Evidence into Clinical Practice

Clinical judgment, expertise, and understanding of the patient's preferences, values, and beliefs must be utilized while integrating evidence into clinical practice. Other considerations relevant to integrative evidence-based practice include assessment of risks and benefits, evaluation of socioeconomic issues' potential impact to adherence, and the organizational culture.

Step 5: Evaluate Patient Outcomes

Any time an intervention is implemented, it is critical to evaluate the effectiveness of the practice change. Outcome measurements should be performed at baseline (prior to implementation), then at set intervals for analysis and comparison. Determining the absence or presence of improved outcomes is followed by evaluation for all the possible reasons an intervention did not work. Such reasons may include nonadherence to treatment plan or varying patient prognostic factors, but could also be related to the nurse practitioner's skill in evidence interpretation or delivery of interventions.

Step 6: Disseminate the Outcomes

Once valuable interventions or changes in practices have been identified, the nurse practitioner may want to disseminate the findings. Identifying the communication mode and type of audience are critical first steps. There are multiple forums to be considered when disseminating information among colleagues, including intradepartmental in-services, journal clubs, lectures, posters, and manuscripts.

Takeaways

- Evidence-based practice allows a provider to implement clinical findings from prior research to an individual patient's plan of care.

- Six steps are involved in the process of acquiring evidence to use in practice (clinical inquiry, literature search, synthesis of the evidence, integrating evidence into practice, evaluating outcomes, and disseminating the outcomes).

LESSON 2: RESEARCH

Learning Objectives
- Identify steps to the research process
- Discuss research designs and the characteristics of each

Nurse practitioners are in the position to bring new research findings into practice (*refer to Chapter 21, Lesson 1, for a discussion on evidence-based practice*). This lesson takes that concept one step further and discusses basic research terminology and design in order to assist the nurse practitioner in identifying quality research and using it in practice.

Research Process

The following steps make up the research process:

- Define the problem
- Generate literature review (justify the research)
- Refine research question and hypotheses
- Select study design and methodology
- Collect and analyze data
- Draw conclusions (interpret data)

Basic Terminology

- **Hypothesis**: provisional (and testable) proposal by a researcher to explain a phenomenon
- **Theory**: well-established model, based on accumulated evidence, to explain a phenomenon
- **Variable**: factor that can be measured, controlled, or altered in a scientific experiment
- **Independent variable**: variable that is manipulated (controlled or altered) by the researcher to produce an effect
- **Dependent variable**: variable that is measured to see if the intervention had an effect
- **Confounding variable**: extraneous variable that was not controlled for by the researcher that can influence the outcome of an experiment
- **Control group**: group that does not receive the intervention (such as a new medication or procedure); this group, for example, may be receiving a placebo
- **Intervention group**: group that receives the intervention (such as a new medication or procedure)
- **Blinding**: concealment of whether or not a subject is placed in a group receiving an intervention or in a placebo-receiving (control) group
- **Double-blinding**: when neither the researcher nor the subjects are aware whether the subject is in the intervention or control group
- **Placebo**: medication or treatment with no actual therapeutic effect
- **Placebo effect**: when subjects who think they are getting a treatment show improvement in their condition though they are receiving a medication or treatment with no actual therapeutic effect
- **Retrospective study**: study evaluating past collected data to identify potential causal factors
- **Prospective study**: study that evaluates subjects who have been separated into an experimental group that is believed to have been exposed to a causal factor vs. a control group that has not been exposed to that factor
- **Longitudinal study**: consists of observational research in which researchers gather data on the same subjects repeatedly over a period of time
- **Cross-sectional study**: observational study of an entire population at a specific point in time; for example, researchers may collate data on how many people in a population have type 2 diabetes at a given time (prevalence)
- **Quantitative analysis**: documenting the meaning of measurable numerical values (such as INR values)
- **Qualitative analysis**: documenting subjective information (such as "burning," "gnawing," or "stabbing" abdominal pain)

Research Designs

There are three major categories of research design: experimental designs, quasi-experimental designs, and non-experimental designs.

Experimental Design

A researcher may wish to use a classic experimental design (a **randomized controlled trial**) by controlling an environment and then introducing an independent variable. An example would be administering a specific dosage of warfarin to subjects (as the **independent variable**) and then measuring the resulting INR in patients (as the **dependent variable**). The point here might be to establish a causal relationship between the warfarin administration and increased INR.

To make an experiment as strong as possible, subjects should be **randomized**—meaning placement of subjects in either the control or intervention group should be left to chance. If subjects are selected (or self-selected in some way), the researcher runs the risk of introducing a **confounding variable**. Confounding variables ultimately impact study results.

Types of Control Groups

Sometimes it would be unethical to present an intervention to one group and withhold that intervention from the other. For example, say a cancer researcher has developed a cancer medication that he/she knows will work to extend the life of breast cancer patients with only minor side effects. It would be unethical to withhold the medication from the control group. Could the researcher still conduct a study?

One way to address this would be to create a **wait list control group**. The idea is to give the control group the cancer medication, but at a later date than the intervention group (note: this solution may still not meet ethical standards—for example, if some members of the wait list died while waiting to receive the intervention).

Another option would be to create a **dose-response control group**, where you give the intervention group a larger dose of the cancer medication than the control group (note: this solution may still be unethical if members of the control group faced poorer outcomes than members of the intervention group).

A third way would to create a **standard treatment control group**, where you give the intervention group the new medication while the control group receives an established older medication (note: this may still be unethical if the newer medication was so superior to the established medication that the control group ends up with poorer outcomes than members of the intervention group).

A fourth possibility would be to offer the control group a **placebo**, a pill that has no active ingredient. This recreates the original problem, however, and amounts to unethically withholding the medication from the control group.

Non-Randomized Study: "Quasi-Experimental" Design

Sometimes a researcher follows an experimental design model, but opts not to randomize subjects into control vs. intervention groups. This is called **quasi-experimental design**.

There are many reasons to do use quasi-experimental design. Examples include cost (it can be costly to randomize subjects) or a small subject pool (perhaps the researcher cannot amass enough subjects to attempt randomization).

Non-Experimental Design

Examples of non-experimental design include observational studies, descriptive/interpretative studies, and surveys.

In an **observational design**, the researcher may simply observe without intervening. An example of observational research is Charles Darwin's studies of finches in the Galapagos Islands, observations that contributed to his theories on evolution. For the kind of research Darwin was attempting—evaluating what kinds of finches existed in this natural habitat—this methodology made sense. He hoped to identify how different kinds of finches had naturally adapted to their environments; it would not have made sense for him to introduce artificial stimuli.

In **descriptive/interpretative design**, the researcher is usually exploring a research question. An example is a phenomenological study in which the researcher explores various patients' experiences of pulmonary hygiene teaching in a COPD support group.

For **surveys**, subjects respond to interviews or written questionnaires.

At the end of a study, the researcher hopes to answer a question about the data collected. After gathering empirical evidence (data gained by observation or experimentation), the researcher evaluates it quantitatively (for example, measuring numerical values such as the international normalized ratio—the INR) or qualitatively (subjective information such as burning, gnawing, or stabbing abdominal pain) to make a clinical assertion.

Takeaways

- Being familiar with the steps of the research process and basic research design allows the nurse practitioner to identify quality research and apply it to practice.

- The research question determines the research design.

- Each design provides findings; a researcher must define if those findings can be generalized to a patient/population.

PRACTICE QUESTIONS

Select the ONE best answer.

Lesson 1: Evidence-Based Practice

1. Sensitivity is the ability of a test to:

    A. Detect true positives

    B. Detect true negatives

    C. Rule in disease

    D. Differentiate between two conditions

2. According to the hierarchy of evidence, which of the following is considered level I (strongest-level) evidence?

    A. A cohort study

    B. An expert opinion

    C. A randomized control trial

    D. A meta-analysis of a randomized control trial

3. The third step involved in the process of evidence-based practice is:

    A. Evaluating patient outcomes before and after implemented practice change

    B. Performing a literature search for the best evidence

    C. Critically appraising and synthesizing the evidential findings

    D. Composing a clinical inquiry

4. The elements of clinical inquiry known as PICO stand for:

    A. Problem, interaction, cause, outcome

    B. Population, intervention, comparison, outcome

    C. Patient, implementation, control, outliers

    D. Prognostic factor, intervention, cause, outcome

Lesson 2: Research

5. The independent variable in an experiment refers to:

    A. The variable that is measured to see if the intervention had an effect

    B. A provisional (and testable) proposal by a researcher to explain a phenomenon

    C. An extraneous variable that was not controlled for by the researcher

    D. The variable that is manipulated by the researcher to produce an effect

6. In a study where a researcher has developed a medication he knows will work to extend the life of lung cancer patients with only minor side effects, it would not be ethical to withhold the medication from the control group. In this instance, the researcher might conduct the study using which type of control group?

    A. Randomized, meaning placement of subjects in either the control or intervention group should be left to chance

    B. Placebo, using a pill that has no active ingredient

    C. Dose-response, where the intervention group receives a larger dose of the cancer medication than the control group

    D. Wait list, where the intervention group receives the new medication while the control group receives an established older medication

7. Which research term is matched correctly with its description?

   A. Hypothesis: a well-established model, based on accumulated evidence, to explain a phenomenon

   B. Theory: a provisional (and testable) proposal by a researcher to explain a phenomenon

   C. Independent variable: an extraneous variable not controlled for by the researcher that can influence the outcome of an experiment

   D. Dependent variable: an extraneous variable not controlled for by the researcher that can influence the outcome of an experiment

8. The nurse practitioner's current research features observational study of an entire population at a specific point in time. This is also known as a:

   A. Cross-sectional study

   B. Longitudinal study

   C. Placebo effect

   D. Randomized controlled trial

ANSWERS AND EXPLANATIONS

Lesson 1: Evidence-Based Practice

1. A

The sensitivity of a test is its ability to detect true positives **(A)**. The ability to detect true negatives (B) and rule in disease (C) are reflected in a test's specificity. There is no measurement available to differentiate between two conditions (D).

2. D

The strongest level of evidence (level I) consists of meta-analysis of RCTs **(D)**, systematic reviews, and clinical practice guidelines based on SRs. Cohort studies (A) are level IV. Expert opinions (B) are level VI. Randomized control trials (C) are level II.

3. C

The third step involved in the process of evidence-based practice is critically appraising and synthesizing the evidential findings **(C)**. The process of evidence-based practice includes: (1) composing a clinical inquiry or guiding question; (2) performing a literature search for the best evidence; (3) critically appraising and synthesizing the evidential findings; (4) implementing and integrating evidence into daily clinical practice; (5) evaluating patient outcomes before and after implemented practice change; and (6) disseminating the outcome.

4. B

PICO stands for: (P) patient, population, or problem; (I) intervention or indicator; (C) comparison or control; and (O) outcome **(B)**.

Lesson 2: Research

5. D

An independent variable is a variable whose presence is manipulated (controlled or altered) by the researcher to produce an effect **(D)**. A dependent variable is the variable that is measured to see if the intervention had an effect (A). A hypothesis is a provisional (and testable) proposal by a researcher to explain a phenomenon (B). Last, a confounding variable is an extraneous variable that was not controlled for by the researcher (C).

6. C

Given this ethical dilemma, the researcher may opt for a dose-response control group **(C)**, where the intervention group is given a larger dose of the cancer medication than the control group. A randomized control group (A) or placebo group (B) are not good options, as each recreates the original problem—withholding the medication from the control group. A wait list group in and of itself is a valid option, but to give the intervention group the new medication while the control group receives an established older medication (D) defines a standard treatment group.

7. D

The dependent variable **(D)** is the variable that is measured to see if the intervention had an effect. A hypothesis (A) is a provisional (and testable) proposal by a researcher to explain a phenomenon. A theory (B) is a well-established model, based on accumulated evidence, to explain a phenomenon. An independent variable (C) is the variable that is manipulated (controlled or altered) by the researcher to produce an effect.

8. A

A cross-sectional study **(A)** is an observational study of an entire population at a specific point in time. A longitudinal study (B) features observational research on data gathered by researchers on the same subjects repeatedly over a period of time. The placebo effect (C) is when subjects who think they are getting a treatment show improvement in their condition even though they are receiving a medication or treatment with no actual therapeutic effect. It is not a research design. A randomized controlled trial (D) features an experimental design achieved by controlling an environment, then introducing an independent variable. It does not seek to study an entire population.